MW00335997

MANAGEMENT OF CARDIAC ARRHYTHMIAS

CONTEMPORARY CARDIOLOGY

CHRISTOPHER P. CANNON, MD
SERIES EDITOR

MANAGEMENT OF CARDIAC ARRHYTHMIAS

Edited by

LEONARD I. GANZ, MD

University of Pittsburgh Medical Center,
Pittsburgh, PA

Foreword by

EUGENE BRAUNWALD, MD

Brigham and Women's Hospital, Partners Health Care System,
and Harvard Medical School, Boston, MA

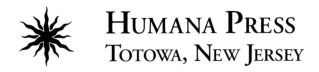

HUMANA PRESS
TOTOWA, NEW JERSEY

© 2002 Humana Press Inc.
999 Riverview Drive, Suite 208
Totowa, New Jersey 07512
humanapr.com

For additional copies, pricing for bulk purchases, and/or information about other Humana titles,
contact Humana at the above address or at any of the following numbers: Tel.: 973-256-1699;
Fax: 973-256-8341, E-mail: humana@humanapr.com; or visit our Website: humanapr.com

Cover design by Patricia F. Cleary.
Cover illustration: Shown are four surface ECG leads (I, III, aVL, and V_2) and an intracardiac recording (proximal
coronary sinus) in a patient with recurrent supraventricular tachycardia due to a manifest right posteroseptal accessory
pathway (Wolff-Parkinson-White Syndrome). Sinus rhythm is present. A delta wave and short PR interval are due to
ventricular pre-excitation; the atrial and ventricular electrograms in the proximal coronary sinus are continuous. At the
left of the figure, radiofrequency energy is applied to a catheter positioned at the site of the accessory pathway in the
posteroseptal tricuspid annulus. After three beats, the delta wave disappears, the PR interval normalizes, and the atrial
and ventricular electrograms separate, signifying successful ablation of the accessory pathway. Wolff-Parkinson-White
Syndrome, supraventricular tachycardia, and radiofrequency catheter ablation are discussed in detail in Chapters 3 and 4.

Production Editor: Kim Hoather-Potter.

This publication is printed on acid-free paper. ∞
ANSI Z39.48-1984 (American National Standards Institute) Permanence of Paper for Printed Library Materials.

Printed in the United States of America. 10 9 8 7 6 5 4 3 2 1

Library of Congress Cataloging-in-Publication Data
Management of cardiac arrhythmias/edited by Leonard I. Ganz.
     p. ; cm. – (Contemporary cardiology)
    Includes bibliographical references and index.
    ISBN 0-89603-846-7 (alk. paper)
    1. Arrhythmia–Treatment. 2. Electric countershock. I. Ganz, Leonard I. II.
    Contemporary cardiology (Totowa, N.J. : unnumbered)
    [DNLM: 1. Arrhythmia–therapy. 2. Electrophysiology. WG 330M266 2002]
    RC685.A65 M337 2002
    616.1'2806–dc21
                                  2001039366

DEDICATION

For my parents, who instilled in me a life-long desire to learn; my wife Sue Ellen, who continues to teach me the most important things; and my children Rachel, Alana, and Michael, who keep me in rhythm.

Leonard I. Ganz, MD

FOREWORD

During the past decade there have been enormous advances in the management of patients with cardiac arrhythmias. Catheter ablation has become a first-line therapy for a growing number of supraventricular tachyarrhythmias and idiopathic ventricular tachycardia. Frequently performed on an outpatient basis, radiofrequency catheter ablation actually cures the majority of patients with these disorders, restoring a normal quality of life.

Implantable cardioverter defibrillators (ICDs) have progressed from a therapy of last resort at the time of FDA approval in 1985, to the preferred therapy in the majority of patients with life-threatening ventricular arrhythmias. ICD implantation, once a morbid cardiothoracic surgical procedure, is now similar to pacemaker implantation. Advances in pacemaker technology have restored normal physiology to many patients; current trials focus on the utility of multisite atrial pacing to prevent atrial fibrillation and biventricular pacing (cardiac resynchronization) in patients with advanced congestive heart failure. For patients with syncope, new diagnostic approaches such as the implantable loop recorder, as well as new therapies, offer improved outcomes.

New nonpharmacologic therapies have been developed for virtually every type of cardiac arrhythmia. Previously the mainstay of therapy for arrhythmia patients, pharmacologic therapies have assumed an adjunctive rather than primary role in many patients. This paradigm shift, from pharmacologic to nonpharmacologic therapies, the proliferation of the types of devices and procedures available, as well as the growing number of patients who may benefit, require that cardiac electrophysiologists keep their colleagues in general cardiology, cardiac surgery, and primary care updated. The purpose of this fine text is to help inform these physicians and surgeons about recent advances in the diagnosis and management of patients with cardiac arrhythmias, and to describe how electrophysiologists can best assist in the care of their patients. Written by leaders in the field of cardiac electrophysiology, and well edited by Leonard I. Ganz, *Management of Cardiac Arrhythmias* provides lucid descriptions of diagnostic and therapeutic strategies in patients with heart rhythm disturbances. Tables, figures, and treatment algorithms are used extensively to make this book a practical clinical guide as well as an excellent reference source. This book will prove to be of enormous value both to specialists and generalists responsible for the care of patients with cardiac arrhythmias.

Eugene Braunwald, MD
Boston, MA

PREFACE

The last ten years have witnessed a tremendous change in the management of patients with cardiac arrhythmias. Cardiac electrophysiology has evolved from a purely descriptive discipline into an interventional field, in which procedures developed over the last fifteen years directly improve the survival and quality of life of a broad population of patients. Radiofrequency catheter ablation and implantable cardioverter defibrillator (ICD) implantation have become standard therapies, and in many cases are performed on an outpatient basis.

A recurring theme has been the development of new nonpharmacologic therapies for virtually every type of cardiac arrhythmia. Unlike in the past, pharmacologic therapies are frequently supplemental rather than primary therapy. Atrial fibrillation, the most common sustained arrhythmia encountered, has recently been the target of a variety of nonpharmacologic therapies. Previously considered unattainable, a curative catheter ablation procedure for atrial fibrillation appears within reach.

This major shift in paradigm—from pharmacologic to nonpharmacologic therapies—has been accompanied by a marked expansion in the pool of patients who may benefit from these therapies. The mission of this text is to help inform our colleagues in general cardiology and primary care about recent advances in the diagnosis and management of patients with cardiac arrhythmias. Written by leaders in the field of cardiac electrophysiology, *Management of Cardiac Arrhythmias* provides both an overview and in-depth discussion of diagnostic and therapeutic strategies in patients with heart rhythm disturbances. Tables, figures, and treatment algorithms are used extensively to make this book a practical clinical guide as well as a reference. After an historical perspective on the development of cardiac electrophysiology is a chapter outlining the evaluation of patients with arrhythmia. From there, supraventricular tachycardia, atrial fibrillation, syncope, ventricular tachycardia, and sudden cardiac death are covered. There are also chapters devoted to specific treatment modalities, including catheter ablation, pacemakers, and implantable cardioverter defibrillators. Finally, the book closes with detailed reviews describing the management of special populations with arrhythmia: children, pregnant and nursing women, and patients suffering acute myocardial infarction.

In editing this text, I have been extremely privileged to have had the opportunity to work with such distinguished colleagues. It has been a pleasure, and I have learned a great deal from the contributors. I would like to thank Kim Potter, Craig Adams, and Paul Dolgert at Humana Press for their hard work and dedication to this project, and to Christopher Cannon, MD, the *Contemporary Cardiology* Series Editor, for giving me this opportunity. Finally, I would like to thank several individuals who have been instrumental in my development as a physician and electrophysiologist. Elliott Antman and Eugene Braunwald triggered my interest in cardiology as well as academic medicine. Peter Friedman and William Stevenson sparked and nurtured my interest in cardiac electrophysiology. Mark Josephson has been and continues to be a tremendous inspiration, instilling in me the desire to take care of patients with arrhythmias, to understand the mechanisms of arrhythmias, and to teach others.

Leonard I. Ganz, MD

CONTENTS

CONTRIBUTORS

KELLEY P. ANDERSON, MD • *Heart Care, Marshfield Clinic, Marshfield, WI*

ELLIOTT M. ANTMAN, MD • *Cardiovascular Division, Brigham and Women's Hospital, Boston, MA*

WALTER L. ATIGA, MD • *Cardiovascular Institute, University of Pittsburgh Medical Center, Pittsburgh, PA*

RALPH S. AUGOSTINI, MD • *Mid Ohio Cardiology Consultants, Columbus, OH*

SUSAN BRODE, MD • *Cardiovascular Institute, University of Pittsburgh Medical Center, Pittsburgh, PA*

HUGH CALKINS , MD • *Johns Hopkins Hospital, Baltimore, MD*

DAVID J. CALLANS, MD • *Cardiology Division, Hospital of the University of Pennsylvania, Philadelphia, PA*

OTTO COSTANTINI, MD • *Heart and Vascular Center, MetroHealth Hospital, Case Western Reserve University, Cleveland, OH*

N. A. MARK ESTES III, MD • *Division of Cardiology, New England Medical Center, Boston, MA*

JOHN K. FINKLE, MD • *Lankenau Hospital, Wynnewood, PA*

RICHARD N. FOGOROS, MD • *MCP-Hahnemann School of Medicine, Pittsburgh, PA*

PETER GALLAGHER, MD • *Division of Cardiology, Duke University Medical Center, Durham, NC*

LEONARD I. GANZ, MD • *Cardiovascular Institute, University of Pittsburgh Medical Center, Pittsburgh, PA*

MICHAEL R. GOLD, MD, PHD • *Division of Cardiology, University of Maryland School of Medicine, Baltimore, MD*

VENKATESHWAR GOTTIPATY, MD, PHD • *South Carolina Heart Center, Columbia, SC*

BLAIR P. GRUBB, MD •*Rupert Health Center, The Medical College of Ohio, Toledo, OH*

REGINALD T. HO, MD • *Cardiology Division, Hospital of the University of Pennsylvania, Philadelphia, PA*

JOSÉ A. JOGLAR, MD • *Cardiovascular Division, University of Texas Southwestern Medical Center, Dallas, TX*

MARK E. JOSEPHSON, MD • *Electrophysiology and Arrhythmia Service, Beth Israel Deaconess Medical Center, Boston, MA*

DANIEL KOSINSKI, MD • *Rupert Health Center, The Medical College of Ohio, Toledo, OH*

PETER R. KOWEY, MD • *Lankenau Hospital, Wynnewood, PA*

MARK S. LINK, MD • *Division of Cardiology, New England Medical Center, Boston, MA*

FRANCIS E. MARCHLINSKI, MD • *Cardiology Division, Hospital of the University of Pennsylvania, Philadelphia, PA*

BRIAN OLSHANSKY, MD • *Cardiac Electrophysiology, University of Iowa Hospitals, Iowa City, IA*

RICHARD L. PAGE, MD • *Cardiovascular Division, University of Texas Southwestern Medical Center, Dallas, TX*

ROBERT W. PETERS, MD • *Department of Veterans' Affairs Medical Center, Baltimore, MD*

KENNETH PLUNKITT, MD • *Lankenau Hospital, Wynnewood, PA*

ERIC J. RASHBA, MD • *Division of Cardiology, University of Maryland School of Medicine, Baltimore, MD*

ROBERT W. RHO, MD • *Cardiology Division, Jefferson Medical College, Philadelphia, PA*

ALLISON W. RICHARDSON, MD • *Electrophysiology and Arrhythmia Service, Beth Israel Deaconess Medical Center, Boston, MA*

DAVID SCHWARTZMAN, MD • *Cardiovascular Institute, University of Pittsburgh Medical Center, Pittsburgh, PA*

ROBERT A. SCHWEIKERT, MD • *The Cleveland Clinic Foundation, Cleveland, OH*

ALAA SHALABY, MD • *Department of Veterans' Affairs Medical Center, Pittsburgh, PA*

VLADIMIR SHUSTERMAN, MD, PHD • *Cardiovascular Institute, University of Pittsburgh Medical Center, Pittsburgh, PA*

BRUCE STAMBLER, MD • *University Hospitals of Cleveland, Case Western Reserve University, Cleveland, OH*

WILLIAM G. STEVENSON, MD • *Harvard Medical School, Cardiac Arrhythmia Program, Brigham and Women's Hospital, Boston, MA*

JOHN K. TRIEDMAN, MD • *Department of Cardiology, Arrhythmia Service, Children's Hospital, Boston, MA*

RAUL WEISS, MD • *Mid Ohio Cardiology Consultants, Columbus, OH*

HEIN J. J. WELLENS, MD • *University Hospital, Maastricht, The Netherlands*

J. MARCUS WHARTON, MD • *Division of Cardiology, Duke University Medical Center, Durham, NC*

BRUCE L. WILKOFF, MD • *The Cleveland Clinic Foundation, Cleveland, OH*

PETER J. ZIMETBAUM, MD • *Electrophysiology and Arrhythmia Service, Beth Israel Deaconess Medical Center, Boston, MA*

COLOR PLATES

Color plates 1–6 appear as an insert following p. 208.

PLATE 1   Fig. 1. (A) Endocardial radiofrequency ablation lesion demonstrating a round shape with sharp borders. (B) Histologic section of lesion in A, demonstrating hemispheric shape and extensive fibrosis. (From Jumrussirikul P, et al. Prospective comparison of temperature guided microwave and radiofrequency catheter ablation in the swine heart. PACE 1998;21[7]:1364–1374. Reproduced with permission.) (*See* full caption on p. 52, Chapter 4.)

PLATE 2   Fig. 4. Electroanatomical map (CARTO™) (Biosense/Webster Inc., Diamond Bar, CA, USA) of ablation lesions encircling a right superior pulmonary vein in a patient in whom AF was consistently triggered by atrial premature beats emanating from myocardium deep within this vein. Each circle (A) represents the site of an individual focal radiofrequency energy application. The summed effect of this series of lesions was "electrical isolation" of the vein. (*See* full caption on p. 149, Chapter 8.)

PLATE 3   Fig. 10. Endocardial view of a 1-d-old lesion (L) deployed in the right atrium percutaneously utilizing radiofrequency energy. Unablated myocardium stains red. (*See* full caption on p. 156, Chapter 8.)

PLATE 4   Fig. 7. Electro-anatomic map of the left ventricle in a patient with infarct-related VT, left anterior oblique (LAO) view. Radiofrequency lesions are depicted by dark red dots. Lesions are delivered in a line connecting densely scarred myocardium (red) to normal myocardium (purple). (*See* full caption on p. 250, Chapter 12.)

PLATE 5   Fig. 4. Mechanism of reentry associated with ventricular scar is illustrated. The schematics show a view of the left ventricle from the apex looking into the ventricle towards the mitral and aortic valves. A region of heterogeneous scar is present in the inferior wall. In (A), the reentry wavefront circulates counterclockwise around and through the scar. Regions of dense scar create an isthmus in the circuit. The QRS onset occurs when the wavefront emerges from the isthmus at the Exit. It then circulates around the border of the scar, returning to the isthmus. Slow conduction through some regions in the scar is caused by discontinuities between myocyte bundles, as illustrated in the magnified image at the right. A wavefront that enters the bottom left myocyte bundles takes a circuitous course to emerge at the superior left bundle. In (B), an ablation catheter has been introduced through the aortic valve and positioned in the reentry circuit isthmus. In (C), following ablation of the isthmus for VT-1, a second VT is still possible because of reentry through an isthmus beneath the mitral valve. This circuit revolves in the opposite direction from the first circuit; the resulting VT has a different QRS morphology. (*See* full caption on p. 367, Chapter 17.)

PLATE 6   Fig. 5. Findings during catheter mapping in a patient with recurrent VT late after anterior-wall MI are shown. In (A) and (B) are shown the right anterior oblique (RAO) and left lateral views, respectively. Electrocardiogram voltage is designated by colors with the lowest voltage shown in red, progressing to greater voltage regions of yellow, green, blue, and purple. In (C), the activation sequence of induced VT is shown in the RAO view of the left ventricle. The colors now indicate the activation sequence, with red being the earliest activation (identifying the reentry circuit exit), progressing to yellow, green, blue, and purple. (D) Shows the effect of pacing during tachycardia (entrainment) in the central common pathway isthmus. (*See* full caption on p. 369, Chapter 17.)

1

Historical Perspectives on Clinical Cardiac Electrophysiology

Mark E. Josephson, MD, Leonard I. Ganz, MD, and Hein J.J. Wellens, MD

CONTENTS

INTRODUCTION

Cardiac electrophysiology is an extremely new and dynamic discipline. Although its roots may be traced to the beginning of the twentieth century, clinical cardiac electrophysiology proper was born in the late 1960s. During this short time period, cardiac electrophysiology has undergone several major paradigm shifts. At the onset, clinical electrophysiologists strove to understand the physiology of the conducting system and cardiac arrhythmias. This initial phase of exploration evolved into a diagnostic field, in which electrophysiologic studies could be used to assess risk and to define the arrhythmia diagnosis, although therapeutic interventions were relatively modest. The past decade has witnessed a virtual explosion in interventional electrophysiology, with an increasing reliance on nonpharmacologic therapies. Throughout this period, cellular electrophysiologists, animal researchers, and more recently, molecular geneticists, have worked to advance our understanding of the mechanisms of arrhythmias at a more basic level than previously appreciated.

HISTORICAL BACKGROUND

Observations describing the effects of electricity on the heart date back to the mid-1800s. Several lines of inquiry, each dating back about 100 years, helped to set the stage for the development of electrophysiology. One important achievement was the development of electrocardiography by Einthoven. Related contributions include the descriptions of conduction block by Wenkebach, Mobitz, and Hay, and the initial

From: *Contemporary Cardiology: Management of Cardiac Arrhythmias*
Edited by: L. I. Ganz © Humana Press Inc., Totowa, NJ

analysis of permanent reciprocating tachycardia by Gallaverdin. The original report by Wolff, Parkinson, and White of the syndrome that bears their names followed shortly thereafter in 1930 *(1)*, although these investigators did not understand the physiology underlying their observation. It was Wolferth and Wood who actually first described the true mechanism of ventricular pre-excitation and reciprocating tachycardia in the Wolff-Parkinson-White Syndrome *(2)*.

Knowledge of the anatomy of the conducting system also grew substantially during this time. The work of His, Kent, and others laid the foundation for the studies in physiology that would follow. The development of arrhythmia surgery and catheter ablation techniques has led to a renewal of interest in the anatomy and histology of the cardiac conducting system.

Another important development during this time period was the initial description of excitable tissues. Mayer, Mines, and Moe explored reentry in various animal tissue models *(3–5)*. Subsequent studies have securely established reentry as the dominant mechanism responsible for clinical arrhythmias.

The development of cardiac pacing also represents an important foundation of cardiac electrophysiology. Hyman developed the "artificial pacemaker" in 1930 *(6)*; this device used a needle to penetrate the heart through the chest wall. Beginning in the late 1950s, a number of advances appeared in rapid succession: epicardial lead systems, transvenous pacing electrodes *(7)*, and a totally implantable pacemaker *(8)*. Advances in battery and electronics technology helped fuel the development of pacing systems. In related work, Zoll introduced the external defibrillator in the mid-1950s *(9)*. This device was used to resuscitate victims of cardiac arrest and cardiovert atrial fibrillation (AF). The ability to resuscitate patients from ventricular tachycardia (VT) and ventricular fibrillation (VF) was certainly a prerequisite to early electrophysiology studies, in which these arrhythmias could be induced.

ORIGINS OF CLINICAL CARDIAC ELECTROPHYSIOLOGY

Clinical cardiac electrophysiology was "born" in the late 1960s. The technique of programmed electrical stimulation of the heart was developed independently by Durrer and colleagues *(10)* in Amsterdam and Coumel and colleagues *(11)* in Paris. Scherlag's technique for transcutaneous recording of the His potential was an invaluable contribution *(12)*, and led to the first systematic evaluation of normal and abnormal function of the A-V node, by Damato and colleagues in Staten Island, NY *(13)*. Another key development was the combination of programmed electrical stimulation with multiple intracardiac recordings by Wellens to discern arrhythmia mechanisms *(14)*. (*see* Fig. 1). Shortly thereafter, three American electrophysiology centers, established by investigators trained in Staten Island, began making important contributions. These centers included Gallagher at Duke, Rosen at the University of Illinois, and Josephson at the University of Pennsylvania. These three centers and the facility established by Wellens in Maastricht have contributed tremendously to the development of electrophysiology, both in terms of scientific discovery, and in training other investigators in cardiac electrophysiology. Wellens and Josephson continue to train electrophysiologists and make major contributions to the field as the twenty-first century begins.

The early years of electrophysiology were largely descriptive. Programmed stimulation was used to define the electrophysiologic parameters of the atria, A-V node, bundle

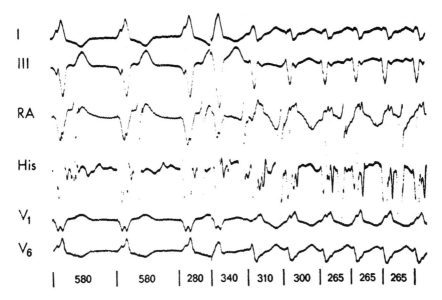

Fig. 1. Figure from the seminal publication of Wellens et al., which first demonstrated the use of programmed stimulation to initiate VT. From top to bottom are surface leads I and III, intracardiac recordings from the right atrium (RA) and His position (HIS), and surface leads V_1 and V_6. Annotated at the bottom are timing intervals in ms. Shown are the last two beats of a right ventricular drive train at 580 ms, and then a single stimulus (coupling interval 280 ms). Monomorphic VT is induced. (With permission from Wellens HJ, Schuilenburg RM, Durrer D. Electrical stimulation of the heart in patients with ventricular tachycardia. Circulation 1972;46:216–226.)

of His, Purkinje system, and the ventricles, and then to assess the effects of various pharmacologic agents on these parameters. The reentrant nature of the vast majority of clinical arrhythmias was established using programmed stimulation. Serial drug testing was the first real therapeutic advance in electrophysiology; the ability of a drug to acutely render an arrhythmia noninducible in the laboratory implied a lower risk of recurrence when the drug was administered chronically. Despite this advance, the limitations of this methodology, in which a clinical recurrence of VT could be fatal, were also recognized.

With increasing experience came the confidence to place multiple electrode catheters in multiple cardiac chambers. Endocardial catheter mapping techniques, in which catheters were sequentially moved to many sites in multiple chambers, allowed identification of the sites of origin of VT, definition of the mechanisms of supraventricular tachycardia (SVT), and delineation of the location of accessory pathways *(15,16)* *(see* Fig. 2). These technologies paved the way for surgical treatment of Wolff-Parkinson-White Syndrome (WPW), VT, and other arrhythmias *(17)*.

INTERVENTIONAL ELECTROPHYSIOLOGY

The successes of arrhythmia surgery using intra-operative mapping, and the realization that the majority of targets for these techniques were subendocardial or could be mapped via an endocardial approach, led to efforts to ablate arrhythmogenic foci using percutaneous, catheter-based techniques. Initial catheter ablation procedures used high-energy direct current to fulgurate endocardial tissue. This technique, initially introduced

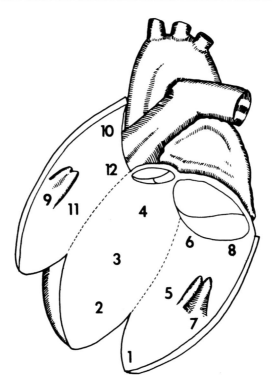

Fig. 2. Left ventricular endocardial mapping schema published by Josephson and colleagues. Left ventricular catheter mapping was initially used to understand the mechanism of VT and plan surgical treatment; catheter ablation is now performed in patients with VT of various etiologies. (With permission from Cassidy DM, Vassallo JA, Buxton AE, Doherty JU, Marchlinski FE, Josephson ME. The value of catheter mapping during sinus rhythm to localize site of origin of ventricular tachycardia. Circulation 1984;69:1103–1110.)

in 1981 by Gonzalez and Scheinman *(18)* and then Gallagher and colleagues *(19)* to create AV block in patients with refractory AF, was extended to relatively small numbers of patients with accessory pathways, other forms of SVT, and VT.

Although it was an important innovation, direct current (DC) shock ablation had a number of features that limited its widespread use. Delivered from a catheter tip, the high-voltage discharge caused local tissue ablation from barotrauma and thermal injury. Because of the relative "brute force" of this technique, the procedure carried the risk of major complications, including cardiac perforation and rupture. In addition, general anesthesia was required for the procedure.

Radiofrequency energy quickly supplanted DC as an energy source for catheter ablation procedures. Huang and colleagues first demonstrated radiofrequency catheter ablation in a canine model in 1985 *(20)*. Unlike direct current, radiofrequency energy created small, discrete lesions, which could be delivered using conscious sedation rather than general anesthesia. This advance ensured the success and widespread acceptance of catheter ablation procedures, and transformed electrophysiology from a descriptive specialty to an interventional field. For the first time, the electrophysiologist could cure patients with Wolff-Parkinson-White Syndrome (WPW) and A-V nodal reentrant tachycardia *(21,22)*. In fact, radiofrequency catheter ablation for SVT was the first and remains the only instance in which a cardiologist cures a patient of disease. Over the last fifteen years, radiofrequency catheter ablation has been applied to an ever-expanding list of arrhythmias, including atrial tachycardia, atrial flutter, VT, and AF.

The development of catheter ablation can be viewed as the coalescence of diagnostic electrophysiology and arrhythmia surgery, with important contributions from a number of investigators. The other important therapeutic advance in electrophysiology was much more the brainchild of a single man. Michel Mirowski first conceived of an implantable defibrillator in the 1970s after witnessing the sudden death of a colleague. Mirowski persevered in developing an automatic implantable defibrillator despite criticism from many colleagues. The first human implant was in 1980 *(23)*, and FDA approval followed in 1985. Though initial systems required a thoracotomy for epicardial lead placement, and abdominal placement of the large generator, it was apparent from the onset that the implantable defibrillator saved lives.

Several technological advances increased the efficacy of these devices, and greatly eased the implantation process. The development of endocardial lead systems *(24)*, biphasic waveforms, and active can technology *(25)* has made epicardial lead systems of primarily historical significance, and has made device implantation only slightly more complicated than pacemaker implantation. Current devices are capable of anti-tachycardia pacing as well as cardioversion and defibrillation therapy, and provide back-up bradycardia pacing, single- or dual-chamber, with rate response if necessary. Multiple clinical trials have demonstrated the effectiveness of the implantable cardio-verter defibrillator (ICD) in saving lives, both in patients who have had ventricular arrhythmias, and in patients at risk for life-threatening ventricular arrhythmias.

ELECTROPHYSIOLOGY TODAY AND TOMORROW

As the 21st century begins, electrophysiology remains a dynamic and expanding field. Catheter ablation and implantable devices (ICD and pacemaker) are first-line therapies for an ever-increasing array of diagnoses. Although antiarrhythmic drugs were initially mainstays of therapy for patients with arrhythmias, currently these drugs have largely been relegated to an adjunctive role in patients treated nonpharmaco-logically.

At present, investigation focuses on the extension of nonpharmacologic therapies to new patient populations. For catheter ablation, the frontiers are AF and VT in patients with chronic coronary artery disease (CAD). Although atrial fibrillation was previously viewed as "nonfocal," recent work suggests that in selected patients, AF is triggered from premature atrial beats, primarily originating in and around the pulmonary veins. Haissaguerre and colleagues *(26)* and others have shown that focal ablation can be curative in these highly selected patients (at least in the short term). Current efforts focus on improving the efficacy and safety of this procedure, and importantly, in developing criteria for selecting patients for whom this procedure should be under-taken. Advances in mapping and imaging—including electroanatomic mapping, noncon-tact mapping, and intracardiac echocardiography—all promise to advance catheter ablation.

Similarly, current device research focuses on identifying new patient populations who may benefit from ICD implantation. Several clinical trials in the 1990s established that ICD therapy is superior to pharmacologic therapy in most patients who have had sustained VT or cardiac arrest. AVID, the largest of these trials, was controversial because many electrophysiologists believed that the superiority of ICDs was well-established, and that a randomized trial was not necessary or even ethical. Two trials, MADIT and MUSTT, demonstrated a survival benefit in high-risk patients with CAD decreased left ventricular function, spontaneous nonsustained VT, and inducible VT/VF at electrophysiologic studies. Ongoing trials, including MADIT 2, SCD-HeFT, and DEFINITE, will assess the efficacy of prophylactic ICDs in various populations.

ICD technology itself is mature, yet it continues to evolve. Current devices are small enough—and lead and waveforms effective enough—to allow subcutaneous pectoral devices to be implanted in nearly all patients. Device advances include combination atrial-ventricular defibrillators for management of patients with atrial arrhythmias with and without accompanying ventricular arrhythmias. Trials that evaluate biventricular pacing with and without ICD backup, in patients with heart failure, show great promise.

In addition to these clinical frontiers is important basic and genetic research. Genetic engineering to create transgenic mice has complemented traditional cellular electrophysiologic techniques in advancing our understanding of ion-channel physiology and pathophysiology (27,28). Genetic mapping has identified the genes responsible for many cases of long QT syndrome, hypertrophic cardiomyopathy, and Brugada syndrome. Technological advances have made the possibility of "real-time" genetic diagnosis not only a possibility, but an expectation, within the next 10 yr.

In summary, cardiac electrophysiology has evolved from a descriptive discipline to an increasingly interventional field. Although less time is spent performing diagnostic electrophysiology studies, all of the basic principles and techniques developed and the tenets established in the early years remain as the foundation for increasingly complex catheter ablation procedures. With the rapid pace of technologic development, cardiac electrophysiology remains a vibrant, rewarding field. Nevertheless, "grandfathers" Wellens and Josephson caution that thoughtful physiologic research rather than technology should drive the field, and that electrophysiologists should adhere to the principles that gave birth to the field:

1. Understanding the pathophysiologic process causing the arrhythmia will lead to more effective therapies.
2. Patients' health and safety remain our first priority.

REFERENCES

1. Wolff L, Parkinson J, White PD. Bundle-branch block with short P-R interval in healthy young people prone to paroxysmal tachycardia. Am Heart J 1930;5:685.
2. Wolferth CC, Wood FC. The mechanism of production of short PR intervals and prolonged QRS complexes in patients with presumably undamaged hearts: hypothesis of an accessory pathway of auricolo-ventricular conduction (Bundle of Kent). Am Heart J 1933;8:298.
3. Mayer AG. Rhythmical pulsation in a scyphomedusae. Carnegie Institution 1906; publication 47.
4. Mines GR. On dynamic equilibrium in a heart. J Physiol 1913;46:349.
5. Mines GR. On circulating excitations in heart muscles and their possible relation to tachycardia and fibrillation. Trans R Soc Can 1914;4:43.
6. Hyman AS. Resuscitation of the stopped heart by intracardial therapy. II Experimental use of an artificial pacemaker. Arch Intern Med 1932;50:283.
7. Furman S, Schwedel JB. An intracardiac pacemaker for Stokes-Adams seizures. N Engl J Med 1959; 261:943.
8. Chardack WM, Gage AA, Greatbatch W. A transistorized, self-contained implantable pacemaker for the long-term correction of complete heart block. Surgery 1960;48:643.

9. Zoll PM, Linenthal AJ, Gibson W, et al. Termination of ventricular fibrillation in man by externally applied electric countershock. N Engl J Med 1956;254:727.

10. Durrer D, Schoo L, Schuilenburg RM, et al. The role of premature beats in the initiation and maintenance of supraventricular tachycardia in the WPW syndrome. Circulation 1967;36:644–662.

11. Coumel P, Cabrol C, Fabiato A, et al. Tachycardiamente par rythme reciproque. Arch Mal Coeur 1967;60:1830.

12. Scherlag BJ, Lau SH, Helfant RA, et al. Catheter technique for recording His bundle stimulation in the intact dog. J Appl Physiol 1968;25:425.

13. Damato AN, Lau SH, Helfant R, et al. Study of heart block in man using His bundle recordings. Circulation 1969;39:297–305.

14. Wellens HJ, Schuilenburg RM, Durrer D. Electrical stimulation of the heart in patients with ventricular tachycardia. Circulation 1972;46:216–226.

15. Josephson ME, Horowitz LN, Farshidi A, et al. Recurrent sustained ventricular tachycardia. 1. Mechanisms. Circulation 1978;57:431–440.

16. Josephson ME, Horowitz LN, Farshidi A, et al. Recurrent sustained ventricular tachycardia. 2. Endocardial mapping. Circulation 1978;57:440–447.

17. Cobb FR, Blumenschein SD, Sealy WC, et al. Successful surgical interruption of the bundle of Kent in a patient with Wolff-Parkinson-White syndrome. Circulation 1968;38:1018–1029.

18. Gonzalez R, Scheinman M, Margaretten W, et al. Closed chest electrode catheter technique for His bundle ablation in dogs. Am J Physiol 1981;241:H283–H287.

19. Gallagher JJ, Svenson RH, Kasell JH, et al. Catheter technique for closed-chest ablation of the atrioventricular conduction system: a therapeutic alternative for the treatment of refractory supraventricular tachycardia. N Engl J Med 1982;306:194–200.

20. Huang SK, Bharati S, Graham AR, Lev M, Marcus FI, Odell RC. Closed chest catheter desiccation of the atrioventricular junction using radiofrequency energy—a new method of catheter ablation. J Am Coll Cardiol 1987;9:349–358.

21. Jackman WM, Wang XZ, Friday KJ, et al. Catheter ablation of accessory atrioventricular pathways (Wolff-Parkinson-White syndrome) by radiofrequency current. N Engl J Med 1991;324:1605–1611.

22. Calkins H, Sousa J, el-Atasi R, et al. Diagnosis and cure of the Wolff-Parkinson-White syndrome or paroxysmal supraventricular tachycardia during a single electrophysiologic test. N Engl J Med 1991;324:1612.

23. Mirowski M, Reid PR, Mower MM, et al. Termination of malignant ventricular arrhythmias with an implanted automatic defibrillator in human beings. N Engl J Med 1980;303:322–324.

24. Saksena S, Parsonnet V. Implantation of a cardioverter/defibrillator without thoracotomy using a triple electrode system. JAMA 1988;259:69–72.

25. Bardy GH, Johnson G, Poole JE, et al. A simplified, single lead unipolar transvenous cardioverter-defibrillator. Circulation 1993;88:543–547.

26. Haissaguerre M, Jais P, Shah DC, et al. Spontaneous initiation of atrial fibrillation by ectopic beats originating in the pulmonary veins. N Engl J Med 1998;339:659–666.

27. Priori SG, Barhanin J, Hauer RNW, et al. Genetic and molecular basis of cardiac arrhythmias: impact on clinical management Parts I and II. Circulation 1999;99:518–528.

28. Priori SG, Barhanin J, Hauer RNW, et al. Genetic and molecular basis of cardiac arrhythmias: impact on clinical management Part III. Circulation 1999;99:674–681.

2

The Diagnosis of Cardiac Arrhythmias

Allison W. Richardson, MD,
and Peter J. Zimetbaum, MD

CONTENTS

INTRODUCTION

Patients with cardiac arrhythmias may come to the attention of their physicians in a variety of ways. An asymptomatic arrhythmia may be fortuitously discovered on a routine electrocardiogram (ECG) or physical exam. Alternatively, a patient may present with a complaint suggestive of arrhythmia, usually palpitations, syncope, or presyncope. Finally, patients who have no history of arrhythmia, but who may be prone to ventricular tachyarrhythmias because of underlying heart disease, may undergo routine testing to evaluate their level of risk. Patients in each category may be evaluated by invasive or noninvasive means. This chapter focuses on the noninvasive evaluation of patients with suspected arrhythmias and discusses indications for invasive testing.

THE INITIAL EVALUATION
OF THE PATIENT WITH PALPITATIONS OR SYNCOPE

The initial evaluation of a patient with palpitations, syncope, or presyncope should include a careful history, physical exam, and baseline ECG, all of which may be helpful in defining the need for further evaluation. A clear description of palpitations may help the physician make a diagnosis. A sensation of the heart stopping and then starting

From: *Contemporary Cardiology: Management of Cardiac Arrhythmias*
Edited by: L. I. Ganz © Humana Press Inc., Totowa, NJ

again, or of a brief "flip-flopping" of the heart, is most often caused by a single premature contraction, either atrial or ventricular in origin. The feeling that the heart has stopped is a result of the pause that follows a premature depolarization, and the "flip-flopping" sensation is caused by the hyperdynamic post-extrasystolic beat *(1)*. Patients often notice these beats, particularly when they are lying on their left side, because of the heart's proximity to the chest wall in that position. A sensation of pulsations in the neck is usually caused by cannon A waves, resulting from contraction of the atria against a closed tricuspid valve. This may occur with a variety of arrhythmias; however, when the pulsations are described as being rapid and regular, the diagnosis of AV nodal reentrant tachycardia (AVNRT) should be considered *(1)*. A sensation of a rapid pounding or fluttering in the chest may be caused by a supraventricular or ventricular arrhythmia. When a patient is able to describe regularity or irregularity of the rhythm, or has taken his or her pulse during an episode, this information may help to narrow the differential diagnosis *(1)*.

Similarly, in patients presenting after a syncopal or presyncopal episode, a careful description of the event may help identify a diagnosis. Vasovagal (neurocardiogenic) syncope is the most common etiology of syncope, particularly among patients with no structural heart disease *(2)*. This is caused by a period of autonomic imbalance during which an excessive vagal response occurs following a period of catecholamine predominance, leading to bradycardia and/or vasodilation. A feeling of warmth, nausea, and lightheadedness classically precedes vasovagal syncope *(3)*. Patients may describe a feeling of fatigue after awakening, and may suffer recurrent syncope if they attempt to arise too quickly. In contrast, arrhythmic syncope often occurs without warning, and a history of injury resulting from syncope may indicate an arrhythmic etiology.

In patients with palpitations or syncope, a situational history may be useful. Vasovagal syncope may occur following a precipitating incident or in a predisposing setting (following a meal, in a restaurant or bar, or another warm, crowded place). Palpitations during exercise or other periods of catecholamine excess may have a triggered mechanism, as occurs with idiopathic ventricular tachycardia (VT) in patients with structurally normal hearts *(4)*. Patients with congenital long QT syndrome (LQTS) may also present with palpitations or syncope, caused by polymorphic VT, during exercise or emotional stress *(5)*.

A personal history of structural heart disease, including prior myocardial infarction (MI), congestive heart failure (CHF), or cardiomyopathy, may identify patients at high risk for ventricular arrhythmias. A family history of sudden death or arrhythmic disease must also be elicited to identify patients with inherited disorders that may predispose them to arrhythmias (*see* Table 1).

The physical exam is used in the evaluation of patients with palpitations or syncope to aid in the diagnosis of structural heart disease. A physical exam suggestive of previously undiscovered hypertrophic obstructive cardiomyopathy (HOCM), CHF, or a valvular abnormality should prompt the physician to further characterize the abnormality with an echocardiogram. The twelve-lead ECG can also be useful in making a diagnosis of structural heart disease in this patient population. In the occasional situation in which an ECG has been obtained when a patient's symptoms occur, a diagnosis may be made based on the ECG *(6)*. More often, the only available ECG is obtained during an asymptomatic period. Even a sinus rhythm ECG may offer clues to the cause of a patient's symptoms. (*see* Table 2) *(1)*.

Table 1
Personal and Familial Disorders that Place Patients at Risk for Ventricular Arrhythmias

Personal Disorders	Familial Disorders
CAD (prior MI)	Congenital LQTS
Dilated cardiomyopathy	Brugada syndrome
HOCM	Arrhythmogenic right ventricular dysplasia
Severe valvular disease	HOCM
Congenital heart disease	Dilated cardiomyopathy
Congenital AV block	

CAD = coronary artery disease, MI = myocardial infarction; HOCM = hypertrophic obstructive cardiomyopathy; LQTS = long QT syndrome.

Table 2
Sinus Rhythm ECG Clues to Arrhythmia Diagnosis in Patients with Palpitations or Syncope

ECG Finding	Suggested Cause of Symptom
Short PR interval/delta wave	AVRT related to Wolf-Parkinson-White syndrome
Q waves	VT or VF related to coronary artery disease/ prior infarct
P mitrale, LVH, frequent atrial ectopy	Atrial fibrillation
Conduction system disease (bundle-branch or fascicular block, PR prolongation)	High-grade or complete heart block
LVH, apical T-wave inversions, prominent septal Q waves	VT or VF caused by hypertrophic cardiomyopathy
Epsilon wave, inverted T waves V1-V3	VT or VF caused by arrhythmogenic right ventricular dysplasia (ARVD)
Monomorphic VPBs, LBBB, positive axis	Idiopathic VT, RVOT type
Monomorphic VPBs, RBBB, negative axis	Idiopathic VT, left ventricular type
Long QT interval	Polymorphic ventricular tachycardia

AVRT = atrioventricular reentrant tachycardia; LVH = left ventricular hypertrophy; VPB = ventricular premature complex; LBBB = left bundle branch block; RBBB = right bundle branch block; VT = ventricular tachycardia; VF = ventricular fibrillation; RVOT = right ventricular outflow tract. Adapted from Zimetbaum et al. (1).

DIAGNOSTIC TESTING

After the initial evaluation has been completed, we recommend further testing for three groups of patients with palpitations: those with structural heart disease or a family history of an arrhythmic disorder, those with frequent symptoms that may be amenable to medical or catheter-based treatment, and those who feel compelled to have a specific explanation for their symptoms. We recommend further testing for patients with syncope or presyncope whose history is consistent with an arrhythmic etiology. We do not routinely recommend further testing for those with a history strongly suggestive of neurocardiogenic syncope.

Ambulatory Monitoring: Technology

Since 1961, when the Holter monitor was introduced, ambulatory monitoring has been used in the evaluation of palpitations and syncope *(7)*. The diagnosis of cardiac arrhythmias can be safely made in many patients using the variety of ambulatory monitoring devices available today. These include continuous electrocardiographic recorders and intermittent recorders with transtelephonic capabilities. The Holter monitor is the prototype for the continuous recorder. These monitors are typically worn for 24–48 h at a time. They record a continuous ECG tracing in two or three bipolar leads. Data is stored on a cassette or compact disk, and is subsequently digitized for analysis. These devices contain patient-activated event markers that allow patients to indicate the occurrence of symptoms. One advantage of Holter monitors is that they do not require patient activation. Thus, they may be successful in capturing arrhythmias that cause loss of consciousness, and can be used by patients who may have difficulty activating a monitor. These devices offer full disclosure, and will record asymptomatic as well as symptomatic arrhythmias that occur during the monitoring period. The major disadvantage of this system is the relatively short time that these devices are worn. In addition, the devices can be cumbersome and may prevent patients from participating in routine activities, such as exercise, that may be arrhythmic triggers. Asymptomatic arrhythmias that are detected may decrease the specificity of the findings of the test. Although patient event markers and diaries allow correlation between recorded arrhythmias and symptoms, patients often forget to accurately record the time of symptoms.

Intermittent recorders, or event recorders, store a brief ECG tracing when activated by the patient. Some of these devices are applied to the chest wall at the time of symptoms, and record information prospectively for approximately 2 min once activated. Other devices, called loop recorders, are worn continuously by the patient. These devices record continuously, but store data only when activated. This process allows storage of data both preceding and subsequent to device activation. Loop recorders usually consist of two or three chest leads attached to a small monitor the size of a beeper that can be worn on the patient's belt. These recorders are often worn for up to 1 mo at a time. They have the ability to transmit stored information over the telephone, so that data can be analyzed and interpreted immediately. Because they can be worn for up to 1 mo, event recorders are more likely than continuous monitors to capture infrequent arrhythmias. Information obtained is correlated with patient symptoms, and is thus very specific. The major disadvantage of this system is that patients may be unable to activate the recorder as a result of loss of consciousness, disorientation, or confusion about the activation process.

Recently, implantable loop recorders (ILRs) have become available. These monitors can be left in place for up to 2 yr, and are particularly useful in diagnosing very infrequent arrhythmias *(8)*. These devices are approximately the size of a pacemaker and are implanted subcutaneously to one side of the sternum. Like external loop recorders, they are patient-triggered, and store both prospective and retrospective data when activated. Recordings are initiated by placement of an activator over the device. Unlike external recorders, ILRs are not yet able to transmit tracings over the telephone. The obvious advantage of these devices is that they can conveniently be used even when symptoms rarely occur (less than once per month). Like other loop recorders, most ILRs require patient activation. The most recent devices contain automatic triggers

Table 3
Percentage of patients with palpitations whose various diagnoses
were made by continuous event recorder

Diagnosis	Percentage of patients	
	Kinlay et al. (14)	Zimetbaum et al. (13)
Sinus rhythm	35%	39%
Ventricular premature depolarizations	12%	36%
Atrial premature depolarizations	0%	13%
Atrial fibrillation	6%	2%
Ventricular tachycardia	0%	1%
Sinus tachycardia	29%	5%
Supraventricular tachycardia	18%	4%

Adapted from Zimetbaum et al. (1).

for prespecified high and low heart rates that will allow storage of data without patient activation.

Ambulatory Monitoring in the Evaluation of Palpitations

Ambulatory monitoring is a safe and effective way of diagnosing the cause of palpitations (9). Palpitations are usually benign, but may occasionally signify the presence of a significant arrhythmia (1). Although some patients identified during their initial visit as being at risk for dangerous arrhythmias may benefit from an aggressive evaluation including an electrophysiology study, most patients do not fall into this category, and are best evaluated by outpatient monitoring. Loop recorders are approximately twice as effective as Holter monitors when used in the evaluation of palpitations (diagnostic yield 66% vs 33%) (10). Two weeks of monitoring is usually adequate, and little is gained by longer periods of monitoring (11,12). Table 3 lists diagnoses made by event recorders used for the evaluation of palpitations by two authors (13,14). Clearly, the majority of patients monitored are found to have a benign cause of palpitations that does not result in specific treatment. In some cases, however, an arrhythmia requiring treatment is discovered, and often a benign diagnosis offers a patient the reassurance they need.

Our strategy for the diagnostic evaluation of patients with palpitations usually involves 2 wk of ambulatory monitoring using a loop recorder (see Fig. 1). If no symptoms occur during the initial 2 wk of monitoring, another 2 wk may be performed. Occasionally we choose a 24-h Holter monitor rather than a loop recorder for a patient who has very frequent palpitations or who is incapable of activating an event recorder. For a patient whose symptoms are rare, we may choose an ILR (10). Patients whose symptoms are sustained or poorly tolerated, especially those who have evidence of underlying heart disease, may warrant initial evaluation with an electrophysiology study (EPS) rather than ambulatory monitoring (1).

Ambulatory Monitoring in the Evaluation of Syncope and Presyncope

Ambulatory monitoring is also indicated in the evaluation of patients with syncope or presyncope (9). Proven cardiac syncope connotes a 24% 1-yr risk of sudden death (2). Thus, patients at high risk for serious arrhythmias who present with syncope are

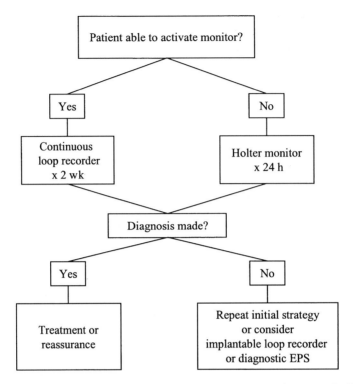

Fig. 1. The evaluation of palpitations. Adapted from Zimetbaum et al. *(10)*.

candidates for invasive evaluation, and in some instances implantable cardioverter defibrillators (ICD) implantation. Syncope is a very common problem, however, and most patients with syncope do not fall into this category. Ambulatory monitoring can be a useful tool in the diagnosis of low-risk patients with syncope. The diagnostic yield of Holter monitoring in the evaluation of syncope is low (15–22%) *(15,16)*. This is a result of the short duration of monitoring and the relative infrequency of symptoms in most cases. Several studies have examined the use of external event recorders in patients with syncope, and have found the diagnostic yield to be similarly low at 6–25% *(13,16–18)*. Some studies have shown event monitors to have a significantly higher yield in the evaluation of presyncope than syncope *(10,13)*.

The ILR has proven more effective than both the Holter monitor and the external loop recorder in diagnosing the cause of syncope. A recently published study of patients with undiagnosed syncope who underwent monitoring by ILR demonstrated a 59% diagnostic yield *(19)*. Of 85 patients, 50 recorded a rhythm corresponding with symptoms, at an average of 2.3 mo after device implantation. Of these, 16 patients had a specific arrhythmia diagnosed, 7 were given the diagnosis of neurocardiogenic syncope, and 27 had an arrhythmic cause of their symptoms excluded. Diagnosis of a specific arrhythmia was more common among patients who had syncope while being monitored than among those who had only presyncope (70% vs 24%). There was no incidence of sudden death during the follow-up period of this study. Another study examined the cost-effectiveness of the ILR, and found that its cost per diagnosis fell within the range of those of other diagnostic tests used commonly in the evaluation of syncope

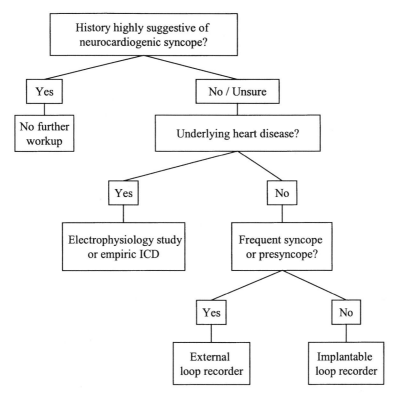

Fig. 2. The evaluation of arrhythmic syncope. Adapted from Zimetbaum et al. *(10)*.

(20). Incorporation of automatic triggers in the new generation of ILRs will likely improve the diagnostic yield of these devices for syncope.

Our strategy for the diagnostic evaluation of the patient with syncope or presyncope involves a careful initial evaluation as described above here (*see* Fig. 2). If the syncope is believed to be arrhythmic, and the history is not highly suggestive of neurocardiogenic syncope, further evaluation is undertaken. If the initial evaluation suggests the presence of underlying heart disease, an aggressive approach is chosen, and the patient is evaluated by EPS. If there is no evidence of underlying heart disease, we generally proceed with ambulatory monitoring using a loop recorder. If the patient's symptoms are frequent, we begin with an external loop recorder; if they are infrequent, we start with an ILR *(10)*.

Ambulatory Monitoring for Other Symptoms

Ambulatory monitoring may occasionally be considered for symptoms other than palpitations or syncope, to "rule out" arrhythmia as a cause for chest pain, diaphoresis, dyspnea, or fatigue. In a retrospective analysis of 729 loop recorder reports, we found no diagnostic yield for studies ordered for this indication *(13)*. As a result, we do not generally recommend ambulatory monitoring for symptoms that are not highly suggestive of arrhythmia. Likewise, the recently published American College of Cardiology/ American Heart Association (ACC/AHA) guidelines for ambulatory electrocardiography list unexplained, episodic shortness of breath, fatigue, or chest pain as a class IIB indication for ambulatory monitoring, or one for which efficacy is not well established *(9)*.

Other Noninvasive Diagnostic Tests

Ambulatory monitoring is the mainstay of the noninvasive diagnosis of symptomatic arrhythmias. However, in certain situations other tests may provide added information. Exercise testing can be useful in the evaluation of patients who present with symptoms during or after exercise. Exercise on a treadmill may provoke a patient's clinical symptoms, and in this case they can be correlated with the obtained rhythm strip. This is particularly useful when the clinical suspicion of a dangerous arrhythmia is not high enough to warrant initial evaluation by EPS, but either the patient or physician feels uncomfortable reinstating an exercise regimen prior to a trial of observed exercise in a controlled setting. In other situations, the use of an event recorder during daily exercise may accomplish the same goals as formal exercise testing.

Tilt table testing can be used to provoke neurocardiogenic syncope, and may be useful in the evaluation of patients with syncope. A test is considered positive if syncope occurs with associated hypotension or bradycardia *(21)*. A positive result may be particularly convincing if a patient reports reproduction of his clinical symptoms during the test. Recently there has been concern about frequent false-positive results in tilt table testing, with some studies finding the specificity of the test to be as low as 50% *(22)*. Kapoor et al. reviewed 23 studies of patients undergoing tilt table testing, and found that specificity varied widely, but seemed to decrease with an increasing tilt angle, and with the use of isoproterenol *(23)*. Reproducibility of positive results varied from 71–87% when tilt table testing was reported after 3 d to 6 wk *(23)*. Because of the relatively low specificity and reproducibility of tilt table testing, and the fact that a diagnosis of neurocardiogenic syncope may not result in specific treatment, tilt table testing is not appropriate for every patient with syncope. Recent ACC guidelines *(21)* state that tilt table testing is indicated in the evaluation of patients with recurrent or high-risk syncope, who have no underlying heart disease or have had other causes of syncope excluded by appropriate testing. In addition, tilt testing is warranted in the evaluation of recurrent exercise-induced syncope after structural heart disease has been excluded *(21)*.

NONINVASIVE RISK STRATIFICATION AND SURVEILLANCE FOR ASYMPTOMATIC ARRHYTHMIAS

The noninvasive determination of a patient's risk for developing life-threatening ventricular arrhythmias may be approached using traditional ambulatory monitoring or one of several newer techniques. Holter monitoring for asymptomatic ventricular ectopy has been used in the evaluation of patients with various forms of underlying heart disease, including coronary artery disease (CAD), dilated cardiomyopathy, hypertrophic cardiomyopathy, congenital heart disease, and primary electrophysiologic abnormalities such as congenital heart block and LQTS.

Post-Myocardial Infarction

Patients with nonsustained ventricular tachycardia (NSVT) and left ventricular dysfunction following MI have a 2-yr rate of up to 30% for sudden death *(24–27)*. The Multicenter Automatic Defibrillator Implantation Trial (MADIT) demonstrated significantly improved survival among CAD patients with left ventricular dysfunction, NSVT, and inducible, drug-unresponsive VT who were treated with ICDs *(28)*. More recently, the Multicenter Unsustained Tachycardia Trial (MUSTT) found that a similar group of patients treated with electrophysiology (EP)-guided therapy (antiarrhythmic medication or ICDs) had decreased mortality compared to those treated with traditional therapy *(29)*. This benefit was entirely attributable to the use of ICDs. These studies, which demonstrate a clear benefit associated with the use of ICDs in the treatment of certain post-MI patients with left ventricular dysfunction, raise the question of whether all such patients should undergo routine ambulatory monitoring to screen for NSVT. Such monitoring would place an enormous burden on the health care system *(28,30)*. It is not clear how many patients enrolled in MADIT and MUSTT were identified by routine ambulatory monitoring. In addition, the optimal timing of initial screening and interval follow-up has not been defined. For these reasons, there are not currently guidelines recommending routine ambulatory monitoring in post-MI patients *(9)*.

Dilated Cardiomyopathy/Congestive Heart Failure

Nonsustained VT can be identified by Holter monitoring in more than 50% of patients with idiopathic dilated cardiomyopathy *(31–34)*. Reports differ as to whether NSVT has any prognostic implication in these patients. Several studies have examined the use of empiric antiarrhythmic therapy in patients with cardiomyopathy, and have shown no consistent benefit *(31,33,35–37)*. The presence of CHF clearly increases the risk of sudden death in patients with dilated cardiomyopathy *(38–41)*. There is conflicting evidence as to whether NSVT further increases the mortality risk in this population. In the GESICA study *(42)*, patients with cardiomyopathy, CHF, and NSVT had a 24% 2-yr mortality as compared to a 9% 2-yr mortality among patients without NSVT. In the CHF STAT study *(43)*, 80% of patients with primarily nonischemic cardiomyopathy and CHF had NSVT. In this study, nonsustained VT was not found to be an independent predictor of mortality. Finally, there is no evidence that the use of antiarrhythmic medication to decrease NSVT in this population leads to improved survival *(44)*. Thus routine ambulatory monitoring is not recommended in adults with dilated cardiomyopathy with or without CHF *(9)*. Children with dilated cardiomyopathy are believed to have a higher risk of sudden death than adults, and periodic Holter monitoring is often recommended. Dilated cardiomyopathy is a class I indication for screening Holter monitoring in the pediatric population, according to the most recent ACC/AHA guidelines *(9)*.

Hypertrophic Cardiomyopathy

Patients with HOCM are at risk for sudden death; yet, predicting which individuals have the highest risk has proven difficult. Established risk factors in this population include history of syncope and history of sudden death in a first-degree relative *(45)*. NSVT was previously believed to be prognostically important in these patients, and guidelines once advocated routine ambulatory monitoring of patients with HOCM *(46)*. Several subsequent studies found that NSVT was not an independent predictor of death in this population *(47–49)*. Importantly, there is no evidence that antiarrhythmic treatment of patients with HOCM and NSVT has any effect on outcome. Maron et al. again raised the issue of screening for NSVT in their recent retrospective analysis of HOCM patients who had been deemed high-risk and treated with ICDs *(50)*. Although there remains some controversy as to whether adults with HOCM should undergo screening for NSVT, the most recent ACC/AHA guidelines for ambulatory monitoring do not recommend routine Holter monitoring in this population (9). Hypertrophic HOCM, like dilated cardiomyopathy, is associated with a higher sudden death rate in children than in adults (51), probably because patients who survive to adulthood are selected survivors. Periodic Holter monitoring of children with HOCM is recommended (9).

Congenital Heart Disease

Patients with complex congenital heart disease who have undergone surgical correction are at risk for ventricular arrhythmias as well as for conduction abnormalities that may lead to heart block (52). It is unclear whether NSVT is prognostically significant in this population (53–55), and there is no data supporting treatment of nonsustained VT once it is discovered. Although some experienced clinicians recommend routine Holter monitoring of patients with corrected tetralogy of Fallot (56), the most recent ACC/AHA guidelines classify asymptomatic corrected congenital heart disease as a class IIB indication for routine monitoring (usefulness not well-established) (9).

It must be emphasized that although routine monitoring of asymptomatic patients with the diseases discussed here is not currently recommended, these patients are at increased risk of dangerous arrhythmias. Palpitations, presyncope, and syncope should be taken very seriously in these populations and should prompt evaluation either with an event recorder or by EPS, depending on the clinical scenario.

Patients With Congenital Electrophysiologic Abnormalities

Patients with congenital LQTS and congenital heart block are at increased risk for arrhythmic death. Patients with LQTS may develop polymorphic VT (torsades de pointes), causing syncope or sudden death (57,58). These patients may benefit from treatment with beta-blockers and/or implantation of permanent pacemakers or ICDs. Patients who have a family history of sudden death or a personal history of syncope are at particularly high risk for sudden death. Ambulatory monitoring can be used to identify patients with significant bradycardia, periods of QT prolongation, or asymptomatic nonsustained polymorphic VT, which may put patients at increased risk for sudden death (59,60). As a result, many clinicians use annual or biannual Holter monitoring to screen patients with LQTS. There is no available data to support this practice. Evaluation of asymptomatic pediatric patients with known or suspected LQTS is a class I indication for Holter monitoring, according to the most recent ACC/AHA guidelines (9). Whether monitoring should be routinely undertaken in asymptomatic adults, who are likely to be selected survivors, is less certain.

Congenital heart block places patients at risk for left ventricular dysfunction, mitral regurgitation resulting from left ventricular dilation, and sudden death. The likelihood of these complications is diminished by ventricular pacing (61). A recent study showed that in 27 asymptomatic patients followed for 8 ± 3 yr, the presence of a daytime heart rate of less than 50 beats per min, or evidence of an unstable junctional escape (junctional exit block or ventricular arrhythmias) predicted an increased likelihood of complications (62). Another recent study followed 102 patients for up to 30 yr (61). In this study, ventricular response rate decreased with age, with associated increases in ventricular ectopy and worsening of left ventricular function and mitral regurgitation. Only a prolonged corrected QT interval was found to be predictive of syncope. Our practice is to screen these patients yearly by Holter monitor to evaluate their ventricular response, corrected QT interval, and ventricular ectopic activity. We recommend placement of a permanent pacemaker when patients develop symptomatic bradycardia, exercise intolerance, QT prolongation, frequent ventricular ectopy, or a wide complex escape rhythm. This practice differs from that outlined in the recent ACC/AHA pacing guidelines *(63)* only because we include QT prolongation among absolute indications for pacing in this population. Holter monitoring is limited by the brief period of time during which the monitor is worn. Consequently, episodic QT prolongation, severe bradycardia, or NSVT may be missed. Patients may develop complications of congenital heart block despite the absence of detectable risk factors, partly because periodic Holter monitoring does not adequately disclose their day-to-day rhythm. As in patients with structural heart disease, palpitations, presyncope and syncope must be taken very seriously in patients who have LQTS or congenital heart block. These conditions should be evaluated by event monitor or invasive testing, depending on the clinical setting.

OTHER TECHNIQUES FOR RISK STRATIFICATION

Several newer techniques, like Holter monitoring, may be useful in predicting the risk of ventricular arrhythmias. These include the signal-averaged ECG (SAECG), heart-rate variability (HRV), T-wave alternans (TWA), and QT dispersion (QTD). There is data to suggest that each of these methods can independently predict risk in certain populations; however, it is not yet clear how information obtained from their use should be clinically applied.

Signal-Averaged ECG

The signal-averaged ECG was developed to identify the existence of substrate for reentrant VT. The goal of the SAECG is to detect late potentials, which represent low amplitude, high-frequency electrical activity occurring in the terminal portion of the QRS. Late potentials are felt to be caused by slow conduction and delayed activation of tissue, and thus to identify the presence of substrate that could potentially cause reentrant ventricular arrhythmias. Because late potentials are very low in amplitude, they are obscured by noise on a regular twelve-lead ECG. Signal averaging improves the signal-to-noise ratio through temporal or spatial averaging, allowing the detection of low-amplitude electrical activity. Unfortunately, the use of this technique is limited because time-domain analysis—the method of analysis most often used—cannot be applied in patients with bundle-branch block or significant intraventricular conduction delay. Atrial fibrillation (AF) and flutter have also been shown to diminish the predictive accuracy of the SAECG *(64)*.

There is strong evidence that the SAECG can identify post-MI patients at risk for ventricular arrhythmias *(64–70)*. There is much less data available on its use in other populations *(70)*. Based on data compiled from 15 studies, 8–48% of post-MI patients who have late potentials detected on SAECG will ultimately experience sustained VT or sudden death *(70)*. A positive SAECG in this population has a positive predictive accuracy of 14–29% when used to predict major arrhythmic events, and a normal SAECG has a negative predictive accuracy of 95–99% *(70)*. Although the presence of late potentials is an independent predictor of major arrhythmic events in the post-MI population, the positive predictive accuracy of the SAECG is not high enough to base clinical decisions regarding treatment of individual patients on this information alone

(70). Eventually, the SAECG may be used in conjunction with other information to determine which post-MI patients may benefit from invasive evaluation. We do not currently obtain SAECGs on our post-MI patients, as there are no data to support basing management decisions on SAECG results.

Heart-Rate Variability

Heart-rate variability analysis is the evaluation of beat-to-beat variability of the R-R interval. Data is obtained from digitized Holter tracings. HRV is believed to be largely a reflection of autonomic tone *(71).* There is evidence for a correlation between the risk of sudden cardiac death and autonomic tone, with relatively decreased vagal activity indicating increased susceptibility to lethal arrhythmias *(72).* Following MI, HRV is decreased. It is lowest soon after MI, and begins to recover within several weeks *(73,74).* HRV is an independent risk factor for mortality post-MI. In 1987, Kleiger et al. demonstrated a 34% mortality over 4 yr among post-MI patients with depressed HRV, as compared to a 12% mortality among patients with normal HRV *(75).* Decreased HRV post-MI has been shown to predict increased mortality, and to specifically predict sudden cardiac death and sustained VT *(76).* Although diminished HRV post-MI is an independent risk factor for ventricular arrhythmias and mortality, its predictive accuracy when used alone is low *(9,71).* Information regarding HRV can be used in conjunction with other tests to increase the accuracy of risk stratification post-MI *(71).* Bigger et al. *(77)* and Farrell et al. *(78)* each demonstrated that the use of multiple risk stratifiers such as left ventricular ejection fraction (LVEF), NSVT, SAECG, and HRV in combination could result in positive predictive accuracy of approx 50%. Thus, HRV analysis may eventually be incorporated into protocols for risk stratification post-MI. It has not yet been determined how HRV analysis should be used in directing therapy to justify its routine use in the post-MI population *(9).* There is conflicting data on the relationship between HRV and arrhythmic events in patients with underlying heart disease other than history of MI. Thus, HRV analysis is not recommended in risk stratification of patients with dilated or hypertrophic cardiomyopathy or other underlying disease *(9,71).*

Microvolt T-Wave Alternans

Electrical alternans is the variability of the ECG waveform on alternate beats. Repolarization alternans (ST- and T-wave alternans) shows promise as a risk stratifier for ventricular arrhythmias associated with various conditions *(79).* T-wave alternans, a marker of heterogeneous electrical repolarization, has been observed on ECG tracings just prior to the onset of ventricular fibrillation (VF) in acutely ischemic animals *(80,81)* and humans *(82–85).* In most cases, however, TWA is too subtle to be seen on a basic surface ECG. Recently, techniques have become available to allow visualization of microvolt TWA, which would otherwise be undetectable. TWA is best measured during exercise or atrial pacing with a target heart rate of approx 100 beats per minute (BPM) *(86).* Slower heart rates and ectopic beats can obscure the detection of alternans *(82).* In 1994, Rosenbaum et al. *(87)* studied TWA during atrial pacing in 83 patients with a variety of underlying conditions who were undergoing EPS. Alternans was predictive of inducibility of VT at EPS, and was also an independent risk factor for spontaneous VT, VF, or sudden cardiac death during 20 mo of follow-up. The relative risk for major arrhythmic events was 9.0 in patients with detectable TWA as compared to those without TWA. Other small-scale studies have similarly demonstrated TWA to be predictive of ventricular arrhythmias *(88)*. The clinical implication of TWA has also been evaluated among groups of patients with specific underlying conditions. In patients with HOCM, exercise-induced TWA has been shown to correlate with the presence of traditional risk factors such as a history of syncope or family history of sudden death *(89)*. There is no information yet as to whether exercise-induced TWA will prove to be an independent predictor for ventricular arrhythmias among these patients. In a pilot study of 70 patients with CHF, the presence of TWA at rest or during exercise appeared to be a strong marker for sustained VT, VF arrest, or death during a 1-yr follow-up *(82)*. Although the measurement of TWA is a promising technique for predicting patients' propensity for ventricular arrhythmias, there is no available information yet as to which patients will benefit from use of this technique, or as to whether patient management should be altered based on a positive test. Thus, we do not currently measure TWA for clinical purposes. In the future, TWA may be used in combination with other markers to improve accuracy in the prediction of ventricular arrhythmias in certain patient populations in order to determine which patients warrant further testing or treatment.

QT Dispersion

QT interval dispersion (QTD) is a measure of variability of the QT interval, which, like TWA, it is a marker of the heterogeneity of ventricular repolarization. The measurement of QTD is made simply by taking the difference between the longest and shortest QT intervals on a 12-lead ECG. QT dispersion has been found an independent predictor of cardiovascular mortality in two large studies, one examining an elderly population in Rotterdam *(90)*, and the other examining middle-aged and elderly native Americans (the Strong Heart study) *(91)*. In each study, abnormal QTD was associated with an approximately twofold increase in the risk of cardiovascular mortality. The research of de Bruyne et al. also demonstrated a 1.4-fold increase in all cause mortality among patients with abnormal QTD *(90)*. In Okin et al., a corrected QT interval was also an independent predictor of cardiovascular mortality, and corrected QT interval and QTD were additively predictive *(91)*. These large studies examined populations in which the majority of patients had no known heart disease. In addition, QTD seems to be useful in risk stratification of patients with LQTS *(92)*. When other groups of patients who have cardiac disease which places them at risk for sudden death have been evaluated, the results have been variable. In 1994, a retrospective case-control study of patients with CAD showed an association between an abnormal QTD and sudden death *(93)*. Subsequent prospective studies have differed as to whether QTD is predictive of cardiovascular mortality post-MI *(94,95)*. In the study by Spargias et al., although QTD was found to be predictive, it was not a very sensitive or specific marker. Studies have also differed as to whether QTD is of prognostic value in patients with CHF. Barr et al. *(96)* showed an association between abnormal QTD and sudden death in patients with CHF. However, a larger study *(97)* failed to demonstrate an independent relationship between QTD and all causes of mortality or sudden death after multivariate analysis. In patients with hypertrophic cardiomyopathy, QTD does not seem to correlate with any of the known risk factors for sudden death *(98)*. Thus, although QTD is predictive of cardiovascular death in a wide population, its clinical usefulness as a risk stratifier in diseases other than LQTS has not yet been demonstrated.

INDICATIONS FOR EPS

When there is high suspicion for a serious arrhythmia, or when an arrhythmia has been diagnosed, but further characterization or catheter-based treatment is desired, invasive testing with an EPS is warranted. Based on the data from MADIT *(28)* and MUSTT *(29)*, EPS is also indicated for risk stratification in patients who have CAD, LVEF less than 40%, and nonsustained VT occurring more than 96 h after an ischemic event or revascularization. During an EPS, intracardiac recordings are made to document conduction intervals and activation patterns, and programmed electrical stimulation is delivered to attempt reproduction of clinical arrhythmias. The information obtained can be useful in the diagnosis of both bradyarrhythmias and tachyarrhythmias. In symptomatic patients with suspected sinus node disease, information regarding sinus node function can be obtained by measuring sinus node recovery time *(99)* or sinoatrial conduction time *(100,101)*. In patients with syncope or presyncope and evidence of conduction system disease on ECG, measurement of the HV interval can be used to estimate the likelihood of progression to a heart block *(102–104)*. Electrical stimulation protocols targeting the atria and/or ventricles can be used for induction of supraventricular or ventricular tachyarrhythmias. Induction of a patient's clinical arrhythmia in the electrophysiology lab enables study of its mechanism, and in some cases catheter ablation of the arrhythmia. Even when the arrhythmia is not ablatable, information obtained during EPS can be used to guide further therapy. In patients with a history of cardiac arrest, EPS can help to define the mechanism for the arrest. Most cardiac arrest patients should be treated with ICDs. Information gathered at EPS can help guide device selection and programming *(105)*. Finally, as previously mentioned, EPS is useful in risk-stratification of post-MI patients with poor left ventricular function and nonsustained VT, and in determining which patients in this category should be treated with ICDs *(28,29)*. Detailed information regarding EPS is beyond the scope of this discussion, but can be found elsewhere *(106)*. Some specific indications for EPS based on the 1995 ACC/AHA guidelines for clinical intracardiac electrophysiological and catheter ablation procedures *(107)* are listed in Table 4.

FUTURE STRATEGIES

Emerging technologies will continue to change the way diagnoses are made in electrophysiology. In particular, advances in ambulatory monitoring will facilitate the diagnosis of arrhythmia in the outpatient setting. As mentioned here, recent technology has allowed loop recorders to self-trigger in the setting of marked changes in heart rate. This feature will likely improve the diagnostic yield of ILRs used in the evaluation of syncope. Systems capable of recording and transmitting blood pressure and oximetry data in addition to ECG data in the ambulatory setting will eventually become available, and will allow more comprehensive monitoring. These systems may provide physicians with an improved understanding of the clinical significance of detected arrhythmias, and will enable more comprehensive monitoring of known disease and prescribed therapy. Increasing information regarding the clinical utility of currently available technology will also change the evaluation of arrhythmias. Emerging techniques for risk stratification such as heart-rate variability, TWA, QTD, and the SAECG may be used routinely once the optimal application of these techniques is understood.

Table 4
Indications for Electrophysiology Study (EPS)

Class I indications for EPS

1. Evaluation of suspected sinus node dysfunction in symptomatic patients
2. Evaluation of suspected His-Purkinje system block in symptomatic patients
3. Evaluation of patients with bifascicular block and unexplained symptoms consistent with arrhythmia
4. Frequent or poorly tolerated SVT not adequately controlled with medication or with patient preference for ablation therapy
5. Wide QRS tachycardia when the diagnosis is unclear or information obtained from EPS will help guide therapy
6. WPW in patients undergoing evaluation for accessory pathway ablation with symptomatic tachycardia, or history of unexplained syncope or cardiac arrest
7. Unexplained syncope in the setting of structural heart disease
8. Survivors of cardiac arrest other than in the setting of acute Q-wave MI
9. Palpitations preceding syncope
10. Palpitations with a documented tachycardia by pulse with no ECG documentation of rhythm
11. Patients with documented ventricular or supraventricular tachycardias in whom EPS findings will help guide medical therapy or programming of ICDs
12. Nonsustained VT occurring>96 h post-MI or revascularization in patients with CAD and EF<40%*

SVT = supraventricular tachycardia; WPW = Wolff-Parkinson-White syndrome; MI = myocardial infarction; ICD = implantable cardioverter-defibrillator; CAD = coronary artery disease; LVEF = left ventricular ejection fraction. Guidelines are adapted from the 1995 ACC/AHA. Guidelines for clinical intracardiac electrophysiological and catheter ablation procedures *(101)*. *This recommendation is based on recent data *(28,29)* and is not included in the 1995 ACC/AHA guidelines.

REFERENCES

1. Zimetbaum P, Josephson ME. Evaluation of patients with palpitations. N Engl J Med 1998;338:1369–1373.
2. Kapoor WN, Karpf M, Wieand S, Peterson JR, Levey GS. A prospective evaluation and follow-up of patients with syncope. N Engl J Med 1983;309:197–204.
3. Day SC, Cook EF, Funkenstein H, Goldman L. Evaluation and outcome of emergency room patients with transient loss of consciousness. Am J Med 1982;73:15–23.
4. Varma N, Josephson ME. Therapy of "idiopathic" ventricular tachycardia. J Cardiovasc Electrophysiol 1997;8:104–116.
5. Schwartz PJ, Priori SG, Napolitano C. The long QT syndrome. In: Zipes DP, Jalife J, eds. Cardiac Electrophysiology: From Cell to Bedside. 3rd ed. Philadelphia, PA, 2000, pp. 597–615.
6. Josephson ME, Wellens HJ. Differential diagnosis of supraventricular tachycardia. Cardiol Clin 1990;8:411–442.
7. Holter NJ. New method for heart studies: continuous electrocardiography of active subjects over long periods is now practical. Science 1961;134:1214–1220.
8. Krahn AD, Klein GJ, Norris C, Yee R. The etiology of syncope in patients with negative tilt table and electrophysiological testing. Circulation 1995;92:1819–1824.
9. Crawford MH, Bernstein SJ, Deedwania PC, et al. ACC/AHA Guidelines for Ambulatory Electrocardiography. A report of the American College of Cardiology/American Heart Association Task Force on Practice Guidelines (Committee to Revise the Guidelines for Ambulatory Electrocardiography). Developed in collaboration with the North American Society for Pacing and Electrophysiology. J Am Coll Cardiol 1999;34:912–948.

10. Zimetbaum PJ, Josephson ME. The evolving role of ambulatory arrhythmia monitoring in general clinical practice. Ann Intern Med 1999;130:848–856.

11. Zimetbaum PJ, Kim KY, Josephson ME, Goldberger AL, Cohen DJ. Diagnostic yield and optimal duration of continuous-loop event monitoring for the diagnosis of palpitations. A cost-effectiveness analysis. Ann Intern Med 1998;128:890–895.

12. Reiffel JA, Schulhof E, Joseph B, Severance E, Wyndus P, McNamara A. Optimum duration of transtelephonic ECG monitoring when used for transient symptomatic event detection. J Electrocardiol 1991;24:165–168.

13. Zimetbaum P, Kim KY, Ho KK, Zebede J, Josephson ME, Goldberger AL. Utility of patient-activated cardiac event recorders in general clinical practice. Am J Cardiol 1997;79:371–372.

14. Kinlay S, Leitch JW, Neil A, Chapman BL, Hardy DB, Fletcher PJ. Cardiac event recorders yield more diagnoses and are more cost-effective than 48-hour Holter monitoring in patients with palpitations. A controlled clinical trial. Ann Intern Med 1996;124:16–20.

15. DiMarco JP, Philbrick JT. Use of ambulatory electrocardiographic (Holter) monitoring. Ann Intern Med 1990;113:53–68.

16. Bass EB, Curtiss EI, Arena VC, et al. The duration of Holter monitoring in patients with syncope. Is 24 hours enough? Arch Intern Med 1990;150:1073–1078.

17. Brown AP, Dawkins KD, Davies JG. Detection of arrhythmias: use of a patient-activated ambulatory electrocardiogram device with a solid-state memory loop. Br Heart J 1987;58:251–253.

18. Linzer M, Pritchett EL, Pontinen M, McCarthy E, Divine GW. Incremental diagnostic yield of loop electrocardiographic recorders in unexplained syncope. Am J Cardiol 1990;66:214–219.

19. Krahn AD, Klein GJ, Yee R, Takle-Newhouse T, Norris C. Use of an extended monitoring strategy in patients with problematic syncope. Reveal Investigators. Circulation 1999;99:406–410.

20. Krahn AD, Klein GJ, Yee R, Manda V. The high cost of syncope: cost implications of a new insertable loop recorder in the investigation of recurrent syncope. Am Heart J 1999;137:870–877.

21. Benditt DG, Ferguson DW, Grubb BP, et al. Tilt table testing for assessing syncope. American College of Cardiology. J Am Coll Cardiol 1996;28:263–275.

22. Kapoor WN, Brant N. Evaluation of syncope by upright tilt testing with isoproterenol. A nonspecific test. Ann Intern Med 1992;116:358–363.

23. Kapoor WN, Smith MA, Miller NL. Upright tilt testing in evaluating syncope: a comprehensive literature review. Am J Med 1994;97:78–88.

24. Anderson KP, DeCamilla J, Moss AJ. Clinical significance of ventricular tachycardia (3 beats or longer) detected during ambulatory monitoring after myocardial infarction. Circulation 1978;57:890–897.

25. Buxton AE, Marchlinski FE, Waxman HL, Flores BT, Cassidy DM, Josephson ME. Prognostic factors in nonsustained ventricular tachycardia. Am J Cardiol 1984;53:1275–1279.

26. Bigger JT, Jr., Fleiss JL, Rolnitzky LM. Prevalence, characteristics and significance of ventricular tachycardia detected by 24-hour continuous electrocardiographic recordings in the late hospital phase of acute myocardial infarction. Am J Cardiol 1986;58:1151–1169.

27. Mukharji J, Rude RE, Poole WK, et al. Risk factors for sudden death after acute myocardial infarction: two-year follow-up. Am J Cardiol 1984;54:31–36.

28. Moss AJ, Hall WJ, Cannom DS, et al. Improved survival with an implanted defibrillator in patients with coronary disease at high risk for ventricular arrhythmia. Multicenter Automatic Defibrillator Implantation Trial Investigators. N Engl J Med 1996;335:1933–1940.

29. Buxton AE, Lee KL, Fisher JD, Josephson ME, Prystowsky EN, Hafley G. A randomized study of the prevention of sudden death in patients with coronary artery disease. Multicenter Unsustained Tachycardia Trial Investigators. N Engl J Med 1999;341:1882–1890.

30. Naccarelli GV, Wolbrette DL, Dell'Orfano JT, Patel HM, Luck JC. A decade of clinical trial developments in postmyocardial infarction, congestive heart failure, and sustained ventricular tachyarrhythmia patients: from CAST to AVID and beyond. Cardiac Arrhythmic Suppression Trial. Antiarrhythmic Versus Implantable Defibrillators. J Cardiovasc Electrophysiol 1998;9:864–891.

31. Huang SK, Messer JV, Denes P. Significance of ventricular tachycadia in idiopathic dilated cardiomyopathy: observations in 35 patients. Am J Cardiol 1983;51:507–512.

32. Suyama A, Anan T, Araki H, Takeshita A, Nakamura M. Prevalence of ventricular tachycardia in patients with different underlying heart diseases: a study by Holter ECG monitoring. Am Heart J 1986;112:44–51.

33. Neri R, Mestroni L, Salvi A, Pandullo C, Camerini F. Ventricular arrhythmias in dilated cardiomyopathy: efficacy of amiodarone. Am Heart J 1987;113:707–715.
34. Meinertz T, Hofmann T, Kasper W, et al. Significance of ventricular arrhythmias in idiopathic dilated cardiomyopathy. Am J Cardiol 1984;53:902–907.
35. Holmes J, Kubo SH, Cody RJ, Kligfield P. Arrhythmias in ischemic and nonischemic dilated cardiomyopathy: prediction of mortality by ambulatory electrocardiography. Am J Cardiol 1985; 55:146–151.
36. Chakko CS, Gheorghiade M. Ventricular arrhythmias in severe heart failure: incidence, significance, and effectiveness of antiarrhythmic therapy. Am Heart J 1985;109:497–504.
37. Wilson JR, Schwartz JS, Sutton MS, et al. Prognosis in severe heart failure: relation to hemodynamic measurements and ventricular ectopic activity. J Am Coll Cardiol 1983;2:403–410.
38. Singh SN, Fletcher RD, Fisher S, et al. Veterans Affairs congestive heart failure antiarrhythmic trial. CHF STAT Investigators. Am J Cardiol 1993;72:99F–102F.
39. Massie BM, Fisher SG, Radford M, et al. Effect of amiodarone on clinical status and left ventricular function in patients with congestive heart failure. CHF-STAT Investigators (published erratum appears in Circulation 1996; Nov 15;94[10]:2668). Circulation 1996;93:2128–2134.
40. Cohn JN, Johnson G, Ziesche S, et al. A comparison of enalapril with hydralazine-isosorbide dinitrate in the treatment of chronic congestive heart failure [see comments]. N Engl J Med 1991;325:303–310.
41. Doval HC, Nul DR, Grancelli HO, Perrone SV, Bortman GR, Curiel R. Randomised trial of low-dose amiodarone in severe congestive heart failure. Grupo de Estudio de la Sobrevida en la Insuficiencia Cardiaca en Argentina (GESICA). Lancet 1994;344:493–498.
42. Doval HC, Nul DR, Grancelli HO, et al. Nonsustained ventricular tachycardia in severe heart failure. Independent marker of increased mortality due to sudden death. GESICA-GEMA Investigators. Circulation 1996;94:3198–3203.
43. Singh SN, Fisher SG, Carson PE, Fletcher RD. Prevalence and significance of nonsustained ventricular tachycardia inpatients with premature ventricular contractions and heart failure treated with vasodilator therapy. Department of Veterans Affairs CHF STAT Investigators. J Am Coll Cardiol 1998;32:942–947.
44. Sim I, McDonald KM, Lavori PW, Norbutas CM, Hlatky MA. Quantitative overview of randomized trials of amiodarone to prevent sudden cardiac death. Circulation 1997;96:2823–2829.
45. Wigle ED, Rakowski H, Kimball BP, Williams WG. Hypertrophic cardiomyopathy. Clinical spectrum and treatment. Circulation 1995;92:1680–1692.
46. Knoebel SB, Crawford MH, Dunn MI, et al. Guidelines for ambulatory electrocardiography. A report of the American College of Cardiology/American Heart Association Task Force on Assessment of Diagnostic and Therapeutic Cardiovascular Procedures (Subcommittee on Ambulatory Electrocardiography). Circulation 1989;79:206–215.
47. Spirito P, Rapezzi C, Autore C, et al. Prognosis of asymptomatic patients with hypertrophic cardiomyopathy and nonsustained ventricular tachycardia. Circulation 1994;90:2743–2747.
48. Fananapazir L, Chang AC, Epstein SE, McAreavey D. Prognostic determinants in hypertrophic cardiomyopathy. Prospective evaluation of a therapeutic strategy based on clinical, Holter, hemodynamic, and electrophysiological findings. Circulation 1992;86:730–740.
49. Cecchi F, Olivotto I, Montereggi A, Squillatini G, Dolara A, Maron BJ. Prognostic value of nonsustained ventricular tachycardia and the potential role of amiodarone treatment in hypertrophic cardiomyopathy: assessment in an unselected non-referral based patient population. Heart 1998; 79:331–336.
50. Maron BJ, Shen WK, Link MS, et al. Efficacy of implantable cardioverter-defibrillators for the prevention of sudden death in patients with hypertrophic cardiomyopathy. N Engl J Med 2000; 342:365–373.
51. McKenna WJ, Franklin RC, Nihoyannopoulos P, Robinson KC, Deanfield JE. Arrhythmia and prognosis in infants, children and adolescents with hypertrophic cardiomyopathy. J Am Coll Cardiol 1988; 11:147–153.
52. Pinsky WW, Arciniegas E. Tetralogy of Fallot. Pediatr Clin N Am 1990;37:179–192.
53. Chandar JS, Wolff GS, Garson A, Jr., et al. Ventricular arrhythmias in postoperative tetralogy of Fallot. Am J Cardiol 1990;65:655–661.
54. Joffe H, Georgakopoulos D, Celemajer DS, Sullivan ID, Deanfield JE. Late ventricular arrhythmia is rare after early repair of tetralogy of Fallot. J Am Coll Cardiol 1994;23:1146–1150.

55. Cullen S, Celermajer DS, Franklin RC, Hallidie-Smith KA, Deanfield JE. Prognostic significance of ventricular arrhythmia after repair of tetralogy of Fallot: a 12-year prospective study. J Am Coll Cardiol 1994;23:1151–1155.

56. Marelli A, Moodie D. Adult congenital heart disease. In: Topol E, ed. Textbook of Cardiovascular Medicine. Lippincott-Raven, Philadelphia, PA, 1998, pp. 769–797.

57. Schwartz PJ. The long QT syndrome. Curr Probl Cardiol 1997;22:297–351.

58. Tan HL, Hou CJ, Lauer MR, Sung RJ. Electrophysiologic mechanisms of the long QT interval syndromes and torsade de pointes. Ann Intern Med 1995;122:701–714.

59. Eggeling T, Osterhues HH, Hoeher M, Gabrielsen FG, Weismueller P, Hombach V. Value of Holter monitoring in patients with the long QT syndrome. Cardiology 1992;81:107–114.

60. Locati EH, Maison-Blanche P, Dejode P, Cauchemez B, Coumel P. Spontaneous sequences of onset of torsade de pointes in patients with acquired prolonged repolarization: quantitative analysis of Holter recordings. J Am Coll Cardiol 1995;25:1564–1575.

61. Michaelsson M, Jonzon A, Riesenfeld T. Isolated congenital complete atrioventricular block in adult life. A prospective study. Circulation 1995;92:442–449.

62. Dewey RC, Capeless MA, Levy AM. Use of ambulatory electrocardiographic monitoring to identify high-risk patients with congenital complete heart block. N Engl J Med 1987;316:835–839.

63. Gregoratos G, Cheitlin MD, Conill A, et al. ACC/AHA Guidelines for Implantation of Cardiac Pacemakers and Antiarrhythmia Devices: Executive Summary—a report of the American College of Cardiology/American Heart Association Task Force on Practice Guidelines (Committee on Pacemaker Implantation). Circulation 1998;97:1325–1335.

64. Borggrefe M, Fetsch T, Martinez-Rubio A, Makijarvi M, Breithardt G. Prediction of arrhythmia risk based on signal-averaged ECG in postinfarction patients. Pacing Clin Electrophysiol 1997;20:2566–2576.

65. Kuchar DL, Thorburn CW, Sammel NL. Prediction of serious arrhythmic events after myocardial infarction: signal-averaged electrocardiogram, Holter monitoring and radionuclide ventriculography. J Am Coll Cardiol 1987;9:531–538.

66. Cripps T, Bennett D, Camm J, Ward D. Prospective evaluation of clinical assessment, exercise testing and signal-averaged electrocardiogram in predicting outcome after acute myocardial infarction. Am J Cardiol 1988;62:995–999.

67. el-Sherif N, Ursell SN, Bekheit S, et al. Prognostic significance of the signal-averaged ECG depends on the time of recording in the postinfarction period. Am Heart J 1989;118:256–264.

68. Breithardt G, Schwarzmaier J, Borggrefe M, Haerten K, Seipel L. Prognostic significance of late ventricular potentials after acute myocardial infarction. Eur Heart J 1983;4:487–495.

69. Gomes JA, Winters SL, Stewart D, Horowitz S, Milner M, Barreca P. A new noninvasive index to predict sustained ventricular tachycardia and sudden death in the first year after myocardial infarction: based on signal-averaged electrocardiogram, radionuclide ejection fraction and Holter monitoring. J Am Coll Cardiol 1987;10:349–357.

70. Signal-averaged electrocardiography. J Am Coll Cardiol 1996;27:238–249.

71. Hohnloser SH, Klingenheben T, Zabel M, Li YG. Heart rate variability used as an arrhythmia risk stratifier after myocardial infarction. Pacing Clin Electrophysiol 1997;20:2594–2601.

72. Schwartz PJ, La Rovere MT, Vanoli E. Autonomic nervous system and sudden cardiac death. Experimental basis and clinical observations for post-myocardial infarction risk stratification. Circulation 1992;85:177–191.

73. Bigger JT, Jr., Kleiger RC, Fleiss JL, Rolnitzky LM, Steinman RC, Miller JP. Components of heart rate variability measured during healing of acute myocardial infarction. Am J Cardiol 1988;61:208–215.

74. Bigger JT, Jr., Fleiss JL, Rolnitzky LM, Steinman RC, Schneider WJ. Time course of recovery of heart period variability after myocardial infarction. J Am Coll Cardiol 1991;18:1643–1649.

75. Kleiger RE, Miller JP, Bigger JT, Jr., Moss AJ. Decreased heart rate variability and its association with increased mortality after acute myocardial infarction. Am J Cardiol 1987;59:256–262.

76. Odemuyiwa O, Malik M, Farrell T, Bashir Y, Poloniecki J, Camm J. Comparison of the predictive characteristics of heart rate variability index and left ventricular ejection fraction for all-cause mortality, arrhythmic events and sudden death after acute myocardial infarction. Am J Cardiol 1991;68:434–439.

77. Bigger JT, Jr., Fleiss JL, Steinman RC, Rolnitzky LM, Kleiger RE, Rottman JN. Frequency domain measures of heart period variability and mortality after myocardial infarction. Circulation 1992;85:164–171.

78. Farrell TG, Bashir Y, Cripps T, et al. Risk stratification for arrhythmic events in postinfarction patients based on heart rate variability, ambulatory electrocardiographic variables and the signal-averaged electrocardiogram. J Am Coll Cardiol 1991;18:687–693.

79. Armoundas AA, Osaka M, Mela T, et al. T-wave alternans and dispersion of the QT interval as risk stratification markers in patients susceptible to sustained ventricular arrhythmias. Am J Cardiol 1998;82:1127–1129.

80. Russell DC, Smith JH, Oliver MF. Transmembrane potential changes and ventricular fibrillation during repetitive myocardial ischemia in the dog. Br Heart J 1979;42:88–96.

81. Downar E, Janse MJ, Durrer D. The effect of acute coronary artery occlusion on subepicardial transmembrane potentials in the intact porcine heart. Circulation 1977;56:217–224.

82. Murda'h MA, McKenna WJ, Camm AJ. Repolarization alternans: techniques, mechanisms, and cardiac vulnerability. Pacing Clin Electrophysiol 1997;20:2641–2657.

83. Salerno JA, Previtali M, Panciroli C, et al. Ventricular arrhythmias during acute myocardial ischaemia in man. The role and significance of R-ST-T alternans and the prevention of ischaemic sudden death by medical treatment. Eur Heart J 1986;(7 Suppl A):63–75.

84. Joyal M, Feldman RL, Pepine CJ. ST-segment alternans during percutaneous transluminal coronary angioplasty. Am J Cardiol 1984;54:915–916.

85. Kleinfeld MJ, Rozanski JJ. Alternans of the ST segment in Prinzmetal's angina. Circulation 1977;55:574–577.

86. Hohnloser SH, Klingeheben T, Zabel M, et al. Heart rate threshold is important for detecting T wave alternans (abstract). PACE 1996;19:II–588.

87. Rosenbaum DS, Jackson LE, Smith JM, Garan H, Ruskin JN, Cohen RJ. Electrical alternans and vulnerability to ventricular arrhythmias. N Engl J Med 1994;330:235–241.

88. Estes MNA, Zipes DP, el-Sherif N, et al. Electrical alternans during rest and exercise as a predictor of vulnerability to ventricular arrhythmias. J Am Coll Cardiol 1995; Special Issue:409A.

89. Murda'h M, Nagayoshi H, Albrecht P, et al. T-wave alternans as a predictor of sudden death in hypertrophic cardiomyopathy (abstract). Circulation 1996;94(Suppl.):I–669.

90. de Bruyne MC, Hoes AW, Kors JA, Hofman A, van Bemmel JH, Grobbee DE. QTc dispersion predicts cardiac mortality in the elderly: the Rotterdam Study. Circulation 1998;97:467–472.

91. Okin PM, Devereux RB, Howard BV, Fabsitz RR, Lee ET, Welty TK. Assessment of QT Interval and QT dispersion for prediction of all-cause and cardiovascular mortality in American Indians: The Strong Heart Study. Circulation 2000 Jan 4;101:61–66.

92. Priori SG, Napolitano C, Diehl L, Schwartz PJ. Dispersion of the QT interval. A marker of therapeutic efficacy in the idiopathic long QT syndrome. Circulation 1994;89:1681–1689.

93. Zareba W, Moss AJ, le Cessie S. Dispersion of ventricular repolarization and arrhythmic cardiac death in coronary artery disease. Am J Cardiol 1994;74:550–553.

94. Zabel M, Klingenheben T, Franz MR, Hohnloser SH. Assessment of QT dispersion for prediction of mortality or arrhythmic events after myocardial infarction: results of a prospective, long-term follow-up study. Circulation 1998;97:2543–2550.

95. Spargias KS, Lindsay SJ, Kawar GI, et al. QT dispersion as a predictor of long-term mortality in patients with acute myocardial infarction and clinical evidence of heart failure [see comments]. Eur Heart J 1999;20:1158–1165.

96. Barr CS, Naas A, Freeman M, Lang CC, Struthers AD. QT dispersion and sudden unexpected death in chronic heart failure. Lancet 1994;343:327–329.

97. Brooksby P, Batin PD, Nolan J, et al. The relationship between QT intervals and mortality in ambulant patients with chronic heart failure. The United Kingdom heart failure evaluation and assessment of risk trial (UK-HEART) [see comments]. Eur Heart J 1999;20:1335–1341.

98. Yi G, Ellioitt P, McKenna WJ, et al. QT dispersion and risk factors for sudden cardiac death in patients with hypertrophic cardiomyopathy. Am J Cardiol 1998;82:1514–1519.

99. Mandel W, Hayakawa H, Danzig R, Marcus HS. Evaluation of sino-atrial node function in man by overdrive suppression. Circulation 1971;44:59–66.

100. Strauss HC, Saroff AL, Bigger JT, Jr., Giardina EG. Premature atrial stimulation as a key to the understanding of sinoatrial conduction in man. Presentation of data and critical review of the literature. Circulation 1973;47:86–93.

101. Strauss HC, Bigger JT, Saroff AL, Giardina EG. Electrophysiologic evaluation of sinus node function in patients with sinus node dysfunction. Circulation 1976;53:763–776.

102. Scheinman MM, Peters RW, Modin G, Brennan M, Mies C, O'Young J. Prognostic value of infranodal conduction time in patients with chronic bundle branch block. Circulation 1977;56:240–244.

103. McAnulty JH, Rahimtoola SH, Murphy E, et al. Natural history of "high-risk" bundle-branch block: final report of a prospective study. N Engl J Med 1982;307:137–143.

104. Dhingra RC, Palileo E, Strasberg B, et al. Significance of the HV interval in 517 patients with chronic bifascicular block. Circulation 1981;64:1265–1271.

105. Myerburg RJ, Castellanos A. Evolution, evaluation, and efficacy of implantable cardioverter-defibrillator technology [editorial; comment]. Circulation 1992;86:691–693.

106. Josephson ME. Clinical Cardiac Electrophysiology: Techniques and Interpretations. 2nd ed. Lea & Febiger, Philadelphia, PA, 1993, pp. 1–839.

107. ACC/AHA Task Force Report. Guidelines for Clinical Intracardiac Electrophysiological and Catheter Ablation Procedures. A report of the American College of Cardiology/American Heart Association Task Force on Practice Guidelines (Committee on Clinical Intracardiac Electrophysiologic and Catheter Ablation Procedures). Developed in collaboration with the North American Society of Pacing and Electrophysiology. J Cardiovasc Electrophysiol 1995;6:652–679.

3

Approach to the Patient with Supraventricular Tachycardia

Leonard I. Ganz, MD

INTRODUCTION

Supraventricular tachyarrhythmias are relatively common, and occur in patients of all ages, with and without structural heart disease. This chapter examines the pathophysiology, epidemiology, and natural history of the supraventricular tachyarrhythmias, and focuses on diagnostic and therapeutic options for these patients *(1)*.

PATHOPHYSIOLOGY

Any tachyarrhythmia that requires atrial and/or AV junctional tissue for its initiation and maintenance can properly be considered a supraventricular tachyarrhythmia. Ventricular tachyarrhythmias, conversely, require only ventricular tissue for their initiation and maintenance. Supraventricular tachyarrhythmias can be divided into those that require only atrial tissue (atrial tachyarrhythmias) and those that require AV junctional tissue (*see* Table 1). Supraventricular tachycardia (SVT) may be paroxysmal (PSVT) or incessant.

Atrial Tachyarrhythmias

ATRIAL TACHYCARDIA

Atrial tachycardia is a supraventricular tachyarrhythmia that arises from atrial muscle tissue *(2)*. Atrial tachycardia, also called unifocal or ectopic atrial tachycardia, is a relatively unusual form of supraventricular tachyarrhythmia, particularly in adults.

From: *Contemporary Cardiology: Management of Cardiac Arrhythmias*
Edited by: L. I. Ganz © Humana Press Inc., Totowa, NJ

Table 1
Classification of Supraventricular Tachycardia

Atrial	A-V Junctional
Ectopic (unifocal) atrial tachycardia	Atrioventricular nodal reentrant tachycardia[a]
Sinus tachycardia	Atrioventricular reentrant tachycardia[b]
Inappropriate sinus tachycardia	Nonparoxysmal junctional tachycardia
Sinus node reentrant tachycardia	Junctional ectopic tachycardia
Multifocal atrial tachycardia	
Atrial fibrillation	
Atrial flutter	

[a]Includes typical and atypical AVNRT.
[b]Includes WPW and concealed accessory pathways, orthodromic and antidromic tachycardia, and PJRT.

Electrocardiographically, atrial tachycardias tend to be "long RP" tachycardias; the P wave is closer to the next QRS complex than to the previous QRS complex. The P-wave morphology depends on the site of the tachycardia focus (see Fig. 1). Atrial tachycardia may arise from a reentrant, automatic, or triggered mechanism. The nonreentrant atrial tachycardias may be incessant rather than paroxysmal, and may pose a risk of tachycardia-induced cardiomyopathy.

SINUS TACHYCARDIA

Sinus tachycardia is a physiologic response to a perturbation. The sinoatrial (SA) node is innervated by sympathetic and vagal nerve endings. Sympathetic stimulation as well as vagal withdrawal increases the sinus rate. Circulating catecholamines also affect the sinus rate. Common causes of sinus tachycardia include pain, anxiety, fever, hypotension, hypoxia, hyperthyroidism, and hypovolemia. Although beta-blockers may blunt the elevated heart rate, since sinus tachycardia is generally a response to some other physiologic derangement, treatment efforts are directed at the underlying cause of tachycardia, rather than the elevated heart rate itself.

INAPPROPRIATE SINUS TACHYCARDIA

In this case, the rhythm is sinus tachycardia, but there is no apparent underlying cause (3). These patients tend to have an elevated resting heart rate, and a marked increase in heart rate with even mild exertion. Hyperthyroidism and pheochromocytoma can mimic inappropriate sinus tachycardia (IST), and should be excluded in this setting. It remains unclear whether IST reflects an underlying abnormality of the sinoatrial (SA) node, the autonomic input to the SA node, or both.

SINUS NODE REENTRANT TACHYCARDIA

This is a form of reentrant atrial tachycardia in which the reentry circuit involves SA nodal or peri-SA nodal tissue (4). Thus, the P waves appear identical or nearly identical to sinus P waves. Unlike sinus tachycardia and inappropriate sinus tachycardia, however, sinus node reentrant tachycardia is distinguished by an abrupt onset and offset, like other reentrant arrhythmias. Sinus node reentrant tachycardia is occasionally induced in the electrophysiology (EP) lab, and is often nonsustained and relatively slow in rate. Clinically, the occurrence of significant sinus node reentrant tachycardia is relatively rare.

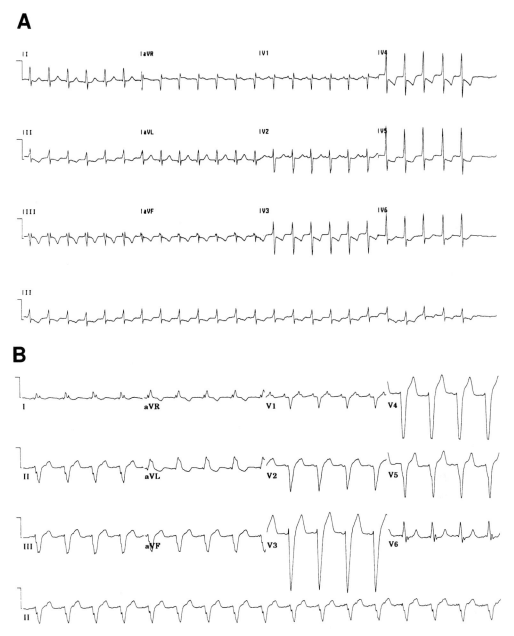

Fig. 1. ECGs in three patients with atrial tachycardia. **(A)** Atrial activity is most prominent in lead V₁. Note that the P wave is closer to the next QRS complex than the previous QRS complex; a so-called "long-RP tachycardia." There is 1:1 conduction until the end of the tracing, when AV nodal block reveals low amplitude P waves. **(B)** Atrial tachycardia with 2:1 A:V conduction, and left bundle-branch block (LBBB) aberrancy in a patient with dilated cardiomyopathy. P-wave activity is most evident in lead V₁. **(C)** Atrial tachycardia with variable A:V conduction. Once again, P-wave activity is most obvious in lead V₁. The atrial rate is 180 BPM; 1:1 conduction occurred with minimal exertion. This tachycardia was incessant, and the patient was referred for cardiac transplantation because of intractable class IV heart failure (left ventricular ejection fraction 9%). Catheter ablation of this left atrial focus led to prompt symptomatic improvement, with normalization of left ventricular function over a six month period.

C

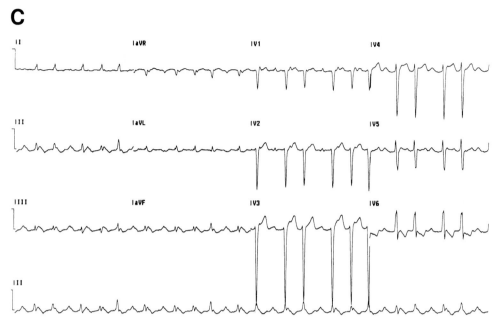

Fig. 1. (*Continued.*)

MULTIFOCAL ATRIAL TACHYCARDIA

This arrhythmia is diagnosed when there are at least three P-wave morphologies, and an irregular atrial rate of at least 100 beats per minute (BPM) (*see* Fig. 2) (*5*). Variability in the PR interval is common. This arrhythmia tends to occur in acutely ill, elderly patients, particularly those with active pulmonary disease. Discrete P waves, with intervening isoelectric segments, distinguish this arrhythmia from atrial fibrillation (AF).

ATRIAL FIBRILLATION (AF)

The most common sustained tachyarrhythmia results from multiple reentrant circuits in the right and left atria. Atrial fibrillation (AF) is discussed in great detail in Chapters 5–8, and thus will not be considered further in this chapter.

ATRIAL FLUTTER

A macroreentrant arrhythmia, atrial flutter may involve a stereotypical right atrial circuit (typical counterclockwise and clockwise isthmus-dependent flutter) or other circuits (atypical flutters). Atypical flutters commonly occur in patients with prior surgical repair of congenital heart disease. Atrial flutter is considered in detail in Chapter 9, and will therefore not be discussed further in this chapter.

A-V Junctional Tachyarrhythmias

AV NODAL REENTRANT TACHYCARDIA (AVNRT)

AVNRT is the most common form of paroxysmal supraventricular tachycardia (PSVT) (*6*). The typical form of AVNRT is a short RP tachycardia; P waves are either buried entirely within the QRS complex, or visible just as a tiny deflection at the

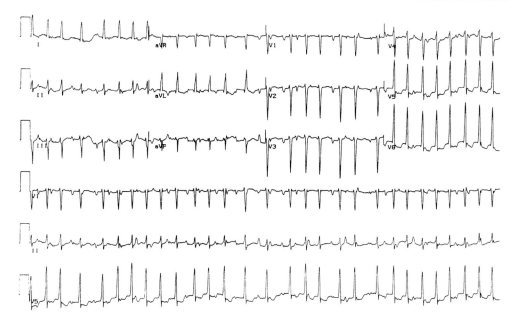

Fig. 2. ECG in a patient with advanced COPD. Multiple P-wave morphologies, most evident in the lead V_1 and lead II rhythm strips, and rapid rate are diagnostic of multifocal atrial tachycardia (MAT). Note the variability in PR interval and occasional blocked P wave.

junction of the QRS complex and ST segment (*see* Fig. 3). Atypical AVNRT is a long RP tachycardia, and electrocardiographically may resemble unifocal atrial tachycardia with 1:1 A:V conduction. AVNRT occurs in patients with dual AV nodal pathways, usually called the fast and slow pathways (*see* Fig. 4). During sinus rhythm, anterograde conduction occurs over the fast pathway. An atrial premature depolarization (APD) may find the fast pathway still refractory from the previous depolarization, and may thus conduct down the slow pathway (*see* Fig. 5). If this conduction is slow enough, the fast pathway may recover excitability, so the impulse can turn around propagate retrogradely up to the atrium over the fast pathway, creating a reentry circuit. Atypical AVNRT is usually initiated by a ventricular premature depolarization (VPD), which conducts retrogradely up the slow pathway, and then turns around and proceeds anterogradely over the fast pathway. Patients tend to have one of these two forms of AVNRT clinically, but occasionally both types are inducible during electrophysiology study (EPS). Because infranodal tissue is not part of the reentry circuit itself, AVNRT occasionally occurs with 2:1 infranodal block, resembling atrial tachycardia with 2:1 A:V conduction.

A-V REENTRANT TACHYCARDIA (AVRT)

Normally, the AV node and His-Purkinje system constitute the only electrical connection between the atria and ventricles. An accessory pathway or bypass tract consists of strands of working myocardium that bridge the mitral or tricuspid annulus, creating an additional electrical connection between atria and ventricles. When an accessory pathway capable of anterograde conduction is present, ventricular pre-excitation and the Wolff-Parkinson-White Syndrome (WPW) are apparent during sinus rhythm (*see* Figs. 6, 7) (*7,8*). The most common arrhythmia in patients with WPW is orthodromic

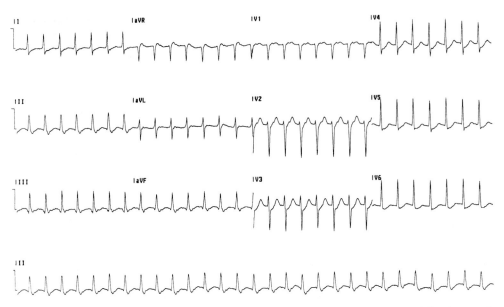

Fig. 3. ECG in a patient with typical AVNRT. Retrograde P waves are evident as deflections at the junction of the QRS complex and ST segment. Pseudo S waves are evident in leads II, III, and aVF, while pseudo R′ waves are seen in aVR and V₁. Since the P waves are much closer to the previous QRS complex compared with the next complex, this is a short RP tachycardia.

AVRT; in this macroreentrant circuit, anterograde conduction is over the AV node, and retrograde conduction is up the accessory pathway. Like AVNRT, this orthodromic AVRT is a short RP tachycardia, and the P wave is sometimes visible superimposed on the ST segment (*see* Figs. 7, 8). Less commonly in patients with WPW, the opposite circuit occurs, inscribing a tachycardia with a wide and bizarre QRS complex called antidromic AVRT (*see* Figs. 7, 9) In WPW patients, atrial fibrillation and atrial flutter are of great concern (*see* Figs. 10, 11). Unlike the AV node, many accessory pathways are capable of rapid, nondecremental conduction. Ventricular rates of 250–300 BPM or higher can occur, with the risk of degeneration into ventricular fibrillation (VF). Thus, there is a risk of sudden death associated with the WPW syndrome.

Some accessory pathways are capable of only retrograde conduction; since there is no evidence of pre-excitation in sinus rhythm, these pathways are said to be concealed. Patients with concealed accessory pathways can have orthodromic but not antidromic AVRT, and are not at risk for sudden death caused by extremely rapid, pre-excited AF or atrial flutter. Some concealed pathways display slow retrograde conduction. These patients have an orthodromic AVRT characterized by a long RP interval called permanent junctional reciprocating tachycardia (PJRT) (*see* Fig. 12) *(9)*. As this tachycardia tends to be incessant, it can lead to tachycardia-induced cardiomyopathy *(10)*.

Nonparoxysmal Junctional Tachycardia (NPJT)

This tachycardia is extremely rare. Unlike AVNRT and AVRT, which are reentrant in nature, NPJT is believed to be caused by enhanced automaticity or triggered activity within the AV junction *(11)*. Electrocardiographically, this may resemble AVNRT, or there may be A-V dissociation during the narrow complex tachycardia (*see* Fig. 13).

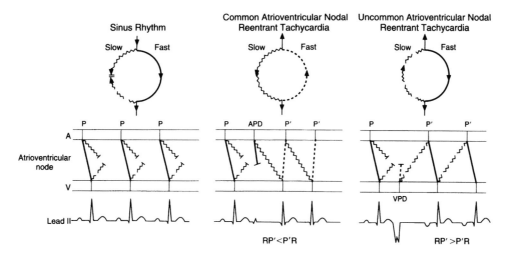

Fig. 4. Mechanism of AVNRT. Each panel shows a diagram of the AV node, a Lewis (ladder) diagram, and surface ECG lead II. Continuous lines represent anterograde conduction; broken lines represent retrograde conduction. Straight lines signify fast pathway conduction; wavy lines slow pathway. P represents sinus P waves, P' A-V nodal echoes, APD-atrial premature depolarization, VPD-ventricular premature depolarization. The left panel represents sinus rhythm, in which anterograde conduction is over the fast pathway. In the middle panel, an APD finds the fast pathway refractory and travels anterograde over the slow pathway. When the impulse has traversed the slow pathway, the fast pathway has recovered; thus the impulse can turn around and travel retrograde up the fast pathway. Note the nearly simultaneous inscription of P' and the QRS complex during common AVNRT. In the right panel, a VPD finds the retrograde fast pathway refractory, and travels up the slow pathway, initiating uncommon AVNRT. Note that in common AVNRT RP' < P'R, while in uncommon AVNRT, RP' > P'R. (Reproduced from Ganz LI, Friedman PL. Supraventricular tachycardia. N Engl J Med 1995;332:162–173. Copyright © 1995 Massachusetts Medical Society.)

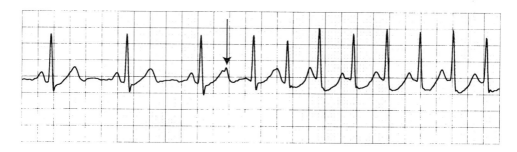

Fig. 5. Event monitor in patient with PSVT. An APD (arrow), conducted with a long PR interval, initiates tachycardia. This is characteristic of typical AVNRT.

This arrhythmia tends to occur in the setting of digitalis toxicity or early after valve surgery; it is also seen rarely in the setting of acute myocardial infarction (MI).

JUNCTIONAL ECTOPIC TACHYCARDIA (JET)

This is also a nonparoxysmal, nonreentrant tachycardia, frequently described in the pediatric literature (12). This arrhythmia may have the same mechanism as NPJT. JET tends to occur following surgical repair of congenital heart disease, has an extremely rapid ventricular response, and is associated with a very high mortality.

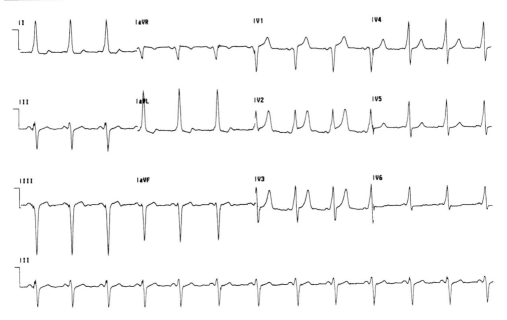

Fig. 6. ECG in a patient with WPW. Note the short PR interval and delta wave reflective of ventricular pre-excitation. In this case, the pathway is right septal.

EPIDEMIOLOGY AND NATURAL HISTORY

Data on the prevalence of supraventricular tachyarrhythmias are extremely scarce. Electrocardiographic (ECG) screening studies of large populations *(13,14)* suggest a prevalence of the WPW pattern on ECG of 1 to 2 per 1000, but not all of these patients have clinical arrhythmia. In a study of the 50,000 residents of the Marshfield Epidemiologic Study Area (MESA) in Wisconsin, the prevalence of symptomatic PSVT was 2.25 per 1000, with an incidence of 35 per 100,000 person-years *(15)*. In this study, PSVT occurred more frequently in women than in men, which is also reflected in series of patients undergoing catheter ablation. Interestingly, episodes of PSVT may occur more during the luteal than the follicular phase of the menstrual cycle in premenopausal women *(16)*.

Notably, PSVT is frequently misdiagnosed as panic disorder. Two-thirds of patients with PSVT fulfill DMS-IV criteria for panic disorder *(17)*. In these patients, the proper diagnosis may be delayed by failure to recognize overt pre-excitation on a baseline ECG, as well as reliance on Holter monitoring rather than event monitoring (*see* Chapter 2).

Natural history data are also lacking in these patients. Except for patients with WPW, the prognosis in most patients with SVT is generally believed to be excellent, with therapeutic measures aimed at improving symptoms. Supraventricular arrhythmias can occur in the presence or absence of structural heart disease. In the absence of WPW and significant structural heart disease, the risk of sudden cardiac death resulting from SVT is extremely low *(18)*. Although mitral valve prolapse is frequently diagnosed in patients with PSVT, evidence of a particular association is lacking thus far *(19)*.

In patients with WPW, the risk of sudden cardiac death is linked to extremely rapid rates during AF/atrial flutter with degeneration into VF. This risk relates to the

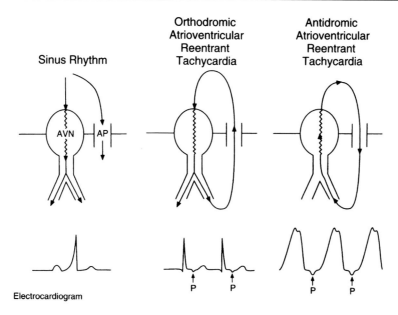

Sinus Rhythm

Orthodromic Atrioventricular Reentrant Tachycardia

Antidromic Atrioventricular Reentrant Tachycardia

Electrocardiogram

Fig. 7. Mechanism of AVRT in WPW. The left panel represents sinus rhythm. The QRS has a slurred upstroke (delta wave), caused by rapid activation (pre-excitation) of the ventricle over the accessory pathway. During orthodromic AVRT (middle panel), there is no delta wave, because ventricular activation occurs entirely over the normal AV node and His-Purkinje system, with retrograde conduction over the accessory pathway. In antidromic AVRT (right panel), the ventricle is activated entirely over the accessory pathway, with retrograde conduction up the AV node (or a second accessory pathway). Thus, the QRS is fully pre-excited and is wide and bizarre appearing, an exaggerated version of the delta wave during sinus rhythm. (Reproduced from Ganz LI, Friedman PL. Supraventricular tachycardia. N Engl J Med 1995;332:162–173. Copyright © 1995 Massachusetts Medical Society.)

anterograde refractory period of the accessory pathway. Because of this risk, EPS and radiofrequency catheter ablation (*see* Chapter 4) are typically recommended as initial therapy in symptomatic patients. The management of asymptomatic patients is frequently debated, as sudden cardiac death can rarely be the initial clinical presentation in patients with the WPW syndrome *(20–22)*. The risk of sudden death in asymptomatic WPW patients is estimated to be about 1 per thousand patient-years; the risk of death during catheter ablation is estimated to be about 1 per thousand. Noninvasive indicators (such as intermittent pre-excitation in sinus rhythm (*see* Fig. 14), or sudden loss of pre-excitation during exercise test or with procainamide infusion) carry some prognostic information, but direct measurements of the accessory pathway anterograde refractory period during EPS and shortest R-R interval during pre-excited AF are more accurate. Yet the specificity of all of these measures, both noninvasive and invasive, is limited. When coupled with a low pretest probability of sudden death in asymptomatic WPW patients, the positive predictive value of these tests remains low *(23)*. In addition, most patients with asymptomatic WPW at initial diagnosis remain asymptomatic during follow-up, and some of these patients lose their capacity for anterograde conduction (and thus risk of sudden death) over time *(24,25)*. For all of these reasons, many electrophysiologists recommend no particular diagnostic testing or treatment for asymptomatic individuals unless they are engaged in high-risk professions, such as the transpor-

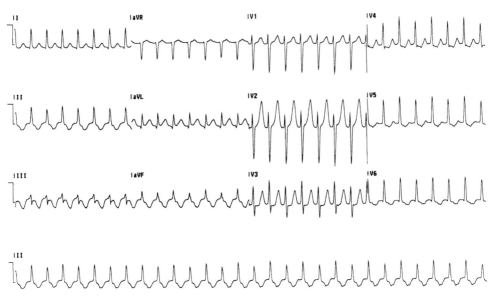

Fig. 8. ECG in the same patient as in Fig. 6, during PSVT. Note that the QRS complex is now normal, with a sharp upstroke, and no evidence of pre-excitation. Retrograde P waves, best seen in leads $V_4 - V_6$ (arrows), fall on the junction of the ST segment and T wave, considerably later than during typical AVNRT. The P waves are still closer to the previous QRS complex compared to the next QRS complex, so like AVNRT, orthodromic AVRT is typically a short RP tachycardia.

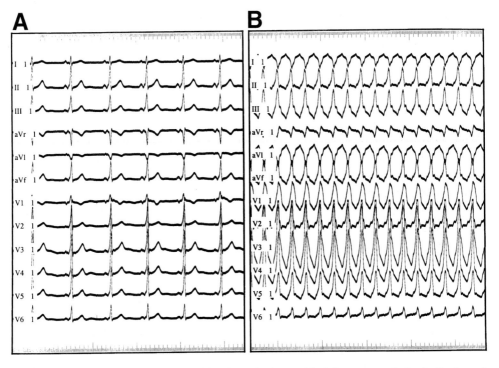

Fig. 9. ECGs in a patient with WPW. **(A)** Sinus rhythm, with delta-wave polarity indicative of a left-free-wall pathway. **(B)** Antidromic AVRT. Note that the QRS morphology is wide and bizarre, an exaggeration of the delta wave seen during sinus rhythm. Retrograde atrial activation is via the AV node, and is not evident in this tracing.

Table 2
Differential Diagnosis of Supraventricular Tachycardia

Short RP	Long RP
Typical AVNRT	Atypical AVNRT
AVRT	PJRT
Nonparoxysmal junctional tachycardia*	Ectopic (unifocal) atrial tachycardia
Junctional ectopic tachycardia*	Sinus tachycardia
	Inappropriate sinus tachycardia
	Sinus node reentrant tachycardia

AVNRT = Atrioventricular nodal reentrant tachycardia; AVRT = Atrioventricular reentrant tachycardia; PJRT = Permanent junctional reciprocating tachycardia.

* Only if 1:1 V:A conduction; if A-V dissociation, RP classification does not apply.

tation industry or elite athletes *(26)*. Other electrophysiologists feel that because of the risk of sudden death, even asymptomatic patients should undergo diagnostic EPS, with catheter ablation if the accessory pathway has a short refractory period and a location that is approachable without posing a high risk of heart block (e.g., left free wall) *(27)*.

Few data are available regarding the natural history of symptomatic PSVT after patients present initially. Among 113 patients with WPW, concealed accessory pathway, or AVNRT initially presenting in the precatheter ablation era, only 10.3% reported spontaneous disappearance of their tachycardia during a mean follow-up of 9 ± 1 yr. Rather, both the symptom score and frequency of episodes tended to increase over time. Moreover, 13.5% developed new tachyarrhythmias during follow-up, most commonly atrial fibrillation (AF). For patients with manifest WPW, 38.5% developed new AF during follow-up *(28)*.

DIAGNOSTIC EVALUATION

The diagnostic approach depends on the manner in which patients present. Patients presenting with palpitations, without documented tachycardia, should have a history and physical examination for signs and/or symptoms of structural heart disease and baseline ECG. In most cases, ambulatory event monitoring will be the most cost-effective means of documenting an arrhythmia (*see* Chapter 2). If WPW is present, documentation of tachycardia is useful, but probably not necessarily imperative if the history is convincing. Patients with a history of syncope and WPW should proceed directly to EPS.

Documentation of tachycardia is useful in differentiating among the types of SVT. Most commonly, if regular P waves are apparent, there is a 1:1 relationship between P waves and QRS complexes. If the ratio of P waves to QRS complexes is greater than one, the diagnosis is almost always atrial tachycardia. Rarely, AVNRT can present with 2:1 infranodal block. AVRT must have a 1:1 A-V relationship. In multifocal atrial tachycardia (MAT), the P-wave morphology is variable, and the ventricular rate is irregular. Tachycardias with a 1:1 A-V ratio may be divided by the relationship between the QRS complex and the next P wave; short RP tachycardias are much more common than long RP tachycardias (*see* Table 2).

The most common short RP tachycardias are AVNRT and AVRT. With AVNRT, atrial and ventricular activation are roughly simultaneous, so the P wave is frequently

Table 3
Electrocardiographic Diagnosis of Supraventricular Tachycardia

Tachycardia	Prevalence	Usual Presentation	Electrocardiographic Characteristics
Atrioventricular nodal reentrant			
Common	Common	Paroxysmal	P waves hidden, pseudo-R in V_1, pseudo-S in II or III
Uncommon	Uncommon	Paroxysmal	Inverted P waves, RP>PR
Accessory-pathway–mediated supraventricular			
Orthodromic atrioventricular reentrant	Common	Paroxysmal	Inverted P waves,* RP<PR, QRS alternans
Atrial fibrillation (Wolff–Parkinson–White)	Common	Paroxysmal	Irregularly irregular, variable QRS configuration
Antidromic atrioventricular reentrant	Rare	Paroxysmal	Inverted P waves, wide and bizarre QRS
Permanent junctional reciprocating	Rare	Incessant	Inverted P waves,* RP>PR
Sinus-node reentrant	Uncommon	Paroxysmal	Upright P waves, RP>PR
Unifocal atrial			
Reentrant	Uncommon	Paroxysmal	Upright, biphasic, or inverted P waves; RP>PR
Automatic	Rare	Incessant	Upright, biphasic, or inverted P waves; RP>PR; variable atrial rate
Multifocal atrial	Common	Incessant	Variable P waves, variable rate, variable PR intervals

*The electrocardiographic lead or leads showing inverted P waves are related to the site of the earliest atrial activation during tachycardia.

Reproduced from Ganz LI, Friedman PL. Supraventricular tachycardia. N Engl J Med 1995;332:162–173. Copyright © 1995 Massachusetts Medical Society.

buried within the QRS complex. If a P wave is visible, it usually manifests as a small deflection at the junction of the QRS complex and the ST segment (*see* Table 3). With orthodromic AVRT, ventricular activation must precede atrial activation, so the P wave may be visible further out on the ST segment. In antidromic AVRT, the QRS complexes are wide and bizarre—an exaggeration of the delta wave seen in sinus rhythm. Typical heart rates of AVNRT and AVRT overlap considerably, making this measure a poor method of discriminating between these diagnoses. QRS alternans is said to be more typical of AVRT than AVNRT, but this can also occur with AVNRT at extremely rapid rates. Patients with AVNRT frequently describe neck pounding during tachycardia, which has been called the "frog sign" *(29)*.

The long RP tachycardias are frequently difficult to distinguish electrocardiographically. With PJRT and atypical AVNRT, the atria are activated in retrograde fashion. Thus, the P waves must be inverted in the inferior leads. In atrial tachycardia, the P-wave axis and morphology depend on the site of the tachycardia focus. Thus, a tachycardia in which the P waves are upright in the inferior leads must be atrial (ectopic, sinus node reentrant, etc.) in origin. Conversely, a long RP tachycardia with inverted P waves can be atrial tachycardia, PJRT, or atypical AVNRT.

If the mechanism of tachycardia cannot be discerned from careful review of the ECG, the response to vagal maneuvers or adenosine infusion (*see* Fig. 15) can be very useful. Tachycardias that continue despite transient AV block are atrial in origin. Although most tachycardias that terminate with adenosine infusion are AVRT or AVNRT, atrial tachycardias are also occasionally adenosine-sensitive *(30)*. Tachycardias that terminate with a nonconducted P wave are much more likely to be AVNRT or AVRT than atrial tachycardia.

Once PSVT is documented, little other diagnostic work-up is necessary in the absence of other cardiovascular disease. An echocardiogram is reasonable to rule out structural heart disease, particularly in patients with recurrent SVT. This is also useful in patients with WPW and apparent right-sided accessory pathways to evaluate for Ebstein's anomaly. Checking for hyperthyroidism is reasonable, although the yield is low. Exercise

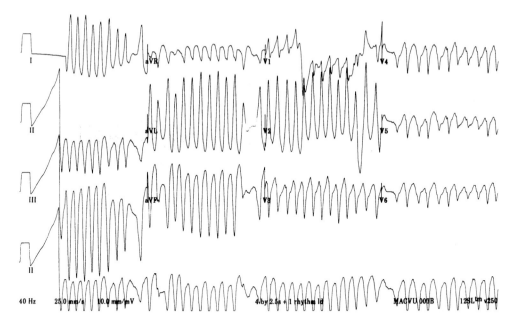

Fig. 10. ECG in a patient with WPW who presented after a syncopal spell. AF is present, with extremely rapid pre-excited QRS complexes. Pre-excited R-R intervals as short as 160 ms are present, suggesting an accessory pathway with an extremely short anterograde refractory period and therefore an extremely high risk. Cardiac arrest occurred moments after this ECG was recorded. The patient was successfully resuscitated, and underwent successful catheter ablation of a left septal pathway the next day.

testing and coronary angiography should not be performed routinely, but rather reserved for patients for whom there is a specific indication.

ACUTE MANAGEMENT

Although direct current cardioversion will terminate most PSVTs, this is rarely necessary, as the vast majority of patients are hemodynamically stable. In stable patients with regular SVTs, vagal maneuvers may be attempted initially *(31)*. If vagal stimuli are unsuccessful in terminating tachycardia, an intravenous (IV) AV-nodal-blocking agent should be administered (*see* Fig. 10). Adenosine *(32)* and verapamil appear to be of similar efficacy in terminating PVSTs that require AV-nodal conduction. Adenosine frequently causes flushing, dyspnea, and chest pain, but these symptoms are fleeting because of the extremely short half-life of this agent. The initial dose of adenosine should be a 6-mg iv push, followed by a rapid flush of fluid; 12-mg or higher doses may be given to nonresponders *(33)*. The initial dose through a central line should generally be 3 mg *(34)*. If adenosine is effective in terminating SVT, it is typically effective at the dose that causes transient symptoms of flushing and chest discomfort. Dipyridamole potentiates adenosine effect, and some cardiac transplant patients seem supersensitive to adenosine. Adenosine can trigger bronchospasm in asthmatics. Theophylline and caffeine counteract the effect of adenosine; frequently patients using these agents are refractory to adenosine, or require higher doses. Finally, adenosine may initiate AF in up to 12% of patients—of particular concern when WPW is present or suspected *(35)*.

Verapamil is also frequently used intravenously for the acute termination of PSVT. Verapamil may be particularly beneficial in patients with recurrent or incessant tachycardia because of its longer half-life, but it can also cause hypotension. Negative inotropic effects are also possible in patients with left ventricular dysfunction. Verapamil is typically administered in 2.5–5.0-mg boluses every 5–10 min until PSVT terminates, with careful monitoring of blood pressure and lung exam. Intravenous calcium-channel blockers (or beta-blockers) may be particularly beneficial in patients with atrial tachycardia; AV nodal blockade may allow control of the ventricular rate even when the tachycardia persists. Intravenous diltiazem and beta-blockers may also be effective in terminating PSVT, although data are fewer than with adenosine or verapamil.

Response to pharmacologic therapy is dependent on the mechanism of the arrhythmia. Approximately 90% or more cases of AVNRT or AVRT can be terminated by adequate iv doses of adenosine or verapamil. For the atrial tachyarrhythmias, response rates are typically lower. Only a minority of ectopic atrial tachycardias are terminated with adenosine; those that do terminate with adenosine tend to be catecholamine-dependent *(30)*.

Patients presenting with well-tolerated PSVT that is terminated in the emergency room do not routinely require admission to the hospital. A sinus-rhythm ECG should always be obtained post-termination, in sinus rhythm, to evaluate for WPW. Stable patients can frequently be discharged from the emergency room, with implementation of a long-term treatment plan as described here. Admission to "rule out" myocardial infarction (MI) is of extremely low yield in young patients with recurrent PSVT and no evidence of structural heart disease.

Management of MAT is usually directed at treating the underlying metabolic and pulmonary abnormalities. Potassium and magnesium supplementation may be helpful *(36,37)*. MAT is rarely associated with theophylline or digitalis toxicity. Calcium-channel blockers may help control both the atrial firing rate and AV-nodal conduction. Beta-blockers may have similar activity, but their use is generally limited by the underlying lung disease *(38)*.

Patients with atrial fibrillation (AF) and/or atrial flutter in the setting of WPW syndrome should follow a different treatment algorithm. AV nodal-blocking agents (calcium-channel blockers, beta-blockers, digoxin, adenosine), can shunt conduction over the accessory pathway, accelerating the ventricular rate and increasing the risk of degeneration into VF *(39,40)*. Thus, these agents are contraindicated in pre-excited AF or atrial flutter. Hemodynamically unstable patients should undergo direct current cardioversion for restoration of sinus rhythm. Patients who are hemodynamically stable should be treated with iv procainamide. This agent slows conduction in the accessory pathway as well as the AV node (and atrial and ventricular myocardium), and helps convert AF of short duration to sinus rhythm.

LONG-TERM MANAGEMENT

The long-term treatment strategy for patients who present with PSVT has changed, because of the remarkable effectiveness of radiofrequency catheter ablation (*see* Chapter 3) in the management of these patients (*see* Fig. 16) *(41,42)*. Patients with WPW who present with aborted sudden cardiac death, unexplained syncope, or pre-excited AF

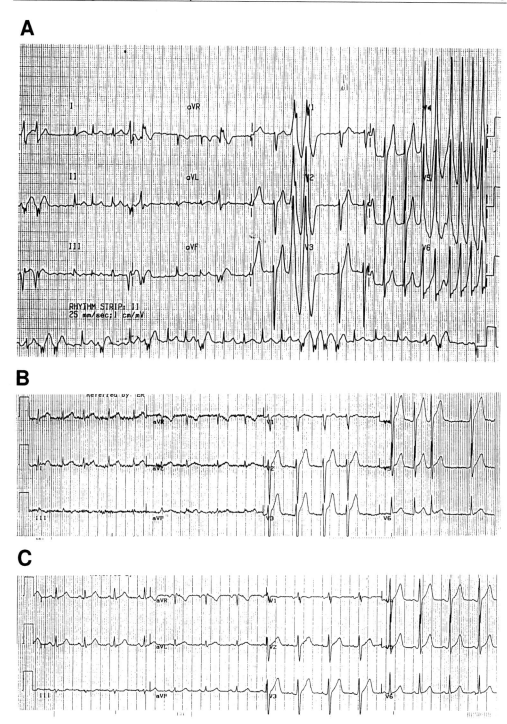

Fig. 11. Serial ECGs in a patient with WPW. **(A)** This initial ECG reveals AF. Although not all of the complexes are pre-excited, pre-excited R-R intervals shorter than 240 ms are evident to the right side of the tracing, suggesting the possibility of high risk. **(B)** After approx 500 mg iv procainamide, AF persists. There is no evidence of pre-excitation because the accessory pathway blocked by procainamide. **(C)** After approx 1000 mg iv procainamide, the patient has converted to sinus rhythm, with no evidence of pre-excitation. The patient underwent a successful ablation of a left posteroseptal pathway the next day.

should undergo catheter ablation prior to hospital discharge unless there is a contraindication to the procedure. Following successful ablation, implantable cardiovascular defibrillator (ICD) therapy is not necessary in patients with WPW and aborted sudden
death. For patients with PSVT in the setting of WPW, catheter ablation is generally
recommended as initial therapy because of the risk of sudden death associated with
this condition. There is also the theoretic risk that long-term therapy with AV nodal-
blocking agents could be detrimental if AF or atrial flutter occurs. Few long-term safety
data exists regarding chronic beta-blocker, calcium-channel blocker, or digoxin therapy
in patients with PSVT caused by WPW. In patients for whom catheter ablation is not
undertaken, the best option may be combination therapy with an AV-nodal blocker
and class I antiarrhythmic drug, to slow accessory pathway conduction.

Although some recommend catheter ablation to all patients with symptomatic PSVT
in the absence of WPW, a reasonable, more conservative stance is to individualize
therapy for each patient (*see* Fig. 16). Patients presenting with a first episode, or rare
recurrences, of well-tolerated PSVT can frequently be observed without chronic therapy.
These patients can be taught vagal maneuvers, which are often effective in terminating
PSVT. If episodes are frequent and/or cause severe symptoms, however, chronic therapy
with an AV-nodal blocking agent is reasonable. Few data are available regarding the
relative efficacy of beta-blockers, calcium-channel blockers, and digoxin in patients
with PSVT. If an AV-nodal blocker is unsuccessful or not tolerated, a different agent
may be tried. We find that about a third of PSVT patients will find an AV-nodal
blocking agent that is both effective and well-tolerated. Alternatively, catheter ablation
may be employed as initial therapy in patients with severely symptomatic PSVT or a
reluctance to take long-term medical therapy. In the case of PSVT refractory to multiple
AV-nodal blocking agents, we generally recommend catheter ablation rather than class
I or III antiarrhythmic therapy, because of the cumulative risk of toxicity and proarrhythmia of these agents. Success rates for catheter ablation of atrial tachycardias
are not quite as high as for AVNRT and AVRT, yet these tachycardias are frequently
extremely refractory to medical therapy, and the same treatment algorithm may be
recommended. An important exception is inappropriate sinus tachycardia. Because the
SA nodal complex constitutes an extensive area of right atrial tissue, catheter ablation
is extremely difficult, and poses a higher risk. For these reasons, aggressive attempts
at pharmacologic suppression with beta-blockers and/or calcium-channel blockers are
usually recommended, with catheter ablation reserved for extremely refractory cases.

In patients who present with incessant tachycardia and nonischemic cardiomyopathy,
the mechanism of myopathy may be tachycardia-induced. In these patients, we typically
recommend catheter ablation as initial therapy, because of the higher likelihood of cure
compared with medical therapy, and the possibility of recovery of ventricular function
following successful treatment.

The cost-effectiveness of catheter ablation for PSVT depends on the frequency and
severity of symptoms, as well as refractoriness to medical therapy. For patients with
frequent emergency-room visits and hospital admissions, radiofrequency ablation results
in relatively rapid cost savings (43,44). Costs are reduced further when ablations are
performed on an outpatient basis, which has proven to be feasible and safe when performed by experienced operators (45). In addition, as initial therapy in patients with
symptomatic SVT, radiofrequency ablation results in more complete resolution of symptoms and health-related quality of life compared with medical therapy (46). Combined

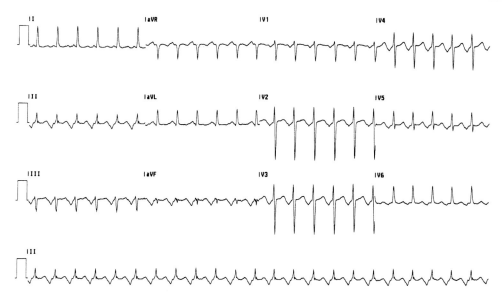

Fig. 12. ECG in patient with nearly incessant PSVT. Note the deeply inverted P waves relatively close to the next QRS complex, a so-called "long RP" tachycardia. EPS confirmed the diagnosis of permanent junctional reciprocating tachycardia (PJRT), caused by a slowly conducting concealed right posteroseptal accessory pathway. This ECG is also consistent with atypical AVNRT, and even a low septal ectopic atrial tachycardia.

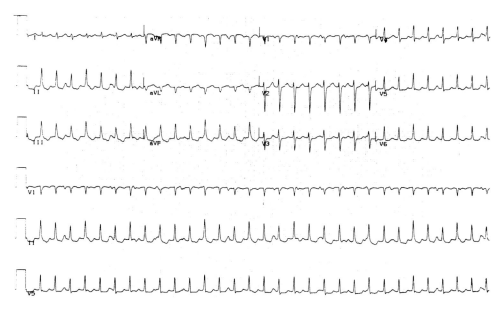

Fig. 13. ECG in a patient with nonparoxysmal junctional tachycardia (NPJT). The tachycardia is regular and narrow complex, though A-V dissociation is clearly present (seen best in the lead V₁ rhythm strip).

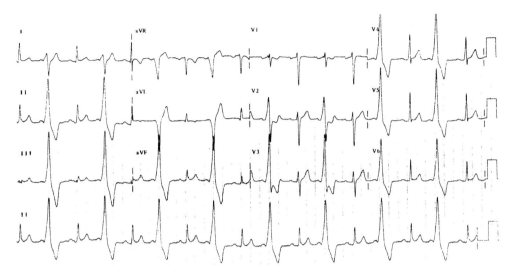

Fig. 14. ECG in a patient with asymptomatic, intermittent pre-excitation. Note that every other beat is pre-excited. This suggests a long anterograde refractory period and therefore low-risk accessory pathway. No further workup was recommended, and the patient remained asymptomatic during follow-up. Note that this ECG is also consistent with sinus rhythm with ventricular bigeminy. At lower rates, however, the short PR interval and delta wave were present on every beat, confirming the diagnosis of ventricular pre-excitation.

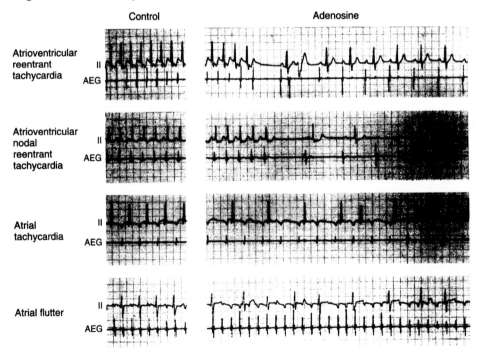

Fig. 15. Response of various SVTs to adenosine infusion. In each panel, surface ECG lead II and an intracardiac right atrial electrogram are depicted. During AVRT, atrial activation clearly follows ventricular activation. During AVNRT, atrial and ventricular activation are nearly simultaneous; in this case, atrial activation precedes ventricular activation. Because AVRT and AVNRT require AV nodal conduction, both are terminated by adenosine. During atrial tachycardia and atrial flutter, adenosine transiently increases the level of AV block, but tachycardia persists in the atrium. However, in some atrial tachycardias, the atrial tachycardia mechanism itself may be susceptible to adenosine termination (not shown). (Reproduced from Ganz LI, Friedman PL. Supraventricular tachycardia. N Engl J Med 1995;332:162–173. Copyright © 1995 Massachusetts Medical Society.)

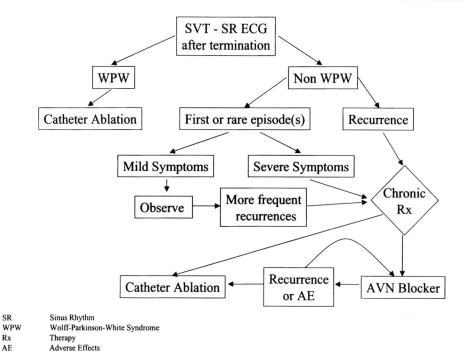

SR   Sinus Rhythm
WPW   Wolff-Parkinson-White Syndrome
Rx   Therapy
AE   Adverse Effects

Fig. 16. Algorithm for long-term management in patients who present with PSVT. For patients with WPW, EPS and radiofrequency catheter ablation are recommended as initial therapy. In the absence of WPW, the long-term treatment strategy depends on the frequency and severity of episodes, as well as patient preference.

with the limited natural history data suggesting a low rate of spontaneous resolution of SVT, these studies would suggest that relatively early intervention with catheter ablation is appropriate, particularly in younger patients.

SUMMARY

SVT is a relatively common medical problem. Although a variety of mechanisms are possible, AVNRT and AVRT using an accessory pathway constitute the majority of cases. Patients with symptomatic WPW should generally undergo catheter ablation as initial therapy. Management of patients with asymptomatic WPW remains controversial. In the absence of WPW, therapy should be individualized for patients with PSVT.

REFERENCES

1. Ganz LI, Friedman PL. Supraventricular tachycardia. N Engl J Med 1995;332:162–173.
2. Lesh MD, Van Hare GF, Epstein LM, et al. Radiofrequency catheter ablation of atrial arrhythmias: results and mechanisms. Circulation 1994;89:1074–1089.
3. Krahn AD, Yee R, Klein GJ, Morillo C. Inappropriate sinus tachycardia: evaluation and therapy. J Cardiovasc Electrophysiol 1995;6:1124–1128.
4. Gomes JA, Mehta D, Langan MN. Sinus node reentrant tachycardia. PACE 1995;18:1045–1057.
5. Kastor RA. Multifocal atrial tachycardia. N Engl J Med 1990;322:1713–1717.
6. Akhtar M, Jazayeri MR, Sra J, Blanck Z, Deshpande S, Dhala A. Atrioventricular nodal reentry: clinical, electrophysiological, and therapeutic considerations. Circulation 1993;88:282–295.

7. Miller JM. Therapy of Wolff-Parkinson-White syndrome and concealed bypass tracts: Part I. J Cardiovasc Electrophysiol 1996;7:85–93.

8. Miller JM. Therapy of Wolff-Parkinson-White syndrome and concealed bypass tracts: Part II. J Cardiovasc Electrophysiol 1996;7:178–187.

9. Critelli G. Recognizing and managing permanent junctional reciprocating tachycardia in the catheter ablation era. J Cardiovasc Electrophysiol 1997;8:226–236.

10. Dorostkar PC, Silka MJ, Morady F, Dick M. Clinical course of persistent junctional reciprocating tachycardia. J Am Coll Cardiol 1999;33:366–375.

11. Rosen KM. Junctional tachycardia: mechanisms, diagnosis, differential diagnosis, and management. Circulation 1973;47:654–664.

12. Walsh EP, Saul JP, Sholler GF, et al. Evaluation of a staged treatment protocol for rapid automatic junctional tachycardia after operation for congenital heart disease. J Am Coll Cardiol 1997;29:1046–1053.

13. Hiss RG, Lamb LE. Electrocardiographic findings in 122,043 individuals. Circulation 1962;25:947–961.

14. Guize L, Soria R, Chaouat JC, Chretien JM, Houe D, Le Heuzey JY. Prevalence et evolution du syndrome Wolff-Parkinson-White dans une population de 138 048 sujets. Ann Med Interne 1985;136:474–478.

15. Orejarena LA, Vidaillet H, DeStefano F, et al. Paroxysmal supraventricular tachycardia in the general population. J Am Coll Cardiol 1998;31:150–157.

16. Rosano GMC, Sarrel PM, Beale CM, DeLuca F, Collins P. Cyclical variation in paroxysmal supraventricular tachycardia in women. Lancet 1996;347:786–788.

17. Lessmeier TJ, Gamperling D, Johnson-Liddon V, et al. Unrecognized paroxysmal supraventricular tachycardia: potential for misdiagnosis as panic disorder. Arch Int Med 1997;157:537–543.

18. Wang Y, Scheinman MM, Chien WW, Cohen TJ, Lesh MD, Griffin JC. Patients with supraventricular tachycardia presenting with aborted sudden death: incidence, mechanism, and long-term follow-up. J Am Coll Cardiol 1991;1711–1719.

19. Chiou C-W, Chen S-A, Chiang C-E, et al. Mitral valve prolapse in patients with paroxysmal supraventricular tachycardia. Am J Cardiol 1995;75:186–188.

20. Klein GJ, Bashore TM, Sellers TD, Pritchett EL, Smith WM, Gallagher JJ. Ventricular fibrillation in the Wolff-Parkinson-White Syndrome. N Engl J Med 1979;301:1080–1085.

21. Montoya PT, Brugada P, Smeets J, et al. Ventricular fibrillation in the Wolff-Parkinson-White syndrome. Eur Heart J 1991;12:144–150.

22. Timmermans C, Smeets JLRM, Rodriguez L-M, Vrouchos G, van den Dool A, Wellens HJJ. Aborted sudden death in the Wolff-Parkinson-White Syndrome. Am J Cardiol 1995;76:492–494.

23. Sharma AD, Yee R, Guiraudon G, Klein GJ. Sensitivity and specificity of invasive and noninvasive testing for risk of sudden death in Wolff-Parkinson-White syndrome. J Am Coll Cardiol 1987;10:373–381.

24. Klein GJ, Yee R, Sharma AD. Longitudinal electrophysiologic assessment of asymptomatic patients with the Wolff-Parkinson-White electrocardiographic pattern. N Engl J Med 1989;320:1229–1233.

25. Munger TM, Packer DL, Hammill SC, et al. A population study of the natural history of Wolff-Parkinson-White syndrome in Olmstead County, Minnesota, 1953–1989. Circulation 1993;87:866–873.

26. Steinbeck G. Should radiofrequency current ablation be performed in asymptomatic patients with the Wolff-Parkinson-White syndrome? PACE 1993;16:649–652.

27. Wellens HJJ, Rodriguez LM, Timmermans C, Smeets JL. The asymptomatic patient with the Wolff-Parkinson-White electrocardiogram. PACE 1997;20:2082–2086.

28. Chen S-A, Chiang C-E, Tai C-T, et al. Longitudinal clinical and electrophysiological assessment of patients with asymptomatic Wolff-Parkinson-White syndrome and atrioventricular node reentrant tachycardia. Circulation 1996;93:2023–2032.

29. Gursoy S, Steurer G, Brugada J, Andries E, Brugada P. The hemodynamic mechanism of pounding in the neck in atrioventricular nodal reentrant tachycardia. N Engl J Med 1992;327:772–774.

30. Kall JG, Kopp D, Olshansky B, et al. Adenosine-sensitive atrial tachycardia. PACE 1995;18:300–306.

31. Mehta D, Wafa S, Ward DE, Camm AJ. Relative efficacy of various physical manoeuvres in the termination of junctional tachycardia. Lancet 1988;1:1181–1185.

32. Camm AJ, Garratt CJ. Adenosine and supraventricular tachycardia. N Engl J Med 1991;325:1621–1629.

33. DiMarco JP, Miles W, Akhtar M, et al. Adenosine for paroxysmal supraventricular tachycardia: dose

ranging and comparison with verapamil: assessment in placebo-controlled, multicenter trials. Ann Int Med 1990;113:104–110.

34. McIntosh-Yellin NL, Drew BJ, Scheinman MM. Safety and efficacy of intravenous bolus administration of adenosine for termination of supraventricular tachycardia. J Am Coll Cardiol 1993;22:741–745.

35. Strickberger SA, Man KC, Daoud EG, et al. Adenosine-induced atrial arrhythmia: a prospective analysis. Ann Int Med 1997;127:417–422.

36. Iseri LT, Fairshter RD, Hardemann JL, Brodsky MA. Magnesium and potassium therapy in multifocal atrial tachycardia. Am Heart J 1985;110:789–794.

37. McCord JK, Borzak S, Davis T, Gheorghiade M. Usefulness of intravenous magnesium for multifocal atrial tachycardia in patients with chronic obstructive pulmonary disease. Am J Cardiol 1998;81:91–93.

38. Arsura E, Lefkin AS, Solar M, Tessler S. A randomized, double-blind, placebo-controlled study of verapamil and metoprolol in treatment of multifocal atrial tachycardia. Am J Med 1988;85:519–524.

39. Exner DV, Muzyka T, Gillis AM. Proarrhythmia in patients with the Wolff-Parkinson-White syndrome after standard doses of intravenous adenosine. Ann Intern Med 1995;122:351–352.

40. Garrat C, Antoniou A, Ward D, Camm AJ. Misuse of verapamil in pre-excited atrial fibrillation. Lancet 1989;1:367–369.

41. Calkins H, Yong P, Miller JM, et al. Catheter ablation of accessory pathways, atrioventricular nodal reentrant tachycardia, and the atrioventricular junction: final results of a prospective, multicenter clinical trial. Circulation 1999;99:262–270.

42. Wellens HJJ. Catheter ablation of cardiac arrhythmias: usually cure, but complications may occur. Circulation 1999;99:195–197.

43. Kalbfleisch SJ, Calkins H, Langberg JL, et al. Comparison of the cost of radiofrequency catheter modification of the atrioventricular node and medical therapy for drug-refractory atrioventricular node reentrant tachycardia. J Am Coll Cardiol 1992;19:1583–1587.

44. Hegenhuis W, Stevens SK, Wang P, et al. Cost-effectiveness of radiofrequency ablation compared with other strategies in Wolff-Parkinson-White syndrome. Circulation 1993;88(part II):437–446.

45. Vora AM, Green MS, Tang ASL. Safety and feasibility of same day discharge in patients undergoing radiofrequency catheter ablation. Am J Cardiol 1998;81:233–235.

46. Bathina MN, Mickelsen S, Brooks C, Jaramillo J, Hepton T, Kusumoto FM. Radiofrequency catheter ablation versus medical therapy for initial treatment of supraventricular tachycardia and its impact on quality of life and healthcare costs. Am J Cardiol 1998;82:589–593.

4

Catheter Ablation
of Supraventricular Tachycardias

Walter L. Atiga, MD, and Hugh Calkins, MD

CONTENTS

INTRODUCTION

Catheter ablation was initially described in 1982 by Gallagher et al. *(1)*. Before 1990, it was performed primarily with high-energy direct-current (DC) shocks using a multipolar electrode catheter positioned in the heart and attached to a standard defibrillator. Under general anesthesia, 100–360 J of direct current energy was delivered between the distal electrode and a patch placed on the patient's chest. This produced an explosive flash, heat, and increased pressure. Myocardial injury resulted from heat, barotrauma, and direct electrical injury.

More recently, DC energy has been largely replaced with radiofrequency energy as the preferred energy source during catheter ablation procedures. As a result of this change in energy source, the use of catheter ablation increased more than 30-fold between 1989 to 1992, from an estimated 450 to 15,000 procedures per year *(2)*.

RADIOFREQUENCY ENERGY ABLATION

Radiofrequency catheter ablation is performed by delivery of a continuous, unmodulated, sinusoidal, high frequency (500,000 cycles per s) alternating electrical current

From: *Contemporary Cardiology: Management of Cardiac Arrhythmias*
Edited by: L. I. Ganz © Humana Press Inc., Totowa, NJ

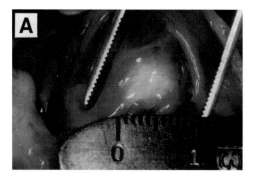 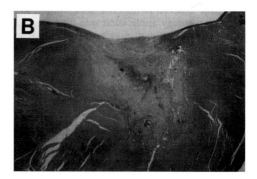

Fig. 1. (A) Endocardial radiofrequency ablation lesion demonstrating a round shape with sharp borders. **(B)** Histologic section of lesion in A, demonstrating hemispheric shape and extensive fibrosis. (From Jumrussirikul P, et al. Prospective comparison of temperature guided microwave and radiofrequency catheter ablation in the swine heart. PACE 1998;21[7]:1364–1374. Reproduced with permission.) (*See* color plate appearing in the insert following p. 208.)

between the tip of an electrode catheter and a ground plate positioned on the back or chest. Because the ground plate has a much larger surface area than the tip, current density is focused at the smaller electrode. Current flows from the active electrode into the underlying tissue in alternating directions at high frequency. As a result of ionic agitation in the tissue, resistive heating ensues. Thus, the tissue underlying the ablation electrode, rather than the electrode itself, is the source of heat generation. This contrasts with a thermal probe or soldering iron, in which a resistive element positioned within the probe is the source of heat generation.

The tissue undergoing resistive heating transfers heat to surrounding tissues by conductive heat transfer. Since direct resistive heating falls precipitously with increasing distance from the ablation electrode, it is responsible for heating only a very narrow rim of tissue extending approx 1 mm beyond the ablation electrode *(3)*. The majority of lesion volume is determined by the relative contributions of conductive heat exchange into surrounding tissue and convective heat loss toward the relatively cooler moving blood.

The principal mechanism of tissue destruction during radiofrequency catheter ablation procedures is thermal injury. Elevation of tissue temperature leads to denaturation of proteins and evaporation of fluids, resulting in subsequent tissue destruction and coagulation of tissue and blood *(4,5)*. Temperature-dependent depolarization of myocardial tissue and loss of excitability occurs at temperatures greater than 43°C. Between tissue temperatures of 43°C and 50°C, there is reversible loss of excitability. Once the tissue reaches a temperature greater than 50°C, irreversible tissue injury occurs *(6)*. Electrode-tissue interface temperatures in excess of 100°C cause tissue desiccation and plasma protein denaturation, which result in the formation of coagulum. The development of a coagulum results in a rapid increase in impedance, which leads to a dramatic decrease in current density, thereby limiting further lesion growth. As a result, the lesions created during radiofrequency catheter ablation procedures have well-demarcated borders and are small: 3–6 mm in width, depth, and length (*see* Fig. 1).

It is well known that deeper ablation lesions can be obtained by increasing the radiofrequency power, since this increases both the volume of resistive heating and the depth of passive conductive heating. However, because coagulation necrosis at the tissue-electrode interface results in a rise in impedance once temperatures reach 100°, the degree to which radiofrequency power can be increased is limited (7). Recently, methods for improved cooling of the electrode have been developed to allow delivery of higher radiofrequency power. These include the use of larger (8-mm) electrodes (7,8), which receive greater convective cooling by the blood, and saline-irrigated electrode tips, in which the electrode is actively cooled (9,10). The use of these catheters has resulted in higher success rates for selected arrhythmias, including ventricular tachycardia (VT) and isthmus-dependent atrial flutter (11–15).

CATHETER ABLATION OF SUPRAVENTRICULAR ARRHYTHMIAS

The goal of catheter ablation is to cure cardiac arrhythmias by destroying small areas of myocardial and/or conducting tissue that is critical to the initiation or maintenance of a cardiac arrhythmia. In general, those arrhythmias that have either a focal origin or involve an anatomically defined narrow isthmus may be cured using radiofrequency catheter ablation techniques. In contrast, arrhythmias that are multifocal in origin are generally not amenable to cure with catheter ablation at the present time using conventional catheter ablation techniques.

Catheter ablation procedures are performed in a catheterization laboratory specifically equipped to perform electrophysiology testing and catheter ablation procedures. Patients receive conscious sedation during the procedure in order to minimize discomfort and movement. Two to five multipolar electrode catheters are inserted percutaneously under local anesthesia into femoral, subclavian, and internal jugular veins and positioned in the heart under fluoroscopic guidance. Each catheter has four or more electrodes, with the most distal electrode pair typically used for pacing and the delivery of critically timed extrastimuli and the proximal electrodes used to record local electrograms. During radiofrequency catheter ablation procedures, radiofrequency energy is delivered using an electrode catheter with a deflectable shaft and a 4-mm distal electrode. Radiofrequency energy is usually delivered for 30–60 s between the distal electrode and a patch placed on the patient's back or chest.

Because tissue-electrode interface temperatures are of critical importance during radiofrequency catheter ablation, recent ablation catheters and radiofrequency generators have been designed to monitor electrode temperature and to help achieve targeted electrode temperatures via automatic power output regulation using a closed-loop control system (16). Knowledge of the electrode temperature at a particular ablation site is useful in determining whether an unsuccessful application of radiofrequency energy failed because of inaccurate mapping or inadequate heating. In the event of inadequate heating, additional applications of energy at the same site with improved catheter stability may result in success. Closed-loop temperature control has been demonstrated to reduce the incidence of coagulum development, which may also facilitate catheter ablation by reducing the number of times the catheter must be withdrawn from the body to have a coagulum removed from the electrode tip.

CATHETER ABLATION IN THE MANAGEMENT
OF SUPRAVENTRICULAR ARRHYTHMIAS

The optimal management of an individual patient depends on many factors, including the type, frequency and duration of arrhythmia, associated symptoms, concomitant disease, and patient preference. Therapeutic options for patients with supraventricular arrhythmias include pharmacologic agents, arrhythmia surgery, and catheter ablation. With the exception of Wolff-Parkinson-White syndrome (WPW), supraventricular arrhythmias are generally not life-threatening. Therefore, the inherent attractiveness of catheter ablation as a curative approach must be tempered with the cost and potential complications associated with an invasive procedure.

From the perspective of catheter ablation, supraventricular arrhythmias can be broadly classified into two groups: paroxysmal supraventricular tachycardias (PSVT), which require the AV node for perpetuation, including accessory pathway-mediated tachycardias; and arrhythmias that are confined to the atrium and do not require the atrioventricular (AV) node for perpetuation.

PAROXYSMAL SUPRAVENTRICULAR TACHYCARDIAS

Paroxysmal supraventricular tachycardias (PSVT) characteristically begin and terminate abruptly. Electrocardiograms (ECGs) obtained during PSVT typically reveal a narrow QRS complex with a rate between 130 and 240 beats per minute (BPM). Atrioventricular nodal reentrant tachycardia (AVNRT) is the most common cause of PSVT, accounting for two-thirds of cases. Atrioventricular reciprocating tachycardias (AVRT), which involve conduction through both the AV node and an accessory pathway, are the second most common cause of PSVT, accounting for approximately one-third of cases. Since PSVT is generally benign, the main indication for treatment is the presence of frequent or severe symptoms.

Electrophysiology testing and catheter ablation are considered early in the management of supraventricular tachycardia (SVT) for patients with significant hemodynamic compromise during tachycardia (syncope or presyncope). Early electrophysiology testing is also considered for patients with PSVT who have evidence of pre-excitation WPW because of the potentially life-threatening nature of this condition *(17)*. Catheter ablation is generally not recommended for patients with asymptomatic pre-excitation *(18)*. An exception may exist for individuals with "high-risk" occupations, such as competitive athletes, airline pilots, and bus drivers. In this group of patients, diagnostic electrophysiology testing can be used to identify the small proportion of patients who have accessory pathways capable of rapid antegrade conduction (refractory period <250 ms), a finding that would confer an increased risk of sudden cardiac death in the event of a rapid atrial arrhythmia *(17)*.

For patients with PSVT in the absence of significant hemodynamic compromise or pre-excitation, catheter ablation can be viewed as one of several potential therapeutic alternatives. Other alternatives include chronic treatment with antiarrhythmic drugs or no therapy. The optimal approach in a given patient varies and is based on several factors, including the patient's frequency and severity of symptoms, prior failure of antiarrhythmic theray, or the anticipation of pregnancy. For instance, no specific therapy other than instructing patients on how to perform the Valsalva maneuver may be preferable in a patient who has experienced only a single episode of self-terminating

PSVT associated with palpitations. In contrast, chronic antiarrhythmic drugs or catheter ablation can be considered in a patient with frequent episodes of tachycardia that do not terminate spontaneously and require emergency-room visits for termination. If antiarrhythmic drug therapy is either ineffective or poorly tolerated, catheter ablation can be reconsidered at a later time.

Atrioventricular Nodal Reentrant Tachycardia

Atrioventricular nodal reentrant tachycardia (AVNRT) is a common arrhythmia, comprising approx 60% of cases of PSVT referred for electrophysiology testing. It occurs in patients with two functionally distinct conduction pathways through the AV node, referred to as the fast and slow pathways. The slow pathway has a shorter refractory period than the fast pathway. Both the fast and slow pathway are necessary to maintain AVNRT.

The common form of AVNRT is typically initiated when an atrial premature beat blocks in the fast pathway, conducts down the slow pathway, and returns via the fast pathway to depolarize the atrium. During the rare form of AVNRT, the wavefront propagates in the opposite direction, conducting down the fast pathway and returning via the slow pathway. The fast pathway is located anteriorly along the septal portion of the tricuspid annulus, near the compact AV node. The atrial insertion of the slow pathway is located more posteriorly along the tricuspid annulus, closer to the coronary sinus ostium.

CATHETER ABLATION OF AVNRT

Indications. Catheter ablation is indicated for patients with symptomatic sustained AVNRT that is drug-resistant or the patient is drug-intolerant or does not desire long-term drug therapy *(18)*. In patients with documented SVT who are found to have dual AV nodal pathway physiology and single AV nodal echoes, but without inducible AVNRT during electrophysiology testing, slow pathway ablation may eliminate the recurrence of symptomatic tachycardia *(19)*. When SVT compatible with AVNRT has not been documented clinically, it remains unclear whether prophylactic catheter ablation of the AV node slow pathway should be performed if sustained AVNRT is identified during electrophysiology study or catheter ablation of another arrhythmia.

Techniques. AVNRT may be cured by ablation of either the fast or the slow pathway. These alternative approaches are referred to as the "anterior" and the "posterior" approaches, respectively.

The anterior approach targets the fast pathway. Catheter ablation is performed by locating an electrogram with a large His potential, and then withdrawing the ablation catheter into the right atrium until the atrial signal is at least twice that of the ventricular signal (A/V ratio >2) with a His potential no larger than 50 microvolts. Twenty-five to 50 W of radiofrequency energy are then applied during sinus rhythm for 30–60 s while watching for prolongation in the PR interval. Energy delivery is immediately terminated if AV block occurs. Successful ablation of AVNRT using the anterior approach is characterized by lengthening of the PR interval and the inability to induce the tachycardia. Typically, either elimination or marked attentuation of retrograde conduction during ventricular pacing will occur. The atrioventricular block cycle length and the AV node effective refractory period are not usually altered during ablation of AVNRT using the anterior approach.

The posterior approach to ablation of AVNRT targets the slow pathway (Fig. 2A). The ablation catheter is directed into the right ventricle near the posterior septum, and is then withdrawn until an electrogram is recorded with a small atrial electrogram and a large ventricular electrogram. (A/V ratio <0.5). Specific ablation sites along the posterior portion of the tricuspid annulus can be selected based on the appearance of the local atrial electrogram or based strictly on anatomic factors. When using the electrogram-guided approach, fractionated atrial electrograms with a late "slow potential" are targeted (Fig. 2B). When using the anatomic approach, the initial applications are delivered at the level of the coronary sinus (CS) ostium, with subsequent applications of energy delivered to more superior sites. With either approach, accelerated junctional beats occurring during the application of radiofrequency energy are a marker for successful ablation. Successful ablation of AVNRT using the posterior approach is characterized by an increase in both the AV block-cycle length and the AV node effective refractory period, as well as the elimination of inducible AVNRT.

Outcomes and complications. Catheter ablation of AVNRT using the anterior approach is successful in approx 90% of patients. Major limitations of the technique are the creation of inadvertent AV block in approx 7% of patients and a 9% incidence of recurrence *(2,20–22)*. The posterior approach for ablation of AVNRT is effective in 95–97% of patients *(11,23–27)* (Fig. 3A). The incidence of recurrence following successful ablation of AVNRT using the posterior approach is 3–5% *(23–27)*. AV block is the most common complication, occurring in 0.5–1% of patients *(23–27)*. Other associated complications may result from obtaining vascular access (hematoma, deep venous thrombosis, arteriovenous fistula, pneumothorax) or catheter manipulation (perforation of the CS or myocardial wall). The long-term patient survival following catheter ablation of AVNRT is excellent (Fig. 4).

Because of the higher efficacy, the lower incidence of AV block and arrhythmia recurrence, and the greater likelihood of maintaining a normal PR interval during sinus rhythm, the posterior approach is now considered the preferred approach to ablation of AVNRT *(2,26)*.

Accessory Pathways

Accessory pathways are anomalous extranodal tissues that connect the epicardial surface of the atrium and ventricle along the atrioventricular groove. Accessory pathways can be classified based on their location along the mitral or tricuspid annulus, type of conduction (decremental or nondecremental), and whether they are capable of antegrade conduction, retrograde conduction, or both. Accessory pathways that conduct only retrogradely are termed "concealed" since they do not cause ventricular preexcitation and cannot be detected by ECG. Accessory pathways that conduct antegradely are termed "manifest" because they are demonstrable on a standard ECG as a short PR interval and a widened QRS complex with a slow and prolonged upstroke, referred to as a delta wave (Fig. 5A). This ECG pattern is termed "preexcitation" because it results in early activation of the ventricle through the accessory pathway that bypasses the normal AV conduction. Patients are diagnosed with WPW syndrome when they have both preexcitation and symptomatic tachyarrhythmias.

Patients with accessory pathways are capable of having atrioventricular reciprocating tachycardia. AVRT accounts for approx 30% of all patients referred for electrophysiology testing for PSVT. Among patients with the WPW, AVRT is the most common

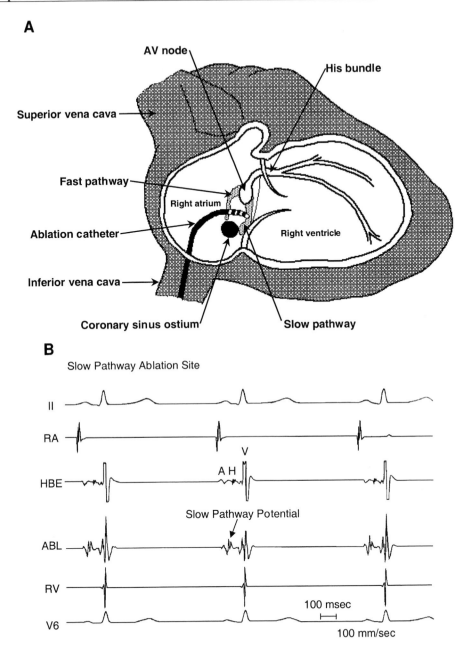

Fig. 2. (A) Schematic drawing of the posterior, or slow pathway, approach to ablation of AVNRT, in which ablation catheter is positioned anterior to the CS ostium. **(B)** Intracardiac electrogram characteristics of a successful slow pathway ablation site. At the ablation site (ABL), the ventricular electrogram is considerably larger than the atrial electrogram, and a slow-pathway potential is seen immediately after the atrial electrogram.

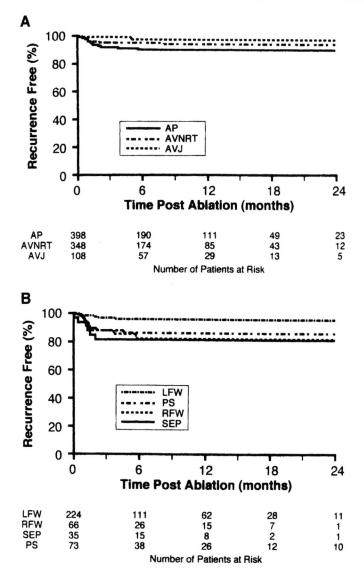

Fig. 3. (**A**) Kaplan-Meier curves demonstrating arrhythmia-free rates for patients who underwent successful ablation of an accessory pathway (AP), atrioventricular nodal reentrant tachycardia (AVNRT), or atrioventricular junction (AVJ). (**B**) Kaplan-Meier curves showing arrhythmia-free rates among patients who underwent successful ablation of a left free-wall (LFW), right free-wall (RFW), septal (SEP) or posteroseptal (PS) accessory pathway. (From Calkins et al. Catheter ablation of accessory pathways, atrioventricular nodal reentrant tachycardia, and the atrioventricular junction: final results of a prospective, multicenter clinical trial. Circulation 1999;99(2):262–270. Reproduced with permission.)

arrhythmia, occurring in 75% of patients. AVRT is further subclassified into orthodromic and antidromic AVRT. During orthodromic AVRT, the reentrant impulse utilizes the AV node and His-Purkinje system for conduction from the atrium to the ventricle, and utilizes the accessory pathway for conduction from the ventricle to the atrium (Fig. 5B). Thus, orthodromic AVRT is typically a narrow-complex tachycardia, unless there

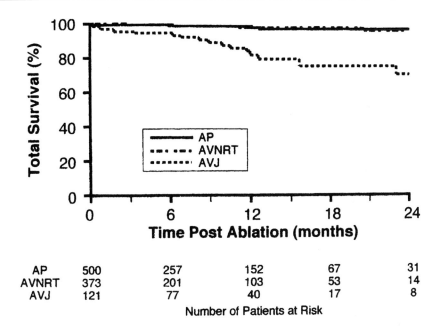

Fig. 4. Kaplan-Meier curves demonstrating survival following radiofrequency ablation of an accessory pathway (AP), AVNRT, or the atrioventricular junction (AVJ). (From Calkins, et al. Catheter ablation of accessory pathways, atrioventricular nodal reentrant tachycardia, and the atrioventricular junction: final results of a prospective, multicenter clinical trial. Circulation 1999;99(2):262–270. Reproduced with permission.)

is preexisting or functional bundle-branch block. In contrast, antidromic AVRT is typically a wide-complex arrhythmia, because the reentrant impulse travels from the atrium to the ventricle via the accessory pathway and then back to the atrium retrogradely through the normal AV conduction system (Fig. 5C). Even in patients with manifest accessory pathways, orthodromic AVRT is the most common form of PSVT.

Atrial fibrillation (AF) is a less common but potentially more serious arrhythmia in patients with WPW. It can result in a very rapid ventricular response through the accessory pathway, with degeneration into ventricular fibrillation (VF) in rare cases. The incidence of sudden cardiac death in patients with WPW has been estimated to be 0.15% per patient year *(28)*.

CATHETER ABLATION OF ACCESSORY PATHWAYS

Indications. Referral for electrophysiology testing and catheter ablation is recommended for all patients with symptomatic WPW, as it is associated with an increased risk of sudden death. Radiofrequency ablation is also recommended for patients with suspected AVRT involving a concealed accessory pathway if it is drug-resistant or the patient is drug-intolerant or does not desire long-term drug therapy *(18)*. There is divided opinion as to whether patients with asymptomatic ventricular pre-excitation should be considered for electrophysiology testing and catheter ablation. At the present time, this approach is generally reserved for patients whose livelihood or profession, important activities, insurability, or mental well being, or the public safety, would be affected by spontaneous tachyarrhythmias or the presence of the ECG abnormality.

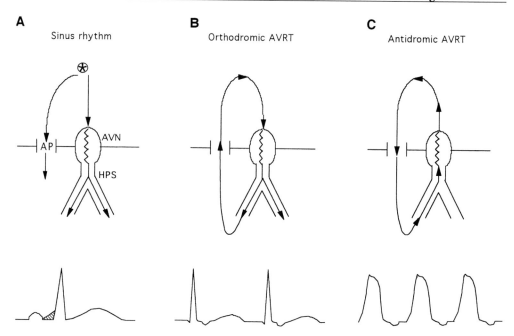

A Sinus rhythm **B** Orthodromic AVRT **C** Antidromic AVRT

Fig. 5. (A) Schematic representation of early activation of part of the ventricle through rapid anterograde conduction over an accessory pathway (AP), resulting in a delta wave (initial shaded portion of QRS). **(B)** Orthodromic atrioventricular reciprocating tachycardia (AVRT), in which no delta waves are seen, because ventricular activation proceeds through the normal conduction system and retrograde through the accessory pathway to the atrium. **(C)** Antidromic AVRT, during which anterograde conduction proceeds to ventricle entirely over AP, resulting in maximal pre-excitation with wide QRS complexes.

Techniques. An important part of catheter ablation of accessory pathways is the diagnostic electrophysiology test, in which the presence of an accessory pathway is confirmed, its conduction characteristics are determined, and the role of the accessory pathway in the patient's clinical arrhythmia is defined *(29)*. Accurate localization of an accessory pathway is critical to the success of catheter ablation procedures. In patients with preexcitation, preliminary localization of the accessory pathway can be determined based on the delta wave and QRS morphologies *(30)*. Mapping of concealed accessory pathways and accurate localization of manifest accessory pathways require analysis of the retrograde atrial activation sequence and/or antegrade ventricular activation sequence. Right-sided and posteroseptal accessory pathways are typically localized and ablated using a steerable catheter with a 4-mm distal electrode positioned along the tricuspid annulus or in the CS ostium. The general location of a left-sided accessory pathway can be determined using a multipolar electrode catheter positioned in the CS, which runs parallel to the left AV groove, or with a steerable catheter positioned on the mitral annulus. Once localized to a region of the heart, more precise mapping and ablation are performed using a steerable 4-mm tip-electrode ablation catheter positioned along the mitral annulus using either the transseptal or retrograde aortic approach. These two approaches for ablation of left-sided accessory pathways are associated with similar rates of success and incidence of complications *(31)*. The decision as to which approach to employ is usually based on physician preference, although the transeptal approach may be preferable in the elderly and in young children. Rarely, left-sided accessory pathways can only be ablated via the CS *(32)*.

Appropriate sites for radiofrequency energy delivery during ablation of manifest accessory pathways are characterized by early ventricular activation, the presence of an accessory pathway potential, and stability of the local electrogram *(33)* (Fig. 6A). Appropriate sites for energy delivery in patients with retrogradely conducted accessory pathways mapped during ventricular pacing or orthodromic AVRT are characterized by continuous electrical activity, the presence of an accessory pathway potential, and electrogram stability *(33)*. Once an appropriate target site is identified, 25–50 W of radiofrequency energy are delivered for 30–60 s with a target electrode temperature of 60–70°C. At successful ablation sites, interruption of conduction through the accessory pathway usually occurs within 10 s, and often within 2 s, of the onset of radiofrequency energy delivery. This is demonstrated by disappearance of the delta wave for manifest pathways (Fig. 6B) and a change in retrograde activation sequence for concealed pathways.

Outcomes and Complications. The reported efficacy of catheter ablation of accessory pathways varies from 89% to 99% with an overall success rate of approx 93–95% *(27,29,34–39)* (Fig. 3A). The success rate for catheter ablation of accessory pathways is highest for left free-wall (95%) and lowest for posteroseptal (88%) and right free-wall (90%) accessory pathways *(27)*. Following an initially successful procedure, recurrence of accessory pathway conduction occurs in approx 7–8% of patients *(27,29,34–39)*. Recurrence of conduction is more common following ablation of septal, right free-wall, and posteroseptal pathways *(27)* (Fig. 3B). Accessory pathways that recur can usually be successfully re-ablated. Complications may result from obtaining vascular access (hematoma, deep venous thrombosis, perforation of the aorta, arteriovenous fistula, pneumothorax), catheter manipulation (valvular damage, microemboli, perforation of the CS or myocardial wall, coronary dissection, and/or thrombosis), or delivery of radiofrequency energy (myocardial perforation, coronary artery spasm or occlusion, transient ischemic attacks, or cerebrovascular accidents). Complete heart block during ablation of an accessory pathway occurs in approx 1%, observed most commonly after ablation of septal (2.5%) and posteroseptal (3%) pathways *(27)*. Overall, the incidence of complications varies from 1–4% *(27,29,34–39)*. The incidence of procedure-related death is estimated to be less than 0.2% *(2)*. Long-term patient survival following catheter ablation of accessory pathways is excellent (Fig. 4).

ATRIAL ARRHYTHMIAS

The traditional approach to treatment of patients with sustained atrial arrhythmias—including atrial tachycardia, atrial flutter, and AF—involves initial attempts to slow the ventricular response to the tachycardia with AV-node blocking agents such as digoxin, calcium antagonists, or beta-blockers. Membrane-active antiarrhythmic agents are then added in an attempt to restore sinus rhythm. If the atrial arrhythmia persists after these measures have been instituted, direct current (DC) cardioversion may be considered. If the arrhythmia recurs, chronic antiarrhythmic therapy is recommended. Limitations of this approach include a high (>50%) incidence of arrhythmia recurrence as well as the expense, inconvenience, side effects, and proarrhythmic risks associated with antiarrhythmic agents *(40–42)*.

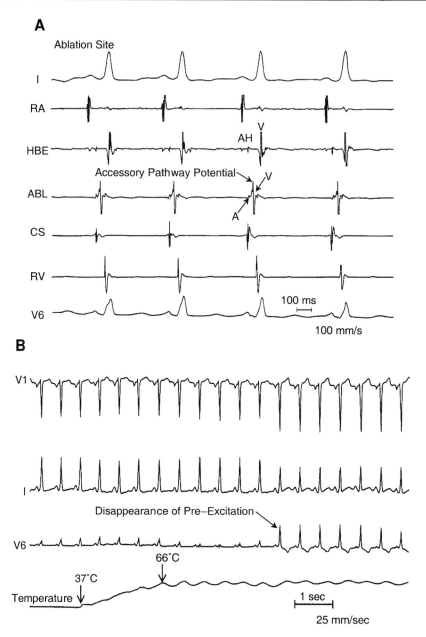

Fig. 6. (A) Typical successful ablation site (ABL) electrograms of an accessory pathway. Also shown are surface leads 1 and V6 and intracardiac recordings obtained from the high right atrium (RA), right ventricle (RV), His bundle (HBE), and CS ostium. The interval from the His bundle (H) recording to the QRS complex is less than 35 ms, confirming the presence of pre-excitation. At the successful ablation site, the ventricular electrogram (V) occurs early relative to the onset of the QRS complex, and a discreet deflection between the atrial (A) and ventricular electrograms is present, consistent with an accessory pathway (or "Kent") potential. **(B)** Within 2 s of radiofrequency energy delivery, the temperature recorded from the ablation catheter reaches 66°C. Several seconds after onset of energy delivery, pre-excitation disappears abruptly, as best seen in surface ECG lead V6.

Patients in whom initial attempts are unsuccessful or whose arrhythmia recurs early after sinus rhythm is restored can be stratified into those in whom a potentially curative approach to catheter ablation exists (focal atrial tachycardia or type 1 atrial flutter) and those in whom curative approaches to catheter ablation do not exist or are currently under investigation (AF or atypical atrial flutter). Patients for whom catheter ablation represents an option for cure may elect to proceed directly to catheter ablation or undergo further trials of antiarrhythmic therapy. Patients for whom catheter ablation does not offer a potential for cure may undergo additional attempts at pharmacologic control. If initial measures are ineffective or poorly tolerated, the alternative therapeutic strategy of ventricular rate control can be employed using beta-blockers, calcium-channel blockers, or digoxin. If control of the ventricular response cannot be achieved with pharmacologic agents, catheter ablation or modification of the AV node can be considered. Under rare circumstances, such as patients with dilated cardiomyopathy resulting from recurring atrial tachycardia or atrial tachycardia presenting with significant hemodynamic compromise, electrophysiology testing and catheter ablation may be recommended as initial therapy. For example, an invasive approach would be recommended for a patient with syncope associated with 1:1 conduction of common atrial flutter.

Atrial Tachycardias

The term "atrial tachycardia" refers to a group of arrhythmias that are confined to the atrium, have a rate <240 BPM, and are often difficult to control with standard antiarrhythmic medications. Atrial tachycardia affects less than 10% of patients presenting with supraventricular tachycardia (SVT). During tachycardia, P waves are usually dissimilar from sinus P waves, with rates between 100 and 240/min. Atrial tachycardias that have a focal site of origin or result from macroentry involving a critical isthmus of atrial tissue are amenable to cure with radiofrequency catheter ablation. From an ablation perspective, three major types of atrial tachycardia can be considered: automatic ectopic atrial tachycardia, sinus node reentrant tachycardia, and reentrant atrial tachycardia. This chapter also examines the role of catheter ablation for "inappropriate" sinus tachycardia.

CATHETER ABLATION FOR AUTOMATIC ECTOPIC ATRIAL TACHYCARDIA

The majority of atrial tachycardias (70–90%) arise from the right atrium, with a particular clustering in the region of the crista terminalis, resulting in the terms "atrial ring of fire" and "cristal tachycardias" *(43–45)*. However, a left atrial origin may be more common in children, and arise most commonly from ostia of the pulmonary veins *(46,47)*.

Indications. Ablation of automatic ectopic atrial tachycardia is recommended for patients when their arrhythmia is drug-resistant, or the patient is drug-intolerant or does not desire long-term drug therapy *(9)*.

Techniques. Catheter ablation is performed by manipulating one or more steerable electrode catheters in the right or left atrium to identify the site of earliest atrial activation, usually at least 30 ms prior to onset of the P wave. Once identified, 25–50 W of radiofrequency energy are delivered for 30–60 s to achieve a target electrode temperature of 60–70°C.

Outcomes and Complications. Although the clinical experience with catheter ablation of automatic atrial and tachycardia is limited, largely because of the rare occurrence of this arrhythmia, the results appear favorable. Among four published series, catheter ablation was successful in 41 of 45 patients (91%), with recurrence of tachycardia in eight patients (17%) *(47–50)*. No complications were reported.

CATHETER ABLATION FOR SINUS NODE REENTRANT TACHYCARDIA

Sinus node reentrant tachycardia is a rare type of atrial tachycardia involving a reentrant circuit completely confined to or partially involving the sinus node. It is characterized by paroxysmal onset and offset, a rate that is often less than 130/min and P waves during tachycardia that are identical or nearly so to those seen in sinus rhythm.

Indications. Ablation of sinus node reentrant tachycardia is recommended for patients when their arrhythmia is drug-resistant, or the patient is drug-intolerant or does not desire long-term drug therapy *(9)*.

Techniques. Catherer ablation is performed by positioning the ablation catheter at the junction of the SVC and right atrium in the region of the sinus node. The ablation catheter is then manipulated to identify the site of earliest atrial activation, typically at least 30 ms prior to onset of the P wave. Fractionated atrial electrograms are commonly observed at successful ablation sites.

Outcomes and Complications. Among three published series, catheter ablation was successful in 17 of 17 patients (100%), with a recurrence of tachycardia reported in one patient (6%) *(48,51,52)*. No complications were reported.

CATHETER ABLATION FOR REENTRANT ATRIAL TACHYCARDIA

Reentrant atrial tachycardia usually occurs in patients with structural heart disease, particularly in patients with prior cardiac surgery.

Indications. Ablation of reentrant atrial tachycardia is recommended for patients when their arrhythmia is drug-resistant, or the patient is drug-intolerant or does not desire long-term drug therapy *(9)*.

Techniques. Frequently, a prior atriotomy scar may serve as an obstacle around which the reentrant wavefront can travel. Optimal ablation sites are those that occur within a protected isthmus of slow conduction. These sites are identified using entrainment mapping techniques, which involve overdrive atrial pacing at multiple atrial sites during tachycardia.

Outcomes and Complications. Because of the rare occurrence of these arrhythmias, the clinical experience with catheter ablation is small. Among two published series, catheter ablation was successful in 14 of 15 patients (93%) with no complications and no late recurrences *(51,52)*.

CATHETER ABLATION FOR INAPPROPRIATE SINUS TACHYCARDIA

"Inappropriate" sinus tachycardia (IST) is a poorly defined and rare clinical syndrome characterized by an increased resting heart rate and an exaggerated response to stress or exercise *(53)*. The mechanism of this tachycardia is unknown, although it may involve a primary abnormality of the sinus node, demonstrating enhanced automaticity or a primary autonomic disturbance with increased sympathetic activity and enhanced sinus node beta-adrenergic sensitivity *(54)*. The diagnosis of IST is one of exclusion. It usually occurs in young women, particularly those employed in the health care field. It is important to distinguish IST from the postural orthostatic tachycardia syndrome (POTS). POTS is a type of dysautonomia that also typically occurs in young women. It is defined as a greater than 30 BPM increase in heart rate on standing with associated symptoms of orthostatic intolerance such as lightheadedness and palpitations. Patients with POTS are treated primarily with increased salt intake, fludrocortisone, and midodrine *(55)*. Catheter ablation does not play a role in the management of these patients.

Indications. There are no specific guidelines to decide which patients with IST should undergo modification of the sinus node. However, this procedure is rarely performed, and should be reserved for the most highly symptomatic of patients (in whom POTS has been excluded) who have failed attempts at pharmacologic therapy—patients who are willing to undergo a procedure with considerable risk of recurrence or the need for a pacemaker, and without assurance that their symptoms will be improved.

Techniques. The sinus-node complex originates at the junction of the superior vena cava (SVC) and right atrial appendage and extends inferiorly along the crista terminalis. Sympathetic activation results in an increase in heart rate accompanied by a shift in earliest activation to the superior portion of the sinus node. Conversely, vagal stimulation results in slowing with a more inferior focus *(56,57)*. Thus, catheter ablation is targeted at the higher rate, superior portion of the crista terminalis at the junction of the right atrium and the SVC. If unsuccessful, progressively inferior applications are given to modify the sinus node until a 25% reduction in the sinus heart rate occurs *(58)*. Total sinus-node ablation is characterized by a reduction in heart rate of >50% of the tachycardia rate, with a junctional escape rhythm *(58)*.

Outcomes and Complications. In a study of 16 patients with IST, the sinus node was modified successfully in 12 patients and totally ablated in four patients, with a slower sinus-node rate corresponding to a caudal shift of the sinus node depolarization origin *(58)*. None of the four patients who underwent total sinus-node ablation had recurrence of IST during a mean follow-up period of 20.5 ± 0.3 mo. However, two patients required permanent pacemaker implantation for symptomatic bradycardias, and one patient had right diaphragmatic paralysis, which resolved within 1 mo. For patients who underwent sinus-node modification, the short-term response appeared to be favorable, with recurrences of IST in only 2 of 12 patients during a follow-up of 7.1 ± 1.7 mo. The procedure was complicated by SVC syndrome in one patient, with resolution within 1 h. However, a subsequent preliminary observation from the same laboratory reported that sustained improvement of tachycardia symptoms was achieved in only 8 of 22 patients (36%) during a mean follow-up of 8 ± 5 mo *(59)*. In a report of three patients, Jayaprakash et al. *(60)* reported a satisfactory outcome for all patients, although one patient required continuation of beta-blocker therapy.

Atrial Flutter

Atrial flutter is an atrial arrhythmia characterized by uniform morphology and a rate that is regular and greater than 240 BPM. It is often accompanied by a fixed 2:1 ventricular response, and it is this rapid ventricular response that results in the majority of symptoms. It may be observed transiently following cardiac surgery, or may persist for months to years. Atrial flutter is generally classified into three types: common, uncommon, and atypical (impure or type 2) atrial flutter. Common atrial flutter (also called typical counterclockwise flutter) is characterized by negative flutter waves in II, III, and aVF and an atrial rate of 250–320 BPM (Fig. 7). Uncommon atrial flutter (also called typical clockwise flutter) is characterized by upright flutter waves in II, III, and aVF and an atrial rate of 250–320 BPM. Atypical atrial flutter demonstrates morphologic features intermediate between AF and atrial flutter with atrial rates greater than 320 BPM.

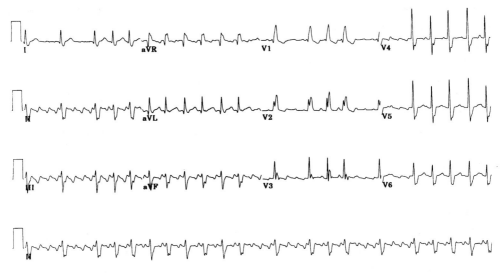

Fig. 7. ECG demonstrating common atrial flutter with characteristic negative "sawtooth" flutter waves in leads II, III, and AVF and positive flutter waves in V1. Atrial rate is 280/min with variable conduction to the ventricle.

CATHETER ABLATION FOR ATRIAL FLUTTER

The common and uncommon forms of atrial flutter are macroreentrant tachycardias confiend to the right atrium, and can potentially be cured with catheter ablation. In the common form of atrial flutter, the reentrant wavefront travels caudo-cranially along the interatrial septum and around the right atrium in a counterclockwise direction through a critical zone of slow conduction in the inferior right atrium between the triscupid annulus, the inferior vena cava (IVC), and the ostium of the CS. Conversely, the wavefront in uncommon atrial flutter travels in the reverse direction, proceeding cranio-caudally down the interatrial septum and around the right atrium in a clockwise direction. In contrast, atypical atrial flutter does not rely on an anatomically defined circuit, and thus is currently not amenable to catheter ablation.

Indications. Ablation of atrial flutter is indicated for patients with atrial flutter that is drug-resistant, or when the patient is drug-intolerant or does not desire long-term drug therapy *(9)*.

Techniques. Catheter ablation of atrial flutter was first reported in 1986, and was performed by employing cryosurgery in the region of the CS ostium *(61)*. Subsequently, success rates of approx 50% were reported for catheter ablation of atrial flutter using DC shock energy delivered in the low posteroseptal right atrium *(62)*. Direct current energy has subsequently been abandoned in favor of radiofrequency energy *(63–67)*.

Catheter ablation of atrial flutter is performed using an anatomic approach *(63–65)*. A series of radiofrequency lesions are delivered along a line connecting the tricuspid annulus and the IVC or connecting the tricuspid annulus, the coronary sinus ostium, and the IVC. Radiofrequency energy (25–50 W) are delivered for 30–60 s at each ablation site either in sinus rhythm or during atrial flutter. The end point for catheter ablation of atrial flutter is the creation of bidirectional block along the ablation line

(68). Since restoration of sinus rhythm may transiently increase a patient's chance for embolic events, anticoagulation with warfarin is recommended for at least 1 mo prior to and following the procedure.

Outcomes and Complications. Although follow-up times are limited, the reported acute efficacy for radiofrequency catheter ablation of atrial flutter exceeds 85% in most series *(64–69)*. Recurrences of atrial flutter or AF following a successful ablation procedure occur in approx 10% of patients using current techniques *(27)*. Techniques to create larger radiofrequency lesions, such as ablation catheters with larger or saline-irrigated electrodes, have recently been shown to be useful in patients who fail ablation with standard radiofrequency catheters *(12–15)*. No significant complications have been reported.

ABLATION OF THE AV JUNCTION

Theoretically, catheter ablation of the AV junction can eliminate any type of supraventricular arrhythmias that utilize the AV node as part of the reentrant circuit and can slow the ventricular response to supraventricular arrhythmias confined to the atrium.

Indications. In practice, catheter ablation of the AV junction is reserved for atrial arrhythmias that cannot be controlled with pharmacologic therapy, and which result in a rapid ventricular response.

Techniques. The procedure is performed by positioning a steerable ablation catheter across the tricuspid annulus to record a His bundle electrogram associated with a large atrial electrogram. A second electrode catheter is placed at the apex of the right ventricle for temporary pacing. Once an appropriate target site is identified, radiofrequency energy is delivered for 30–60 s. If AV conduction remains unchanged, the catheter is repositioned and a repeat attempt is made. If unsuccessful, a left-sided approach can be used *(54)*. The ablation catheter is passed retrogradely across the aortic valve into the left ventricle and positioned immediately below the aortic valve to record a His bundle electrogram. Radiofrequency energy is then delivered in a standard fashion.

Outcomes and Complications. The overall efficacy of catheter ablation of the AV junction using these two approaches is nearly 100% *(27,70–72)*. The recurrence rate is approx 2% (Fig. 3A) *(27)*. In one recent series, the 1-yr survival following catheter ablation of the AV junction was 86% *(27)* (Fig. 4). Prior to or following ablation of the AV junction, a permanent rate-responsive pacemaker is inserted. For patients with drug-refractory AF, AV junction ablation with implantation of a DDDR pacemaker has been shown to be superior to drug therapy in controlling symptoms and improving quality of life *(73)*. Complication rates are generally less than 2%, with an estimated incidence of procedure-related death of 0.2% *(2,27)*. Late, sudden death has been reported following both DC or radiofrequency ablation of the AV junction *(27,74)*. Because many of these patients have severe underlying heart disease, it is difficult to attribute these late, sudden deaths directly to the ablation procedure *(27)*.

Recent studies have demonstrated the feasibility of slowing the ventricular response during AF by delivering radiofrequency energy along the posteroseptal portion of the tricuspid annulus, using a technique similar to the posterior approach to ablation of AVNRT *(75,76)*. Although the initial results appear promising, the long-term safety and efficacy of this procedure remain uncertain and await the results of larger studies. This procedure has not gained widespread acceptance.

SPECIAL CONSIDERATIONS DURING CATHETER ABLATION OF SUPRAVENTRICULAR ARRHYTHMIAS IN CHILDREN

The technique, results, complications, and clinical role of catheter ablation in children are generally similar to that in adults. However, several important differences exist. First, the incidence of major complications during catheter ablation procedures is significantly increased in infants. Second, accessory pathways are the most common cause of PSVT in children. Significant proportions of accessory pathways resolve spontaneously during the first several years of life. Because of the increased incidence of complications and the potential for accessory pathways to resolve spontaneously, catheter ablation should be avoided in favor of pharmacologic therapy in very small children.

Recently, the results of multicenter catheter ablation registry in 652 pediatric patients were reported (77). The median patient age was 13.5. Forty-one percent of patients were less than 13 yr of age, and 8% of patients were less than 4 yr of age. The two most common indications for catheter ablation were patient preference in 30% of patients and failure of antiarrhythmic therapy in 39% of patients. Successful ablation was accomplished in 83% of patients with an accessory pathway, 83% of patients with AVNRT, and 92% of patients with atrial tachycardia. The incidence of complications was 3.7%. A body wt of less than 15 kg was identified as an independent risk factor.

Somewhat more favorable results were reported by Calkins et al. (27). Among 1050 patients undergoing ablation of AVNRT, an accessory pathway or the AV junction, 326 (31%) were less than 20 yr of age with 133 (13%) younger than 13 yr. No difference in success (95%), recurrence (6%), or complication (3%) rates were observed in children as compared with adults (27).

COST-EFFECTIVENESS OF CATHETER ABLATION

The cost of catheter ablation procedures compares favorably with the cost of arrhythmia surgery or lifelong antiarrhythmic therapy. In one study, the cost of arrhythmia surgery in patients with WPW was estimated to be $53,000 vs. $15,000 for catheter ablation (78). Another study compared the costs of medical management vs. catheter ablation for treatment of patients with AVNRT. The cost of catheter ablation was $16,000, compared with an estimated annual health care cost of $7,600 prior to catheter ablation. When compared with the annual medical costs of a patient whose tachycardia is effectively controlled with a medication such as verapamil, for example, it was estimated that the cumulative costs of medications and an annual office visit would equal the cost of catheter ablation after approx 15 yr (79). Thus, in a young patient, the costs of catheter ablation are justifiable from an economic perspective. The cost-effectiveness of catheter ablation has recently been further improved by shorter hospital stays and the elimination of routine echocardiograms and electrophysiology testing following catheter ablation procedures. The feasibility of performing catheter ablation procedures on an outpatient basis has been demonstrated and has gained widespread acceptance, which is likely to further reduce the costs associated with catheter ablation therapy (80,81).

FUTURE DEVELOPMENTS IN CATHETER ABLATION
OF SUPRAVENTRICULAR ARRHYTHMIAS

The single greatest limitation of current ablation technologies is the inability to cure AF with catheter ablation. A surgical technique to cure AF, called the Maze procedure, has been developed *(82)*. The procedure is performed by creating multiple linear incisions in the right and left atrium to interrupt conduction through the most common reentrant circuits during AF. Among 164 patients, followed for at least 3 mo, AF was eliminated in 152 (93%). Recently, preliminary reports have described successful radiofrequency catheter ablation of AF in humans by creating a series of linear lines, similar to the Maze procedure *(83–85)*. There is also increasing evidence that in some patients, paroxysmal AF may be cured by targeting the site or origin of atrial premature beats, which are often localized in the pulmonary veins *(86)*. A great deal of additional research is needed, both to determine the optimal technique and tools required for these procedures and also to better define the safety, efficacy, and hemodynamic consequences of radiofrequency catheter ablation of AF.

Although the majority of research today is being focused on developing new tools to cure AF, there also are ongoing efforts to improve the safety and efficacy of other types of supraventricular arrhythmias. These efforts include the development of advanced mapping systems aimed at reducing fluoroscopy and procedure times, as well as the development of new tools to image radiofrequency lesions and the arrhythmia substrate, such as intracardiac ultrasound *(87)* and MRI *(88,89)*.

REFERENCES

1. Gallagher JJ, Svenson RH, Kassell HJ, German LD, Bardy GH, Broughton A, et al. Catheter technique for closed-chest ablation of the atrioventricular conduction system: a therapeutic alternative for the treatment of refractory supraventricular tachycardia. N Engl J Med 1982;306:194–200.
2. Scheinman, Melvin M. NASPE Survey on Catheter Ablation. From the Cardiac EP Service, University of California, San Francisco, CA, PACE. 1995;18:1474–1478.
3. Haines DE, Watson DD, Verow AF. Electrode radius predicts lesion radius during radiofrequency energy heating: validation of a proposed thermodynamic model. Circ Res 1990;67:124–129.
4. Erez A, Shitzer A. Controlled destruction and temperature distributions in biological tissues subjected to monoactive electrocoagulation. Trans ASME. 1980;102:42–49.
5. Avitall B, Khan M, Krum D, Hare J, Lessila C, Dhala A, Deshpande S, Jazayeri M, Sra J, Akhtar M. Physics and engineering of transcatheter cardiac tissue ablation. J Am Coll Cardiol 1993;22:921–32.
6. Nath S, DiMarco JP, Haines DE. Basic aspects of radiofrequency catheter ablation. J Cardiovasc Electrophysiol 1994;5:863–876.
7. Nath S, Lynch C III, Whayne JG, Haines DE. Cellular electrophysiology effects of hyperthermia on isolated guinea pig papillary muscle: implications for catheter ablation. Circulation 1993;88(part 1):1826–1831.
8. Haines DE, Verow AF. Observations on electrode-tissue interface temperature and effect on electrical impedance during radiofrequency ablation of ventricular myocardium. Circulation 1990;82:1034–1038.
9. Nakagawa H, Wittkampf FH, Yamanashi WS, Pitha JV, Imai S, Capmbell B, Arruda M, Lazzara R, Jackman WM. Inverse relationship between electrode size and lesion size during radiofrequency ablation with active electrode cooling. Circulation 1998;5:458–465.
10. Otomo K, Yamanashi WS, Tondo C, Antz M, Bussey J, Pitha JV, et al. Why a large tip electrode makes a deeper radiofrequency lesion: effects of increase in electrode cooling and electrode-tissue interface area. J Cardiovasc Electrophysiol 1998;9:47–54.
11. Ruffy R, Imran MA, Santel DJ, Wharton JM. Radiofrequency delivery through a cooled catheter tip allows the creation of larger endomyocardial lesions in the ovine heart. J Cardiovasc Electrophysiol 1995;6:1089–1096.

12. Nakagawa H, Yamanashi WS, Pitha JV, Arruda M, Wang X, Ohtomo K, et al. Comparison of in vivo tissue temperature profile and lesion geometry for radiofrequency ablation with a saline-irrigated electrode versus temperature control in a canine thigh muscle preparation. Circulation 1995;91:2264–2273.

13. Calkins H, Epstein A, Packer D, Arria AM, Hummel J, Gilligan DM, Trusso J, Carlson M, Luceri R, Kopelman H, Wilber D, Wharton JM, Stevenson W. Catheter ablation of ventricular tachycardia in patients with structural heart disease using cooled radiofrequency energy: results of a prospective multi-center study. Cooled RF Multi Center Investigators Group. J Am Coll Cardiol 2000;35(7):1905–1914.

14. Jais P, Haissaguerre M, Shah DC, Taqkahashi A, Hocini M, Lavergne T, et al. Successful irrigated-tip catheter ablation of atrial flutter resistant to conventional radiofrequency ablation. Circulation 1998; 98:835–838.

15. Delacretaz E, Stevenson WG, Winters GL, Mitchell RN, Stewart S, Lynch K, et al. Ablation of ventricular tachycardia with a saline-cooled radiofrequency catheter: anatomic and histologic character-istics of the lesions in humans. J Cardiovasc Electrophysiol 1999;10(6):860–856.

16. Tsai C-F, Tai C-T, Yu W-C, Chen Y-J, Hsieh M-H, Chiang C-E, et al. Is 8-mm more effective than 4-mm tip electrode catheter for ablation of typical atrial flutter? Circulation 1999;100:768–771.

17. Atiga WL, Worley SJ, Hummel J, Berger RD, Gohn DC, Mandalakas NJ, et al. Prospective randomized comparison of cooled RF versus standard RF energy ablation of typical atrial flutter. PACE 2001, (in press).

18. Calkins H, Prystowsky E, Carlson M, Klein LS, Saul JP, Gillette P: the Atakr Multicenter Investigators Group. Temperature monitoring during radiofrequency catheter ablation procedures using closed loop control. Circulation 1994;90:1279–1286.

19. Klein GJ, Bashore TM, Sellers TD, Pritchett ELC, Smith WM, Gallagher JJ. Ventricular fibrillation in the Wolff-Parkinson-White syndrome. N Engl J Med 1979;301:1080–1085.

20. Zipes DP, DiMarco JP, Gillette PC, Jackman WM, Myerburg RJ, Rahimtoola SH, et al. Guidelines for clinical intracardiac electrophysiology and catheter ablation procedures: a report of the American College of Cardiology/American Heart Association Task Force on Practice Guidelines. Circulation 1995;92:673–691.

21. Bogun F, Knight B, Weiss R, Bahu M, Goyal R, Harvey M, et al. Slow pathway ablation in patients with documented but noninducible paroxysmal supraventricular tachycardia. J Am Coll Cardiol 1996; 28:1000–1004.

22. Jazayeri MR, Hempe SL, Sra JS, Dhala AA, Blanck Z, Deshpande SS, et al. Selective transcatheter ablation of the fast and slow pathways using radiofrequency energy in patients with atrioventricular nodal reentrant tachycardia. Circulation 1992;85:1318–1328.

23. Lee MA, Morady F, Kadish A, Schamp DJ, Chin MC, Scheinmann MM, et al. Catheter modification of the atrioventricular junction with radiofrequency energy in patients with atrioventricular nodal reentry tachycardia. Circulation 1991;83:827–835.

24. Kottkamp H, Hindricks G, Willems S, Chen X, Reinhardt L, Haverkamp W, et al. An anatomically and electrogram-guided stepwise approach for effective and safe catheter ablation of the fast pathway for elimination of atrioventricular node reentrant tachycardia. J Am Coll Cardiol 1995;25:974–983.

25. Haissaguerre M, Gaita F, Fischer B, Commenges D, Montserrat P, d'Ivernois C, et al. Elimination of atrioventricular nodal reentrant tachycardia using discrete slow potentials to guide application of radiofrequency energy. Circulation 1992;85:2162–2175.

26. Jackman WM, Beckman KJ, McClelland JH, Wang X, Friday KJ, Roman CA, et al. Treatment of supraventricular tachycardia due to atrioventricular nodal reentry by radiofrequency catheter ablation of slow-pathway conduction. N Engl J Med 1992;327:313–318.

27. Calkins H, Prystowsky E, Berger RD, Saul JP, Klein LS, Liem LB, et al. Recurrence of conduction following radiofrequency catheter ablation procedures: relationship to ablation target and electrode temperature. J Cardiovasc Electrophysiol 1996;7:704–712.

28. Kalbfleisch SJ, Strickberger SA, Williamson B, Vorperian VR, Man C, Hummel JD, et al. Randomized comparison of anatomic and electrogram mapping approaches to ablation of the slow pathway of atrioventricular node reentrant tachycardia. J Am Coll Cardiol 1994;23:716–723.

29. Calkins H, Yong P, Miller JM, Olshansky B, Carlson M, Saul JP, et al. Catheter ablation of accessory pathways, atrioventricular nodal reentrant tachycardia, and the atrioventricular junction: final results of a prospective, multicenter clinical trial. Circulation 1999;99:262–270.

30. Munger TM, Packer DL, Hammill SC, Feldman BJ, Bailey KR, Ballard DJ, et al. A population study

of the natural history of Wolff-Parkinson-White syndrome in Olmsted County, Minnesota, 1953–1989. Circulation, 1993;87:866–873.

31. Calkins H, Sousa J, El-Atassi R, Rosenheck S, DeBuitleir M, Kou WH, et al. Diagnosis and cure of the Wolff-Parkinson-White syndrome or paroxysmal supraventricular tachycardias during a single electrophysiology test. N Engl J Med 1991;324:1612–1618.

32. Fitzpatrick AP, Gonzales RP, Lesh MD, Modin GW, Lee RJ, Scheinman MM. New algorithm for the localization of accessory atrioventricular connections using a baseline electrocardiogram. J Am Coll Cardiol 1994;23:107–116.

33. Lesh MD, Van Hare G, Scheinman MM, Ports TA, Epstein LA. Comparison of the retrograde and transseptal methods for ablation of left free-wall accessory pathways. J Am Coll Cardiol 1993;22:542–549.

34. Langberg JJ, Man C, Vorperian VR, Williamson B, Kalbfleisch SJ, Strickberger SA, et al. Recognition and catheter ablation of subepicardial accessory pathways. J Am Coll Cardiol 1993;22:1100–1104.

35. Calkins H, Kim Y-N, Schmaltz S, Sousa J, El-Atassi R, Leon A, et al. Electrogram criteria for identification of appropriate target sites for radiofrequency catheter ablation of accessory atrioventricular connections. Circulation 1992;85:565–573.

36. Calkins H, Langberg J, Sousa J, El-Atassi R, Leon A, Kou W, et al. Radiofrequency catheter ablation of accessory atrioventricular connections in 250 patients: abbreviated therapeutic approach to Wolff-Parkinson-White syndrome. Circulation 1992;85:1337–1346.

37. Jackman WM, Wang X, Friday KJ, Roman CA, Moulton KP, Beckman KJ, et al. Catheter ablation of accessory atrioventricular pathways (Wolff-Parkinson-White syndrome) by radiofrequency current. N Engl J Med 1991;324:1605–1611.

38. Kuck KH, Schluter M, Geiger M, Siebels J, Duckeck W. Radiofrequency current catheter ablation of accessory atrioventricular pathways. Lancet 1991;337:1557–1561.

39. Kay GN, Epstein AE, Dailey SM, Plumb VJ. Role of radiofrequency ablation in the management of supraventricular arrhythmias: experience in 760 consecutive patients. J Cardiovasc Electrophysiol 1993;4:371–389.

40. Swartz JF, Tracy CM, Fletcher RD. Radiofrequency endocardial catheter ablation of accessory atrioventricular pathway atrial insertion sites. Circulation 1993;87:487–499.

41. Twidale N, Wang X, Beckman KJ, McClelland JH, Moulton KP, Prior MI, et al. Factors associated with recurrence of accessory pathway conduction after radiofrequency catheter ablation. PACE 1991; 14(Part 2):2042–2048.

42. Antman EM, Beamer AD, Cantillon C, McGowan N, Friedman PL. Therapy of refractory symptomatic atrial fibrillation and atrial flutter: a staged care approach with new antiarrhythmic drugs. J Am Coll Cardiol 1990;15:698–707.

43. Crijns HJ, Van Gelder IC, Van Gilst WH, Hillege H, Gosselink AM, Lie KI. Serial antiarrhythmic drug treatment to maintain sinus rhythm after electrical cardioversion for chronic atrial fibrillation or atrial flutter. Am J Cardiol 1991;68:335–341.

44. Coplen SE, Antman EM, Berlin JA, Hewitt P, Chalmers TC. Efficacy and safety of quinidine therapy for maintenance of sinus rhythm after cardioversion. Circulation 1990;82:1106–1116.

45. Wharton JM. Atrial tachycardia: advances in diagnosis and treatment. Cardiol Rev 1995;3:332–342.

46. Shenasa H, Merrill JJ, Hamer ME, Wharton JM. Distribution of ectopic atrial tachycardias along the crista terminalis: an atrial ring of fire? (abstract) Circulation 1993;88(2):1–29.

47. Kalman JM, Olgin JE, Karch MR, Hamdan M, Lee RJ, Lesh MD. "Cristal tachycardias": origin of right atrial tachycardias from the crista terminalis identified by intracardiac echocardiography. J Am Coll Cardiol 1998;31:451–459.

48. Hatala R, Weiss C, Koschyk DH, Siebels J, Cappato R, Kuck K-H. Radiofrequency catheter ablation of left atrial tachycardia originating within the pulmonary vein in a patient with dextrocardia. PACE 1996;19:999–1002.

49. Walsh EP, Saul JP, Hulse JE, Rhodes LA, Hordof AJ, Mayer JE, et al. Transcatheter ablation of ectopic atrial tachycardia in young patients using radiofrequency current. Circulation 1992;86:1138–1146.

50. Kay GN, Chong F, Epstein AE, Dailey SM, Plumb VJ. Radiofrequency ablation for treatment of primary atrial tachycardias. J Am Coll Cardiol 1993;21:901–909.

51. Tracy CM, Swartz JF, Fletcher RD, Hoops HG, Solomon AJ, Karasik PE et al. Radiofrequency catheter ablation of ectopic atrial tachycardia using paced activation sequence mapping. J Am Coll Cardiol 1993;21:910–917.

52. Lesh MD, Van Hare GF, Epstein LM, Fitzpatrick AP, Scheinman MM, Lee RJ, et al. Radiofrequency catheter ablation of atrial arrhythmias: results and mechanisms. Circulation 1994;89:1074–1089.

53. Sanders WE, Sorrentino RA, Greenfield RA, Shenasa H, Hamer ME. Wharton JM. Catheter ablation of sinoatrial node reentrant tachycardia. J Am Coll Cardiol 1994;23:926–934.

54. Chen S-A, Chiang C-E, Yang C-J, Cheng C-C, Wu T-J, Wang S-P, et al. Radiofrequency catheter ablation of sustained intra-atrial reentrant tachycardia in adult patients: Identification of EP characteristics and endocardial mapping techniques. Circulation 1993;88:578–587.

55. Krahn AD, Yee R, Klein GJ, Morillo C. Inappropriate sinus tachycardia: evaluation and therapy. J Cardiovasc Electrophysiol 1995;6:1124–1128.

56. Morillo CA, Klein GJ, Thakur RK, Li H, Zardini M, Yee R. Mechanism of "inappropriate" sinus tachycardia. Role of sympathovagal balance. Circulation 1994;90:873–877.

57. Low PA, Opfer-Gehrking TL, Textor SC, Benarroch EE, Shen W-K, Schondorf R, et al. Postural orthostatic tachycardia syndrome (POTS). Neurology 1995;45(Suppl 5):S19–S25.

58. Randall WC, Rinkema LE, Jones SB, et al. Functional characterization of atrial pacemaker activity. Am J Physiol 1982;242:H98–106.

59. Boineau JP, Scheussler RB, Hackel DB, et al. Widespread distribution and rate differentiation of the atrial pacemaker complex. Am J Physiol 1980;239:H406–415.

60. Lee RJ, Kalman JM, Fitzpatrick AP, Epstein LM, Fisher WG, Olgin JE, et al. Radiofrequency catheter modification of the sinus node for "inappropriate" sinus tachycardia. Circulation 1995;92:2919–2928.

61. Shinbane JF, Lesh MD, Scheinman MN, Wood K, Evans GT Jr, Saxon LA, et al. Long-term follow up after radiofrequency sinus node modification for inappropriate sinus tachycardia. (abstract) J Am Coll Cardiol 1997;29(Suppl A):199A.

62. Jayaprakash S, Sparks PB, Vohra J. Inappropriate sinus tachycardia (IST): management by radiofrequency modification of sinus node. Aust N Z J Med 1997;27:391–397.

63. Klein GJ, Guiraudon GM, Sharma AD, Milstein S. Demonstration of macroreentry and feasibility of operative therapy in the common type of atrial flutter. Am J Cardiol 1986;57:587–591.

64. Saoudi N, Atallah G, Kirkorian G, Touboul P. Catheter ablation of the atrial myocardium in human type I atrial flutter. Circulation 1990;81:762–771.

65. Calkins H, Leon AR, Deam AG, Kalbfleisch SJ, Langberg JJ, Morady F. Catheter ablation of atrial flutter using radiofrequency energy. Am J Cardiol 1994;73:353–356.

66. Feld GK, Fleck RP, Chen P-S, Boyce K, Bahnson TD, Stein JB, et al. Radiofrequency catheter ablation for the treatment of human type I atrial flutter: identification of a critical zone in the reentrant circuit by endocardial mapping techniques. Circulation 1992;86:1233–1240.

67. Kirkorian G, Moncada E, Chevalier P, Canu G, Claudel J-P, Bellon C, et al. Radiofrequency ablation of atrial flutter: efficacy of an anatomically guided approach. Circulation 1994;90:2804–2814.

68. Poty H, Saoudi N, Aziz AA, Nair M, Letac B. Radiofrequency catheter ablation of type I atrial flutter: prediction of late success by electrophysiology criteria. Circulation 1995;92:1389–1392.

69. Cosio FG, Lopez-Gil M, Goicolea A, Arribas F, Barroso JL. Radiofrequency ablation of the inferior vena cava-tricuspid valve isthmus in common atrial flutter. Am J Cardiol 1993;71:705–709.

70. Sousa J, El-Atassi R, Rosenheck S, Calkins H, Langberg J, Morady F. Radiofrequency catheter ablation of the atrioventricular junction from the left ventricle. Circulation 1991;84:567–571.

71. Morady F, Calkins H, Langberg JJ, Armstrong WF, DeBuitleir M, El-Atassi R, et al. A prospective randomized comparison of direct current and radiofrequency ablation of the atrioventricular junction. J Am Coll Cardiol 1993;21:102–109.

72. Trohman RG, Simmons TW, Moore SL, Firstenberg MS, Williams D, Maloney JD. Catheter ablation of the atrioventricular junction using radiofrequency energy and a bilateral cardiac approach. Am J Cardiol 1992;70:1438–1443.

73. Brignole M, Gianfranchi L, Menozzi C, Alboni P, Musso G, Bongiorni MG, et al. Assessment of atrioventricular junction ablation and DDDR mode-switching pacemaker versus pharmacological treatment in patients with severely symptomatic paroxysmal atrial fibrillation: a randomized controlled study. Circulation 1997;96:2617–2624.

74. Evans GT Jr, Scheinman MM, Zipes DP, Benditt D, Breithardt G, Camm AJ, et al. The percutaneous cardiac mapping and ablation registry: final summary of results. PACE 1988;11:1621–1626.

75. Feld GK, Fleck RP, Fujimura O, Prothro DL, Bahnson TD, Ibarra M. Control of rapid ventricular response by radiofrequency catheter modification of the atrioventricular node in patients with medically refractory atrial fibrillation. Circulation 1994;90:2299–2307.

76. Williamson BD, Man KC, Daoud E, Niebauer M, Strickberger SA, Morady F. Radiofrequency catheter

modification of atrioventricular conduction to control the ventricular rate during atrial fibrillation. N Engl J Med 1994;331:910–917.

77. Kugler JD, Danford DA, Deal BJ, Gillette PC, Perry JC, Silka MJ, et al. Radiofrequency catheter ablation for tachyarrhythmias in children and adolescents. N Engl J Med 1994;330:1481–1487.

78. De Buitleir M, Sousa J, Bolling SF, El-Atassi R, Calkins H, Langberg JJ, et al. Reduction in medical care cost associated with radiofrequency catheter ablation of accessory pathways. Am J Cardiol 1991; 68:1656–1661.

79. Kalbfleisch SJ, Calkins H, Langberg JJ, El-Atassi R, Leon A, Borganelli M, et al. Comparison of the cost of radiofrequency catheter modification of the atrioventricular node and medical therapy for drug-refractory atrioventricular node reentrant tachycardia. J Am Coll Cardiol 1992;19:1583–1587.

80. Kalbfleisch SJ, El-Atassi R, Calkins H, Langberg JJ, Morady F. Safety, feasibility and cost of outpatient radiofrequency catheter ablation of accessory atrioventricular connections. J Am Coll Cardiol 1993;21:567–570.

81. Man KC, Kalbfleisch SJ, Hummel JD, Williamson BD, Vorperian VR, Strickberger SA, et al. Safety and cost of outpatient radiofrequency ablation of the slow pathway in patients with atrioventricular nodal reentrant tachycardia. Am J Cardiol 1993;72:1323–1324.

82. Cox JL, Schuessler RB, Lappas DG, Boineau JP. An 8 1/2-year experience with surgery for atrial fibrillation. Ann Surg 1996;224(3):267–273.

83. Swartz JF, Pellersels G, Silvers J, et al. A catheter-based curative approach to atrial fibrillation in humans (abstract) Circulation 1994;90.

84. Haissaguerre M, Marcus FI, Fischer B, Clementy J. Radiofrequency catheter ablation in unusual mechanisms of atrial fibrillation: report of three cases. J Cardiovasc Electrophysiol 1994;5:743–751.

85. Calkins H, Hall J, Ellenbogen K, Walcott G, Sherman M, Bowe W, et al. A new system for catheter ablation of atrial fibrillation. Am J Cardiol 1999;83:227D–236D.

86. Haissaguerre M, Jais P, Shah DC, Takahashi A, Hocini M, Quiniou G, et al. Spontaneous initiation of atrial fibrillation by ectopic beats originating in the pulmonary veins. N Engl J Med 1998;339:659–666.

87. Chu E, Fitzpatrick AP, Chin MC, Sudhir K, Yock PG, Lesh MD. Radiofrequency catheter ablation guided by intracardiac echocardiography. Circulation 1994;89:1301–1305.

88. Lardo AC, McVeigh ER, Jumrussirikul P, Berger RD, Calkins H, Lima J, Halperin HR. Visualization and temporal/spatial characterization of cardiac radiofrequency ablation lesions using magnetic resonance imaging. Circulation 2000;102(6):698–705.

89. Halperin H, Lardo A, McVeigh E, Calkins H, Lima J, Berger R. Catheter navigation and high fidelity intracardiac electrophysiologic signal acquisition during magnetic resonance imaging (abstract) PACE 1999;22(4)pt 2:491.

5

Approach to the Patient with Atrial Fibrillation

Otto Costantini, MD, and Bruce Stambler, MD

CONTENTS

INTRODUCTION
EPIDEMIOLOGY
CLASSIFICATION AND ETIOLOGY
DIAGNOSTIC EVALUATION
THERAPEUTIC OPTIONS
NONPHARMACOLOGICAL TREATMENT
SUMMARY
REFERENCES

INTRODUCTION

At the dawn of the twenty-first century, atrial fibrillation (AF), recognized as a distinct rhythm since the first decade of the twentieth century *(1)*, remains one of the greater challenges facing physicians in the future. An aging population and the association of AF with several cardiac and noncardiac conditions makes this arrhythmia a problem to be confronted not only by cardiologists, but by all physicians, from general internists to surgeons. Over the last several years, important advancements have been made in both the understanding of mechanisms and in the therapeutic management of this condition. Many controversies regarding mechanisms are unresolved, and a cure is still elusive *(2a)*. This chapter provides an overview of the scope of the problem, the most common etiologies, and the appropriate diagnostic evaluation and optimal therapeutic management. It should be emphasized that because of varied presentations, etiologies, and associated conditions, therapy must often be individualized, and presents more difficult challenges than other supraventricular tachycardias (SVTs). A detailed discussion regarding the different treatment modalities follows in subsequent chapters.

EPIDEMIOLOGY

Prevalence and Demographics

AF affects an estimated 1–2 million people in the United States alone *(3,4)*, but this number may be an underestimate because of the difficulty in identifying patients with

From: *Contemporary Cardiology: Management of Cardiac Arrhythmias*
Edited by: L. I. Ganz © Humana Press Inc., Totowa, NJ

paroxysmal asymptomatic episodes. The prevalence of this rhythm rises significantly with age; it is less common among individuals 25–35 years old (<0.5%) (5). However, the incidence is 2–4% in patients over the age of 60, and approximately doubles with each decade of life thereafter (6). Data from the Framingham study show that the prevalence of chronic AF is higher in all age groups in men than it is in women. This arrhythmia is clearly a disease of the elderly—the median age of affected patients is 75 years, more than 60% of patients affected are older than 65, and as many as 9–10% of octogenarians are affected. The prevalence has increased and is likely to increase further in future years as the population continues to age and the "baby-boomer" generation approaches the retirement age. The problem will be compounded by the fact that more patients are living longer with other cardiovascular problems, such as hypertension, coronary disease, and cardiomyopathy, all of which predispose to the development of AF.

Cost and Outcomes

The cost of AF to the health care system as a whole is difficult to measure. The staggering cost of hospital admissions and outpatient visits for the treatment of AF itself must be considered, as well as the cost of complications directly related to the disease, especially those of debilitating strokes. In an attempt to estimate only a portion of total costs, Geraets et al. (7) found that between 1985 and 1990 patients with AF had an average length of stay of 5 d per admission, with an average cost of $4800 per admission, adding up to an annual expense of one billion dollars in the United States alone. More recently, Dell'Orfano et al. (8) found that in patients admitted via the emergency department, the length of stay was 4 d, but the average cost was approx $6,700 per admission. These figures, of course, do not take into account the annual cost of over 75,000 strokes believed to be directly attributable to AF.

Based on these data, it is clear that a cost-effective strategy of treating patients with AF must be found. However, studies have not determined which of the many approaches to therapy is the most cost-effective.

Anticoagulation of patients with AF has clearly been shown to provide health benefits at a decreased cost (9). The cost-effectiveness of other aspects of AF therapy remains uncertain. For example, the optimal strategy following cardioversion remains unclear. In a study by Eckman et al. (10), cardioversion followed by aspirin therapy alone yielded a gain in quality-adjusted life years (QALYs) of 1.2 yr at a cost of $10,800 per QALY. On the other hand, cardioversion followed by amiodarone and warfarin therapy, although the most effective therapy in the model, yielded a gain of 2.3 QALYs at the relatively high cost of $92,400 per QALY.

Another management option of uncertain cost-effectiveness is the use of transesophageal echocardiography to expedite cardioversion, rather than the traditional approach of waiting for at least 3 wk of therapeutic anticoagulation prior to the restoration of normal sinus rhythm. One study suggests that this is an effective approach to therapy, especially in patients admitted to the hospital and at a high risk of hemorrhagic complications (11). Another issue which has spawned much debate, is whether hospitalization is needed for the initiation of antiarrhythmic therapy for acute pharmacological cardioversion or immediately following electrical cardioversion. Some studies, especially in Europe, suggest that this is not necessary for all antiarrhythmic drugs (12). Unfortunately, all of these cost-effective analyses use decision-analysis models, which make several important assumptions (based on sometimes limited data) to obtain their conclusions. It is uncertain how applicable these models and their conclusions are to cohorts of "real" patients. The relative merit of maintaining sinus rhythm over rate control alone, for example, is being evaluated by several large multicenter trials in the United States and Europe. More studies are needed to establish the most cost-effective strategies for the management of this disease, bearing in mind that the well-being and safety of the patient should always be the top priority.

In terms of long-term outcomes, most longitudinal studies have demonstrated an increase in total and cardiovascular mortality in patients with AF compared to those without it *(13,14)*. However, whether the increased mortality is causally related to the presence of AF, or whether AF is simply a marker of advanced cardiovascular disease, remains to be established. Contradictory data can be found in the literature in this regard in all patients, including those post-myocardial infarction (MI) *(15,16)* and those with congestive heart failure (CHF) *(17,18)*.

Although there is some controversy on whether AF confers an increased mortality risk, there is no doubt that it increases the risk of cerebral thromboembolic events *(19)*. Epidemiological and clinical studies have shown a 4–5% risk per yr, which constitutes a four-to-fivefold increased risk compared to the population at large. The risk is clearly increased in all subsets of patients, except for those who are of a young age and have "lone" AF. "Lone" AF is defined as AF in the absence of any structural heart disease, including hypertension. For example, Kopecky et al. *(20)* found that in Olmsted County, MN, patients less than 60 yr old and with no structural heart disease (including no hypertension), had a risk of a cerebral thromboembolic event of only 1.3% after 15 yr of follow-up. Based on these and other studies, it is now widely believed that young patients without structural heart disease do not need chronic anticoagulation with warfarin.

Despite the increased risk of stroke and the possible increase in total mortality, AF is often considered a benign rhythm. Physicians often tend to settle for rate-control management, especially in patients with minimal symptoms. However, one should consider other important effects of AF on both atrial and ventricular tissue. Recently, for example, the concept of "atrial remodeling" was elucidated in an elegant study by Wijffels et al. *(21)*. In a goat model, the authors demonstrated that paroxysms of AF lead to persistent AF through a progressive shortening of the atrial refractory periods. They also showed that the longer these episodes were allowed to persist, the more difficult it was to maintain a normal sinus rhythm post-cardioversion. Atrial dilatation and chronically elevated left atrial pressures have also been shown to occur when AF becomes persistent *(22,23)*. "Atrial stunning" is a delay in the return of atrial mechanical function post-cardioversion; the return of atrial mechanical systole may lag from a few hours to 6 wk after restoration of sinus rhythm. This effect on atrial mechanical function can be associated with significant morbidity if the patient is not appropriately anticoagulated post-cardioversion.

The effects of AF on the ventricular tissue can be dramatic. A reduction in left ventricular function, and an improvement in function after restoring sinus rhythm, has been demonstrated in several studies *(24)*. This entity has been termed a "tachycardia mediated cardiomyopathy" because the poor left ventricular function results primarily from poor ventricular rate control, and the process is usually reversible by restoring sinus rhythm. However, an improvement in left ventricular function has also been shown in patients with a well-controlled ventricular response, raising the possibility that other mechanisms, such as the irregularity of the rhythm *(25)*, may contribute to the ventricular dysfunction.

CLASSIFICATION AND ETIOLOGY

Although AF affects mostly an elderly population, the etiology of the disease is varied, and it is likely that several mechanisms play a role in its development. Because of this, a common classification of AF has been difficult *(26)*. Some authors have attempted to classify the disease based on its underlying mechanisms and clinical associations, whereas others have promoted an electrocardiographic classification based on the degree of organization of the atrial activity shown on the 12-lead electrocardiogram (ECG) *(27)*. Neither of these classifications is entirely adequate because of overlap of clinical conditions and types of AF, as well as limitations in our understanding of mechanisms. More recently, an attempt at a more clinically useful classification has divided patients into three groups: paroxysmal, self-terminating episodes of AF; persistent episodes requiring termination with electrical or pharmacological cardioversion; and permanent episodes which cannot be terminated by any available means *(28)*. Limitations also exist for this type of classification. Some patients experience very frequent paroxysmal episodes, and others may present with episodes that are many months or even years apart. Others may present with paroxysmal episodes that quickly become persistent or even permanent. This type of classification also does not take into account the electrophysiologic mechanism of initiation, which in the future may have important implications in terms of therapy, especially for a possible cure. Although imperfect, when combined with the underlying substrate, this classification system provides an easy framework to guide therapeutic intervention, both in the short term and on a more long-term basis.

From the standpoint of etiology, we have divided AF into three subsets of patients: those who develop AF without any obvious clinically associated disease ("lone" AF), those who develop it in the setting of disease (cardiac or noncardiac), which is known to be associated with this rhythm, and those who develop it in the postoperative period.

"Lone" Atrial Fibrillation

"Lone" or idiopathic AF *(29)*, occurs in a small percentage (5–20%) of all patients with AF. As the term implies, this entity corresponds to AF in the absence of any clinical entity associated with the disease, and is therefore a diagnosis of exclusion. Excluded from this category are patients with structural heart disease, including hypertension alone, or with noncardiac diseases that have been associated with AF (*see* Table 1); this diagnosis is usually reserved for patients less than 65 yr of age. Patients with "lone" AF are therefore more likely to be younger and to present with paroxysmal or persistent, rather than permanent, episodes of AF. While the mechanism remains unclear, some authors have suggested that a subset of these patients may have a familial predisposition *(30,31)*, and other reports imply atrial myocarditis as a possible cause *(32)*, but these underlying associations are likely not to be causal in the vast majority of patients with "lone" AF. The mode in which initiation occurs in patients with lone AF may shed some light on the underlying mechanism and provide a guide for future therapeutic intervention. Modulation of the autonomic system, for example, is often

Table 1
Conditions Associated with Atrial Fibrillation

Cardiac Disease	Non-Cardiac Disease
Primary Atrial Disease	Endocrine Disease
Fibrosis	Hyperthyroidism
Myocardial degeneration with aging	Diabetes Mellitus
Atrial Scar post myocarditis	Pheochromocytoma
Atrial infarction	
Post atriotomy scar	
Infiltrative/Inflammatory Disease	Pulmonary Disease
Sarcoidosis	Chronic Obstructive Lung Disease
Hemochromatosis	Pulmonary Hypertension
Amyloidosis	Pulmonary Embolism
Acute pericarditis or myocarditis	Neoplasm
Valvular Heart Disease	High Adrenergic Tone
Mitral Stenosis/Regurgitation	Post non-cardiothoracic surgery
Aortic Stenosis/Regurgitation	Systemic infection
Congenital Heart Disease	Electrolyte abnormalities
Cardiomyopathy	Other
Dilated	Familial
Hypertrophic	High Vagal Tone
Infiltrative	
Ischemic	
Acute Coronary syndromes	
Ventricular MI	
Acute ventricular ischemia	
Hypertension	
Post Coronary Artery Bypass Graft Surgery	

implicated as the possible precipitant of AF in subsets of this patient population. Some patients, such as young males and athletes, show a tendency to develop paroxysms of lone AF when vagal tone is enhanced *(33)* (at night, or post-prandially), while other patients, usually older, seem to develop AF in the face of adrenergic stimulation. Finally, the patients with lone AF should be carefully screened for other atrial arrhythmias, which may be the precursors to AF. If arrhythmias such as atrial flutter, AV reciprocating tachycardia, AV nodal reentrant tachycardia (AVNRT) and atrial tachycardia are recognized as the precipitants of AF, curing these may also eliminate AF. It is of particular interest that even unifocal premature atrial beats may be the target of ablative therapy to cure lone AF in a subset of patients with this disease *(34)*.

Atrial Fibrillation and Associated Diseases

Lone AF represents only a small subset of all patients with AF. The overwhelming majority of patients with AF have an associated underlying illness, which—some better understood than others—affect the electrophysiologic characteristics of the atria to promote the initiation of this rhythm. Several disease states have been linked to the development of AF. For simplicity, we will divide them into cardiac and extra-cardiac disease (Table 1). The extra-cardiac disease most commonly screened for, with new onset of AF, is hyperthyroidism. This disease entity should always be part of the initial differential diagnosis of AF, especially in the elderly, in whom the symptoms and signs of AF may be the only manifestation of hyperthyroidism. AF complicates approx 10–15% of all cases of hyperthyroidism, occurring more frequently in the elderly *(35,36)*. The mechanism by which hyperthyroidism precipitates AF is poorly understood, but it is likely related to alterations in the autonomic system. An increased adrenergic state in these patients favors an increase in automatic and triggered activity and a decrease in action potential duration in the atria, which promotes microreentry. Another endocrine disease associated with an increased risk of AF is pheochromocytoma. Diabetes has also been associated with the development of AF, imparting a twofold increased risk in the Framingham population *(37)*, but whether this association is real or just related to the cardiovascular conditions often present in diabetes has not been elucidated *(38)*. Alcohol intoxication, the so-called "holiday heart syndrome," and/or alcohol withdrawal represent another important extra-cardiac risk factor for the development of AF. This can occur in young patients with no obvious structural heart disease, as well as in those with an overt alcoholic cardiomyopathy. Chronic alcohol intake has been shown to decrease atrial refractory periods *(39)* favoring reentry, while alcohol withdrawal is associated with high adrenergic tone. Other possible causes of adrenergically driven AF include anxiety and stress, hypoxia, severe infections, and electrolyte disturbances. Finally, there is a significant association between pulmonary diseases and AF. In one series of patients presenting with AF, 2–3% of patients had pulmonary disease *(40)*. The mechanisms behind this association are most likely multifactorial and include hypoxia, sympathetic hyperstimulation, the use of sympathomimetic drugs, involvement of the pericardium by the disease process, and right atrial pathology in the presence of cor pulmonale. Notably, despite the widespread belief of clinicians, which links caffeine to palpitations and SVT, evidence in the literature of such an effect is lacking. Caffeine has multiple effects on myocytes, and one recent animal study suggests that more studies are needed to elucidate the answer to this age-old question *(41)*.

Cardiac disease is associated with the majority of the cases of AF, but whether this is a causal association is often difficult to determine. Hypertension alone is the most common cardiac precursor, increases the risk of developing AF fourfold, and is associated with more than 14% of all cases. Coronary artery disease (CAD), acute or chronic, is associated with approx 8% of AF cases. In acute MI, the development of AF portends a poorer prognosis and is associated with left ventricular failure. However, AF alone is very rarely the only presenting sign of an acute coronary syndrome, and other signs and symptoms of ischemia should be sought in this setting. Chronic ischemic syndromes are more rarely associated with AF. It is more likely that in this setting, left ventricular dysfunction and chamber dilatation play a much larger role. In fact, AF is commonly associated with cardiomyopathies, both ischemic and nonischemic. In the Framingham study, patients with CHF had a fivefold increased risk of developing the arrhythmia. In this setting, AF can cause significant hemodynamic compromise and worsen heart failure symptoms, and may be associated with increased mortality. Patients with AF and CHF often pose an important therapeutic dilemma. Because of the significant symptoms, clinicians most often attempt to maintain sinus rhythm with antiarrhythmic drugs in these patients. However, studies such as the one by Flaker et al. *(42)* suggest that treatment with antiarrhythmic drug therapy may be most dangerous in the very patients perceived to need it the most, those with a cardiomyopathy and CHF symptoms.

Other cardiac causes of AF include acute inflammatory syndromes such as myocarditis and pericarditis and valvular heart disease (2.5-fold increased risk in the Framingham study), particularly mitral stenosis and regurgitation, and aortic stenosis, which elevate atrial pressures significantly and predispose the patient to this arrhythmia. Mitral-valve prolapse without mitral regurgitation has been associated with several atrial arrhythmias, but whether the incidence of AF is increased in the presence of mitral-valve prolapse remains unclear. Also, other SVTs, including the Wolff-Parkinson-White (WPW) syndrome increase the risk of AF. It is important to search for these, as curing them via radiofrequency ablation may greatly reduce the occurrence of paroxysms of AF or even eliminate them. In elderly patients, AF is often associated with clinically important bradycardias, such as long sinus pauses upon spontaneous conversion from AF, sinus bradycardia, and junctional rhythms. It is important to recognize this form of sick sinus syndrome, often termed "tachy-brady" syndrome, because conjunctive therapy with a pacemaker may be required. Finally, infiltrative diseases of the myocardium—such as sarcoidosis and amyloidosis—have been associated with the increased risk of developing both bradyarrhythmias and tachyarrhythmias, including AF.

Perioperative Atrial Fibrillation

One specific type of AF is that which occurs postoperatively. The overwhelming majority of episodes occur in patients who have undergone cardiothoracic surgery. AF is said to complicate 25–30% of all coronary-artery bypass surgery and up to 40% of all valvular surgery. The peak incidence of AF occurs most often on day 2 or 3 after surgery. The mechanism for its development in this setting is poorly understood, but potential causes include inflammation of the pericardium, elevated atrial pressures, atrial stretch, atrial ischemia, and high catecholamine tone. The treatment of AF in this setting is highly controversial; the benefits and risk of maintaining sinus rhythm with antiarrhythmic drugs vs rate control and anticoagulation, which clearly has higher risks in patients with recent surgery, must be weighed carefully. Recently, two large prospective studies have suggested that prophylaxis of this difficult problem with amiodarone therapy significantly reduces the incidence of postoperative AF *(43,44)*. Moreover, in the study using prophylactic oral amiodarone, the length of stay was significantly shorter, which translated into a lower cost of care *(43)*. Neither of the studies, however, compared amiodarone to beta-blockers, a less expensive prophylactic strategy also known to reduce the prevalence of AF after cardiac surgery *(45,46)*.

Cardiothoracic surgery patients are not the only ones who suffer from the occurrence of AF postoperatively. The arrhythmia can occur in all patients postoperatively, typically in procedures requiring general anesthesia such as vascular, abdominal, and orthopedic surgery. The etiology of AF in this setting is believed to be the high adrenergic state present in the first 48–72 h postoperation. In this setting as well as post-cardiothoracic surgery, the prophylactic use of beta-blockers pre- and post-procedure has been shown to be of value.

DIAGNOSTIC EVALUATION

Patients who present with the first episode of AF should undergo a thorough evaluation to check for the presence of any of the conditions discussed here. In most cases, this requires a comprehensive history and physical examination to rule out precipitating factors such as diabetes and hypertension, a few simple chemical assays including thyroid function tests, and a surface ECG. A transthoracic echocardiogram is also of paramount importance, as AF can be the sole presenting sign of several underlying cardiac diseases—such as cardiomyopathy—as discussed here. Only if all of this diagnostic evaluation is negative, should the patient be given the diagnosis of "lone" AF. If the patient simply has a history of hypertension, for example, this should be considered a sign of structural heart disease. These patients, regardless of age, are at a higher risk for embolic complications, and should be treated differently than patients with true "lone" AF. Other tests that may be useful in the diagnosis and in the management of this arrhythmia are 24-h ambulatory recordings and 30-d event monitors. These tests may help to determine the frequency and duration of asymptomatic episodes of AF which, if present, may impact on therapeutic management. In addition, ambulatory monitoring may determine whether the patient's symptoms are truly secondary to the arrhythmia. Importantly, they may also give the physician a very good idea of how the rhythm begins and terminates, and whether it would be amenable to ablative therapy for a possible cure. For example, if all of the patient's events initiated with atrial flutter degenerating to AF, one may be more prone to treating this patient with radiofrequency ablation of the atrial flutter circuit. On the other hand, if all of the episodes initiated with single premature atrial stimuli that are unifocal in origin, one may consider ablation of the atrial focus. After the diagnosis is made and treatment is initiated, 24-h recordings and event monitors are an essential tool, together with symptom recurrence, to assess the efficacy of therapy.

Tests that generally have limited usefulness in the diagnostic evaluation of AF include stress testing and cardiac catheterization. The yield of these tests is extremely low, and they should not be routinely ordered unless there are other signs and symptoms of CAD. One possible indication for a stress test is for those patients in whom treatment with a class IC antiarrhythmic drug is contemplated. In such patients it is important to rule out significant, unrecognized CAD before starting treatment. It is also important to do a stress test after initiation of therapy, to rule out exercise induced proarrhythmia. In addition to atrial tachycardia or flutter with 1:1 A-V conduction, patients on these agents can develop a wide QRS tachycardia which manifests itself at faster heart rates (a concept known as "use dependence").

THERAPEUTIC OPTIONS

Pharmacological Therapy

In considering pharmacological therapy for the management of AF, one must consider that there are several facets to the management of this arrhythmia. The initial consideration is the need for anticoagulation therapy. Following the decision on anticoagulation, ventricular rate control is the next most pressing therapeutic issue, as a fast ventricular response is the most common cause of symptoms. Finally, acute restoration and long-term maintenance of sinus rhythm vs chronic rate control and anticoagulation in the patient who presents with frequent persistent episodes must be addressed. The pattern of the arrhythmia varies significantly between patients, and this should be considered in the acute management of such patients. A general approach to the management of AF is presented in Fig. 1. The patient who presents with frequent paroxysms that spontaneously terminate within 24 h should generally not be referred for electrical or

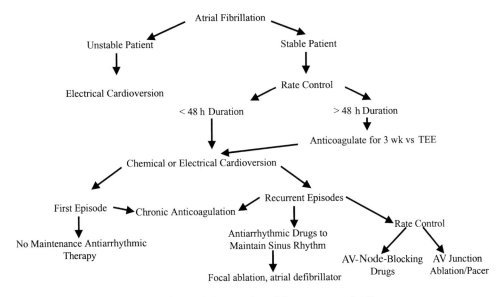

Fig. 1. General Approach to Management of AF.

pharmacological cardioversion unless this pattern changes over the long term. In these patients, the more difficult decisions are determining when and whether to start antiarrhythmic therapy vs rate control, and when the episodes are frequent and prolonged enough to warrant initiation of anticoagulation therapy. These decisions should be dictated by the patient's symptomatology and by the presence or absence of clinical and echocardiographic risk factors for thromboembolism. In patients with higher thromboembolic risk and with severe symptoms, the option of restoring and maintaining sinus rhythm may, at least initially, be preferred.

Once the episodes become persistent, the patient must be informed of the fact that the window to restore sinus rhythm without concomitant anticoagulation is fairly narrow. If the pattern is one of a few episodes per yr, acute pharmacological or electrical cardioversion, within the first 24–48 h of the onset of arrhythmia, may be the treatment of choice if the patient is very symptomatic. This may be done without concomitant rate-controlling agents and without anticoagulation. In these patients, the anticoagulation issue is a difficult one, as one must consider that patients may have some episodes that are asymptomatic and therefore go unrecognized. If these episodes become "too frequent," one must consider using antiarrhythmic drugs to eliminate or at least to decrease the number of episodes vs treating the patient with rate-controlling agents. In the absence of clinical data, we would recommend continuing anticoagulation in these patients even if a strategy of rhythm control is chosen, as the risk of asymptomatic recurrences is fairly high. The decision of when to consider the episodes "too frequent," however, is a difficult one. It is one that should be made in agreement with the patient's wishes, and by considering the clinical circumstances that may place the patient at a higher risk of complications, such as worsening heart failure, worsening angina, and thromboembolic complications.

If the AF becomes permanent despite attempts at restoration of sinus rhythm with drugs and direct current (DC) cardioversion—external and internal—then antiarrhythmic therapy should be abandoned. Further management should be aimed at controlling symptoms with pharmacological and nonpharmacological means for rate control, and at protecting the patients with clinical and echocardiographic risk factors from the risk of thromboembolism.

Historically, because of the theoretical and physiological advantages of maintaining sinus rhythm and because of several experimental animal studies that support the concept of AF spawning AF, most physicians have attempted the restoration of normal sinus rhythm in virtually all patients with a new onset of this arrhythmia. However, the difficulty in maintaining sinus rhythm over the long term and the dangers of antiarrhythmic therapy must be recognized, as well as the absence of data supporting this approach in the asymptomatic patient, or in the one whose symptoms are easily controlled by rate-controlling drugs. Multicenter randomized trials, such as the Atrial Fibrillation Follow-up Investigation of Rhythm Management (AFFIRM) trial *(47)* and the Pharmacological Intervention in Atrial Fibrillation (PIAF) trial, will hopefully shed some light on the advantages of one management strategy over the other.

Anticoagulation Therapy

Therapy for the prevention of thromboembolic complications in patients with AF has been studied extensively over the last several years. In the late 1980s and early 1990s, five randomized clinical trials clearly established the efficacy of warfarin to reduce the risk of stroke in patients with AF *(48)* (Fig. 2). Although the majority of patients enrolled in these trials had chronic AF, patients with paroxysmal AF benefited as well. The relative merits of warfarin therapy vs aspirin were examined in these and later trials. A superior benefit of warfarin compared with aspirin was established in these trials, especially in patient populations with clinical risk factors for stroke, other than AF itself. These risk factors were determined by the trials in "post hoc" analyses.

These clinical trials prompted the publication of practice recommendations by the American College of Chest Physicians (ACCP) in 1996 and most recently in 2001 *(49)*. Today, there is no controversy regarding whether the majority of patients with AF should be anticoagulated. Rather, debate persists on how to best identify the subset of patients in whom the risks, expense, and inconvenience of anticoagulation outweigh the benefits. The group at lowest risk for thromboembolic events are young (<60–65 yr old) patients without clinical and echocardiographic risk factors for thromboembolism, as determined by the pooled data from the prevention trials. Risk factors for stroke include prior stroke/transient ischemic attack (TIA), hypertension, diabetes, CHF, an enlarged left atrium, mitral stenosis, hyperthyroidism, and a depressed left ventricular systolic function. The patients who are younger than 65 yr of age and free of all of these risk factors usually fall into the category of "lone" AF. Their risk of stroke appears to be similar to the general population (approx 1%/yr or less).

The patients at high risk of stroke are the elderly (>75 yr old) and those who are 60–75 yr old, with one or more of the other clinical or echocardiographic risk factors. Their risk of stroke is, on average, approx 5% per yr, but it has been shown to be as high as 12% per yr in those with a prior history of stroke or transient ischemic attack. Unless there are clear contraindications to anticoagulation, such as bleeding diathesis, active gastrointestinal bleeding, and a propensity to falls or trauma (such as seizures, or gait disturbance), these patients should be anticoagulated with warfarin.

A

	AFASAK	SPAF	BAATAF	CAFA	SPINAF
number	1007	1330	420	383	571
Age	75	66	68	67	67
Paroxysmal AF(%)	0	34	16	7	0
CHF(%)	51	19	28	20	30
HTN(%)	31	55	51	34	58

B

	Control	Warfarin	Risk Reduction	P
AFASAK	5.5%	1.9%	58%	0.03
SPAF	7.4%	2.3%	67%	0.01
BAATAF	2.9%	0.1%	86%	0.002
CAFA	3.8%	2.1%	42%	0.2
SPINAF	4.3%	0.9%	79%	0.002
TOTAL	4.5%	1.4%	68%	0.001

C

	Aspirin	Warfarin	Risk Reduction	P
AFASAK	4%	1.9%	51%	NS
SPAF II	2.9%	1.8%	32%	NS
SPAF II (on treatment)	3.6%	1.5%	53%	0.03
EAFT	10.5%	4%	62%	0.001

NS = nonsignificant

Fig. 2. (A) AF Trials: Patient Characteristics. **(B)** Thromboembolic Complications in AF Trials: Warfarin vs Control. **(C)** Thromboembolic Complications in AF Trials: Warfarin vs Aspirin.

All patients with AF (and with atrial flutter) in whom electrical or pharmacological cardioversion is planned should be anticoagulated prior to the procedure if their arrhythmia is of more than 48 h duration or if it is of unclear duration. The patient should have a therapeutic International Normalized Ratio (INR) for at least 3 wk (target INR 2.5; range 2.0–3.0) prior to cardioversion, whether electric or pharmacologic. Because the contractile activity of the atria can take up to 4 wk to return to normal after cardioversion, the recommendations of the American College of Chest Physicians

(ACCP) are to continue warfarin for at least 4 wk. Some experts, however, will continue therapy for as long as 6 mo to 1 yr to protect the patient from early recurrences, and others will recommend chronic anticoagulation even after the first episode of AF.

Ventricular Rate Control

As the natural history of AF progresses from brief paroxysms to persistent episodes and on to permanent AF, often despite the physician's attempts at maintenance of sinus rhythm, rate control is of paramount importance. Failure to maintain reasonable rate control is associated with significant morbidity, disabling symptoms, and a very poor quality of life for the patient. Hemodynamic and structural changes occur within a few weeks when median heart rates are elevated—generally above 100 BPM—although the exact heart-rate threshold is unknown. These changes result in increased ventricular filling pressure *(50),* decreased left and right ventricular systolic function, *(51),* and decreased cardiac output *(52).* Although the mechanisms for these changes, the time course needed to observe them, and the relative importance of rate vs the degree of irregularity of the rhythm *(53)* must be better elucidated, it is clear that most of these changes are reversible in hearts that were normal prior to the onset of AF. Therefore, all efforts should be made to control the ventricular response in the acute setting and especially in the chronic setting, as this will have a significant beneficial effect for the patient's sense of well-being and for the long-term prognosis. In general, achieving a heart rate of less than 100 BPM is the goal of ventricular rate control. In order to assure appropriate rate control with daily activities, one should ascertain the ventricular response not only at rest, but also with mild to moderate exercise. This can be evaluated either with a 24-h ambulatory recording or with an exercise treadmill. In the acute setting, when the patient presents to the office or to the emergency room with new-onset AF and a rapid ventricular response, if he/she is hemodynamically stable, and there is no evidence of active ischemia or worsening pulmonary edema, the drugs most often used to achieve rate control have been digitalis, beta-blockers, or calcium-channel blockers. In this setting, the usefulness of digitalis alone has not been demonstrated. Its effectiveness on rate reduction in the presence of a high sympathetic tone is often called into question. Digitalis therapy may be most beneficial in patients with significant left ventricular dysfunction. In these patients, beta-blockade or calcium-channel block-ade may acutely worsen heart failure. For the same reason, digitalis should be used as initial therapy in patients who experience AF after cardiothoracic surgery, if these patients have decreased left ventricular function and signs and symptoms of overt heart failure or fluid overload. In patients with left ventricular dysfunction and compensated heart failure, beta blockers should be considered first-line treatment in light of recent data.

In most patients, calcium-channel blockers and beta-blockers are the drugs of choice to achieve adequate AV-node blockade, with or without the addition of a cardiac glycoside. In terms of efficacy, these two classes of drugs are equivalent both in the intravenous (iv) form for the acute setting and in the oral form for the chronic setting. Therefore, the choice of which agent to use should be made on the basis of tolerability and other medical conditions. For example, in patients with prior MI, in those with left ventricular dysfunction and compensated CHF and in those with hyperthyroidism, beta-blockers should be the treatment of choice. In patients with significant reactive airway disease or peripheral vascular disease, on the other hand, calcium-channel blockers should be used as first-line therapy. Recently, Farshi et al. *(54)* demonstrated that the combination of diltiazem plus digitalis or the combination of atenolol plus digitalis, are equivalent and superior to any of the three drugs alone in controlling ventricular response. Very recent experimental data suggest that verapamil may prevent or delay atrial remodeling when given early after the onset of AF *(55)*. The significance of this finding in long-term maintenance of normal sinus rhythm and whether it should influence the choice between calcium-channel blockers and beta-blockers remain to be studied.

Acute Conversion to Sinus Rhythm

It is said that approx 50–60% of new onset (<72 h) episodes of AF terminate spontaneously. Excellent placebo-controlled studies have shown that when the episodes change from paroxysmal to persistent, AV-node-blocking agents such as digitalis, calcium-channel blockers, and beta-blockers do not improve the chances of cardioversion when compared to placebo. These drugs should therefore be used only to control heart rate, and to prepare for other means of cardioversion, either electrical (as discussed in the nonpharmacological therapy section) or pharmacological. It should be noted here that the likelihood of a successful cardioversion, electrical or pharmacological, generally decreases as the episode of AF becomes more prolonged. Thus, it is more difficult to cardiovert a patient with more than 12 mo of continuous AF than a patient who has had AF for only a few days or weeks. It should also be clear that any patient who is hemodynamically unstable because the rapid ventricular response precipitates an ischemic event, pulmonary edema, or significant hypotension, should be cardioverted urgently with DC countershock. This method is successful in 80–90% of cases, as compared to drug cardioversion, which is successful in 40–80% of cases and may take much longer than electrical cardioversion.

Several antiarrhythmics have been used for the acute conversion of a persistent episode of AF to normal sinus rhythm. Class IA drugs such as quinidine and procainamide have been used for several decades with acute conversion rates of 40–60% for procainamide and up to 80% with quinidine, although many of the older studies were not randomized or placebo-controlled. These drugs have more recently been supplanted by the use of the class IC drugs flecainide and propafenone and the class III drug ibutilide, all approved by the FDA for use in patients with AF, with ibutilide indicated specifically for the acute conversion of AF to sinus rhythm. Although it has not been approved by the FDA for this use, procainamide continues to be used, especially as an iv drug in patients after cardiothoracic surgery *(56)*. However, the efficacy and safety of procainamide in this setting should be scrutinized carefully by prospective studies, given the high incidence of ventricular arrhythmias and left ventricular dysfunction in this population. In fact, amiodarone may be a safer drug for the short term in this subset of patients.

Class IC drugs such as flecainide and propafenone, in oral or iv form, are very effective drugs for the acute cardioversion of AF because of their low side-effect profile compared to class III drugs, which have an inherent risk of QT prolongation and ventricular arrhythmias. They have been used extensively in Europe, with good results. The advantage of these drugs is that they can be given as a single oral dose (300 mg of flecainide or 600 mg of propafenone) with very little risk of hypotension and proarrhythmia, especially in patients with no significant structural heart disease. The rate of conversion with these drugs is reported to be as high as 80%. In one study comparing placebo vs amiodarone, flecainide, and propaferone, the placebo group converted 37% of the time, the amiodarone group converted 43% of the time, and the oral propafenone and flecainide groups converted 76% and 75% of the time respectively after eight hours *(57)*. In another study by Capucci et al. *(58)* oral propafenone in combination with digoxin converted 50% of patients after 3 h and 80% of patients after 12 h. All of these patients had AF for less than 48 h. However, it seems clear that the effectiveness of these drugs, as well as others, decreases sharply depending on the duration of AF. In one study by Carr et al. *(59)*, flecainide converted 95% of patients with onset < 72 h and only 11% of those with onset longer than 72 h but less than 1 mo.

For the purpose of acute conversion to normal sinus rhythm, class III drugs have also been used to convert patients to normal sinus rhythm. The FDA has recently approved iv ibutilide for this purpose. It has been shown to acutely convert 30–50% of AF and up to 60–80% of atrial flutter in a single iv dose or in two repeated doses given 10 min apart *(60,61)*. The effects of ibutilide are short-term, but the most serious side effect is a 1–2% occurrence of sustained polymorphic ventricular tachycardia (VT) requiring countershock. This is caused by the QT prolongation observed with this drug and with other class III agents. Ibutilide has recently been shown to be superior to procainamide for acute cardioversion, and to significantly reduce the energy requirement for transthoracic electrical cardioversion, thus offering a new option to patients who fail transthoracic cardioversion alone and may have been referred for internal cardioversion. However, its efficacy has not been tested prospectively against class IC drugs, which may be at least as effective and free of the dangerous proarrhythmic effects related to QTc prolongation. The advantage of ibutilide over the IC drugs may be its more rapid time to cardioversion and a higher success rate in patients with atrial flutter. Intravenous sotalol is not available in the United States for acute conversion to normal sinus rhythm, but in a placebo-controlled trial in Europe, it was no more effective than placebo after 30 min *(62)*.

Dofetilide is another class III antiarrhythmic recently approved for the acute termination of AF and atrial flutter. Conversion rates are similar to ibutilide *(63)*, although the iv formulation is not available in the United States, and the long period to conversion with oral dofetilide makes this application impractical. One advantage of dofetilide is that it is available in oral form as a maintenance drug, and that it has recently been shown to be safe in patients with left ventricular dysfunction *(64)*.

The experience with amiodarone has generally been disappointing. Both in the oral form and in the iv form, this drug has not yielded rates of cardioversion that significantly differ from placebo. The role of amiodarone seems most significant in the maintenance of sinus rhythm and in prophylaxis of AF occurrences and rate control in high-risk patients, especially in patients in the intensive care unit during the perioperative period after cardiothoracic surgery. In this setting, two studies have shown a significant decrease in AF postoperatively compared with placebo in patients loaded with the drug orally over the course of 1 wk preoperatively *(43)*, or in those loaded with an iv infusion for 48 h postoperatively *(44)*. Given its high cost, it remains to be determined whether this drug is superior in efficacy and is safer in the short term compared to other drugs traditionally used in the postoperative setting, such as beta-blockers or procainamide.

Maintenance of Normal Sinus Rhythm

Although acute cardioversion can generally be achieved pharmacologically or electrically most of the time, the task of maintaining sinus rhythm is far more daunting. The first decision facing the clinician, especially following cardioversion of a first persistent episode of AF is whether to treat the patient longitudinally with an antiarrhythmic drug. Given that 25–30% of patients will not experience new episodes of AF for more than 1 yr, it is reasonable to withhold such therapy for the first episode of AF. It should be noted that this decision may be influenced by the initial clinical presentation of the patient and by the presence or absence of underlying structural heart disease. For example, if the patient has had syncope or an exacerbation of CHF or ischemic symptoms, the benefits of using an antiarrhythmic drug may outweigh its risks. In general, the patient with a mildly or moderately symptomatic first episode of AF requiring cardioversion should be treated with AV-nodal-blocking agents and anticoagulation for a period of at least 4 wk postcardioversion. It should be emphasized that patients are likely to experience recurrences. As early as the first episode of AF, it is useful to talk with the patient about the fact that they are facing a disease, which, although not life-threatening, is difficult to suppress or cure over the long term, and therefore may represent a life-long problem.

In the case of early recurrences and the frequent need for cardioversion, the decision facing the clinician is whether to aggressively try to maintain sinus rhythm with antiarrhythmic drugs or to use rate control and anticoagulation. Especially in patients whose symptoms are crippling and whose quality of life is significantly impaired, antiarrhythmic drugs should be considered the therapy of choice. Unfortunately, antiarrhythmic drugs are at best moderately effective in maintaining sinus rhythm over the long term. Most studies have followed patients for 6–12 mo, and have found that the rate of AF recurrence decreases from approx 75% with placebo to approx 50% with an antiarrhythmic drug. This holds true with most antiarrhythmics, including flecainide, propafenone, quinidine, disopyramide, and sotalol. In fact, when tested against each other, rather than against placebo, all of these drugs appear to be equivalent *(65,66)*. The only drug that appears to be more effective is amiodarone. In most studies it seems to maintain sinus rhythm in approx 60–70% of patients at the 12–18 mo follow-up end point. Newer class III drugs, such as dofetilide and azimilide, have shown promise and will be tested *(67)* prospectively in the future.

Based on this discussion, the efficacy of an antiarrhythmic drug should be measured in two different ways. One, of course, is the total prevention of AF recurrences—a goal that is difficult to achieve and may require several trials of different antiarrhythmics. A more practical goal of therapy may be to reduce the frequency, duration, and symptomatic severity of recurrent episodes to a level more acceptable to the patient. For example, a drug may be considered successful if it reduces persistent episodes requiring cardioversion from once per mo to once per yr, or even once every few months. This treatment objective should be discussed with the patient prospectively, so that expectations can be adjusted accordingly, taking into account the patient's current and desired quality of life and symptomatology.

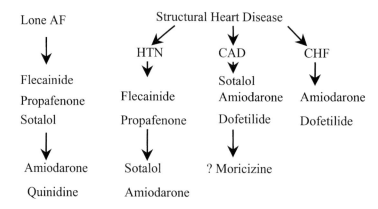

Fig. 3. Drugs for Maintenance of Normal Sinus Rhythm after Cardioversion of AF.

The theoretical advantages of maintaining normal sinus rhythm with an anti-arrhythmic drug, such as decreased symptomatology, improved hemodynamics, decreased electrical remodeling, and a possible decrease in the thromboembolic risk, should be weighed against the risk of drug side effects. The choice of antiarrhythmic drug, given the equivalent efficacy, should be made on the basis of safety (Fig. 3). It is premature to conclude that all patients should receive amiodarone because of its increased efficacy. In fact, because of its cost, its high incidence of drug withdrawal because of side effects, and its risk for severe organ toxicity, amiodarone should be used with caution, especially in the younger population. In patients with structurally normal hearts, the risk of proarrhythmia from class IC drugs is low. Therefore, given their excellent side-effect profile, flecainide and propafenone should be considered the first line of therapy in patients with lone AF. These drugs should also be considered first-line therapy in patients with hypertension, even with mild to moderate left ventricular hypertrophy (LVH). In these patients, drugs that prolong repolarization may be more arrhythmogenic because of a baseline QT-interval prolongation, and thus an increased risk of torsades de pointes. In patients with structural heart disease, for whom the class I drugs are absolutely contraindicated because of their risk of proarrhythmia and the increased mortality shown in some studies (68,69), the class III drugs are clearly the treatment of choice. If the patient can tolerate it, sotalol is often a good first choice in these cases because of its beta-blocking effects. Otherwise, amiodarone has quickly become the drug of choice because of its increased efficacy and its low risk of proarrhythmia. Dofetilide, given its safety profile in patients with left ventricular dysfunction, and in the future possibly azimilide, are likely to play a larger role in the management of these patients.

NONPHARMACOLOGICAL TREATMENT

Because of the inadequacy of medical treatments at maintaining normal sinus rhythm, the significant morbidity to the patient, and the significant cost of hospitalizations for the health care system, invasive treatments have been developed in the hope of treating this arrhythmia more effectively. A nonpharmacologic cure for AF would avoid multiple risks to the patient, including those related to long-term anticoagulation and antiarrhythmic therapy. Nonpharmacologic therapies, including those that are not curative, can also improve quality of life in patients in whom rate control cannot be adequately achieved with medications.

External and Internal Cardioversion, and the Atrial Defibrillator

Transthoracic cardioversion of AF has been achieved successfully for several decades, with success rates reported to be from 70–95%. However, in a small minority of patients, even with the addition of antiarrhythmic drugs to lower the defibrillation threshold, this strategy can fail. More recently, new techniques have been developed to "rescue" the patients who have failed conventional cardioversion. Externally, one can attempt to increase the current delivered to overcome the high transthoracic impedance seen in some patients. Two recently published studies suggest that by delivering 720 J simultaneously over four patches, one can restore sinus rhythm in 75–85% of patients who have failed conventional cardioversion with up to 360 J (70,71). Recently, external defibrillators that deliver biphasic rather than monophasic shocks have been shown to be more effective in cardioverting both ventricular arrhythmias and AF (72).

For patients in whom external cardioversion is unsuccessful, low-energy internal cardioversion is a viable alternative (73). Sinus rhythm can be restored in 70–80% of patients who have failed external cardioversion, by delivering energy between electrodes in the lateral right atrium and the coronary sinus (CS) or the left pulmonary artery.

Because of the success of low-energy internal cardioversion, an implantable atrial defibrillator (IAD) has been studied extensively. In a recent multicenter trial, the atrial defibrillator proved to be safe and efficacious in terminating episodes of AF (74). However, 48 of 51 patients were receiving an antiarrhythmic at the end of the trial, and there was a 2–4% risk of complications, including cardiac tamponade, infection, lead repositioning, and subclavian-vein thrombosis. Larger studies are needed to address the problem of high atrial defibrillation thresholds, which excluded >50% of the patients screened. One of the main advantages of the atrial defibrillator may be the fact that early cardioversion may lead to decreased frequency and duration of the paroxysmal episodes by virtue of a "reverse remodeling" process that decreases left atrial size and improves atrial electrophysiologic parameters (75). Device companies have decided not to market a "stand-alone" atrial defibrillator, but the FDA recently approved an arrhythmia management device capable of both atrial and ventricular defibrillation.

Atrial Pacing for the Prevention of AF

There are many theoretical and experimental reasons to support the belief that permanent atrial pacing may prevent episodes of AF. Suppression of premature atrial beats, elimination of pauses, and reduction in intra-atrial conduction delay and in dispersion of refractoriness are all possible mechanisms by which atrial pacing may reduce the incidence of AF. In fact, recent data support the notion that in order to decrease intra-atrial conduction delay and to limit anisotropy, multisite atrial pacing may be superior to right atrial pacing alone (76). Although prospective trials exist to support the use of atrial pacing vs ventricular pacing to prevent recurrences of AF in patients with sick sinus syndrome (77), data are lacking to support pacing vs no pacing in patients with AF alone, who do not otherwise need a pacemaker. Several multicenter trials are now underway to assess the usefulness of pacing to prevent episodes of AF in patients with paroxysmal or persistent episodes of AF. As of now, the strategy of pacing to prevent AF episodes remains largely unproven, and preliminary results from larger multicenter trials have been disappointing *(78,79)*.

Surgical and Catheter-Based Ablation

As catheter-based radiofrequency ablation has become first-line therapy for other supraventricular arrhythmias, including atrial flutter, the cure of AF with this procedure remains elusive and limited to a small subset of patients. In the late 1980s, Cox et al. developed a surgical Maze procedure, which aims to interrupt all macroreentrant circuits which initiate and perpetuate AF. In its latest iteration, this procedure isolates the pulmonary veins, removes the left and right atrial appendages, and creates several lesions in the right atrium *(80)*. Of the patients followed for longer than 3 mo, 92% remain in sinus rhythm without the need for antiarrhythmic drugs. Although efficacious, this procedure requires open-heart surgery, with all of its inherent risks. Using the same principles, Swartz et al. *(81)* demonstrated that a catheter-based Maze procedure, which created linear lesions in the right and left atrium, was also feasible and efficacious. The difficulties with this procedure include the challenge of delivering long continuous lesions in the atria, the prolonged procedure time, the fluoroscopy times, and the need for a second intervention in 55% of patients. Most recently, Haissaguerre et al. *(82)* have shown that the initiation of AF in some patients is secondary to "focal triggers" that usually originate in the pulmonary veins and are amenable to radiofrequency ablation. Much work needs to be done in this area before this technique becomes widely available, as new catheter technology is being developed, the identification of the most appropriate patients needs to be refined, and the long-term complications of these procedures need to be elucidated.

Although radiofrequency ablation for a cure is in its early clinical stage, the role of AV-node ablation in combination with pacing therapy for the palliative treatment of refractory AF is well-established. In patients who have failed both rhythm control and rate-control therapy, results are remarkably effective in decreasing health care resource utilization, improving symptoms, increasing exercise tolerance, and improving left ventricular function *(83)*. Given the failures of antiarrhythmic drugs in maintaining sinus rhythm and the difficulty of controlling symptoms related to a fast and irregular ventricular response, this approach can improve the quality of life of many patients *(84)*, and may be used not only in patients with permanent AF but also in those with frequent, very symptomatic persistent or paroxysmal episodes. In such patients, the use of dual-chamber pacemakers with "mode-switch" capabilities may be superior to ventricular pacing alone *(85)*.

One concern related to this approach is the increased risk of sudden cardiac death noted in some early studies *(86)* in the first 6–12 mo post-procedure. Whether the increased risk is secondary to myocardial injury post-procedure, or to autonomic dys-regulation after the creation of complete heart block, or simply to the fact that these patients often have underlying structural heart disease, is unclear. Some experts have advocated setting the pacing rate at 80–90 beats per minute (BPM) to avoid bradycardia-related "torsades de pointes" ventricular tachycardia (VT). More recent studies have shown no increase in clinical events in patients treated with AV-nodal ablation and pacing compared to patients treated medically *(87)*. Although it is a palliative measure, which does not obviate the need for chronic anticoagulation, AV-nodal ablation with pacing remains the most commonly used nonpharmacological approach for the long-term treatment of AF.

SUMMARY

Despite the recent advances in our understanding of mechanisms, in our catheter-based therapies, and in our antiarrhythmic drug choices, AF remains a public health problem of epidemic proportions. The cost to society is enormous, and the morbidity is related to thromboembolic complications that are often devastating to the patient. Our therapy is still mostly focused on palliating symptoms with rate-controlling drugs, reducing recurrences with antiarrhythmic drugs, and preventing thromboembolic complications with anticoagulation. Thanks to important recent advances in catheter-based interventions, it is now possible to at least attempt to cure a small subset of patients with this arrhythmia. Much work needs to be done in the future, with the hope of achieving cure rates for AF similar to other SVTs.

REFERENCES

1. Lewis T. Auricular fibrillation: a common clinical condition. Br Med J 1909;2:1528.
2. Fuster V, Rydén LE, Asinger RW, et al. ACC/AHA/ESC guidelines for the management of patients with atrial fibrillation: A report of the American College of Cardiology/American Heart Association Task Force on Practice Guidelines and the European Society of Cardiology Committee for Practice Guidelines and Policy Conferences. J Am Coll Cardiol 2001;38.
2a. Falk RH. Atrial fibrillation. N Engl J Med 2001;344(14):1067–1078.
3. Dalen JE. Atrial fibrillation and stroke. Arch Intern Med 1991;151:1922–1924.
4. Blackshear JL, Kopecky SL, Litin SC, et al. Management of atrial fibrillation in adults: prevention of thromboembolism and symptomatic treatment. Mayo Clin Proc 1996;71:150–160.
5. Kerr C, Chung D. Atrial fibrillation: fact, controversy, and future. Clin Prog Electrophysiol Pacing 1991;3:319–337.
6. Martin A, Benbow LJ, Butrous GS, Leach C, Camm AJ. Five year follow-up of 101 elderly subjects by means of long term ambulatory cardiac monitoring. Eur Heart J 1984;5:592–596.
7. Geraets DR, Kienzle MG. Atrial fibrillation and atrial flutter. Clin Pharm 1993;12:721–735.
8. Dell'Orfano JT, Hemantkumar P, Wolbrette DL, et al. Acute treatment of atrial fibrillation: spontaneous conversion rates and cost of care. Am J Card 1999;83:788–790.
9. Gage BF, Cardinalli AB, Albers GW, et al. Cost-effectiveness of warfarin and aspirin for prophylaxis of stroke in patients with nonvalvular atrial fibrillation. JAMA 1995;274:1839–1845.
10. Eckman MH, Falk RH, Pauker SG. Cost effectiveness of therapies for patients with nonvalvular atrial fibrillation. Arch Intern Med 1998;158:1669–1677.
11. Seto TB, Taira DA, Tsevat J, et al. Cost effectiveness of transesophageal echocardiographic-guided cardioversion: a decision analytic model for patients admitted to the hospital with atrial fibrillation. JACC 1997;29:122–130.
12. Botto GL, Bonini W, Broffoni T, et al. Conversion of recent onset atrial fibrillation with single oral loading dose of propafenone: is in-hospital admission absolutely necessary? PACE 1996;19:1939–1943.
13. Kannel WB, Abbott RD, Savage DD, et al. Epidemiologic features of chronic atrial fibrillation: the Framingham study. N Engl J Med 1982;306:1018–1022.
14. Gajewski J, Singer RB. Mortality in an insured population with atrial fibrillation. JAMA 1981;245:1540–1545.
15. Crenshaw BS, Ward SR, Granger CB, et al. Atrial fibrillation in the setting of acute myocardial infarction: the GUSTO I experience. JACC 1997;30:406–413.
16. Goldberg RJ, Seeley D, Becker RC, et al. Impact of atrial fibrillation on the in-hospital and long term survival of patients with acute myocardial infarction: a community wide perspective. Am Heart J 1990;119:996–1001.

17. Middlekauff HR, Stevenson WG, Stevenson LW. Prognostic significance of atrial fibrillation in advanced heart failure: a study of 390 patients. Circulation 1991;84:40–48.

18. Carson PE, Johnson GR, Dunkman WB, et al. The influence of atrial fibrillation on prognosis in mild to moderate heart failure. The VHeFT Studies. 1993;87:VI 102–VI 110.

19. Singer DE. Anticoagulation to prevent stroke in atrial fibrillation and its implications for managed care. Am J Cardiol 1998;81:35C–40C.

20. Kopecky SL, Gersh BJ, McGoon MD, et al. The natural history of lone atrial fibrillation, a population based study. N Engl J Med 1987;317:669–674.

21. Wijffels MCEF, Kirchhof CJHJ, Dorland R, Allessie MA. Atrial fibrillation begets atrial fibrillation: a study in awake chronically instrumented goats. Circulation 1995;92:1954–1968.

22. Sanfilippo AJ, Abascal VM, Sheehan M, et al. Atrial enlargement as a consequence of atrial fibrillation: a prospective echocardiographic study. Circulation 1990;82:792–797.

23. Leistad E, Christensen G, Ilebekk A. Effects of atrial fibrillation on left and right atrial dimensions, pressures, and compliances. Am J Physiol 1993;264:H1093–H1097.

24. Van Gelder IC, Crijns HJ, Blanksma PK, et al. Time course of hemodynamic changes and improvement of exercise tolerance after cardioversion of chronic atrial fibrillation unassociated with cardiac valve disease. Am J Cardiol 1993;72:560–566.

25. Olsson SB, Carlson J, Holm M, et al. Atrioventricular nodal function in atrial fibrillation: what is the optimal ventricular rate? In: Murgatroyd FD, Camm AJ, eds. Nonpharmacological Management of Atrial Fibrillation. Futura Publishing, Armonk, NY, 1996, pp. 55–64.

26. Gallagher MM, Camm AJ. Classification of atrial fibrillation. Am J Cardiol 1998;82:18N–28N.

27. Wells JL, Karp RB, Kouchoukos NT, MacLean WAH, James TN, Waldo AL. Characterization of atrial fibrillation in man: studies following open heart surgery. PACE: 1978;1:426–428.

28. Gallagher MM, Camm AJ. Schemes of classification. Replace a number of complicated systems with a simple division of atrial fibrillation (AF) based on temporal pattern. PACE 1998;21:776–777.

29. Evans W, Swann P. Lone auricular fibrillation. Br Heart J 1954;16:189–194.

30. Gould WL. Auricular fibrillation: report on a familial tendency. Arch Intern Med 1957;100:916–926.

31. Brugada R, Tapscott T, et al. Identification of a genetic locus for familial atrial fibrillation. N Engl J Med 1997;336:905–911.

32. Frustaci A, Chimenti C, Bellocci F, Morgante E, Russo MA, Maseri A. Histologic substrate of atrial biopsies in patients with lone atrial fibrillation. Circulation 1997;96:1180–1184.

33. Waxman MB, Cameroon D, Wald RW. Role of the autonomic nervous system in atrial arrhythmias. In: DiMarco JP, Prystowsky EN, eds. Atrial Arrhythmias: State of the Art. Futura, Armonk, NY, 1995.

34. Jais P, Haissaguerre M, Shah D, Chouairi S, Gencel L, Hocini M, et al. A focal source of atrial fibrillation treated by discrete radiofrequency ablation. Circulation 1997;95:572–576.

35. Scott GR, Forfar JC, Toft AD. Graves disease in atrial fibrillation: the case for even higher doses of therapeutic iodine-131. Br Med J 1984;289:399–400.

36. Camm AJ, Evans KE, Ward DE, Martin A. The rhythm of the heart in active elderly subjects. Am Heart J 1980;99:598–603.

37. Benjamin EJ, Levy D, Vaziri SM, et al. Independent risk factors for atrial fibrillation in a population based cohort. The Framingham heart study. JAMA 1994;271:840–844.

38. Kannell WB, Abbott RD, Savage DD, McNamara PM. Epidemiologic features of atrial fibrillation. The Framingham study. N Engl J Med 1982;306:1018–1022.

39. Luca C. Electrophysiological properties of right heart and atrioventricular conduction system in patients with alcoholic cardiomyopathy. Br Heart J 1979;42:274–281.

40. Schlofmitz RA, Hirsch BE, Meyer BR. New onset atrial fibrillation. Is there a need for emergency hospitalization? J Gen Intern Med 1986;1:139–142.

41. Mehta A, Jain AC, Mehta MC, et al. Caffeine and cardiac arrhythmias. An experimental study in dogs with review of the literature. Acta Cardiol 1997;52:273–283.

42. Flaker GC, Blackshear JL, McBride R, et al. Antiarrhythmic drug therapy and cardiac mortality in atrial fibrillation. JACC 1992;20:527–532.

43. Daoud EG, Strickberger SA, Man KC, et al. Preoperative amiodarone as prophylaxis against atrial fibrillation after heart surgery. N Engl J Med 1997;337:1785–1791.

44. Guarnieri T, Nolan S, Gottlieb SO, et al. Intravenous amiodarone for the prevention of atrial fibrillation after open heart surgery. The ARCH Trial. JACC 1999;34:343–347.

45. Andrews TC, Reimold SC, Berlin JA, Antman EM. Prevention of supraventricular arrhythmias

after coronary artery bypass surgery. A meta-analysis of randomized control trials. Circulation 1991; 84(Suppl):III236–III244.

46. Kowey PR, Taylor JE, Rials SJ, et al. Meta-analysis of the effectiveness of prophylactic drug therapy in preventing supraventricular arrhythmias early after coronary artery bypass grafting. Am J Cardiol 1992;69:963–965.

47. The planning and steering committees of the AFFIRM study for the NHLBI AFFIRM investigators. Atrial fibrillation follow-up investigation of rhythm management: the AFFIRM study. Am J Cardiol 1997;79:1198–1202.

48. Atrial Fibrillation Investigators. Risk factors for stroke and efficacy of anti-thrombotic therapy in atrial fibrillation. Analysis of pooled data from five randomized controlled trial. Arch Intern Med 1994;154:1449–1457.

49. Laupacis A, Albers G, Dalen J, et al. Antithrombotic therapy in atrial fibrillation. Chest 1998;114:579S–589S.

50. Shannon RP, Komamura K, Stambler BS, et al. Alterations in Myocardial Contractility in Conscious Dogs with Dilated Cardiomyopathy. Am J Cardiol 1991;260:H1903–H1911.

51. Ohno M, Cheng CP, Little WC. Mechanisms of altered patterns of left ventricular filling during the development of congestive heart failure. Circulation 1994;89:2241–2250.

52. Morgan DE, Tomlinson CW, Qayumi AK, et al. Evaluation of ventricular contractility indexes in the dog with left ventricular dysfunction induced by rapid atrial pacing. JACC 1989;14:489–495.

53. Clark DM, Plumb VJ, Epstein AE, et al. Hemodynamic effects of an irregular sequence of ventricular cycle lengths during atrial fibrillation. JACC 1997;30:1039–1045.

54. Farshi R, Kistner D, Sarma JS, et al. Ventricular rate control in chronic atrial fibrillation during daily activity and programmed exercise: a crossover open-label study of five drug regimens. JACC 1999;33:304–310.

55. Tieleman RG, Delangen D, VanGelder IC, et al. Verapamil reduces tachycardia induced electrical remodeling of the atria. Circulation 1997;95:1945–1953.

56. Gold MR, O'Gara PT, Buckley MJ, et al. Efficacy and safety of procainamide in preventing arrhythmias after coronary artery bypass surgery. Am J Cardiol 1996;78:975–979.

57. Boriani G, Capucci A, Botte GC, et al. Different pharmacological treatment for converting recent-onset atrial fibrillation: evaluation in 377 patients. JACC 1996;27:80A.

58. Capucci A, Villani GQ, Aschieri D, et al. Safety of oral propafenone in the conversion of recent onset atrial fibrillation to sinus rhythm: a prospective, parallel placebo-controlled multicenter study. Int J Cardiol 1999;68:187–196.

59. Carr B, Hawley K, Channer KS. Cardioversion of atrial fibrillation of recent onset with flecainide. Postgrad Med J 1991;67:659–662.

60. Stambler BS, Wood MA, Ellenbogen KA, et al. Efficacy and safety of repeated doses of ibutilide for rapid conversion of atrial flutter and atrial fibrillation. Circulation 1996;94:1613–1621.

61. Ellenbogen KA, Stambler BS, Wood MA, et al. Efficacy of intravenous ibutilide for acute termination of atrial fibrillation and flutter: a dose response study. JACC 1996;28:130–136.

62. Sung RJ, Tan HL, Karagounis L, et al. Intravenous sotalol for the termination of supraventricular tachycardia and atrial fibrillation and flutter: a multicenter, randomized, double-blind, placebo-controlled study. Am Heart J 1995;129:739–748.

63. Falk RH, Pollack A, Singh SN, et al. Intravenous dofetilde, a class III antiarrhythmic agent for the termination of sustained atrial fibrillation or flutter. JACC 1997;29:385–390.

64. Torp-Pedersen C, Moller M, Bloch-Thomsen PE, et al. Dofetilde in patients with congestive heart failure and left ventricular dysfunction. N Engl J Med 1999;341:857–865.

65. Juul-Moller S, Edvardsson AN, Rehnqvist-Ahlberg N. Sotalol v quinidine for the maintenance of sinus rhythm after direct current cardioversion of atrial fibrillation. Circulation 1990;82:1932–1939.

66. Reimold SC, Cantillon C, Friedman PL, et al. Propafenone vs. Sotalol for suppression of recurrent symptomatic atrial fibrillation. Am J Cardiol 1993;71:558–563.

67. Roy D, Talajic M, Dorian P, et al. Amiodarone to prevent recurrence of atrial fibrillation. N Engl J Med 2000;342:913–920.

68. Cardiac Arrhythmia Suppression Trial (CAST) investigators. Effect of encainide and flecainide on mortality in a randomized trial of arrhythmia suppression after myocardial infarction. N Engl J Med 1989;321:406–412.

69. Coplen SE, Antman EM, Berlin JA, et al. Efficacy and safety of quinidine therapy for maintenance of sinus rhythm after cardioversion. Circulation 1990;82:1106–1116.

70. Saliba WI, Juratli N, Chung MK, et al. High energy synchronized external DC cardioversion for refractory atrial fibrillation. JACC 1999;34:2031–2034.

71. DeLurgio DB, Hanson KJ, Mera F, et al. Simultaneous transthoracic shocks from two defibrillators for conversion of refractory atrial fibrillation. Circulation 1998;98:I-425 (Abstract).

72. Mittal S, Ayati S, Stein KM, et al. Transthoracic cardioversion of atrial fibrillation: comparison of a rectilinear biphasic versus damped sine wave monophasic shocks. Circulation 2000;101:1282–1287.

73. Levy S, Lauribe P, Dolla E, et al. A randomized comparison of external and internal cardioversion of atrial fibrillation. Circulation 1992;86:1415–1420.

74. Wellens HJJ, Lau CP, Luderitz B, et al. Atrioverter: an implantable device for the treatment of atrial fibrillation. Circulation 1998;98:1651–1656.

75. Tse HF, Lau CP, Yu CM, et al. Effect of the atrial defibrillator on the natural history of atrial fibrillation. J Cardiovasc Electrophysiol 1999;10:1200–1209.

76. Delfault P, Saksena S, Prakash A, et al. Long term outcome of patients with drug refractory atrial flutter and fibrillation after single and dual-site right atrial pacing for arrhythmia prevention. JACC 1998;32:1900–1908.

77. Andersen HR, Nielsen JC, Bloch Thomsen PE, et al. Long term follow-up of patients from a randomized trial of atrial versus ventricular pacing for sick sinus syndrome. Lancet 1997;350:1210–1216.

78. Mabo P, Daubert C, Bouhour A. Biatrial synchronous pacing for atrial arrhythmia prevention: the SYNBIAPACE Study. PACE 1999;22:755 (Abstract).

79. Gillis AM, Connolloy SJ, Lacombe P, et al. Randomized crossover comparison of DDDR versus VDD pacing after atrioventricular junction ablation for preventin of atrial fibrillation. Circulation 2000;102:736–741.

80. Sundt TM, Camillo CJ, Cox JL. The MAZE Procedure for Cure of Atrial Fibrillation. Cardiol Clin 1997;15:739–748.

81. Swartz JF, Perrersels G, Silvers J, et al. A Catheter-based curative approach for atrial fibrillation in humans. (Abstr) Circulation 1994;90:I-335.

82. Haissaguerre M, Jais P, Shah DC, et al. Spontaneous initiation of atrial fibrillation by ectopic beats originating in the pulmonary veins. N Engl J Med 1998;339:659–666.

83. Wood MA, Brown-Mahoney Chris, Kay GN, et al. Clinical outcomes after ablation and pacing therapy for atrial fibrillation. A meta-analysis. Circulation 2000;101:1138–1144.

84. Fitzpatrick AP, Kourouyan HD, Siu A, et al. Quality of life and outcomes after radiofrequency hi-bundle catheter ablation and permanent pacemaker implantation: impact of treatment in paroxysmal and established atrial fibrillation. Am Heart J 1996;131:499–507.

85. Marshall HJ, Harris ZI, Griffith MJ, et al. Prospective randomized study of ablation and pacing versus medical therapy for paroxysmal atrial fibrillation. Effects of pacing mode and mode-switch algorithm. Circulation 1999;99:1587–1592.

86. Darp B, Walfridsson H, Aunes M, et al. Incidence of sudden death after radiofrequency ablation of the atrioventricular junction for atrial fibrillation. Am J Cardiol 1997;80:1174–1177.

87. Brignole M, Menozzi C, Gianfranchi L, et al. Assessment of atrioventricular junction ablation and VVIR pacemaker versus pharmacological treatment in patients with heart failure and chronic atrial fibrillation. Circulation 1998;98:953–960.

6

Pharmacologic Management of Atrial Fibrillation

John K. Finkle, MD, FACC,
Kenneth Plunkitt, MD,
and Peter R. Kowey, MD, FACC

CONTENTS

INTRODUCTION
ANTICOAGULATION IN PATIENTS WITH AF
ATRIAL FLUTTER
RATE CONTROL IN AF—OVERVIEW
RHYTHM CONTROL
CHRONIC SUPPRESSION OF AF
OVERALL SUCCESS OF CHRONIC ANTIARRHYTHMIC THERAPY
SPECIAL SITUATIONS
CONCLUSION
REFERENCES

INTRODUCTION

The pharmacological approach to atrial fibrillation (AF) involves heart-rate control, anticoagulation, and restoration of normal sinus rhythm. Whereas there is strong evidence demonstrating a reduction in morbidity and mortality using anticoagulation for AF, there are no large-scale prospective studies demonstrating a similar benefit for using antiarrhythmic drugs to maintain sinus rhythm. This chapter reviews the data regarding anticoagulation, and presents an approach to managing clinical scenarios involving rate-slowing drugs and antiarrhythmic therapy.

ANTICOAGULATION IN PATIENTS WITH AF

Firm data now exist for the use of anticoagulation in patients with AF. It is a well-established fact that AF leads to thrombus formation in the heart. Initially, it was believed that thrombus formation in the atria took several days to develop. More recent studies utilizing transesophageal echocardiography have demonstrated that in the absence of anticoagulation, the incidence of left atrial appendage thrombus formation

From: *Contemporary Cardiology: Management of Cardiac Arrhythmias*
Edited by: L. I. Ganz © Humana Press Inc., Totowa, NJ

within 72 h of the onset of AF is 14%. One-half of the thrombi were mobile. Among patients with a recent thromboembolic event, the prevalence of left atrial thrombus did not differ between the group of patients with new-onset AF and those patients with AF of greater than 3 d duration. There was no significant difference between the incidence of left atrial thrombus formation in patients with AF of less than 2 d duration and those in individuals whose arrhythmia was present for 2–3 d *(1)*.

Acute Anticoagulation for AF

Anticoagulation is a two-step process involving acute and chronic treatment. The risk of cardioversion in the absence of anticoagulation increases proportionally with the time an individual is in AF. Although it is generally considered to be safe to cardiovert an unanticoagulated patient who has been in AF for less than 48 h, left atrial thrombus, spontaneous echo contrast, and stroke have been reported to occur within this 48-h window. Weigner et al. *(2)* retrospectively identified 375 patients with AF lasting less than 48 h. They found the incidence of thromboembolic events after resumption of normal sinus rhythm to be 0.8%. Interestingly, these individuals who had thromboembolic events had normal left ventricular function and no history of AF or prior thromboembolism, and would not have been traditionally characterized as "high risk" for embolism. Although this incidence of clinical thromboembolism is low compared to the 5–7% risk of stroke in unanticoagulated patients who have AF for greater than 48 h who undergo cardioversion, it is nevertheless a significant problem given the overall prevalence of AF in the population. Additionally, there is no difference in atrial mechanical function in patients who cardiovert spontaneously, pharmacologically, or electrically *(3)*. Therefore, it would not be unreasonable to anticoagulate an individual as soon as AF is initially documented if you plan to cardiovert the patient or the patient is at high risk of thromboembolism.

Given the risk of thromboembolism with cardioversion—whether spontaneous, pharmacologic, or electrical—in patients with AF of greater than 48–72 h duration, anticoagulation is needed prior to and after cardioversion. Two approaches are currently acceptable. One method is to place the patient on warfarin and maintain an International Normalized Ratio (INR) of 2 or greater for at least 3–4 wk prior to cardioversion. After cardioversion, the patients need to remain on warfarin for at least 3 wk prior to discontinuing anticoagulation, since there can be a significant lag between the restoration of sinus rhythm and resumption of normal atrial mechanical function. This can lead to thromboembolism after cardioversion if the patient is not adequately anticoagulated. The importance of maintaining strict anticoagulation has been demonstrated in a study performed at the Ochsner Medical Institutions *(4)*. One hundred and fifty patients with AF underwent elective electrical cardioversion. All patients were anticoagulated for at least 3 wk with weekly blood tests to ensure an INR of 2 or greater. If the patient's INR dipped below 2, the "clock" was restarted and the patient would have to demonstrate three more consecutive weeks of therapeutic INRs. Ninety-five percent of the patients were successfully cardioverted, and there were no thromboembolic events. Therefore, by maintaining a very strict level of precardioversion anticoagulation (INR greater than or equal to two or three consecutive weekly measurements) restoration of sinus rhythm can be achieved with minimal morbidity. In clinical practice, this can translate into several weeks or months for an individual patient to achieve this goal. This scenario can potentially result in a decreased effectiveness of cardioversion and antiarrhythmic therapy. The longer a patient is in AF, the more remodeling (i.e., dilatation and fibrosis) can occur, decreasing the likelihood of restoring sinus rhythm.

An alternative abbreviated approach to cardioversion in a patient with AF of greater than 2 d duration is to perform a transesophageal echocardiogram (TEE). If the TEE does not demonstrate left atrial thrombus, the patient can undergo cardioversion followed by anticoagulation for several weeks. Ideally, the patient would receive simultaneous warfarin and intravenous (iv) unfractionated heparin until the INR is therapeutic in order to minimize the time the patient has subtherapeutic levels of anticoagulation. The use of low mol-wt heparins as a substitute for iv heparin in this population is currently being studied in the ACUTE 2 trial.

TEE-expedited cardioversion has been compared to the traditional approach in the ACUTE pilot and main trials. In the pilot study, which was reported by Manning et al. (5), 230 patients with AF of greater than 2 d duration were placed on iv heparin and underwent TEEs. A total of 196 patients without thrombi underwent cardioversion (95% successful) and no patients had thromboembolism. The results of the main ACUTE trial were recently presented (5a). Among 1,222 patients randomized, the risk of stroke and transient ischemic attack was 0.6%, with no statistically significant difference between the TEE-expedited and traditional groups.

There may be a significant lag between the restoration of sinus rhythm as manifested by the presence of P waves on an electrocardiogram and the return of normal atrial transport function after a cardioversion is performed. This atrial electromechanical dissociation may place the patient at risk of thromboembolism in the period after successful cardioversion is performed. Therefore, it is recommended to maintain the patient at therapeutic levels of anticoagulation for at least 3–4 wk after cardioversion. In patients in whom the risk of recurrence of AF is high, anticoagulation may need to be used for several months until adequate assessment of arrhythmia suppression is determined.

Often, a physician or patient cannot determine the onset or duration of the arrhythmia. If the decision is made to cardiovert the patient in this situation, then either of these two approaches is a viable option. The major advantage of the TEE approach is that it reduces the duration of the waiting period prior to cardioversion. In a highly symptomatic patient, this may be the preferred option. Currently, the decision to proceed with cardioversion is based on clinical judgement without morbidity or mortality data to support this approach over rate control and long-term anticoagulation. Dense, spontaneous echo contact is a risk factor for subsequent thromboembolism (6), and it is not well-established when to proceed with cardioversion after TEE when dense, spontaneous echo contrast is seen. There is also uncertainty regarding when a patient in whom TEE has documented atrial thrombus can safely be cardioverted.

Chronic Anticoagulation in AF

In patients with paroxysmal or permanent AF, extensive data supports the use of anticoagulation to prevent thromboembolism (7–11). In a recent meta-analysis (12) of five major studies on 3706 patients with AF (462 patients of whom had paroxysmal AF) the annual risk of stoke in control (unanticoagulated) patients was 4.5%, whereas those patients treated with warfarin had an annual risk of 1.4%. This is a dramatic difference—especially considering that 47% of all strokes were either fatal or caused significant functional impairment. The risk of stroke increases in an individual patient as the number of risk factors (such as diabetes, hypertension, or a previous thromboembolic event) increases. This compares to an annual rate of major bleeding (intracranial hemorrhage or bleeding requiring transfusion) of 1% per yr in patients treated with warfarin.

Aspirin and Chronic Anticoagulation

Aspirin, however, does not appear to offer the same protection that warfarin provides. Only in the SPAF study did aspirin, at the dose of 325 mg per d, provide a significant decrease in the incidence of stroke in certain populations—patients without risk factors for thromboembolism such as recent congestive heart failure (CHF), reduced left ventricular function, hypertension, previous thromboembolism, or female gender greater than 75 yr of age. This may be a result of the low, 1% baseline risk of stroke that this specific population has at baseline. If one or more of these thromboembolic risk factors were present, than the risk of stroke was high (averaging 8% per year) even when aspirin was combined with low-dose warfarin *(13)*. The AFASAK and BAATAF studies *(14)* did not demonstrate a benefit from aspirin at doses of 75 mg or 325 mg per d.

The only group of patients who did not demonstrate a clear benefit from anticoagulation was the group with "lone" AF. Lone AF is defined as AF in patients <65 yr old with no structural heart disease, or other risk factors for stroke such as prior stroke or TIA, hypertension, CHF, diabetes, angina, or prior myocardial infarction (MI). These patients, at baseline, have a low risk of stroke. In the pooled data from the five anticoagulation studies, there were no strokes among 112 patients less than 60 yr old with lone AF. This risk increased to 1.6% in patients 60–69 yr old, 2.1% in patients 70–79 yr old, and 3% in patients over 80 yr old *(12)*. Therefore, before withholding anticoagulation from an individual with AF, one must ensure that all of the criteria for "lone" AF are fulfilled, including the age cut-off. Additionally, given the relatively low risks of aspirin, it would be reasonable (but not mandatory) to treat younger patients with lone AF with aspirin *(15)*. For all other patients with advanced age, risk factors for thromboembolism, or structural heart disease, warfarin is the standard of care if there are no contraindications to anticoagulation.

Unfortunately, not all patients at risk for thromboembolism are suitable candidates for anticoagulation with warfarin. A history of bleeding problems, high fall or injury risk, medical noncompliance, or poor follow-up may preclude the use of warfarin. When possible, empiric use of aspirin and/or other antiplatelet drugs may be considered, although the data supporting this is lacking. Although maintenance of sinus rhythm with antiarrhythmic drugs is practiced as an alternative approach to patients who cannot be anticoagulated, this has not yet been validated in large-scale trials to prevent thromboembolism. Additionally, for patients with AF that only occur for brief periods of time or very infrequently (e.g., 1–2 h every few months), it is not yet clear that this population will benefit from long-term anticoagulation given the risks associated with warfarin. Therefore, there are still many patients with AF for whom the decision to use antithrombotic therapy must be made on an individual basis (Fig. 1).

ATRIAL FLUTTER

Atrial flutter, once believed not to promote thrombus, has subsequently been demonstrated to be associated with thromboembolism. This can occur for three reasons: first,

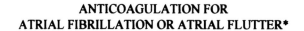

**ANTICOAGULATION FOR
ATRIAL FIBRILLATION OR ATRIAL FLUTTER***

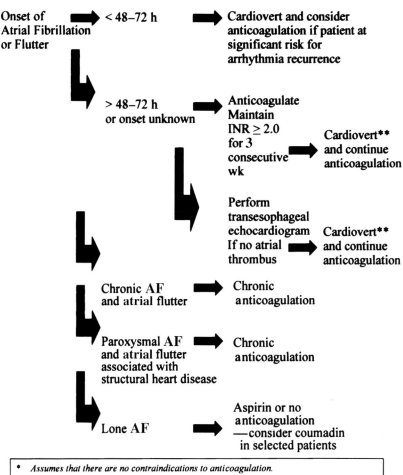

Fig. 1. Anticoagulation Algorithm.

atrial transport function can be significantly impaired during atrial flutter. Secondly, intracardiac electrograms taken during atrial flutter have demonstrated that although certain areas of the atria demonstrate clear flutter waves—and this is the dominant arrhythmia seen on a surface 12-lead electrocardiogram (ECG)—other areas of the atrium may demonstrate simultaneous fibrillatory activity. Thirdly, patients who have documented atrial flutter at office visits may also have unrecognized AF at other times. One study *(16)* demonstrated a 5% incidence of intracardiac thrombi and a 20% incidence of spontaneous echo contrast (a risk factor for thromboembolism) in patients with atrial flutter. Another study *(17)* of unanticoagulated patients undergoing transesophageal echocardiograms had an 11% incidence of left atrial thrombus. Additionally, after cardioversion was performed, 28% of the patients had absence of atrial transport function. In a study of 191 patients with atrial flutter followed for a mean of approx 2 yr, the incidence of thromboembolism was 7% (18). Therefore, the surface electrocardiogram may not be a reliable indicator of intracardiac electrophysiology. The American College of Chest Physicians (AACP) has suggested that atrial flutter should be treated in the same fashion as AF with regards to anticoagulation (19).

RATE CONTROL IN AF—OVERVIEW

In addition to anticoagulation, control of the ventricular rate is necessary in the acute and chronic management of patients with AF. The spectrum of ventricular response varies greatly. On one end of the spectrum are patients with resting ventricular rates of <100 beats per minute (bpm) off AV-node-blocking agents—indicative of intrinsic atrioventricular conduction system disease or excessive resting vagal tone. Other patients can present with severe CHF and a reversible cardiomyopathy (20–21) because of excessive ventricular rates. Currently available medications include beta-adrenergic blockers, calcium-channel blockers (verapamil and diltiazem), digoxin, certain antiarrhythmics such as iv amiodarone, clonidine, and pronestyl (in pre-excited AF). There is little data that definitely demonstrates the superiority of one medication over another, and the decision to use an individual agent is often dictated by the clinical scenario.

Digoxin was the first agent used to control ventricular rates. This medication is generally the least effective. Digoxin has several mechanisms of action. The most prominent effect in controlling the ventricular response is to increase parasympathetic tone. Increased vagal tone shortens the refractory period of the atria, increases the atrial rate in AF, and thus slows conduction over the AV node (resulting from the decremental conduction properties of the AVN). Therefore, at rest, when vagal tone is elevated, ventricular response may be slow. With exertion, when parasympathetic tone is withdrawn, the effect of digoxin is diminished, and the ventricular response may become rapid. In the hospital setting, AF often occurs as a comorbid event—postoperatively, or because of hypoxia or infection. In these settings, when catecholamine levels are elevated, the negative chronotropic effects of digoxin are diminished (22). Although in some patients, digoxin is adequate for rate control, we believe that it is a second-line agent or best used in conjunction with other rate-slowing drugs. The two major uses of digoxin as a first-line agent are in patients with CHF or in patients with paroxysmal AF who also demonstrate sinus-node dysfunction, since it tends not to depress the sinus rate as much as calcium-blocking or beta-blocking agents.

Beta-blockers and calcium-blockers are generally equally effective in controlling the ventricular rate. Specific clinical scenarios should determine the use of a particular medication. Given the hypercatecholamine state of postoperative patients, beta-blockers are very effective in blunting the heart rate response. Patients with a history of MI should be considered for beta-blocker therapy, given the mortality benefit of this medication in this population. Hyperthyroid patients also demonstrate a good clinical response to beta-blockers, because the major abnormality is an exaggerated response to catecholamines. Certain situations, such as bronchospasm or severe left ventricular dysfunction, may preclude the use of beta-blockers to acutely control ventricular rate. Chronically, metoprolol may be used orally for rate control when doses are titrated upwards over the course of several weeks in patients with heart failure. Another drawback is that, with the exception of esmolol, beta-blockers can only be given acutely in intermittent doses when administered intravenously. In patients who manifest both very rapid and slow rates in AF, beta-blockers with intrinsic sympathomimetic activity (ISA) such as acebutolol or pindolol can be used. These agents increase sympathetic tone at slow heart rates—thus minimizing bradycardia—and exert predominant beta-blocking effects at faster heart rates *(23)*.

Acute Rate Control in AF

Verapamil and diltiazem are generally well-tolerated nondihydropyridine calcium-channel blockers used for rate control in AF. The oral forms of these medications can depress left ventricular function. Intravenous verapamil and diltiazem are generally equally effective *(24)* for acute heart-rate control, but iv diltiazem has been demonstrated to be safe to use in patients with moderate to severe CHF *(25–27)*. Intravenous diltiazem or digoxin are the preferred agents in patients with severe left ventricular dysfunction. Intravenous diltiazem has the additional benefit of more rapid heart rate control than digoxin in the setting of CHF.

Often, the dose of iv calcium-channel blockers or beta-blockers is limited by hypotension. In this circumstance, digoxin can be used to control heart rates. If this is not adequate, vasoconstrictors such as neosynephrine may need to be combined with calcium-blockers or beta-blockers to maintain hemodynamic stability if electrical cardioversion cannot be performed. Amiodarone can also be used to control rate in AF in critically ill patients. In one study *(28)* of 8 patients with ejection fractions <15%, iv amiodarone decreased the mean ventricular response by 28%. In another study *(29)* comparing amiodarone to digoxin, amiodarone was more effective in decreasing heart rates at 1 h and at 6 h from onset on infusion compared to digoxin. Amiodarone decreased the mean heart rates from 157 to 92 bpm over 6 h. In this study, over one-half of the patients had class 3 or 4 CHF, again demonstrating that iv amiodarone can be used with caution in critically ill patients.

Clonidine, a central-acting sympatholytic medication has been shown in small series to aid in slowing ventricular response to AF both acutely and chronically *(30–31)*. Intravenous procainamide is used to reduce the ventricular response in patients with hemodynamically stable pre-excited AF (i.e., AF with rapid conduction of atrial impulses to the ventricle over an accessory pathway) by increasing the refractory period of the accessory pathway.

Chronic Rate Control in AF

For rate control in the outpatient setting, calcium-channel blockers and beta-blockers are first-line agents for most patients. In patients with a history of MI, beta-blockers are preferred because of the mortality benefit. Exercise-induced AF is another strong indication for the use of beta-blockers. Diabetic patients and patients with peripheral vascular disease—provided that they do not manifest severe limb ischemia—can be placed on beta-blockers safely. Beta-blockers are frequently associated with symptoms of fatigue and lethargy, necessitating a change to other agents. In patients with severe bronchospastic disease, calcium-blockers are the mainstay of treatment. Digoxin is generally used in addition to these agents when monotherapy is inadequate. An individ-

Table 1
Rate Control for Atrial Fibrillation or Atrial Flutter

Structural heart disease	Drug therapy
None	Beta-blockers or > digoxin Ca-blockers
(CHF)	Digoxin or > amiodarone > Beta-blockers Diltiazem
Post-MI	Beta-blockers > Ca-blockers > digoxin
Postoperative	Beta-blockers > Ca-blockers > digoxin
Vagally mediated AF	Ca-blockers > Beta-blockers > digoxin
Severe LVH	Beta-blockers or > digoxin Ca-blockers
Sinus-node dysfunction	Pindolol or > digoxin > Ca-blockers Acebutolol
Severe obstructive lung disease	Ca-blockers > digoxin > Beta-blockers
Pre-excited atrial fibrillation or flutter	Intravenous procainamide
Thyrotoxicosis	Beta-blockers > Ca-blockers > digoxin
Severe peripheral vascular disease	Ca-blockers > digoxin > Beta-blockers

ual agent should be increased to the maximal dose before a second agent is added. All too often, patients are placed on low doses of two or three AVN-blocking drugs, which decreases compliance in taking the medications and thus effectiveness (Table 1).

RHYTHM CONTROL

Antifibrillatory Agents—An Overview of Pro-arrhythmia

There are no large prospective studies demonstrating a reduced morbidity or mortality for the use of antifibrillatory agents to maintain normal sinus rhythm. In fact, there are very few antiarrhythmic agents which have demonstrated "mortality-neutral" effects when given to patients with significant structural heart disease. Much of the concern in using drugs to suppress AF started in the late 1980s and early 1990s. The Cardiac Arrhythmia Suppression Trial (32) demonstrated an increased mortality in the use of encainide and flecainide to suppress ventricular ectopy in patients with a history of MI. This was the first major large-scale trial to demonstrate an increased mortality in patients despite effective suppression of a clinical arrhythmia (in this case ventricular ectopy as opposed to AF). In 1990, Coplen et al. (33) published a meta-analysis of six trials that used quinidine to maintain sinus rhythm after cardioversion. Although quinidine was twice as effective at maintaining sinus rhythm at 1-yr follow-up, the total mortality of the quinidine-treated patients was 2.9% compared to 0.8% in control patients. In the Stroke Prevention and Atrial Fibrillation Study, (34,35) there was nearly a 2.5-fold increase in cardiac and arrhythmic death in patients treated with antiarrhythmic drugs. This risk was even higher in patients with CHF (36). Interestingly, those patients without a history of CHF had no increase in cardiac mortality. Even as early as 1933,

Sir Thomas Lewis, in discussing the use of quinidine in the treatment of AF wrote, "It is agreed that it is only justifiable to use it in cases that are carefully selected and not as a remedy for fibrillation cases in general. Its administration is definitely forbidden in patients who have experienced haemoptysis or who present venous engorgement or great cardiac enlargement" *(37)*. Given CAST, SPAF and other studies, the use of antiarrhythmic agents to suppress AF fell out of favor.

Many of these studies, though, were not applicable to the general population of patients with AF. The CAST trial examined patients with a history of MI and high-grade ventricular ectopy who were at increased risk for sudden death. The Coplen meta-analysis only demonstrated an increased total mortality, but not cardiac or arrhythmic mortality in patients treated with quinidine. The Atrial Fibrillation Follow-up In Rhythm Management (AFFIRM) trial is currently attempting to answer the question regarding the mortality risk of arrhythmia suppression vs rate control and anticoagulation *(37a)*. Additionally, there are many patients who do not tolerate AF from a hemodynamic or symptomatic standpoint. For this group of patients, rate control alone is not adequate to maintain quality of life. At present, given the absence of data regarding survival and risk of thromboembolism in patients treated with antiarrhythmic drugs, symptoms are typically the main indication for this type of treatment in patients with AF. Careful selection of an antiarrhythmic agent is needed to avoid proarrhythmia and minimize side effects of the drugs.

Currently available drugs that have antifibrillatory action include quinidine, disopyramide, procainamide, flecainide, propafenone, sotalol, ibutilide, dofetilide, and amiodarone. Another agent that is available, but not yet commonly used in clinical practice, is moricizine. In this section, we will assume that the decision has been made to pharmacologically cardiovert or suppress AF, and drug selection will be based on minimizing the risk of proarryhthmia.

It is clear that the risk of proarrhythmia increases with the severity of the patient's heart disease. Proarrhythmia can occur for several reasons. In patients who are placed on antifibrillatory drugs for AF, the rhythm can develop into atrial flutter. If there is not adequate blockage of the AV node, patients can develop one-to-one conduction of the atrial flutter impulses to the ventricle. Drugs can also slow the rate of atrial flutter. A patient may have atrial flutter impulses at a rate of 300 BPM, and only every other beat can conduct to ventricle because of the refractory period of the AV node. Antifibrillatory agents can slow the conduction of the flutter circuit and reduce the flutter rate—for example—240 BPM. This rate may be shorter than the refractory period of the AV node, and can cause one-to-one conduction of atrial impulses to the ventricle and result in extremely rapid heart rates with hemodynamic compromise. Certain drugs with intrinsic vagolytic properties, such as quinidine and disopyramide, can facilitate this proarrhythmic effect by shortening the effective refractory period of the AV node. Therefore, adequate AV-nodal blockade must be present prior to starting an antiarrhythmic agent for AF or atrial flutter.

Other forms of proarrhythmia occur when ventricular arrhythmias arise in patients treated with drugs for AF. Anti-arrhythmic drugs slow conduction and prolong the refractory nature of the myocardium. This can facilitate reentrant ventricular tachycardia (VT) or fibrillation. Medications which prolong refractoriness (and increase the QT interval) can promote the formation of early afterdepolarizations and lead to torsades de points *(38)*. Many of these agents, such as sotalol, have a more pronounced potassium-

Table 2
Drug Regimens for Acute Conversion of Atrial Fibrillation/Flutter

Procainamide:	iv 15 mg/kg over 45 min to 1 h
	PO 1 g Q4–6 h
Quinidine:	PO 200 mg quinidine sulfate Q 2 h × 4 doses, or quinidine gluconate
	324 mg Q 3 h × 3 doses
Propafenone:	PO 450–600 mg single oral dose
	iv 2 mg/kg bolus, then 0.0078 mg/kg/min
Flecainide:	PO 300 mg single oral dose
	iv 2 mg/kg over 10 min; maximum 150 mg
Amiodarone:	iv 5 mg/kg over 30 min, then 2 mg/min for 12 h then 0.7 mg/min thereafter
Ibutilide:	iv 1 mg over 10 min, wait 10 min and repeat dose if patient has not returned
	to sinus rhythm

channel-blocking effect at slower heart rates—an effect known as "reverse use dependence." When sotalol is used in patients who develop bradycardia because of concomitant use of other rate-slowing drugs, baseline slow heart rates, or because of the intrinsic beta-blocking effects of DL-sotalol itself, dangerous ventricular proarrhythmia can result from excessive QT prolongation. Patients with significant structural heart disease, such as hypertrophy or scarring, are much more prone to develop proarrhythmia from these mechanisms *(39)*. Therefore, careful selection of antifibrillatory agents is essential in patients with heart disease to minimize the risk of dangerous ventricular arrhythmias.

Finally, bradycardia secondary to depression of the sinus node or to prolongation of atrioventricular conduction can occur from antiarrhythmic agents. Although this can be treated with pacing, careful selection of a particular drug for an individual may avoid this problem.

Acute Pharmacologic Cardioversion

Antifibrillatory drugs can be used to pharmacologically cardiovert patients as well as to maintain normal sinus rhythm chronically. The success rate for both of these clinical effects is similar for most medications, and generally depends on the duration of the arrhythmia and any underlying heart disease that exists prior to starting the drug. Multiple comparison trials between different medications as well as between active drug vs placebo have been performed *(40–70)*.

For acute pharmacologic cardioversion, several common strategies have been employed *(71–74) (see* Table 2). The success rates for these medications have ranged from no better than placebo to greater than 80–90%. In studies on patients with AF <48 h, there was a relatively high spontaneous conversion rate in placebo-treated patients. Although some studies did not demonstrate an improvement in the overall rate of cardioversion of medically treated patients vs placebo, patients treated with antifibrillatory agents resumed sinus rhythm more rapidly. For patients with a history of infrequent atrial arrhythmias, single, high oral doses of either propafenone or flecainide may be useful if no structural heart disease is present. These drugs have an extremely low rate of life-threatening ventricular arrhythmias. Patients who receive class IC drugs may be prone to a unique form of proarrhythmia. These medications have "use-dependent" effects with increased blockade of sodium channels at faster heart rates. In rare instances, this effect can result in unusual wide-complex tachycardias—either supraventricular tachycardia (SVT) with abnormal ventricular conduction, or ventricular tachycardia (VT)—resulting from diffuse slowing of conduction in the myocardium. At toxic doses, patients with malignant ventricular arrhythmias can be treated with hypertonic $NaHCO_3$ *(75–76)*. The other drugs mentioned (procainamide, quinidine, disopyramide, sotalol, ibutilide, and dofetilide) all have the potential for QT prolongation, and thus should only be initiated with continuous electrocardiographic monitoring. In patients with structural heart disease, all medications used for pharmacologic cardioversion should be administered in the hospital setting.

Recently, iv ibutilide has been used to treat acute-onset AF and atrial flutter. Ibutilide is unique because it blocks potassium channels (IKr) and enhances the slow inward sodium current to prolong the action potential duration. Because of the risk of torsades, potassium and magnesium should be repleted prior to ibutilide administration. Additionally, the risk of ventricular arrhythmias is enhanced in the setting of heart failure, and ibutilide should not be used in decompensated CHF. Patients who receive ibutilide must be monitored for at least 4 h postinfusion with immediate access to defibrillation equipment. We usually perform electrical cardioversion within 30 min after the second mg of ibutilide has been infused if sinus rhythm has not been restored because blood levels of this drug are high at this stage. The success rate for cardioversion is approx 30% for AF and 60% for atrial flutter *(71,72,77)*. Ibutilide pretreatment also increases the efficacy of direct current (DC) cardioversion. (*See* below.)

CHRONIC SUPPRESSION OF AF

Amiodarone in Patients with Structural Heart Disease

Since many of the patients who have AF have significant structural heart disease, attempts should be made to use drugs with mortality-neutral effects. Currently, amiodarone has the largest clinical experience in patients with structural heart disease. The South American GESICA trial *(78)* demonstrated a reduced morbidity and mortality in patients treated with amiodarone who had severe CHF. Although CAMIAT *(79)* and EMIAT trials *(80)* demonstrated a reduced risk of sudden death in patients treated with amiodarone, there was no significant difference in overall mortality compared to patients treated with placebo. The CASCADE trial *(81)* demonstrated an improved survival in patients who survived sudden death when treated with amiodarone vs electrophysiologic-guided standard antiarrhythmic therapy. In a meta-analysis *(82)* of over 6500 patients in 20 trials utilizing amiodarone, post-MI or in CHF, there was a 13% decrease in total mortality in treated patients. Although these trials were not designed to test the safety of amiodarone in the control of AF, they nevertheless demonstrated that amiodarone does not increase mortality in patients with severe structural heart disease or CHF who are at high risk of sudden death. A recent Canadian trial showed amiodarone to be more effective than either sotalol or propafenone in the long-term suppression of AF *(82A)*.

Amiodarone, from a mortality standpoint, appears to be the drug of choice in patients with heart failure or cardiomyopathy. Unfortunately, it has the most significant organ-toxicity profile of any drug. The incidence of severe hepatotoxicity is <3%, neurotoxicity is approx 20%, pulmonary toxicity is 0.5–10%, and thyroid toxicity is 2–24% *(83)*. Therefore, careful initial screening of liver, thyroid, and pulmonary tests as well as long-term serial follow-up of the various organ toxic effects are mandatory. The toxic effects are dose-related and cumulative. The decision to use amiodarone should take into account the age of the patients and the expected number of years that it will be used. The term "low-dose" amiodarone has been coined for the use of doses less than or equal to 200 mg per d to treat AF (less than the typical dose for treating VT). For patients being treated de novo for AF, maintenance doses of this quantity are often adequate. In patients who have failed other antiarrhythmics agents, higher doses are often required to maintain normal sinus rhythm, thus increasing the risk of organ toxicity.

Sotalol in Patients With Structural Heart Disease

Other agents such as racemic or DL-sotalol have demonstrated no increased mortality in patients post-MI (84). When used in the dextrorotatory optical isomer form, d-sotalol, an increased mortality was seen in patients with an ejection fraction greater than 30% (85). Ventricular hypertrophy predisposes the heart to the formation of early afterdepolarizations, which can lead to torsades de pointes. For post-MI patients without left ventricular hypertrophy (LVH) or CHF, racemic d,l-sotalol is a reasonable first-time agent for AF, and avoids the potential organ toxicity of amiodarone (86).

Dofetilide in Patients With Structural Heart Disease

Recently, dofetilide, a pure class III agent devoid of beta-blocker activity, has been shown to have a mortality-neutral effect in patients with low ejection fractions. A recent placebo-controlled trial of over 1500 patients with severe left ventricular dysfunction and CHF demonstrated that dofetilide was effective in converting patients to sinus rhythm, maintaining sinus rhythm, and reducing the risk of hospitalizations for CHF with no increase in mortality (87–88). There is, however, a significant risk of torsades de pointes with dofetilide. Dofetilide is eliminated through the kidneys, and dosage adjustments must be made in patients with even minor renal insufficiency. Patients must be hospitalized with continuous cardiac telemetry to monitor for proarrhythmia when initiating or making upward dose adjustments with this medication (88a). Intravenous dofetilide, currently in clinical investigations, can be used to acutely terminate both AF and atrial flutter (89). This drug must also be used with caution (or not at all) in patients who are concurrently receiving QT-prolonging medications.

Patients With Minimal Structural Heart Disease or With LVH

In patients with minimal or no significant structural heart disease, any antifibrillatory agent can be employed. A specific agent should be selected by its side-effect profile. Class IC agents such as propafenone and flecainide have an extremely low incidence of ventricular proarrhythmia in normal hearts, and are generally well-tolerated. Sotalol and class IA agents such as disopyramide and procainamide can be used safely in this setting if careful attention is given to the dose-dependent QT-prolonging effects of these drugs. Quinidine is the exception, because it has both a dose-dependent and an idiosyncratic QT-prolonging effect in certain individuals. Periodic complete blood counts should be performed on patients who are taking either procainamide or quinidine because of the rare occurrence of blood dyscrasias. Disopyramide is well-tolerated in younger patients, but because of its significant anticholinegic effects, caution should be used in men with symptoms of an enlarged prostate in whom urinary retention may occur. Pyridostigmine, an acetylcholinesterase inhibitor (90–91), can be given in conjunction with disopyramide to mitigate the anticholinergic effects. Patients who are taking these medications should be advised to contact their physician for dosage adjustments during any acute gastrointestinal illness (diarrhea or vomiting), which can alter serum concentrations of potassium or magnesium and thus promote proarrhythmia. Both disopyramide and propafenone exhibit nonlinear pharmacokinetics, in which small increments in dosages can lead to significantly higher serum concentrations. Therefore, dosage increases should be undertaken after the patient has had time to achieve a steady state. Finally, drug selection also depends on pharmacologic interactions with other medications that the patient is taking as well as drug metabolism in patients with underlying renal or hepatic disease. Sotalol, flecainide, and dofetilide need dosage adjustment in patients with renal insufficiency. Quinidine, propafenone, ibutilide, and amiodarone are all metabolized by the liver. Dosage adjustments or complete avoidance of these drugs in patients with hepatic dysfunction is essential. With procainamide and disopyramide, both renal and hepatic metabolism, and elimination occur, and caution should be used in patients with either renal or hepatic dysfunction.

In patients with ventricular hypertrophy and normal left ventricular function, drugs that prolong the QT interval should be used with caution. Class IC agents such as propafenone are safe in this group of patients because there is no prolongation of the QT interval. Amiodarone is also acceptable. Flecainide can be used to suppress atrial arrhythmias in structurally normal hearts. Whether flecainide is safe in patients with minimal LVH vs those patients with severe LVH has yet to be determined (Table 3).

It has been our practice to initiate QT-prolonging drugs while the patient is in the hospital on telemetry. Even in patients with structurally normal hearts, there is a small risk of ventricular proarrhythmia. We are now learning that certain individuals may have a "channelopathy"—they demonstrate abnormalities in sodium or potassium channels that only become manifest when challenged with certain drugs. In patients with structural heart disease or those who may be prone to sinus-node dysfunction or atrioventricular conduction disturbances, in-hospital drug initiation is mandatory. In this manner, prompt drug discontinuation, defibrillation, or pacing can be undertaken if proarrhythmia occurs.

OVERALL SUCCESS OF CHRONIC ANTIARRHYTHMIC THERAPY

The success rate of an antifibrillatory agent to maintain sinus rhythm in patients with a history of paroxysmal or chronic AF ranges significantly. The two factors that have the most influence on maintaining normal sinus rhythm (NSR) in patients with AF are the degree of underlying structural heart disease and the duration of arrhythmia prior to starting the drug. In a summary published by Kassotis et al. (49), there is a wide variation in drug effectiveness in maintaining NSR between various studies. Overall, with antifibrillatory drugs, approx 50% of patients will maintain NSR at 1 yr after initiating therapy. Therefore, the choice of a particular agent should initially be made based on a safety profile with respect to underlying heart disease and drug metabolism, and based secondly on drug tolerance based on side effects.

Studies now indicate that there may be very different mechanisms for paroxysmal vs chronic AF. It has been demonstrated that focal tachycardias from the pulmonary veins may initiate and sustain AF, especially in patients with paroxysmal AF. Chronic AF may result from multiple wavelets of reentry in the atria. The percentage of patients with AF who have focal initiation sites in the pulmonary veins has not yet been

Table 3
Chronic Antiarrhythmic Therapy for Atrial Fibrillation or Flutter

Structural heart disease	Drug therapy		
None	Flecainide Propafenone Sotalol Amiodarone*	>	Procainamide Quinidine Disopyramide
Cardiomyopathy or CHF	Amiodarone or possibly Dofetilide	>	Sotalol Procainamide
	Avoid disopyramide, quinidine, propafenone, flecainide		
Post MI	Sotalol or Amiodarone	> Procainamide	Avoid flecainide or propafenone
Postoperative AF/flutter/prophylaxis	Beta-blockers or possibly sotalol or amiodarone		
Vagally Mediated AF/flutter or patients with sinus-node dysfunction	Disopyramide		
LVH	Amiodarone Procainamide or possibly flecainide or propafenone		Sotalol** (in mild LVH)
Patients with elevated defibrillation threshold for AF or patients with defibrillators with elevated thresholds for ventricular defibrillation	Sotalol Dofetilide		

* Amiodarone should be avoided as first line agent in younger patients due to life-long accumulated risk of end organ toxicity. It can be used as first line agents in patients of advanced age.

** Avoid Sotalol in moderate to severe LVH.

established. Additionally, there have been no studies to specifically evaluate whether any particular antiarrhythmic drugs are more efficacious in patients with "focal" AF. Hopefully, as more insight is gained about the mechanisms of these arrhythmias, drug therapy can be directed to treat a specific subtype of AF.

Adjunctive Therapy in Failed Cardioversions

In a small percentage of patients, electrical cardioversion is unsuccessful. It has been demonstrated that in patients with implantable defibrillators, the energy required to defilbrillate the heart can be reduced by the use of class III antiarrhythmics (92). This property is unique to these drugs. Recently, ibutilide has been used to successfully reduce the AF threshold in patients undergoing cardioversion. Oral et al. (93) randomized patients to cardioversion with and without ibutilide. The mean energy requirement for cardioversion was significantly reduced in patients receiving ibutilide (166 ± 80 J) versus 228 ± 93 J in the placebo group. Whereas 72% of the patients in the placebo group could be successfully cardioverted, 100% of the ibutilide patients were able to achieve NSR. Interestingly, in this trial, ibutilide was given to patients who were on chronic amiodarone, sotalol, or class I agents without an excess incidence of torsades de pointes. Profound left ventricular dysfunction was a risk factor for torsades de pointes in this study. Sotalol may also decrease the energy requirement in patients with AF undergoing cardioversion *(94)*. In one study of failed cardioversions, amiodarone appeared to be effective as an adjunct to electrical therapy *(95)*. Forty-nine patients with chronic AF who had failed electrical cardioversion were given large-dose oral amiodarone 10–15 mg/kg/d for cumulative doses of >6 g. Subsequently, 23 of these patients underwent successful cardioversion after this loading dose. Therefore, consideration can be given to adding a class III agent or amiodarone prior to cardioversion in patients who cannot be successfully cardioverted.

When performing a cardioversion, it is important to establish whether the patient has had brief conversion to NSR. Certain individuals may demonstrate a few sinus depolarizations after electrical cardioversion, and then immediately revert to AF. This phenomenon has been called "early recurrence of atrial fibrillation (ERAF)." In these patients, repeat attempts at cardioversion are usually unsuccessful unless antifibrillatory agents are administered. Therefore, when performing a cardioversion, one must pay particular attention to whether the cardioversion failed because of a high defibrillation threshold (which can be treated acutely with ibutilide or changing the amount or vectors of energy delivery) vs transient success, which would require the long-term administration of drugs to maintain NSR.

SPECIAL SITUATIONS

Vagally Mediated AF

In certain individuals, AF can be precipitated by an increase in vagal tone *(96)*. These episodes are often characterized by onset during sleep or after meals, and are usually preceded by bradycardia. Treatment with vagolytic drugs such as disopyramide may be particularly effective in this situation by preventing the initiating event. Digoxin, by enhancing vagal tone, may actually facilitate the induction of AF in these patients, and should therefore be avoided. Beta-blockers should also be avoided, because they may slow the heart rate and allow the vagal tone to predominate.

Patients With Chronotropic Incompetence

Patients with paroxysmal AF often manifest sinus bradycardia and chronotropic incompetence. All antifibrillatory agents have the ability to further depress sinus-node function and result in symptomatic bradycardia. In this setting, a vagolytic agent such as disopyramide can be used, since it can suppress AF and will often avoid further sinus slowing. If the patient also exhibits rapid rates during paroxysms of AF, pindolol or acebutolol can be added to disopyramide *(97)*. The intrinsic sympathomimetic activity of these agents helps to prevent resting bradycardia, and the beta-blocking properties prevent rapid rates when AF occurs. In patients with permanent AF and wide swings in heart rates, pindolol or acebutolol may be preferred over other agents, because of their unique ability to reduce bradycardic episodes. In many patients with the tachycardia-bradycardia syndrome, a permanent pacemaker facilitates administration of both rate control and antiarrhythmic drug therapy.

Postoperative AF

AF is a major cause of morbidity and increased health care cost after heart surgery. The overall incidence of postoperative AF is approx 30% *(98)*, and may be significantly higher in certain subgroups. In several trials, beta-blockers, by reducing the effect of elevated circulating catecholamines, appear to reduce the incidence of postoperative AF. In a meta-analysis of 2482 patients post-coronary bypass surgery, beta-blockers significantly decreased the incidence of supraventricular arrhythmias compared to digoxin or placebo *(99)*. Digoxin and calcium-channel blockers do not appear to have any significant effect in preventing AF in this setting. Prophylactic treatment with beta-blockers reduces the incidence of postoperative supraventricular arrhythmias. Various antifibrillatory agents have been evaluated in this regard. One large meta-analysis *(100)* of 24 randomized controlled trials demonstrated that beta-blockers significantly reduced the incidence of postoperative supraventricular arrhythmias to 8.7% from 34% in control-treated patients. No beneficial effect was seen in patients treated with verapamil or digoxin. This beneficial effect was seen in patients treated preoperatively or postoperatively with beta-blockers of any type. Therefore, whenever there are no strong contraindications, beta-blockers should be used in patients after cardiac surgery.

Recently, several studies have been published regarding the prophylactic use of antifibrillatory agents after cardiac surgery. When compared to metoprolol after coronary-artery bypass surgery, DL-sotalol reduced the incidence of AF by one-half when started on the first postoperative morning *(101)*. In another study, DL-sotalol, when initiated prior to cardiac surgery, reduced the incidence of postoperative AF by 67% compared to placebo *(102)*. Therefore, in the absence of severe left ventricular dysfunction, renal insufficiency, CHF, or severe bronchospastic lung disease, sotalol is a reasonable agent for the prevention of postoperative AF.

Amiodarone also has been successful in preventing postoperative AF. In the ARCH trial *(103)*, 1 g per d for 2 d of iv amiodarone was given immediately postoperatively. This reduced the incidence of AF by 26% compared to controls. In another trial by Daoud and colleagues *(104)*, amiodarone was administered orally a minimum of 7 d prior to heart surgery. A dose of 600 mg was given preoperatively per d, and 200 mg per d after surgery until the day of discharge. Overall, the incidence of AF was reduced by more than 50% compared to controls, and there was a significant decrease in number of days of hospitalization and total hospital costs. As with any patient receiving amiodarone, caution should be used to ensure that sinus bradycardia or heart block does not develop in individuals susceptible to these adverse events. In patients who are given warfarin postoperatively after valve surgery, close monitoring of the INR is needed to avoid coagulopathy from developing from a warfarin-amiodarone interaction.

Implantable Defibrillators and Anti-arrhythmic Medications

The use of antifibrillatory agents in patients with implantable cardioverter defibrillators (ICDs) represents a unique problem. Many patients who have ICDs for ventricular arrhythmias require drugs for suppression of supraventricular arrhythmias. Antifibrillatory agents can have three major adverse effects on patients. First, these agents have the propensity to raise the defibrillation threshold. For example, a patient with a history of ischemic heart disease and CHF has a baseline defibrillation threshold of 15 J. This patient then develops symptomatic AF, and is placed on amiodarone because of the mortality-neutral effects in this patient population. Repeat defibrillation threshold testing

1 wk after starting amiodarone reveals that the defibrillator cannot reliably rescue the patient from ventricular fibrillation (VF), even at maximum energy. This patient then requires an insertion of a subcutaneous (SC) array lead system to modify the defibrillator and to reduce the defibrillation threshold to an acceptable level. An important exception is sotalol, which may actually lower the defibrillation threshold in some patients. The second major effect is that antifibrillatory agents can slow the rate of an individual's VT. In certain cases, this can result in the failure of the ICD to recognize VT, depending on how the rate detection criteria are programmed. Therefore, it is critical to perform a defibrillation threshold test, and possibly noninvasive programmed stimulation, whenever starting or changing an antifibrillatory agent in a patient. Finally, antifibrillatory agents can increase the pacing threshold in patients with implantable devices, and threshold checks should be undertaken, especially in patients with baseline-elevated thresholds *(105)*.

CONCLUSION

Anticoagulation is recommended for almost all patients presenting with AF. Rate control is essential to alleviate symptoms and prevent deterioration in cardiac function or clinical status. The decision to initiate antifibrillatory agents should be made on an individual case-by-case basis. When drugs are used to convert or suppress atrial arrhythmias, factors such as structural heart disease, comorbid diseases, drug metabolism and elimination, and drug-drug interactions must be considered to reduce the risk of proarrhythmia. Even when these factors are taken into account, medication side effects often limit the use of an individual agent. With the future availability of novel antifibrillatory agents, drug therapy may be safer and more easily tolerated. In highly symptomatic individuals who "fail" antifibrillatory agents and cannot tolerate rate control (with anticoagulation), consideration should be given to either ablation of the AV node and insertion of a permanent pacemaker or primary atrial flutter or fibrillation ablation.

REFERENCES

1. Stoddard MF, Pawking PR, Prince CK, and Ammash NM, et al. Left atrial appendage thrombus is not uncommon in patients with acute atrial fibrillation and a recent embolic event: a transesophageal echocardiographic study. JACC 1995;25:452–459.
2. Weigner N, Caulfield TA, Danias PG, Silverman DJ, and Manning WJ. Risk for clinical thromboembolism associated with conversion to sinus rhythm in patients with atrial fibrillation lasting less than 48 hours. Ann Intern Med 1997;126:615–620.
3. Botto GL et al. Atrial mechanical function after conversion of recent onset atrial fibrillation to sinus rhythm. PACE 1998;21:813 part II.
4. Abi-Samra F, et al. Would a stricter regimen of anticoagulation be effective in further reducing the risk of thromboembolic events following electrical cardioversion for atrial fibrillation? PACE 1998;21:930 Part II.
5. Manning WJ, Silverman DI, Keighley CS, Oettgen P, and Douglas PS. Transesophageal echocardiographically facilitated early cardioversion from atrial fibrillation using short-term anticoagulation: final results of a prospective 4.5 year study. JACC 1995;25:1354–1361.
5a. Klein AL, Grimm RA, Murray RD, Apperson-Hansen C, Asinger RW, Black IW, Davidoff R, Erbel R, Halperin JL, Orsinelli DA, Porter TR, Stoddard MF. The Assessment of Cardioversion Using Transesophageal Echocardiography Investigators. N Engl J Med 2001;344:1411–1420.
6. The Stroke Prevention in Atrial Fibrillation Investigators Committee on Echocardiography. Transesophageal Echocardiographic Correlates of Thromboembolism in High-Risk Patients with Nonvalvular Atrial Fibrillation. Ann Intern Med 1998;128:639–647.
7. Petersen P et al. Placebo controlled, randomized trial of warfarin and aspirin for prevention of

thromboembolic complications in chronic atrial fibrillation: the Copenhagen AFASAK study. Lancet 1989;1:175–178.

8. Stroke Prevention in Atrial Fibrillation Investigators. Stroke prevention in atrial fibrillation study: final results. Circulation 1991;84:527–539.

9. The Boston Area Anticoagulation Trial for Atrial Fibrillation Investigators (BAATAF). The effect of low-dose warfarin on the risk of stroke in patients with nonrheumatic atrial fibrillation. N Engl J Med 1990;323:1505–1511.

10. Connolly SJ, Laupacis A, Gent M, Roberts RS, Cairns JA, and Joyner C. Canadian Atrial Fibrillation Anticoagulation (CAFA) Study. JACC 1991;18:349–355.

11. Ezekowitz MD. Warfarin in the prevention of stroke associated with nonrheumatic atrial fibrillation. N Engl J Med 1992;327:1406–1412.

12. Investigators of 5 studies. Risk factors for stroke and efficacy of antithrombotic therapy in atrial fibrillation. Arch Intern Med 1994;154:1449–1457.

13. The SPAF III Writing Committee. Patients with nonvalvular atrial fibrillation at low risk of stroke during treatment with aspirin. JAMA 1998;279:1273–1279.

14. Singer DE, Hughes RA, Gregg DR, Sheehan MA, Oertel LB, Meraventano SW, et al. The effect of aspirin on the risk of stroke in patients with nonrheumatic atrial fibrillation: the BAATAF study. Am Heart J 1992;124:1567–1573.

15. Stroke Prevention in Atrial Fibrillation Investigators. Warfarin versus aspirin for prevention of thromboembolism in atrial fibrillation: stroke prevention in atrial fibrillation II study. Lancet 1994;343:687–691.

16. Black IW, et al. Thromboembolic risk of atrial flutter. JACC 1992;19:314A.

17. Irani WN, Brayburn PA, Afridi L. Prevalence of thrombus, spontaneous echo contrast, and atrial stunning in patients undergoing cardioversion of atrial Flutter. Circulation 1997;95:962–966.

18. Seidl K, Haper B, Schwick NG, Zellneu D, Zahn K, and Senges J. Risk of thromboembolic events in patients with atrial flutter. Am J Cardiol 1998;82:580–583.

19. Albers GW, Dalen JE, Laupacis A, Manning WJ, Petersen P, Singer DE. Antithrombotic Therapy in Atrial Fibrillation. Chest 2001;119:194S–206S.

20. Fenelon G, Wijns W, Andries E, and Brugada P. Tachycardiomyopathy: Mechanisms and Clinical Implications. PACE 1996;19:95–106.

21. Packer DL, Bardy GH, Worley SJ, Smith MS, Cobb FR, Coleman RE, et al. Tachycardia-induced cardiomyopathy: a reversible left ventricular dysfunction. Am J Cardiol 1986;57:563–570.

22. Blitzer M. Rhythm management in atrial fibrillation—with a primary emphasis on pharmacological therapy. Part 1. PACE 1998;21:590–602.

23. Channer KS, James MA, MacConnell T, and Kees JR. Beta-adrenoceptor blockers in atrial fibrillation: the importance of partial agonist activity. Br J Clin Pharmacol 1994;37:53–57.

24. Philips BG. Comparison of intravenous diltiazem and verapamil for the acute treatment of atrial fibrillation and atrial flutter. Pharmacotherapy 1997;17(6):1238–1245.

25. Grant AO. Mechanisms of atrial fibrillation and action of drugs used in its management. Am J Cardiol 1998;82:43N–49N.

26. Heywood JT, Graham B, Marais GE, and Jutzy KR. Effects of intravenous diltiazem on rapid atrial fibrillation accompanied by congestive heart failure. Am J Cardiol 1991;67:1150–1152.

27. Goldenberg IF, Lewis WR, Dias VC, Heywood JT, and Pedersen WK. Intravenous diltiazem for the treatment of patients with atrial fibrillation or flutter and moderate to severe congestive heart failure. Am J Cardiol 1994;74:884–889.

28. Kumar A. Intravenous amiodarone for therapy of atrial fibrillation and flutter in critically ill patients with severely depressed left ventricular function. South Med J 1996;89:779–785.

29. Hou ZY, Chang MS, Chen CY, Tu MS, Lin SL, Chiang HT, and Woosley RL. Acute treatment of recent-onset atrial fibrillation and flutter with a tailored dosing regimen of intravenous amiodarone. Eur Heart J 1995;16:521–528.

30. Roth A, Kaluski E, Felner S, Heller K, and Lanindo S. Clonidine for patients with rapid/atrial fibrillation. Ann Intern Med 1992;116:388–390.

31. Scardi S, Humar F, Pandullo C, and Poletti A. Oral clonidine for heart rate control in chronic atrial fibrillation. Lancet 1993;341:1211–1212.

32. The Cardiac Arrhythmia Suppression Trial Investigators. Preliminary report: effect of encainide and flecainide on mortality in a randomized trial of arrhythmia suppression after myocardial infarction. N Engl J Med 1989;321:406–413.

33. Coplen SE, Antman EM, Berlin JA, Hewitt P, and Chalmas TC. Efficacy and safety of quinidine therapy for maintenance of sinus rhythm after cardioversion. Circulation 1990;82:1106–1116.

34. Stroke Prevention in Atrial Fibrillation Investigators. Preliminary report of the stroke prevention in atrial fibrillation study. N Engl J Med 1990;322:863–868.

35. Antman EM. Maintaining sinus rhythm with antifibrillatory drugs in atrial fibrillation. Am J Cardiol 1996;78:67–72.

36. Flaker GC, Blackshear JL, McBride R, Kuonmal RA, Halperin JL, and Hart RG. Antiarrhythmic drug therapy and cardiac mortality in atrial fibrillation. JAC 1992;20:527–532.

37. Sir Thomas Lewis, in *Diseases of the Heart,* Macmillan and Co., 1933, 1st ed., p. 90.

37a.The Planning and Steering Committees of the AFFIRM study for the NHLBI AFFIRM investigators. Atrial fibrillation follow-up investigation of rhythm management—the AFFIRM study design. Am J Cardiol 1997;79:1198–1202.

38. Friedman PL and Stevenson WG. Proarrhythmia. Am J Cardiol 1998;82:50N–58N.

39. Reiffel JA. Impact of structural heart disease on the selection of class III antiarrhythmics for the prevention of atrial fibrillation and flutter. Am Heart J 1998;135:551–556.

40. Boriani G, Biffi M, Capucci A, Botto GL, Brottoni T, Rubino J, et al. Oral loading with propafenone: a placebo-controlled study in elderly and nonelderly patients with recent onset atrial fibrillation. PACE 1998;21:2465–2469.

41. Boriani G, Biffi M, Capucci A, Botto G, Brottoni T, Ongari M, et al. Conversion of recent-onset atrial fibrillation to sinus rhythm: effects of different drug protocols. PACE 1998;21:2470–2474.

42. Kochiadakis GE, Egaumenidis NE, Simantirakis EN, Marketov ME, Vorthenakis FJ, Mezilis NE, et al. Intravenous propafenone versus intravenous amiodarone in the management of atrial fibrillation of recent onset: a placebo-controlled study. PACE 1998;21:2475–2479.

43. Botto GL, Bonini W, Brottoni T, Espureo M, Cappelletti G, Lombardi R, et al. Randomized, crossover, controlled comparison of oral loading versus intravenous infusion of propafenone in recent-onset atrial fibrillation. PACE 1998;21:2480–2484.

44. Crijns HJ, Gosselink AT, and Lie KI. Propafenone versus disopyramide for maintenance of sinus rhythm after electrical cardioversion of chronic atrial fibrillation: a randomized, double-blind study. Cardiovasc Drugs Ther 1996;10:145–152.

45. Chimienti M, Cullen MT Jr., and Casadei G. Safety of flecainide versus propafenone for the long-term management of symptomatic paroxysmal supraventricular tachyarrhythmias. Eur Heart J 1995;16:1943–1951.

46. Azpitarte J, Alvarez M, Baun O, Garcia R, Moreno E, Martin F, et al. Value of single oral loading dose of propafenone in converting recent-onset atrial fibrillation. Eur Heart J 1997;18:1649–1654.

47. Steinbeck G, Remp T, and Hoffmann E. Effects of class I drugs on atrial fibrillation. JCE 1998;9:S104–S108.

48. Costeas C, Kassotis J, Blitzer M, and Keiffel JA. Rhythm management in atrial fibrillation—with a primary emphasis on pharmacological therapy: part 2. PACE 1998;21:742–752.

49. Kassotis J, Costens C, Blitzer M, and Keiffel JA. Rhythm management in atrial fibrillation—with a primary emphasis on pharmacologic therapy: part 3. PACE 1998;21:1133–1145.

50. Hopson JR, Buxton AE, Rinkenberger RL, Nademanee K, Heilman JM, and Kienzle MG. Safety and utility of flecainide acetate in the routine care of patients with supraventricular tachyarrhythmias: results of a multicenter trial. Am J Cardiol 1996;77:72A–82A.

51. Chimienti M, Cullen MT Jr., and Casadei G. Safety of long-term flecainide and propafenone in the management of patients with symptomatic paroxysmal atrial fibrillation: report from the flecainide and propafenone Italian study investigators. Am J Cardiol 1996;77:60A–75A.

52. Aliot E and Penjoy I. Comparison of the safety and efficacy of flecainide versus propafenone in hospital outpatients with symptomatic paroxysmal atrial fibrillation/flutter. Am J Cardiol 1996;77:66A–71A.

53. Boriani G, Biffi M, Capucci A, Botto GL, Brottoni T, Rubino I, et al. Oral propafenone to convert recent-onset atrial fibrillation in patients with and without underlying heart disease. Annals Int Med 1997;126:621–625.

54. Lee SH, Chen SA, Tai CT, Chiang CE, Wen ZE, Chen YJ, et al. Comparisons of oral propafenone and sotalol as an initial treatment in patients with symptomatic paroxysmal atrial fibrillation. Am J Cardiol 1997;79:905–908.

55. Kochiadakis GE, Isoumenidis NE, Marketov ME, Solomon ML, Kanoupakis EM, and Vardas, PE. Low-dose amiodarone versus sotalol for suppression of recurrent symptomatic atrial fibrillation. Am J Cardiol 1998;81:995–998.

56. Reisinger J, Gattevev E, Heinze G, Wiesinger K, Zeindlhofer E, Gottermeier M, et al. Prospective comparison of flecamide versus sotalol for immediate cardioversion of atrial fibrillation. Am J Cardiol 1998;81:1450–1454.

57. Bianconi L and Mennuni M. Comparison between propafenone and digoxin administered intravenously to patients with acute atrial fibrillation. Am J Cardiol 1998;82:584–588.

58. Donovan KD, Power BM, Hockings BE, Dobb GJ, and Lee KY. Intravenous flecainide versus amiodarone for recent-onset atrial fibrillation. Am J Cardiol 1995;75:693–697.

59. Sung RJ, Tan HL, Karagounis L, Honyok JJ, Falk R, Platia E, et al. Intravenous sotalol for the termination of supraventricular tachycardia and atrial fibrillation and flutter: a multicenter, randomized, double-blind, placebo-controlled study. Am Heart J 1995;129:739–748.

60. Naccarelli GV, Dorian P, Hohnloser SH, and Coumel P. Prospective comparison of flecainide versus quinidine for the treatment of paroxysmal atrial fibrillation/flutter. Am J Cardiol 1996;77:53A–59A.

61. Ferreira E, Sunderji R, and Gin K. Is oral sotalol effective in converting atrial fibrillation to sinus rhythm?. Pharmacotherapy 1997;17:1233–1237.

62. Galve E, Rius T, Ballester R, Artazn MA, Arnau JM, Garcia-Vovado P, et al. Intravenous amiodarone in treatment of recent-onset atrial fibrillation: results of a randomized controlled study. JACC 1996; 27:1079–1082.

63. Kochiadakis GE, Joumenidis NE, Solomov MC, Kaleboubas MD, Chlouverakis GJ, and Vardas PE. Efficacy of amiodarone for the termination of persistent atrial fibrillation. Am J Cardiol 1999;83:58–61.

64. Kochiadakis GE, Joumenidis NE, Solomov MC, Kaleboubas MD, Chlouverakis GJ, and Vardas PE. Amiodarone versus propafenone for conversion of chronic atrial fibrillation: results of a randomized, controlled study. JACC 1999;33:966–971.

65. Tieleman RG, Gosselink AT, Crijns HJ, van Gelder JC, Van den Berg MP, de Kom PJ et al. Efficacy, safety, and determinants of conversion of atrial fibrillation and flutter with oral amiodarone. Am J Cardiol 1997;79:53–57.

66. Derin NZ et al. The efficacy of intravenous amiodarone for the conversion of chronic atrial fibrillation. Arch Intern Med 1996;156:49–53.

67. Reimold SC, Maisel WH, and Antman EM. Propafenone for the treatment of supraventricular tachycardia and atrial fibrillation: a meta-analysis. Am J Cardiol 1998;82:66N–71N.

68. Rae AP. Placebo-controlled evaluations of propafenone for atrial tachyarrhythmias. Am J Cardiol 1998;82:59N–65N.

69. Ganau G and Lenzi T. Intravenous propafenone for converting recent onset atrial fibrillation in emergency departments: a randomized placebo-controlled multicenter trial. J Emerg Med 1998;16:383–387.

70. Kochiadakis GE, Igoumenidis NE, Solomov MC, Partheunkis FJ, Christakis-Hampsis MG, Chloverakis GJ, et al. Conversion of atrial fibrillation to sinus rhythm using acute intravenous procainamide infusion. Cardiovasc Drugs Ther 1998;12:75–81.

71. Volgman AS, Corberry PA, Stambler B, Lewis WR, Dunn GH, Perry KT, et al. Conversion efficacy and safety of intravenous ibutilide compared with intravenous procainamide in patients with atrial flutter or fibrillation. JACC 1998;31:1414–1419.

72. Stambler BS, Wood MA, Ellenbogen KA, Perry KT, Wakefield LK, and VanderLugt JT. Efficacy and safety of repeated intravenous doses of ibutilide for rapid conversion of atrial flutter or fibrillation. Circulation 1996;94:1613–1621.

73. Stambler BS, Wood MA, and Ellenbogen KA. Antiarrhythmic actions of intravenous ibutilide compared with procainamide during human atrial flutter and fibrillation. Circulation 1997;96:4298–4306.

74. Vos MA, Golitsyn SR, Staugl K, Kudn MY, Van Wijk LV, Harry JD, et al. Superiority of ibutilide (a new class III agent) over DL-sotalol in converting atrial flutter and atrial fibrillation. Heart 1998;79:568–575.

75. Lovecchio F, Berlin R, Brubacher JR, and Sholer JB. Hypertonic sodium bicarbonate in an acute flecainide overdose. Am J Emerg Med 1998;16:534–537.

76. Kerns W, English B, and Food M. Propafenone overdose. Ann Emerg Med 1994;24:98–103.

77. Obel OA and Camm AJ. The use of drugs for cardioversion of recent onset atrial fibrillation and flutter. Drugs Aging 1998;12:461–476.

78. Doval HC, Nul DR, Grancelli HO, Perrone SV, Bortman GR, and Curiel R. Randomized trial of low-dose amiodarone in severe congestive heart failure. Lancet 1994;344:493–498.

79. Cairns JA, Connolly SJ, Roberts R, and Gent M. Randomized trial of outcome after myocardial infarction in patients with frequent or repetitive ventricular premature depolarizations: CAMIAT. Lancet 1997;349:675–682.

80. Julian DG, Camm AJ, Fraugin G, Jruse MJ, Munoz A, Schwartz PJ, and Simon P. Randomized trial of effect of amiodarone on mortality in patients with left-ventricular dysfunction after recent myocardial infarction: EMIAT. Lancet 1997;349:667–674.

81. The CASCADE Investigators. Randomized Antiarrhythmic Drug Therapy in Survivors of Cardiac Arrest. Am J Cardiol 1993;72:280–287.

82. Amiodarone Trials Meta-Analysis Investigators. Effect of prophylactic amiodarone on mortality after acute myocardial infarction and in congestive heart failure: meta-analysis of individual data from 6500 patients in randomized trials. Lancet 1997;350:1417–1424.

82a. Roy D, Talajic M, Dorian P, et al. Amiodarone to prevent recurrences of atrial fibrillation. N Engl J Med 2000;342:913–920.

83. Jafari-Fesharaki M, et al. Adverse effects of amiodarone. PACE 1998;21:108–120.

84. Julian DG, Prescott RJ, Jackson FS, et al. Controlled trial of sotalol for one year after myocardial infarction. Lancet 1982;1:1142–1147.

85. Waldo AL, Camm JA, deRuyter H, et al. Effect of d-sotalol on mortality in patients with left ventricular dysfunction after recent and remote myocardial infarction. Lancet 1996;348:7–12.

86. Reiffel JA. Selecting an antiarrhythmic agent for atrial fibrillation should be a patient-specific, data-driven decision. Am J Cardiol 1998;82:72N–81N.

87. The DIAMOND Study Group. Dofetilide in patients with left ventricular dysfunction and either heart failure or acute myocardial infarction: rationale, design, and patient characteristics of the DIAMOND studies. Clin Cardiol 1997;20:704–710.

88. Torp-Pedersen C, Moller M, Bloch-Thomsen PE, Kober L, Sandoe E, Egstrup K, et al. Dofetilide in patients with congestive heart failure and left ventricular dysfunction. N Engl J Med 1999;341:857–865.

88a. Singh S, Zoble RG, Yellen L, Brodsky MA, Feld GK, Beck M, Billing CB, Jr. Efficacy and safety of oral dofetilide in converting to and maintaining sinus rhythm in patients with chronic atrial fibrillation or atrial flutter: The symptomatic atrial fibrillation investigative (SAFIRE-D) study. Circulation 2000;102:2385–90.

89. Falk RH, Pollak KA, Singh SN, Friedrich T. Intravenous dofetilide, a class III antiarrhythmic agent, for the termination of sustained atrial fibrillation or flutter. JACC 1997;29:385–390.

90. Teichman SL, Fisher JD, Matus JA, and Kim SG. Disopyramide-pyridostigmine: report of a beneficial drug interaction. J Cardiovasc Pharmacol 1985;7:108–113.

91. Teichman SL, Ferrick A, Kim SG, Matus JA, Wasje LE, and Fisher JD. Disopyramide-pyridostigmine interaction: selective reversal of anticholinergic symptoms with preservation of antiarrhythmic effect. JACC 1987;10:633–641.

92. Jung W, Manz M, and Luderitz B. Effects of antiarrhythmic drugs on defibrillation threshold in patients with the implantable cardioverter defibrillator. PACE 1992;15:645–648.

93. Oral H, Souza JJ, Michaud GF, Knight BP, Goya IR, Strickberger SA, et al. Facilitating transthoracic cardioversion of atrial fibrillation with ibutilide pretreatment. N Engl J Med 1999;340:1849–1854.

94. Lau CP and Lok NS. A comparison of transvenous atrial defibrillation of acute and chronic atrial fibrillation and the effect of intravenous sotalol on human atrial defibrillation threshold. PACE 1997;20:2442–2452.

95. Opolski G, Stanislawska J, Gorecki A, Swiecicka G, Toubicki A, and Kroska T. Amiodarone in restoration and maintenance of sinus rhythm in patients with chronic atrial fibrillation after unsuccessful direct-current cardioversion. Clin Cardiol 1997;20:337–340.

96. Prystowsky EN, Benson DW Jr., Fuster V, Hart KG, Kay GN, Myerburg RJ, et al. Management of patients with atrial fibrillation. Circulation 1996;93:1262–1277.

97. Channer KS, James MA, MacConnell T, and Kees JB. Beta-adrenoceptor blockers in atrial fibrillation: the importance of partial agonist activity. Br J Pharmacol 1994;37:53–57.

98. Almassi GH, Schowalter T, Nicolosi AC, Aggarwal A, Moritz TE, Henderson WG, et al. Atrial fibrillation after cardiac surgery. Ann Surg 1997;226:501–513.

99. Kowey PR, Taylor JE, Kinls SJ, and Mariuchok RA. Meta-analysis of the effectiveness of prophylactic drug therapy in preventing supraventricular arrhythmia early after coronary artery bypass grafting. Am J Cardiol 1992;69:963–965.

100. Andrews TC, Reimold SC, Berlin JA, and Antman EM. Prevention of supraventricular arrhythmias after coronary artery bypass surgery. Circulation 1991;84:III-236–III-244 (Suppl).

101. Parikka H, Toivonen L, Heikkila L, Vivtanen K, and Jnvinen A. Comparison of sotalol and metoprolol

in the prevention of atrial fibrillation after coronary artery bypass surgery. J Cardiovasc Pharmacol 1998;31:67–73.

102. Gomes JA, Ip J, Santoni-Rugiv F, Mehta D, Evgin A, Lansman S, et al. Oral d,l-sotalol reduces the incidence of postoperative atrial fibrillation in coronary artery bypass surgery patients: a randomized, double-blind, placebo-controlled study. JACC 1999;34:334–339.

103. Guarnieri T, Nolan S, Gottlieb SO, Dudek A, and Lowry DR. Intravenous amiodarone for the prevention of atrial fibrillation after open heart surgery: the amiodarone reduction in coronary heart (ARCH) trial. JACC 1999;34:343–347.

104. Daoud EG, Strickberger SA, Man KC, Goyal R, Deeb GM, Bolling SF, et al. Preoperative amiodarone as prophylaxis against atrial fibrillation after heart surgery. N Engl J Med 1997;337:1785–1791.

105. Brode SE, Schwartzman D, Cattans DJ, Gottlieb CD, and Marchlinski FE. ICD-antiarrhythmic drug and ICD-pacemaker interactions. Cardiovasc Electrophysiol 1997;8:830–842.

7

Nonpharmacologic Treatment of Atrial Fibrillation

Peter Gallagher, MD,
and J. Marcus Wharton, MD

INTRODUCTION

The prevalence of atrial fibrillation (AF) *(1)* has risen as the population of individuals over 60 years old has increased, fostering a growing need to develop better and more cost-effective means of controlling and preventing AF. Although pharmacological rate control, suppression of recurrent AF, and stroke prevention are the principal therapeutic strategies *(2)*, these approaches have significant limitations. Pharmacological control of the ventricular rate is achievable in most patients with AF; however, many patients may have rapid rates during portions of the day, particularly during exertion or stress *(3,4)*. If unrecognized and uncontrolled, these rapid ventricular rates may result in a tachycardia-induced cardiomyopathy over a period of months to years *(5)*. Pharmacologic approaches to maintain sinus rhythm in patients with AF are even less effective, with arrhythmia recurrence rates of approx 50% at 6–12 mo of follow-up, regardless of the antiarrhythmic drug used *(6–9)*. Pharmacologic maintenance of sinus rhythm may be considered a palliative rather than curative approach, with efficacy now determined as the median time to AF recurrence rather than the number of patients without recurrence, since the latter approaches zero in long-term follow-up *(2)*. All drugs are associated with the risk of serious and troubling side effects. With the atrioventricular (AV)-nodal-blocking agents and class I and III antiarrhythmic drugs, these side effects include

From: *Contemporary Cardiology: Management of Cardiac Arrhythmias*
Edited by: L. I. Ganz © Humana Press Inc., Totowa, NJ

Table 1
Nonpharmacologic Approaches to AF

Rate control	Restoration/maintenance of sinus rhythm
AV-junction ablation	DC cardioversion (e.g., biphasic external, intracardiac)
AV-junction modification	Single- and dual-site atrial pacing
	Implantable atrial defibrillator (IAD)
	Surgical ablation
	Focal and linear catheter ablation

fatigue, decreased exercise capacity, depression, symptomatic bradycardia, worsening heart failure, and, more rarely, organ toxicity. Amiodarone may have greater efficacy than other class I and III antiarrhythmic drugs (9), but is associated with higher rates of discontinuation—about 35% after several years—because of organ toxicity (10,11). Furthermore, all antiarrhythmic drugs have an associated risk of proarrhythmia, which may be life-threatening. Rates of proarrhythmia vary from 1–4%, depending upon the specific class I or III antiarrhythmic drug used and the associated patient risk factors related to that drug (2,6–9). Even amiodarone may have up to a 1.5% risk of serious proarrhythmia, mostly related to profound bradycardia (10,11). Class I and III anti-arrhythmic drugs are used only rarely during pregnancy because of their uncertain teratogenic effects. In addition, class I and III antiarrhythmic drugs are expensive, with current costs in excess of $100 per mo even with generic drugs. Cost and other factors limit compliance, which in turn limits efficacy. Therefore, alternatives to antiarrhythmic drug approaches or methods to reduce dosage and side effects are greatly needed. Several nonpharmacological approaches to AF management have emerged as a result of the failure of medical approaches. These nonpharmacological approaches include techniques to control the rate and to maintain sinus rhythm (Table 1). This chapter addresses all of these nonpharmacological approaches. Curative radiofrequency catheter ablation is considered in additional detail in Chapter 8.

AV-NODAL MODIFICATION AND ABLATION

One of the principal goals of AF management is ventricular rate control. Rapid ventricular rates may cause palpitations, acute hemodynamic decompensation, angina, and, over a sufficient period of time, tachycardia-induced cardiomyopathy (5). The mainstay of rate control is medical therapy with calcium-channel blockers, beta-blockers, and/or digoxin (3,4). However, in a small percentage of patients, adequate rate control cannot be achieved. Much more commonly, these drugs are associated with troubling side effects that may decrease quality of life and activity levels. As an alternative to pharmacological therapy, rate control may be achieved by AV-junction ablation or modification.

The technique of AV-junction ablation involves creating complete heart block by ablating the distal AV node, and requires implanting a permanent pacemaker for ventric-ular rate support. If AF is chronic, a single-chamber ventricular pacing (VVIR) pace-maker is implanted; if AF is paroxysmal, a physiologic pacing (DDDR) pacemaker with mode-switching capability is used. After an AV-junction ablation, AV-nodal blockers can be stopped, but class I and III antiarrhythmic drugs may need to be

Table 2
**Prospective Comparison of Changes in Symptom Scores, Quality of Life Indices, and
Development of Persistent AF with AV-Junction Ablation and Dual-Chamber Pacing vs
Antiarrhythmic Drug Treatment in Patients with Paroxysmal AF**

	AVJ Ablation + DDDR	*Drugs*	*p Value*
Overall symptom	−48%	−4%	<0.005
Palpitations	−62%	−5%	<0.001
Dyspnea	−44%	−3%	<0.005
General well-being	+12%	+0.5%	<0.005
Patients with persistent AF	12/37 (32%)	0/19 (0%)	<0.01

Adapted from Marshall HJ, et al. Circulation 1999;99: 1587–1592 *(19)*.
Abbreviations: AVJ = atrioventricular junction; DDDR = dual-chamber, rate-responsive pacing mode.

continued if sinus rhythm is to be maintained *(12)*. Anticoagulation for stroke prevention is still required.

Multiple retrospective studies and a recently published meta-analysis have shown a dramatic decrease in symptoms and improvements in quality of life, exercise tolerance, and left ventricular function after AV-junction ablation *(13–16)*. Symptomatic improvement has also been specifically documented in the subset of patients with chronic AF and congestive heart failure (CHF) *(17)*. The loss of rapid rates—particularly during exertion or stress—and rate irregularity result in dramatic control of symptoms during rest and exertion. Although the effects on exercise performance have been variable, there have been general improvements in the appropriate programming of rate-response parameters on the pacemaker *(14,15)*. Improvement in quality of life after an AV-junction ablation is related to better rate control and a decreased usage of antiarrhythmic drugs with their inherent side effects. A recent report from the Mayo clinic confirmed that AV-junctional ablation and permanent pacing does not adversely affect patients' long-term survival *(18)*.

In general, patients with depressed left ventricular function prior to the procedure have an increase in ejection fraction over the next 6 mo following the procedure, presumably because of the resolution of a component of tachycardia-induced cardiomyopathy *(14,15)*. However, patients with normal ejection fractions prior to the procedure have no significant change. Unfortunately, the benefit of restoring adequate rate control may be offset by the impairment in ventricular function and worsening of mitral regurgitation induced by right ventricular (RV) pacing *(15)*.

A recent meta-analysis of 21 trials of ablation and pacing revealed improvements in quality of life, left ventricular function, and exercise duration as well as a decrease in health care utilization *(16)*. Only a limited number of prospective, controlled trials regarding the utility of AV-junction ablation and pacing are available *(12,17,19)*. Controlled, randomized trials comparing AV-junction ablation with no antiarrhythmic drug therapy to medical therapy for patients with paroxysmal AF have shown that AV-junction ablation and pacing were associated with a decrease in symptoms of palpitations, chest pain, exertional dyspnea, and fatigue, and improved quality of life *(12,17,19)* (Table 2). However, the withdrawal of antiarrhythmic drugs was associated with a greater probability of developing chronic AF. Thus, when sinus rhythm is desired for patients with paroxysmal or persistent AF undergoing AV-junction ablation, class I or

III antiarrhythmic drugs will need to be continued, which may diminish some benefits seen in quality of life or associated symptoms.

The success rate for AV-junction ablation exceeds 95% *(12,14,17,18)*. Occasional recurrences after apparent successful ablation have been observed, and are amenable to repeat ablation attempts. Patients with AV junctions that cannot be easily ablated from the right atrial approach may be ablated from the left side of the septum via a retrograde aortic or trans-septal approach *(20)*. AV-junction ablation has an acceptably low risk of complications. Since the goal of the procedure is the creation of complete heart block, the patient will be pacemaker-dependent after the procedure. Most patients have been shown to have some type of either junctional or idioventricular escape rhythm after the procedure. In the Ablate and Pace Trial, 67% of patients had some type of escape rhythm after successful AV-junction ablation *(21)*. However, the average heart rate of these escape arrhythmias was 39 ± 10 beats per minute (BPM), and only 31% had a rate greater than 40 BPM. Thus after AV-junction ablation, patients should be considered to be truly pacemaker-dependent, and pacemaker function should be appropriately monitored during the follow-up.

Specific complications associated with AV-junction ablation rarely occur. Polymorphic ventricular tachycardia (PVT) may occur after the procedure *(22–24)*, and appears to be related to absolute or relative bradycardia (compared to the ventricular rate during AF). Pacing at relatively rapid rates for the first several months after the procedure appears to dramatically decrease this risk *(24)*. Another potential explanation involves changes in autonomic tone and action potential duration following AV-junction ablation *(25)*. Hamdan and colleagues recently demonstrated that AV-junction ablation and pacing at 60 BPM was associated with an increase in sympathetic nerve activity, which was attenuated by pacing at 90 BPM. Moreover, they found that potential cardiac action duration increases after AV-junction ablation. For all of these reasons, standard practice involves initially programming the pacemaker's lower rate limit to 90–100 BPM in patients who have been chronically tachycardic, and then decreasing the rate by approx 10 BPM every 2 wk, with a lower target rate of 70 BPM. Overall, the ablate-and-pace strategy does not seem to increase mortality in patients with AF *(18)*.

In rare instances, heart failure may be dramatically worsened, especially in patients with chronic AF and severe mitral regurgitation, where RV apical pacing may exacerbate the mitral regurgitation *(15)*. Right ventricular outflow tract or biventricular pacing may reduce this risk *(26)*.

When AF is poorly controlled on medical therapy, the AV-junction ablation procedure and placement of a permanent pacemaker offers a reliable, effective, and time-tested treatment. Potential candidates for this procedure include patients with symptomatic AF resulting from poor rate control despite medical treatment, intolerance to rate-controlling medications, rapid hemodynamic deterioration, syncope, or ischemia during AF episodes, and tachycardia-induced cardiomyopathy. In addition, AV-junction ablation should be considered for patients with complicating comorbid illnesses that limit medical therapy for AF. An excellent example of this latter indication includes severe chronic obstructive pulmonary disease (COPD) in which AF therapies are limited (digoxin is usually ineffective and beta-blockers are contraindicated) and beta-adrenergic agonist for bronchodilatation may increase the frequency of AF episodes and the ventricular rate during the episodes. In this situation, AV-junction ablation allows

Table 3
Prospective Comparison of AV-Junction Ablation and Pacemaker Placement to AV-Junction Modification

	AV junction ablation		AV junction modification	
	Before	6 mo	Before	6 mo
General QOL	3.2 ± 1.2	1.0 ± 0.8*	3.1 ± 1.1	1.7 ± 0.7*†
Symptom frequency	2.2 ± 1.2	0.7 ± 0.8*	2.3 ± 0.8	1.4 ± 0.9*†
Symptom score	12.9 ± 2.0	6.4 ± 1.7*	13.1 ± 2.1	9.0 ± 2.1*†
Palpitations	2.4 ± 0.9	0.5 ± 0.5*	2.3 ± 0.9	1.3 ± 0.7*†
Syncope	0.7 ± 0.5	0.2 ± 0.4*	0.8 ± 0.6	0.6 ± 0.5*†
Hospital admissions	2.5 ± 2.5	0.2 ± 0.5*	2.9 ± 3.5	0.3 ± 0.6*
ER visits	3.0 ± 3.8	0.3 ± 0.6*	2.9 ± 3.5	0.3 ± 0.6*
Anti-arrhythmic drugs	4.7 ± 3.2	0.3 ± 0.5*	5.4 ± 2.7	0.4 ± 0.5*

Adapted from Lee SH, et al. J Am Coll Cardiol 1998;31:637–644 *(28)*.
*$p < 0.05$ compared to baseline in same treatment group; †$p < 0.05$ compared to 6 mo follow-up for AV junction ablation group.
Abbreviations: QOL = quality of life; ER = emergency room.

discontinuation of AV-nodal-blocking agents, and bronchodilators can be used in the dosages needed for treatment of bronchospasm.

Modification (rather than complete destruction) of the AV junction is a recently developed alternative to AV-junction ablation, which can be used for the same indications. However, an AV-nodal modification procedure *may* circumvent the need for a permanent pacemaker. An AV-junction modification attempts to selectively damage the AV node to slow the ventricular rate during AF, thus eliminating or decreasing the need for AV-nodal-blocking drugs without causing complete heart block *(27,28)*. Similar to AV-junction ablation, the patient will continue to have AF, but in contrast to AV-junction ablation, the ventricular response remains irregular, and the disadvantages of permanent pacing is potentially eliminated. The targeted decrease in ventricular rate is <100 BPM in the baseline state and <120 BPM during adrenergic stimulation. The end point for AV-junction ablation (complete heart block) is easier to achieve, and success rates are higher than for AV-nodal modification *(29,30)*. Thus, the clinical success rate is generally higher with the former, with ineffective AV-junction modifications occurring in up to 25% of procedures *(28,29)*. Late recurrence of rapid rates requiring repeat ablation attempts is common, so patients need to be appropriately monitored several months after AV-junction modification to ensure that adequate rate control has indeed been obtained. In addition, in up to 20% of patients undergoing AV-junction modification, the procedure results in complete heart block, requiring permanent pacing either acutely or during follow-up *(27–30)*. Williamson et al. were able to show a significant decrease in heart rates and an improvement in left ventricular function and functional status after AV-nodal modification in patients with chronic AF *(28)*. In trials comparing AV-junction ablation and modification, both approaches resulted in symptomatic improvement, but this seemed to be more dramatic with AV-junction ablation *(30,31)* (Table 3). Hospital admissions, emergency room visits, and antiarrhythmic drug usage are decreased by both procedures *(31)*. Knight et al. demonstrated that AV-junction modification was more cost-effective than AV-junction ablation, even when the costs for repeat procedures and eventual permanent pacemaker implantation were included *(32)*. The decrease in cost was primarily explained by the fact that, even with the limitations of AV-junction modification, most patients still avoid a permanent pacemaker with its attendant cost.

ADJUNCTIVE ATRIAL PACING

Holter monitor recordings from patients with AF have revealed that episodes may be initiated by absolute or relative bradycardia, by postectopic pauses, and/or by increasing atrial ectopy *(33,34)*. However, the prevalence of bradycardia- or pause-dependent AF onset in patients with AF may be relatively low in untreated patients *(34)*. Regardless of the prevalence, relatively rapid atrial pacing may prevent bradycardia-dependent onsets for AF and overdrive suppress atrial ectopy *(34,35)*. In addition, relatively rapid atrial pacing rates may decrease the dispersion of atrial refractoriness which electrically stabilizes the atria and facilitate rate-dependent antiarrhythmic drug effects *(34,35)*. Thus, there are several reasons that pacing the atria at relatively rapid rates (60–80 BPM) or consistently faster than the underlying sinus rate could result in a decreased frequency of AF.

Previous retrospective studies and some prospective studies comparing single-chamber ventricular pacing (VVI) vs physiologic pacing (DDD or AAI) in patients with sick sinus syndrome (most of whom do not have AF) have suggested that physiologic pacing approaches decrease the likelihood of AF developing during long-term follow-up *(36–40)*. However, the retrospective trials are limited by a number of methodological flaws *(40)*. Only one prospective trial has shown a clinically significant benefit to physiologic pacing *(41,42)*. Other prospective trials have shown only modest benefits *(43)* or no advantage *(44,45)* (Fig. 1). These studies have not confirmed whether the decrease, if any, in AF is a result of a beneficial effect of physiologic pacing or the negative effects of ventricular pacing in facilitating the occurrence of AF. Ventricular pacing may cause manifest or occult pacemaker syndrome *(46)*, exacerbate mitral regurgitation *(15)*, and cause electrical and mechanical remodeling of the atria that facilitate the genesis of AF *(47)*.

Recent prospective trials targeting patients with AF have raised serious questions regarding the benefit of right atrial pacing for prevention of AF *(45,48)*. In the Atrial Pacing Periablation for Prevention of Atrial Fibrillation Trial, patients with planned AV-junction ablation had a dual-chamber pacemaker implanted 3 mo prior to ablation. Patients were randomized to continue their medical management of AF or to receive aggressive atrial pacing in addition to the medical therapy *(48)*. Recurrence rates of AF were identical in paced and nonpaced patients (Fig. 2), indicating no benefit when single-site pacing is used for AF suppression for patients with no bradycardia-pacing indication.

Several innovative pacing algorithms for the prevention of AF recurrences have been proposed. Overdrive atrial pacing simply involves pacing the atrium at a rate higher than would be typical. Consistent atrial pacing involves increasing the atrial rate in response to premature atrial contractions (PACs), in an effort to suppress atrial ectopy. Current clinical trials are addressing these algorithms. More sophisticated pacing prevention algorithms have been incorporated in the Medtronic Jewel AF 7250 atrial/ventricular defibrillator, although efficacy data are not yet available.

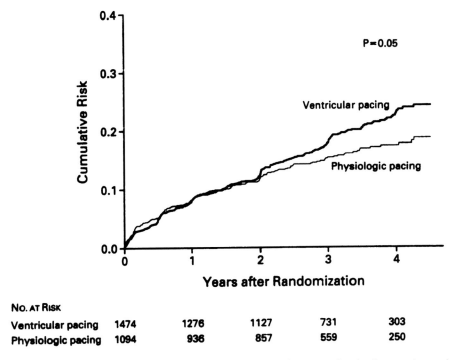

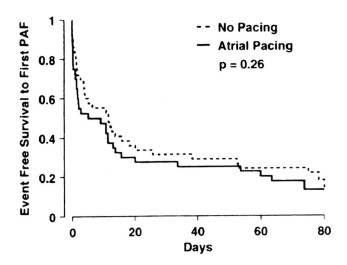

Fig. 1. Cumulative risk of AF in patients with sick sinus syndrome randomized to receive a single-chamber ventricular pacemaker (VVI) or an atrial-based pacemaker (either AAI or DDD) in the Canadian Trial of Physiological Pacing. Note that there is no difference in AF occurrence until after 2 yr of follow-up, at which point atrial-based pacing is associated with a small, decreased risk of AF. (Reproduced with permission from ref. *43*.)

Fig. 2. Survival free of recurrent AF in patients with AF and no indication for pacing randomized to DDD-R pacing or no pacing in the Atrial Pacing Periablation for Prevention of Atrial Fibrillation Trial. There is no difference in risk of recurrent AF in either group. (Reproduced with permission from ref. *48*.)

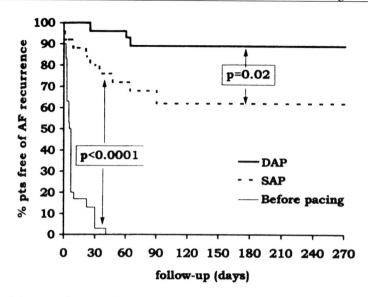

Fig. 3. Actuarial curves demonstrating the percentage of patients free of recurrent AF with dual-atrial-site pacing (DAP) and single-atrial-site pacing (SAP) from the high right atrium compared to the baseline before pacing. Note that both decrease the risk of recurrent atrial fibrillation, but that dual-site pacing is more effective in preventing AF than single-site pacing in this study. (Reproduced with permission from ref. *53a*.)

The site of pacing within the right atrium may also be important. In a retrospective study, Seidl et al. demonstrated that AF occurred in 28% of patients in whom the atrial lead was placed along the right atrial freewall, compared to only 5% when the lead was placed in the right atrial appendage *(49)*. More recent prospective studies have demonstrated a decreased incidence of AF with septal atrial pacing, presumably a result of the rapid and more simultaneous activation of both atria *(50)*. More uniform activation of both atria may decrease the dispersion of electrical refractoriness, decrease intra-atrial conduction, and decrease AV mechanical dys-synchrony, and concomitantly decrease compensatory sympathetic stimulation, all of which may prevent AF initiation or maintenance. Papageorgiou et al. demonstrated that there may be key zones of slow conduction along the tricuspid valve, inferior vena caval isthmus, and intra-atrial septum, which greatly facilitate AF maintenance *(50)*. More uniform activation of these regions may decrease the probability of creating conditions appropriate for intra-atrial reentry and AF initiation maintenance.

Another means of achieving more uniform atrial activation is to pace two atrial sites simultaneously. Dual-site atrial pacing has been clinically evaluated, either by pacing the right atrial appendage and distal coronary sinus (CS) or pacing the right atrial appendage and CS ostium. Preliminary data suggests that either form of dual-site pacing may decrease the risk of AF as compared to the unpaced state and, to a lesser extent, to single-site pacing (Fig. 3) *(51–53)*. This effect may be more dramatic for patients with marked intra-atrial conduction delay *(52)*. However, others have found a benefit to dual-site pacing, even for AF patients with no detectable profound atrial conduction delays *(53)*. Studies have not yet revealed which patient characteristics (if any) suggest a high rate of response to dual-site atrial pacing for suppression of AF in conjunction

Table 4
Factors Relevant to Direct Current Cardioversion Success

Procedural	*Patient-specific*
Waveform (biphasic vs monophasic)	Chronicity of AF
Pad/paddle position	Left atrial size
Electrode size	Body habitus
Energy	Hemodynamic/metabolic issues
Conductive medium	Mitral-valve disease
	Left ventricular dysfunction

with continued antiarrhythmic drug therapy. Multicenter prospective, randomized trials DAPPAF (dual-atrial vs single-atrial) and SYNBIAPACE (dual-atrial vs single-atrial vs no atrial) are currently being performed to further address the preventative role of multi-site pacing in larger patient populations with AF *(54,55)*. However, given the uncertainties surrounding adjunctive pacing for AF suppression, studies should still be considered investigational unless the patient has an established indication for pacemaker insertion.

Atrial fibrillation may occur in up to 40% of patients after open-heart surgery. Temporary single- or dual-site pacing using epicardial wires placed at the time of open-heart surgery may also be useful for prevention of postoperative AF. However, the results of published studies to date are conflicting, with some showing no benefit to pacing and some showing benefit only with dual-site or with single-site pacing *(56–60)*.

DIRECT CURRENT CARDIOVERSION

Direct current (DC) cardioversion, initially introduced by Lown and colleagues for AF in the early 1960s, remains the most effective means of restoring sinus rhythm *(61)*. DC cardioversion is generally performed using transient intravenous (iv) deep sedation or general anesthesia. Success rates for external cardioversion using standard monophasic energies up to 360 J have varied. Lown's initial series reported a success rate of 89% *(62)*, but more recent series have typically reported success rates of 80% or less *(63)*. One of the problems with external cardioversion is that only about 4% of the delivered current passes through the heart *(64)*. For this reason, a number of related approaches have been developed, including internal cardioversion, intracardiac cardioversion, external cardioversion using sequential shocks, and pharmacologic pretreatment prior to cardioversion. The incorporation of biphasic waveforms in external defibrillators has markedly increased the efficacy of external cardioversion, limiting the necessity of these adjunctive techniques. The increased efficacy offered by biphasic external cardioversion and the option to cardiovert internally if necessary have changed the focus from whether or not sinus rhythm can be restored to whether sinus rhythm can be maintained.

A number of variables may affect the success of DC cardioversion, including both patient-specific and procedure-specific issues *(63)* (*see* Table 4). An anterior-posterior pad placement appears optimal; it remains uncertain whether the best initial choice is right anterior-left posterior or left anterior-left posterior. If the initial electrode position is unsuccessful, cardioversion can be reattempted following a change in electrode position. The need for an adequacy of anticoagulation should be considered in any patient undergoing cardioversion; this issue is explored in Chapter 6.

Just as a biphasic waveform markedly improved the ventricular defibrillation efficacy of implantable cardioverter defibrillators (ICD), biphasic cardioversion is more effective at restoring sinus rhythm than monophasic waveforms. In a randomized trial, Mittal and colleagues found that rectilinear biphasic shocks restored sinus rhythm in 94% of patients, compared to 79% of patients receiving damped sine-wave monophasic shocks *(65)*. This increased efficacy was noted even though the maximum biphasic shock was 170 J, compared with a maximum monophasic shock of 360 J.

Internal cardioversion refers to a high-energy discharge between an intracardiac electrode in the right atrium (cathode) and a skin electrode (anode). Internal cardioversion allows greater energy delivery directly to the atrial myocardium. Initial trials of internal atrial defibrillation were performed by discharging high-energy shocks (up to 360 J) between a relatively small surface area electrode in the right atrium and a skin-patch electrode in patients refractory to external cardioversion *(66,67)*. A randomized trial of 112 patients who had at least one prior failed cardioversion revealed a higher success rate with high-energy internal cardioversion than external cardioversion *(62)*. However, the utility of high-energy internal cardioversion was limited by the relatively high rate of complete heart block, and the need for deep sedation to block the pain associated with the procedure.

Many subsequent studies have reported success with low-energy intracardic cardioversion (<10 J) using high-surface-area electrode catheters placed in the right atrial appendage and either the CS or left pulmonary artery *(68–71)*. These catheter configurations allow the best current distribution between the two atria *(68)*.

Patients who are refractory to high-energy external cardioversion can be defibrillated with a couple of J internally using these electrode configurations *(68)*. Although internal defibrillation with a couple of joules is perceived to be painful by most patients *(68,71)*, mild—rather than deep—sedation is all that is required. There is a wide range of variability in pain perception of internal shocks, with a general increase in pain awareness as energy increases *(71)*. In general, patients with chronic AF or AF of longer duration require higher energies for cardioversion compared to patients with paroxysmal or short durations of AF *(71)*. This probably reflects another adverse remodeling effect caused by long durations of AF.

The present techniques for low-energy internal cardioversion require placement of relatively stiff electrophysiology catheters with multiple electrodes and cannulation of either the CS or left pulmonary artery, thus restricting this technique to trained interventionalists. However, soft balloon-flotation pulmonary-artery catheters with defibrillation electrode elements on the distal and proximal (right atrial) portion of the catheter are under clinical evaluation at this time, and should allow more widespread application of internal cardioversion *(72)* (Fig. 4). In the initial experience with the ALERT catheter (EP Medical, Inc., Budd Lake, NJ), sinus rhythm could be restored in 25 of 27 patients with a mean energy of 6.7 ± 4.5 J. The catheter is also capable of right atrial and ventricular pacing immediately after cardioversion, either for overdrive arterial pacing for prevention of post-shock AF or ventricular pacing for bradycardia *(72)*. Another application of internal cardioversion has been the development of temporary epicardial atrial electrodes applied to the left and right atrium at the time of cardiac

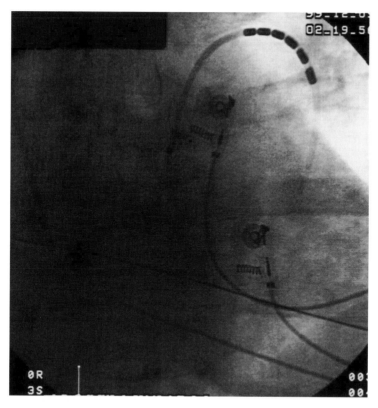

Fig. 4. Radiograph of a balloon flotation catheter with proximal and distal-shock electrode segments in the right atrium and left pulmonary artery used for internal cardioversion. The catheter is under clinical investigation at the present time.

surgery. Besides their use for temporary atrial pacing in the postoperative setting, low-energy cardioversion through the epicardial atrial electrodes successfully terminated AF in 80–89% of patients *(73,74)*. When no longer needed, the temporary electrodes could be removed through the skin by traction. Although potentially very useful for treatment of postoperative AF, these temporary pacing/defibrillation wires are still considered investigational in the United States.

Another alternative in patients refractory to standard external cardioversion is the use of two external defibrillators, either simultaneously or nearly simultaneously *(75,76)*. For this technique, two sets of adhesive skin pads are placed on the patient. Simultaneous delivery offers the obvious advantage of increasing the energy applied. Nearly simultaneous sequential delivery may be successful if the first shock lowers the chest wall impedance, so that more of the energy of the second shock penetrates to the myocardium. If the two discharges are not timed appropriately, there is a risk of inducing ventricular fibrillation (VF).

Although some antiarrhythmic drugs have anecdotally been associated with increasing the efficacy of cardioversion, few data are available. Oral and colleagues studied the use of the iv class III agent ibutilide as an adjunct to cardioversion using a monophasic waveform *(77)*. This randomized trial demonstrated that this drug significantly improved the efficacy of cardioversion, and significantly reduced the energy requirement for restoration of sinus rhythm. Three percent of patients who received ibutilide developed PVT requiring ventricular defibrillation.

As techniques to restore sinus rhythm have improved, it has become clear that in many patients, sinus rhythm can be transiently restored, with then an immediate or early recurrence of AF (ERAF). This may be caused by AF-induced atrial electrophysiologic remodeling *(78)*. Preliminary evidence suggests that verapamil pretreatment may attenuate the risk of ERAF *(79)*.

INTERNAL ATRIAL DEFIBRILLATORS

The success and safety of using low-energy internal cardioversion for AF led to the development of the implantable atrial defibrillator (IAD). The IAD could operate automatically in a manner similar to a ventricular defibrillator, but since AF is rarely an emergency, cardioversion could be delayed for hours, allowing for spontaneous termination of AF, an attempt at pharmacological conversion, and/or patient sedation. The typical candidate for an IAD is a patient with persistent and symptomatic AF occurring relatively infrequently despite treatment with antiarrhythmic medications. Patients with paroxysmal AF, which always spontaneously resolves, are not candidates because electrical cardioversion is not required. Two types of IADs have been developed: one is capable of atrial defibrillation only ("atrioverter"), whereas the other is capable of both atrial and ventricular defibrillation.

The Metrix system (InControl Inc., Redmond WA) was the first IAD tested in clinical trials on patients with persistent AF. It utilized defibrillation leads in the right atrial appendage and CS, and had a ventricular sensing/pacing lead in the right ventricle. In an international multicenter trial, the Metrix system with a maximum output of 6 J, was able to achieve sinus rhythm in 96% of patients *(80)*. However, 27% had an ERAF within minutes of cardioversion, and approximately one-half of the patients required either iv antiarrhythmic drug therapy, repeat internal cardioversion, or external cardioversion. The overall success rate of the atrial defibrillator with and without antiarrhythmic drugs was reported as 86%, but some patients required as many as 8 shocks to treat episodes of recurrence *(80)*. There were no reports of induced ventricular arrhythmias in this trial. The Metrix IAD recognized AF with a very high sensitivity and high specificity, and no inappropriate shocks were delivered. The internal cardioversion was generally well-tolerated by the patients, with only mild sedation required for most cases *(80)*. Although the Metrix IAD has been shown to be effective and safe in appropriately selected patients, it will not be made commercially available in the United States because of the concern that inappropriate timing of an atrial defibrillation shock could induce VF.

Because of this concern, the alternative design of the combined atrial and ventricular defibrillator has gained broader acceptance. These systems usually use a lead system identicial to that of the simpler ventricular defibrillator—typical shocking surfaces including leads in the right ventricle and right atrium and the defibrillator canister in the left pectoral region. An additional CS defibrillation electrode can also be placed if desired to lower the atrial defibrillator threshold. The Jewel AF (model 7250, Medtronic Inc., Minneapolis, MN) is the first of this type of IAD to have undergone clinical testing (Fig. 5). It was originally approved by the FDA for patients with ventricular

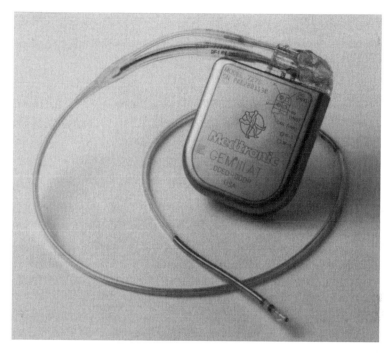

Fig. 5. The GEM III AT IAD system, which is an improved version of the JEWEL AF device. (Courtesy of Medtronic; Inc., Minneapolis, MN.)

tachycardia (VT) or VF who also have—or are at risk for—AF or other atrial tachyar-rhythmias. In April of 2001, this device was approved for the treatment of patients with AF in the absence of ventricular tachyarrhythmias, the so-called "AF only" indica-tion. Unlike a sole atrial defibrillator, the combined atrial and ventricular defibrillator can provide multiple levels of tiered and preventative therapy. As with a ventricular defibrillator, it can provide antitachycardia pacing (ATP) and low- and high-energy shocks for the treatment of VT and VF. If an inappropriately timed atrial defibrillation shock induces VF, then the device could rescue the patients from this potentially lethal complication. Three therapies for atrial tachyarrhythmias are available: ATP, 50-Hz-burst pacing, and cardioversion (shock). Although significant efficacy of overdrive pacing was expected in atrial flutter and other organized atrial tachyarrhythmias, 50-Hz pacing terminated 18% of episodes classified by the device as AF *(81)*. This finding may indicate that AF frequently begins with organized atrial tachyarrhythmias, which are susceptible to pace termination if delivered very early. The Jewel AF was reported to terminate organized atrial tachyarrhythmias with ATP or high-frequency-burst pace in over 85% of the detected atrial tachyarrhythmias *(82)*. This may dramatically reduce the number of shocks a patient receives over time. First-shock cardioversion efficacy was 91%, although ERAF occurred within 1 min of 20% of episodes *(81)*.

Atrial shock therapies may be programmed in three modes: automatic (as in ventricu-lar ICDs), timed (to delay a shock for AF until a programmed time, typically during sleep), or patient-activated using a separate activator device. The nonautomatic modes have dominated, both because of patient preference and to allow episodes an opportunity to convert simultaneously. Lastly, the device has dual-chamber pacemaker capability, and importantly, can utilize pacing algorithms that may be useful for prevention of AF, again potentially limiting the frequency of painful shocks. Because the atrial/ventricular defibrillator has ventricular defibrillation capabilities, it may allow higher dosing of antiarrhythmic drugs and use of the atrial defibrillator in high-risk patients, such as patients with heart failure, cardiac disease, and ventricular arrhythmias, all of whom were excluded in trials with the Metrix IAD. Among 146 patients implanted for AF only with the Jewel AF device, the mean atrial defibrillation threshold was 6.8 J. Symptom scores and quality of life improved over the course of the trial *(81)*.

An interesting inference regarding pathophysiology has been gleaned from the follow-up of patients implanted with either the Metrix or Jewel AF device. There is a subset of patients in whom the frequency and duration of AF episodes, or "AF burden," decreases with time. The explanation of this is a reverse remodeling effect of sinus rhythm: just as AF is accompanied by atrial electrophysiologic remodeling which makes the atria more conducive to maintaining AF, restoration and maintenance of sinus rhythm fosters reversal of these changes. It remains to be seen how complete this remodeling can be, and how to select refractory AF patients for whom aggressive efforts to maintain sinus rhythm will ultimately be successful.

Finally, an unexpected benefit has been noted in a significant proportion of patients who received the Jewel AF device in the "AF only" trial. Although patients had no history of a sustained ventricular tachyarrhythmia prior to implant, 11 of the 144 patients in the trial (7.6%) had a total of 67 spontaneous episodes of VT or VF during follow-up *(81)*. Of these, 10 episodes reverted spontaneously, and 57 (85%) were successfully treated by the device. This relatively high incidence of ventricular tachyarrhythmias during follow-up probably stems from the fact that thus far, the device has been implanted primarily in patients with significant structural heart disease.

Although the IAD appears to be efficacious and safe in the selected patients from initial studies *(82,83)*, the limitations of the IADs include pain from atrial cardioversion, inappropriate shocks from lead damage, dislodgment, or oversensing, early recurrence of AF after a shock resulting in multiple shocks, and the high cost. However, the pain associated with shocks is probably the most important factor limiting the widespread use of IADs. Since patients usually do not tolerate frequent shocks, the device is limited to patients with relatively rare episodes of persistent AF.

SURGICAL THERAPY OF AF

The first nonpharmacologic attempts to ameliorate symptoms and reduce AF recurrence rates were cardiac surgical procedures. In the 1960s, cryoablation of the AV junction via thoracotomy was performed to control rapid ventricular rates in drug-refractory AF. This was replaced by catheter DC shock ablation (fulguration) in the 1980s *(84)*, and by radiofrequency ablation or modification in the 1990s *(12,14,16)*. In the 1980s, various novel surgical approaches were tried, including left atrial isolation and Corridor procedures *(85,86)*. For left atrial isolation, the left atrium was incised along the atrial septum and reconnected, electrically isolating the left atrium from the right atrium *(85)*. However, this resulted in asystole or chronic AF in the left atrium and loss of left atrial-left ventricular synchrony. For the Corridor procedure, a channel of right atrial myocardium was incised between the sinus node and the AV node, allowing sinus nodal activity to drive ventricular activation *(86)*. However, both the

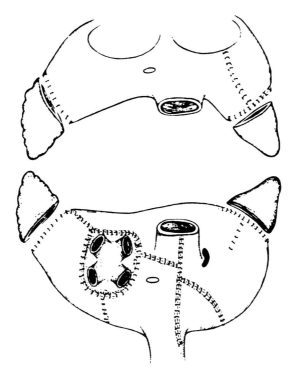

Fig. 6. Diagram of the incisions made for the surgical Maze III operation. (Reproduced with permission from ref. *90a.*)

right and left atria outside of the corridor remained in AF, and AV synchrony was not maintained. Although these surgical procedures improved subsequent quality of life, they were at best palliative procedures with no significant benefit—and certainly greater risks—than transcatheter AV-junction ablation.

Cox described the first curative approach for AF, the Maze procedure, in 1987 *(87,88)*. This surgical procedure uses extensive right and left atriotomies, in combination with cryoablation, to create channels which direct the initial atrial impulse from the sinoatrial (SA) node toward the AV node and across the left atrium. All of the channels end in "blind alleys," so that the reentrant circuits required to generate AF cannot propagate because of the spatial restrictions imposed by the surgical boundaries *(87,88)*. Briefly, the atriotomies involve the superior vena cava (SVC), the right atrium and left atrium, isolation of the pulmonary veins, amputation of both atrial appendages, and cryoablation (Fig. 6). The location of the incisions allows for maintenance of sinus rhythm with intact right-to-left atrial conduction and atrioventricular synchrony. Since right and left atrial transport are restored, the risk of thromboembolism appears to be decreased *(89)*. The Maze procedure has been modified over the years to improve results and decrease risks, particularly those of sinus-node dysfunction and left-atrial mechanical dysfunction *(88)* (Table 5). The most recent version, the Maze III procedure, has a 90% success rate of restoring sinus rhythm *(88,90,90a)*.

The initial eight-year experience with 178 patients was reported by Cox et al. in 1996 *(90)*. The most common indications for the procedure were medically refractory AF, previous thromboembolic complications and drug intolerance. The operative mortal-

Table 5
Results and Complications with Consecutive Versions of the Surgical Maze Procedure

	Maze I (n = 32)	Maze II (n = 15)	Maze III (n = 143)
Successful	81%	79%	97%
Resting sinus tachycardia	13%	21%	6%
Blunted sinus response	88%	21%	4%
Pacemaker-implanted	56%	29%	22%
Normal RA/LA function	100%/73%	100%/64%	98%/92%
Operative mortality	0%	7%	2%
Major complications	14%	53%	3%

Adapted from Sundt TM, III, et al. Cardiol Clin 1997;15:739–748.
Abbreviations: RA = right atrial; LA = left atrial.

ity was 2.2%, in patients with significant cardiac and pulmonary comorbidities. Patients were not routinely anticoagulated postoperatively, and only one perioperative stroke was reported with two late transient ischemic attacks *(90)*. The Maze III procedure has been performed safely and successfully as an adjunctive procedure for patients undergoing mitral-valve repair/replacement *(91,92)*. Recently, simpler procedures have been shown to be highly effective for patients with chronic AF who are undergoing mitral-valve surgery *(93)*. One procedure requires only isolation of the pulmonary-vein ostia with two linear lesions—one septally and one laterally in the left atrium—to connect the pulmonary vein ostia to the mitral annulus, and a third lesion across the roof of the left atrium to connect the two superior pulmonary-vein ostia (Fig. 7). This upside-down "U" lesion can prevent recurrent AF in approx 70% of patients with chronic AF undergoing surgery *(93)*. Tuinenburg and colleagues performed an alternative procedure called the "Mini-Maze" procedure in 13 patients with AF (8 persistent) undergoing concomitant mitral-valve surgery *(94)*. The procedure consisted primarily of biatrial appendectomy, and pulmonary-vein isolation. Although biatrial appendectomy is unlikely to impact on the likelihood of AF during follow-up, it may reduce the risk of thromboembolism, as most left atrial thrombi are detected in the appendage. During follow-up, the maintenance of sinus rhythm was markedly improved, compared to a historical control group that had AF and mitral-valve surgery without a Mini-Maze procedure.

The current indications for surgical ablation procedures include patients who present reasonable operative risk and have medically refractory, symptomatic, paroxysmal, persistent, or permanent AF. The greatest limitation of surgical ablation procedures is the obvious fact that open-chest procedures are required, with their attendant morbidity and mortality. Thus, surgical ablation approaches have the greatest application for patients scheduled to undergo cardiac surgical procedures for other indications. At present, many advocate a limited left atrial maze-type procedure, with left atrial appendectomy, at the time of mitral-valve surgery.

CATHETER ABLATION OF ATRIAL FIBRILLATION

Catheter ablation is rapidly becoming an effective method to cure or palliate selected patients with AF. Two approaches have evolved. The first strategy involves trying to

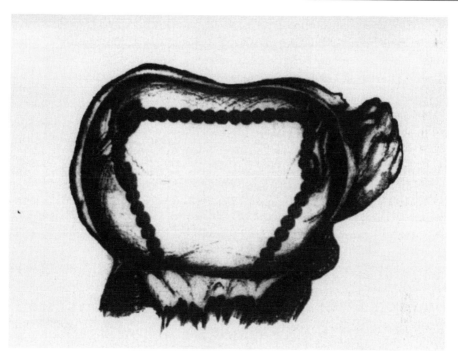

Fig. 7. Diagram of linear lesions made by intra-operative cryoablation for pulmonary-vein isolation in patients with chronic atrial fibrillation undergoing mitral valvular repair. (Reproduced with permission from ref. *93.*)

simulate the surgical maze procedure by trans-catheter placement of multiple left and right atrial linear lesions. The first study using catheter ablation to treat chronic AF was reported by Swartz et al. in 1994 *(95)*. A traditional ablation catheter was used to create a series of long, linear lesions in the right and left atria. AF was terminated and sinus rhythm was maintained in 87% of cases *(95,96)*. Others have subsequently reproduced this work, with success rates ranging from 0–89% *(95–100)*. Several investigators have shown that the left atrial lesion set is critical for curing these patients. In the study by Haissaguerre et al., right atrial-only lesions resulted in cure (no antiarrhythmic drug requirement) in only about 15% of patients; however, palliation (AF controlled with continued antiarrhythmic drugs) was achieved in approx 40% of patients *(97,99)*. Other studies used various other right atrial-only lesion sets, with similar results *(96,101,102)*. In the study by Haissaguerre et al., the addition of left atrial lesions, either with the other right atrial linear lesions or with an atrial flutter ablation only, resulted in cure rates of approx 50%, and 85% cure or palliation rates *(97,99)*. Thus, for catheter-based maze procedures to affect a cure of AF, the left atrium must be ablated in most cases. However, right atrial-only procedures may result in substantial rates of palliation. At the present time, the optimal locations for the lesion sets have not been determined.

Ablating consecutive points with a 4–5 mm tip catheter to create continuous linear lesions is technically difficult, time-consuming, and potentially dangerous. Right and left atrial maze procedures may take over more than 12 h to perform. In addition, the initial linear lesions that are created often have gaps of incompletely ablated tissue, and these gaps may result in recurrent AF or reentrant atrial tachycardias revolving around the linear lesions and through the gaps. Thus, second or even third procedures are often required to fill in these gaps to obtain optimal results. Extensive lesioning may also result in cardiac perforation and tamponade, thrombus formation and thrombo-embolic complications, pulmonary-vein stenosis, sinus-node dysfunction, and left or right atrial mechanical dysfunction. The rates of major complications in retrospective studies have generally been less than 18% *(96)*. However, ongoing prospective studies have demonstrated considerably higher rates of major complications, and even a small risk of death. Although catheter-based maze procedures were initially greeted with great enthusiasm, the technical difficulty and relatively high risk of major complications have made the procedure rare at the present time. Because of the risks to the patient, catheter-based maze procedures should still be considered investigational. New catheters designed to make transmural and continuous linear lesioning easier and safer are now being evaluated *(103)*.

It has long been known that focal atrial tachycardias could simulate AF in animal models *(104)*, and the AF in humans frequently begins with a regular rapid rhythm *(105)*. In 1994, Haissaguerre et al. localized and ablated focal initiators of AF in 3 patients *(106)*. Since that time, Haissaguerre, Chen, and their colleagues have rapidly expanded this observation to a large number of patients *(107–109)*. Premature atrial contractions (PACs) and rapid atrial tachycardias arising predominantly within the atrial muscular sleeve surrounding the pulmonary veins as they insert into the left atrium may generate AF in susceptible patients (Fig. 8). If the site of origin of these initiating arrhythmias can be localized and ablated, then AF can be cured. However, this approach required frequent spontaneous atrial ectopy to facilitate localization of the AF initiators. Given the observation that most (>70%) of the initiators arise from the pulmonary-vein musculature *(107–109)* (Fig. 9), approaches to disconnect the atrial myocardium of the pulmonary veins from the left atrium have evolved to provide an empiric anatomic ablation approach in patients without frequent atrial ectopy *(110)*. Both mapping guided (directed) and empiric pulmonary-vein isolation procedures have current success rates exceeding 70% *(107–110)*. Rates of palliation and cure exceed 90% in appropriately selected patients. Patients who are most likely to benefit from the procedure include patients with paroxysmal or persistent (but not chronic) AF with minimal or no structural heart disease. Given the excellent long-term results in these patients, focal AF ablation approaches have become a reasonable therapeutic option when medical approaches have failed. Patients with chronic AF and extensive cardiac disease may still benefit *(111)*—usually in a palliative rather than curative fashion—from a focal AF ablation procedure, but data are still limited and this approach is probably investigational at this time.

Guided focal AF ablation and pulmonary-vein isolation procedures have success rates considerably less than ablation of other SVTs. This may be a result of the inability to ablate the identified sites of AF initiation, or the failure to identify all the sites responsible for AF initiation. Since up to 30% of triggering sites may occur outside of the pulmonary veins, empirical pulmonary-vein isolation procedures do not affect these individuals. In addition, significant pulmonary-vein stenosis may occur in 1–3% of cases and result in significant dyspnea or hemoptysis *(107–110)*. Lesser degrees of asymptomatic pulmonary-vein stenosis may occur in up to 40% of patients *(108)*. Although these less severe pulmonary-vein stenoses do not result in symptoms, their

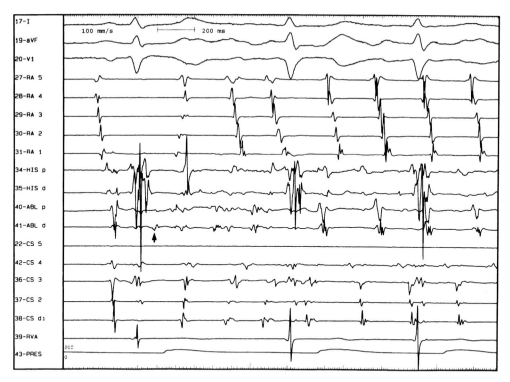

Fig. 8. Intracardiac recordings during the onset of AF from the left upper pulmonary vein. Shown are surface electrocardiographic leads I, aVF, and V$_1$ and multiple intracardiac recordings from the right atrium (RA), His bundle region (HBE), coronary sinus (CS), ablation catheter within the left upper pulmonary vein, and the right ventricular apex (RVA). The first atrial activation is sinus rhythm, followed by ventricular activation. Shortly after the end of the QRS complex, an atrial premature complex (arrow) originates at the site recorded by the distal (d) electrode of the ablation catheter. This premature atrial contraction (PAC) (arrow) initiates AF.

long-term consequences are unknown. In particular, it is not known if these subclinical stenoses may progress and result in occlusion and pulmonary venous hypertension over the years. In cases with symptomatic pulmonary-vein stenosis after ablation, percutaneous stenting may effectively restore pulmonary blood flow *(112)*. Newer ablation energies such as ultrasound *(113)* or cryoablation may be less likely to cause pulmonary-vein stenosis. Clearly, catheter ablation of AF holds enormous potential for the management of patients with refractory AF. As catheter design, energy technology, mapping technique, and knowledge of the underlying pathophysiology of AF improve, catheter ablation will become safer, more reliable, and faster to perform.

HYBRID APPROACHES

Although medical therapy remains the initial treatment of choice for AF, other nonmedical options are becoming available. As discussed here, despite the advances in nonpharmacological approaches, medical therapy must frequently be continued in conjunction with them. Thus, antiarrhythmic drugs must be continued after AV-junction ablation and pacing for patients with paroxysmal AF, if maintenance of sinus rhythm is desired, and they must be continued in most patients receiving IADs to limit the

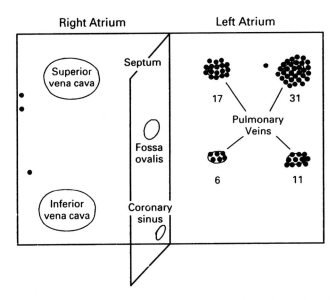

Fig. 9. Distribution of focal initiators of AF in the left and right atrium. (Reproduced with permission.)

frequency of painful shocks. Combined atrial-ventricular ICDs would offer more freedom in choosing and dosing antiarrhythmic drug therapy, because ventricular proarrhythmia can be treated with the ventricular defibrillator. These approaches can be considered "hybrid approaches," because they combine pharmacological and nonpharmacological therapies. Ablation approaches may also result in palliation of AF in conjunction with continued medical therapy. Hybrid ablation approaches include ablation of typical atrial flutter in patients with AF and antiarrhythmic drug-induced atrial flutter *(114)*, focal AF ablation in patients with persistent AF and early recurrence of AF after cardioversion (ERAF) *(111)*, and right-sided maze procedures *(96,97,101,102)*. Ablation approaches can also be used in patients with persistent AF to decrease the frequency of AF and to increase the acceptance of an IAD. The myriad possibilities of hybrid therapy are just beginning to be evaluated, but may provide many potential useful options in the future.

Substantial progress has been made in the last decade in providing a number of nonpharmacological options for treating AF. As it is recognized that AF is a chronic illness and that "atrial fibrillation begets atrial fibrillation," *(115)* efforts to maintain sinus rhythm will become more aggressive. The role of each of the nonpharmacological options discussed in this chapter relative to each other has not been determined, and the optimal patient groups for each approach have not been fully established. It is possible that some types of AF will respond to one approach and not another. However, further progress must be made in understanding the various pathogenetic factors responsible for the syndrome of AF before optimal nonpharmacological therapy can be prescribed.

REFERENCES

1. Bialy DLM, Schumacher DN, Steinman RT, Meissner MD. Hospitalization for arrhythmias in the United States: the importance of atrial fibrillation. J Am Coll Cardiol 1992;19 (Abst).

2. Falk RH. Atrial fibrillation. N Engl J Med 2001;344(14):1067–1078.
3. Farshi R, Kistner D, Sarma JSM, Longmate JA, Singh BN. Ventricular rate control in chronic atrial fibrillation during daily activity and programmed exercise: a crossover open-label study of five drug regimens. J Am Coll Cardiol 1999;33:304–310.
4. Roth A, Harrison E, Mitani G, Cohen J, Rabimtoola SH, Elkayam U. Efficacy and safety of medium and high-dose diltiazem alone and in combination with digoxin for control of heart rate at rest and during exercise in patients with chronic atrial fibrillation. Circulation 1986;73:316–324.
5. Rodriguez LM, Smeets JL, Xie B, deChillou C, Cheriex E, Pieters F, et al. Improvement in left ventricular function by ablation of atrioventricular nodal conduction in selected patients with lone atrial fibrillation. Am J Cardiol 1993;72:1137–1141.
6. Juul-Moller S, Edvardsson N, Rehnqvist-Ahlberg N. Sotalol versus quinidine for the maintenance of sinus rhythm after direct current conversion of atrial fibrillation. Circulation 1990;82:1932–1939.
7. Lee SH, Chen SA, Tai CT, Chiang CE, Wen ZC, Chen YJ, et al. Comparison of oral propafenone and sotalol as an initial treatment in patients with symptomatic atrial fibrillation. Am J Cardiol 1997;79:905–908.
8. Crijns HJ, Van Gelder IC, Van Gilst WH, Hillege H, Gosselink AM, Lie KI. Serial antiarrhythmic drug treatment to maintain sinus rhythm after electrical cardioversion for chronic atrial fibrillation or atrial flutter. Am J Cardiol 1991;68:335–341.
9. Roy D, Taljic M, Dorian P, Newman D, Couturier A, Yang C, et al. Amiodarone to prevent recurrence of atrial fibrillation. Canadian Trial of Atrial Fibrillation Investigators. N Engl J Med 2000;342:913–920.
10. Cairns JA, Connolly SJ, Roberts R, Gent M. Randomised trial of outcome after myocardial infarction in patients with frequent or repetitive ventricular premature depolarisations: CAMIAT. Canadian Amiodarone Myocardial Infarction Arrhythmia Trial Investigators. Lancet 1997;349:675–682.
11. Julian DG, Camm AJ, Frangin G, Janse MJ, Munoz A, Schwartz PJ, et al. Randomised trial of effect of amiodarone on mortality in patients with left-ventricular dysfunction after recent myocardial infarction: EMIAT. European Myocardial Infarct Amiodarone Trial. Lancet 1997;349:667–674.
12. Brignole M, Gianfranchi L, Menozzi C, Alboni P, Musso G, Bongiorni MG, et al. Assessment of atrioventricular junction ablation and DDDR mode-switching pacemaker versus pharmacological treatment in patients with severely symptomatic paroxysmal atrial fibrillation. A randomized controlled study. Circulation 1997;96:2617–2624.
13. Kay GN, Bubien RS, Epstein AE, Plumb VJ. Effect of catheter ablation of the atrioventricular junction on quality of life and exercise tolerance in paroxysmal atrial fibrillation. Am J Cardiol 1988;62:741–744.
14. Kay GN, Ellenbogen KA, Giudici M, Redfield MM, Jenkins LS, Mianu M, et al. The Ablate and Pace Trial: a prospective study of catheter ablation of the AV conduction system and permanent pacemaker implantation for treatment of atrial fibrillation. APT Investigators. J Intervention Cardiac Electrophysiol 1998;2:121–135.
15. Vanderheyden M, Goethals M, Anguera I, Nellens P, Andries E, Brugada J, et al. Hemodynamic deterioration following radiofrequency ablation of the atrioventricular conduction system. PACE 1997;20:2422–2428.
16. Wood MA, Brown-Mahoney C, Kay GN, Ellenbogen KA. Clinical outcomes after ablation and pacing therapy for atrial fibrillation: a meta-analysis. Circulation 2000;101:1138–1144.
17. Brignole M, Menozzi C, Gianfranchi L, Musso G, Mureddu R, Bottoni Lolli G. Assessment of atrioventricular junction ablation and VVIR pacemaker versus pharmacological treatment in patients with heart failure and chronic atrial fibrillation: a randomized, controlled study. Circulation 1998;98:953–960.
18. Ozcan C, Jahangir A, Friedman PA, et al. Long-term survival after ablation of the atrioventricular mode and implantation of a permanent pacemaker in patients with atrial fibrillation. N Engl J Med 2001;344:1043–1051.
19. Marshall HJ, Harris ZI, Griffith MJ, Holder RL, Gammage MD. Prospective, randomized study of ablation and pacing versus medical therapy for paroxysmal atrial fibrillation: effect of pacing mode and mode-switch algorithm. Circulation 1999;99:1587–1592.
20. Sousa J, el-Atassi R, Rosenheck S, Calkins H, Langberg J, Morady F. Radiofrequency catheter ablation of the atrioventricular junction from the left ventricle. Circulation 1991;84:567–571.
21. Curtiss AB, Kutalek SP, Prior M, Newhouse TT. Prevalence and characteristics of escape rhythms

after radiofrequency ablation of the atrioventricular junction: results from the registry for AV junction ablation and pacing in atrial fibrillation. Am Heart J 2000;139:122–125.

22. Peters RH, Wever EF, Hauer RN, Wittkampf FH, Robles de Medina EO. Bradycardia dependent QT prolongation and ventricular fibrillation following catheter ablation of the atrioventricular junction with radiofrequency energy. PACE 1994;17:108–112.

23. Bharati S, Scheinmann NM, Morady F, Hess DS, Lev M. Sudden death after catheter-induced atrioventricular junctional ablation. Chest 1985;88:883–889.

24. Geelen P, Brugada J, Andries E, Brugada P. Ventricular fibrillation and sudden death after radiofrequency catheter ablation of the atrioventricular junction. PACE 1997;20:343–348.

25. Hamdan MH, Page RL, Sheehan CJ, Zagrodzky JD. Increased sympathetic activity after atrioventricular junction ablation in patients with chronic atrial fibrillation. J Am Coll Cardiol 2000;36:151–158.

26. Cazeau S, Leclerq C, Levergne T, Walker S, Varma C, Linde C, et al. Effects of multisite biventricular pacing in patients with heart failure and intraventricular conduction delay. N Engl J Med 2001;344:873–880.

27. Feld GK, Fleck RP, Fujimura O, Prothro DL, Bahnson TD, Ibarra M. Control of rapid ventricular response by radiofrequency catheter modification of the atrioventricular node in patients with medically refractory atrial fibrillation. Circulation 1994;90:2299–2307.

28. Williamson BD, Man KC, Daoud E, Niebauer M, Strickberger SA, Morady F. Radiofrequency catheter modification of atrioventricular conduction to control the ventricular rate during atrial fibrillation. N Engl J Med 1994;331:910–917.

29. Feld GK. Radiofrequency catheter ablation versus modification of the AV node for control of rapid ventricular response in atrial fibrillation. J Cardiovasc Electrophysiol 1995;6:217–228.

30. Proclemer A, Della Bella P, Tondo C, Facchin D, Carbucicchio C, Riva Fioretti P. Radiofrequency ablation of atrioventricular junction and pacemaker implantation versus modulation of atrioventricular conduction in drug refractory atrial fibrillation. Am J Cardiol 1999;83:1437–1442.

31. Lee SH, Chen SA, Tai CT, Chiang CE, Wen ZC, Cheng JJ, et al. Comparisons of quality of life and cardiac performance after complete atrioventricular junction ablation and atrioventricular junction modification in patients with medically refractory atrial fibrillation. J Am Coll Cardiol 1998;31:637–644.

32. Knight BP, Weiss R, Bahu M, Souza J, Zivin A, Goyal R, et al. Cost comparison of radiofrequency modification and ablation of the atrioventricular junction in patients with chronic atrial fibrillation. Circulation 1997;96:1532–1536.

33. Coumel P. Cardiac arrhythmias and the autonomic nervous system. J Cardiovasc Electrophysiol 1993;4:338–355.

34. Murgatroyd F. Modes of onset of spontaneous episodes of atrial fibrillation: implications for the prevention of atrial fibrillation by pacing. In: Daubert JC, Prystowsky EN, Ripart A, eds. Prevention of Tachyarrhythmias with Cardiac Pacing. Futura Publishing Co., Inc., Armonk, NY, 1997;53–65.

35. Mehra R. How might pacing prevent atrial fibrillation? In: Murgatroyd FD, Camm AJ, eds. Nonpharmacological Management of Atrial Fibrillation. Futura Publishing Co., Inc., Armonk, NY, 1997;283–307.

36. Rosenqvist M, Brandt J, Schüller H. Long-term pacing in sinus node disease: effects of stimulation mode on cardiovascular morbidity and mortality. Am Heart J 1988;116:16–22.

37. Hesselson AB, Parsonnet V, Bernstein AD, Bonavita GJ. Deleterious effects of long-term single-chamber ventricular pacing in patients with sick sinus syndrome: the hidden benefits of dual-chamber pacing. J Am Coll Cardiol 1992;19:1542–1549.

38. Sgarbossa EB, Pinski SL, Maloney JD, Simmons TW, Wilkoff BL, Castle LW, et al. Chronic atrial fibrillation and stroke in paced patients with sick sinus syndrome. Relevance of clinical characteristics and pacing modality. Circulation 1993;88:1045–1053.

39. Connolly SJ, Kerr C, Gent M, Yusuf S. Dual-chamber versus ventricular pacing: critical appraisal of current data. Circulation 1996;94:578–583.

40. Lamas GA, Estes NM, III, Schneller S, Flaker GC. Does dual chamber pacing prevent atrial fibrillation? The need for a randomized controlled trial. PACE 1992;15:1109–1113.

41. Andersen HR, Thuesen L, Bagger JP, Vesterlund T, Thomsen PEB. Prospective randomized trial of atrial versus ventricular pacing in sick-sinus syndrome. Lancet 1994;344:1523–1528.

42. Andersen HR, Nielsen JC, Thomsen PEB, Thuesen L, Mortensen PT, Vesterlund T, et al. Long-term follow-up of patients from a randomized trial of atrial versus ventricular pacing for sick-sinus syndrome. Lancet 1997;350:1210–1216.

43. Connolly SJ, Kerr CR, Gent M, Roberts RS, Yusuf S, Gillis AM, et al. Effects of physiologic pacing versus ventricular pacing on the risk of stroke and death due to cardiovascular causes. Canadian Trial of Physiologic Pacing Investigators. N Engl J Med 2000;342:1385–1391.

44. Lamas GA, Orav EJ, Stambler BS, Ellenbogen KA, Sgarbossa EB, Huang SKS, et al. Pacemaker Selection in the Elderly Investigators, Quality of life and clinical outcomes in elderly patients treated with ventricular pacing compared with dual-chamber pacing. N Engl J Med 1998;338:1097–1104.

45. Wharton JM, Sorrentino R, Campbell P, Gonzalez-Zuelgaray J, Keating E, Curtis A, et al. PAC-A-TACH Investigators, Effect of pacing modality on atrial tachyarrhythmia recurrence in the tachycardia-bradycardia syndrome: preliminary results of the pacemaker atrial tachycardia trial. Circulation 1998;98:I–494 (Abstract).

46. Ellenbogen KA, Gilligan DM, Wood MA, Morillo C, Barold SS. The pacemaker syndrome—A matter of definition. Am J Cardiol 1997;79:1226–1229.

47. Sparks PB, Mond HG, Vohra JK, Jayaprakash S, Kalman JM. Electrical remodeling of the atria following loss of atrioventricular synchrony. A long-term study in humans. Circulation 1999;100:1894–1900.

48. Gillis AM, Wyse DG, Connolly SJ, Dubuc M, Philippon F, Yee R, et al. Atrial pacing periablation for prevention of paroxysmal atrial fibrillation. Circulation 1999;99:2553–2558.

49. Seidl K, Drogemuller K, Hauer B, Schwick N, Zahn R, Senges I. The relationship of atrial electrode position and atrial fibrillation in dual chamber pacing. Z Kardiol 1998;87:471–477.

50. Papageorgiou P, Anselme F, Kirchhof CJ, Monahan K, Rasmussen CAF, Epstein LM, et al. Coronary sinus pacing prevents induction of atrial fibrillation. Circulation 1997;96:1893–1898.

51. Saksena S, Prakash A, Hill M, Krol RB, Munsif AN, Mathew PP, et al. Prevention of recurrent atrial fibrillation with chronic dual-site right atrial pacing. J Am College Cardiol 1996;28:687–694.

52. Daubert C, Mabo P, Berder V. Arrhythmia prevention by permanent atrial resynchronization in advanced interatrial block. Eur Heart J 1990;11:237–242.

53. Saksena S, Delfaut P, Prakash A, Kaushik RR, Krol RB. Multisite electrode pacing for prevention of atrial fibrillation. J Cardiovasc Electrophysiol 1998;9:S155–S162.

53a. Delfaut P, Saksena S, Prakash A, Krol RB. Long-term outcome of patients with drug-refractory atrial flutter and fibrillation after single- and dual-site right atrial pacing for arrhythmia prevention. J Am Coll Cardiol 1998;32:1900–1908.

54. Fitts SM, Hill MR, Mehra R, Friedman P, Hammill S, Kay GN, et al. Design and implementation of the Dual Site Atrial Pacing to Prevent Atrial Fibrillation (DAPPAF) clinical trial. J Interv Card Electrophysiol 1998;2:139–144.

55. Sopher SM, Camm AJ. New trials in atrial fibrillation. J Cardiovasc Electrophysiol 1998;9 (Suppl. 8):S211–S215.

56. Kurz DJ, Naegeli B, Kunz M, Genoni M, Niederhauser U, Bertel O. Epicardial, biatrial synchronous pacing for prevention of atrial fibrillation after cardiac surgery. PACE 1999;22:721–726.

57. Gerstenfeld EP, Hill MR, French SN, Mehra R, Rofino K, Vander Salm TJ, et al. Evaluation of right atrial and biatrial temporary pacing for the prevention of atrial fibrillation after coronary artery bypass surgery. J Am Coll Cardiol 1999;33:1981–1988.

58. Chung MK, Augostini RS, Asher CR, Pool DP, Grady TA, Zikri M, et al. Ineffectiveness and potential proarrhythmia of atrial pacing for atrial fibrillation prevention after coronary artery bypass grafting. Ann Thorac Surg 2000;69:1057–1063.

59. Daoud EG, Dabir R, Archambeau M, Morady F, Strickberger SA. Randomized, double-blind trial of simultaneous right and left atrial epicardial pacing for prevention of post-open heart surgery atrial fibrillation. Circulation 2000;102:761–765.

60. Levy T, Fotopoulos G, Walker S, Rex S, Octave M, Paul V, et al. Randomized controlled study investigating the effect of biatrial pacing in prevention of atrial fibrillation after coronary artery bypass grafting. Circulation 2000;102:1382–1387.

61. Lown B. Electrical reversion of cardiac arrhythmias. Br Heart J 1967;29:469–489.

62. Lown B, Perlroth MG, Kaidbey S, Abe T, Harken DE. Cardioversion of atrial fibrillation: a report on the treatment of 65 episodes in 50 patients. New Engl J Med 1963;269:325–331.

63. Ewy GA. Optimal technique for electrical cardioversion of atrial fibrillation. Circulation 1992;86:1645–1647.

64. Deale OC, Lerman BB. Intrathoracic current flow during transthoracic defibrillation in dogs. Transcardiac current fraction. Circ Res 1990;67:1405–1419.

65. Mittal S, Ayati S, Stein KM, Schwartzman D, et al. Transthoracic cardioversion of atrial fibrillation:

comparison of rectilinear biphasic versus damped sine wave monophasic shocks. Circulation 2000;101:1282–1287.

66. Kumagai K, Yamanouchi Y, Hiroki T, Arakawa K. Effects of transcatheter cardioversion on chronic lone atrial fibrillation. PACE 1991;14:1571–1575.

67. Levy S, Lauribe P, Dolla E, Kou W, Kadish A, Calkins H, et al. A randomized comparison of external and internal cardioversion of chronic atrial fibrillation. Circulation 1992;86:1415–1420.

68. Hillsley RE, Wharton JM. Implantable atrial defibrillators. J Cardiovasc Electrophysiology 1995;6:634–648.

69. Levy S, Ricard P, Gueunoun M, Yapo F, Trigano J, Manscouri C, et al. Low-energy cardioversion of spontaneous atrial fibrillation. Immediate and long-term results. Circulation 1997;96:253–259.

70. Schmitt C, Alt E, Plewan A, Ammer R, Leibig M, Karch M, et al. Low energy intracardiac cardioversion after failed conventional external cardioversion of atrial fibrillation. J Am Coll Cardiol 1996;28:994–999.

71. Levy S, Ricard P, Lau CP, Lok NS, Camm AJ, Murgatroyd FD, et al. Multicenter low energy transvenous atrial defibrillation (XAD) trial results in different subsets of atrial fibrillation. J Am Coll Cardiol 1997;29:750–755.

72. Plewan A, Valina C, Hermann R, Alt E. Initial experience with a new balloon-guided single lead catheter for internal cardioversion of atrial fibrillation and dual chamber pacing. PACE 1999;22:228–232.

73. Liebold A, Wahba A, Birnbaum DE. Low-energy cardioversion with epicardial wire electrodes: new treatment of atrial fibrillation after open heart surgery. Circulation 1998;98:883–886.

74. Kleine P, Blommaert D, van Nooten G, Blin O, Haisch G, Stoffelen W, et al. Multicenter results of TADpole heart wire system used to treat postoperative atrial fibrillation. Eur J Cardiothorac Surg 1999;15:525–526.

75. Saliba W, Juratli N, Chung MK, et al. Higher energy synchronized external direct current cardioversion for refractory atrial fibrillation. J Am Coll Cardiol 1999;34:2031–2034.

76. Bjerregaard P, El-Shafei A, Janosik DL, Schiller L, Quattromani A. Double external direct-current shocks for refractory atrial fibrillation. Am J Cardiol 1999;83:972–974.

77. Oral H, Souza JJ, Michaud GF, Knight BP, et al. Facilitating transthoracic cardioversion of atrial fibrillation with ibutilide pretreatment. N Engl J Med 1999;340:1849–1854.

78. Tieleman RG, Van Gelder I, Crijns HJGM, et al. Early recurrences of atrial fibrillation after electrical cardioversion: a result of fibrillation-induced electrical remodeling of the atria? Circulation 1998;31:167–173.

79. Daoud EG, Hummel JD, Augostini R, Williams R, Kalbfleisch SJ. Effect of verapamil on immediate recurrence of atrial fibrillation. J Cardiovasc Electrophys 2000;11:1231–1237.

80. Wellens HJ, Lau CP, Luderitz B, Akhtar M, Waldo AL, Camm AJ, et al. Atrioverter: an implantable device for the treatment of atrial fibrillation. Circulation 1998;98:1651–1656.

81. Jewel AF/AF-only Clinical Study, unpublished data, Medtronic, Inc.

82. Jung W, Wolpert C, Esmailzadeh B, Spehl S, Herwig S, Schumacher B, et al. Clinical experience with implantable atrial and combined atrioventricular defibrillators. J Intervent Cardiac Electrophysiol 2000;4 Suppl. 1:185–195.

83. Swerdlow CD, Schsls W, Dijkman B, Jung W, Sheth NV, Olson WH, et al. Detection of atrial fibrillation and flutter by a dual-chamber implantable cardioverter-defibrillator. For the Worldwide Jewel AF Investigators. Circulation 2000;101:878–885.

84. Scheinman MM, Morady F, Hess DS, Gonzalez R. Catheter-induced ablation of the atrioventricular junction to control refractory supraventricular arrhythmias. JAMA 1982;248:851–855.

85. Williams JM, Ungerleider RM, Lofland GK, Cox JL. Left atrial isolation. New technique for the treatment of supraventricular arrhythmias. J Thorac Cardiovasc Surg 1990;49:466–468.

86. Defauw JJ, Guiraudon GM, van Hemel NM, Vermeulen FE, Kingma JH, de Bakker JM. Surgical therapy of paroxysmal atrial fibrillation with the "corridor" operation. Ann Thorac Surg 1992;53:564–570.

87. Cox JL, Boineau JP, Schuessler RB, Kater KM, Lappas DG. Five-year experience with the maze procedure for atrial fibrillation. Ann Thorac Surg 1993;56:814–823.

88. Sundt TM, Camillo CJ, Cox JL. The maze procedure for cure of atrial fibrillation. Cardiol Clin 1997;15:739–748.

89. Cox JL, Ad N, Palazzo T. Impact of the maze procedure on the stroke rate in patients with atrial fibrillation. J Thorac Cardiovasc Surg 1999;118:833–840.

90. Cox JL, Schuessler RB, Lappas DG, Boineau JP. An 8 1/2-year clinical experience with surgery for atrial fibrillation. Ann Surg 1996;224:267–273.

91. Isobe F, Kawashima Y. The outcome and indications of the Cox maze III procedure for chronic atrial fibrillation with mitral valve-disease. J Thorac Cardiovasc Surg 1998;116:220–227.

92. Izumoto H, Kawazoe K, Kitahara H, Kamata J. Operative results after the Cox/maze procedure combined with a mitral valve operation. Ann Thorac Surg 1998;66:800–804.

93. Gaita F, Gallotti R, Calo L, Manasse E, Riccardi R, Garberoglio L, et al. Limited posterior left atrial cryoablation in patients with chronic atrial fibrillation undergoing valvular heart surgery. J Am Coll Cardiol 2000;36:159–166.

94. Tuinenburg AE, van Gelder IC, Tieleman RG, Grandjean JG, et al. Mini-maze suffices as adjunct to mitral valve surgery in patients with preoperative atrial fibrillation. J Cardiovasc Electrophysiol 2000;960–967.

95. Swartz JF, Pelersels G, Silvers J, Patten L, Cervantez D. A catheter-based curative approach to atrial fibrillation in humans. Circulation 1994;90 (Suppl 1):I–335.

96. Cannom DS. Atrial fibrillation: nonpharmacologic approaches: An evolving era. Am J Cardiol 2000;85:25D–35D.

97. Haissaguerre M, Jais P, Shah DC, Gencel L, Pradeau V, Garrigues S, et al. Right and left atrial radiofrequency catheter therapy of paroxysmal atrial fibrillation. J Cardiovasc Electrophysiol 1996;7:1132–1144.

98. Maloney JD, Milner L, Barold S, Czerska B, Markel M. Two-staged biatrial linear and focal ablation to restore sinus rhythm in patients with refractory chronic atrial fibrillation: procedure experiences and follow-up beyond 1 year. PACE 1998;21:2527–2532.

99. Jais P, Shah DC, Haissaguerre M, Takahashi A, Lavergne T, Hocini M, et al. Efficacy and safety of septal and left-atrial linear ablation for atrial fibrillation. Am J Cardiol 1999;84 (9A):139R–146R.

100. Ernst S, Schluter M, Ouyang F, Khanedani A, Cappato R, Hebe J, et al. Modification of the substrate for maintenance of idiopathic human atrial fibrillation: Efficacy of radiofrequency ablation using nonfluoroscopic catheter guidance. Circulation 1999;100:2085–2092.

101. Gaita F, Riccardi R, Calo L, Scaglione M, Garberoglio L, Antolini R, et al. Atrial mapping and radiofrequency catheter ablation in patients with idiopathic atrial fibrillation. Electrophysiological findings and ablation results. Circulation 1998;97:2136–2145.

102. Natale A, Leonelli F, Beheiry S, Newby K, Pisano E, Potenza D, et al. Catheter ablation approach on the right side only for paroxysmal atrial fibrillation therapy: long-term results. PACE 2000;23:224–233.

103. Calkins J, Hall J, Ellenbogen K, Walcott G, Sherman M, Bowe W, et al. A new system for catheter ablation of atrial fibrillation. Am J Cardiol 1999;83:227D–236D.

104. Scherf D. Studies on auricular tachycardia caused by aconitine administration. Proc Soc Exp Biol Med 1947;64:233–239.

105. Bennett MA, Pentecost BL. The pattern of onset and spontaneous cessation of atrial fibrillation in man. Circulation 1970;41:981–988.

106. Haissaguerre M, Marcus FI, Fischer B, Clementy J. Radiofrequency catheter ablation in unusual mechanisms of atrial fibrillation: report of three cases. J Cardiovasc Electrophysiol 1994;5:743–751.

107. Haissaguerre M, Jais P, Shah DC, Takahashi A, Hocini M, Quiniou G, et al. Spontaneous initiation of atrial fibrillation by ectopic beats originating in the pulmonary veins. N Engl J Med 1998;339:659–666.

108. Chen SA, Hsieh MH, Tai CT, Tsai CF, Prakash VS, Yu WC, et al. Initiation of atrial fibrillation by ectopic beats originating from the pulmonary veins: electrophysiological characteristics, pharmacological responses, and effects of radiofrequency ablation. Circulation 1999;100:1879–1186.

109. Haissaguerre M, Jais P, Shah DC, Arentz T, Kalusche D, Takahashi A, et al. Catheter ablation of chronic atrial fibrillation targeting the reinitiating triggers. J Cardiovasc Electrophysiol 2000;11:2–10.

110. Pappone C, Rosanio S, Oreto G, Tocchi M, Gugliotta F, Vicedomini G, et al. Circumferential radiofrequency ablation of pulmonary vein ostia: an anatomic approach for curing atrial fibrillation. Circulation 2000;102:2619–2628.

111. Natale A, Pisano E, Beheiry S, Richey M, Leonelli F, Fanelli R, et al. Ablation of right and left atrial premature beats following cardioversion in patients with chronic atrial fibrillation refractory to antiarrhythmic drugs. Am J Cardiol 2000;85:1372–1375.

112. Scanavacca MI, Kajita LJ, Vieira M, Sosa EA. Pulmonary vein stenosis complicating catheter ablation of focal atrial fibrillation. J Cardiovasc Electrophysiol 2000;11:677–681.

113. Lesh MD, Diederich C, Guerra PG, Goseki Y, Sparks PB. An anatomic approach to prevention of

atrial fibrillation: pulmonary vein isolation with through-the-balloon ultrasound ablation. Thorac Cardiovasc Surg 1999;47 (Suppl. 3):347–351.

114. Nabar A, Rodriguez LM, Timmermans C, van den Dool A, Smeets JL, Wellens HJ. Effect of right atrial isthmus ablation on the occurrence of atrial fibrillation: observations in four groups having type I atrial flutter with or without associated atrial fibrillation. Circulation 1999;99:1441–1445.

115. Wijffels MC, Kirchhof CJ, Dorland R, Allessie MA. Atrial fibrillation begets atrial fibrillation. A study in awake chronically instrumented goats. Circulation 1995;92:1954–1968.

8

Percutaneous Catheter Ablation to Cure Atrial Fibrillation

David Schwartzman, MD

CONTENTS

"I have opinions of my own—strong opinions—but I don't always agree with them."
George H. Bush

INTRODUCTION

Much of the material in this chapter represents my opinion; it is not even clear that a percutaneous catheter ablation procedure will ever be developed which will cure atrial fibrillation (AF) with an acceptable level of safety and reliability. As with any worthwhile biomedical pursuit, the road to an ablative cure has thus far been paved with both science and serendipity. While years of bench-to-bedside atrial electroanatomical research has provided the basis for this pursuit, the stunning advances in catheter ablation have emboldened clinical investigators to "learn while they burn," yielding critical clues. While technology has to date played a limited role in the process, it is becoming an increasingly important factor.

In this chapter, the state-of-the-art techniques in percutaneous catheter ablation for the cure of AF are summarized. Although it is continually developing, a cognitive framework has been established that is likely to remain fairly constant, which hypothesizes three aspects of AF: initiation, transition, and sustenance. Although this chapter follows this format, it is important to note that these areas are not mutually exclusive, and the necessary designation of certain approaches into a single category is arbitrary.

INITIATION

It is a well-established fact that the electrocardiographic initiation of AF is associated with atrial premature beats *(1)* (Fig. 1). If they are successful in initiating AF, these

From: *Contemporary Cardiology: Management of Cardiac Arrhythmias*
Edited by: L. I. Ganz © Humana Press Inc., Totowa, NJ

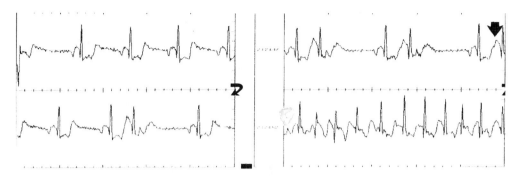

Fig. 1. Electrocardiographic events prior to spontaneously occurring AF. The recording is a modified MCL lead, obtained from a subcutaneously implanted loop recorder. The continuous recording initially demonstrates sinus rhythm. Atrial premature beats intercede in a bigeminal pattern, eventually initiating AF (arrow).

beats likely instigate, either immediately or eventually—multiple wavelet reentry *(2)*. In what appears to be a distinct minority of cases, APDs arise rapidly and persistently, associated with atrial conduction patterns which vary, yielding the electrocardiographic appearance of AF *(3a)*. Regardless, the hypothesis that ablating AF-initiating APDs will eliminate AF makes two assumptions: that their number is limited, and that the sites of origin are constant over time. This hypothesis has yet to be validated, but a remarkable amount of information has recently been accumulated. The "proof of concept" came first from the group in Bordeaux. Haissaguerre et al. described a cohort of patients with a clinical atrial arrhythmia syndrome including AF interspersed with atrial tachycardia and frequent ambient atrial ectopy *(4,5)*. In each of these patients, the entire syndrome was the result of one or more "focal" (capable of being resolved by a single radiofrequency lesion deployed using standard ablation electrode) sites of origin, invariably associated with the myocardium investing the pulmonary veins. Ablation of these sites resulted in a cure, which has largely been maintained in follow-up *(5,6)*. Other atrial areas have been documented to spawn AF-initiating APDs in the context of this syndrome, and these are also amenable to catheter ablation *(7,8)*. Although this syndrome is rare, a growing body of data is addressing the initiation of AF in more common syndromes. The focus remains on the posterior left atrium and the pulmonary veins.

We have systematically catalogued the "sites of origin" (SOO) of AF-initiating APDs utilizing simultaneous multielectrode mapping *(9)* (Fig. 2). Forty-nine patients with antiarrhythmic drug-refractory AF, including paroxysmal, (including patients with frequent and infrequent ambient atrial ectopy), persistent, and permanent syndromes, have thus far been studied. In 38 of these patients, one or more spontaneous AF initiations were recorded (Fig. 3). In 28 patients, a single SOO was responsible for all observed AF events; in the remaining patients, 2–4 SOO were observed. Among 54 total SOO, 49 (91%) were pulmonary-vein-based. Pulmonary-vein SOO were approximately equally divided between intravenous (iv) (emanating from deep within a vein) and ostial (emanating from at/near a vein ostium) types, emphasizing the potential importance of posterior left atrial myocardium near the vein orifices. The clinical AF syndrome appeared to have little impact on the features of initiation.

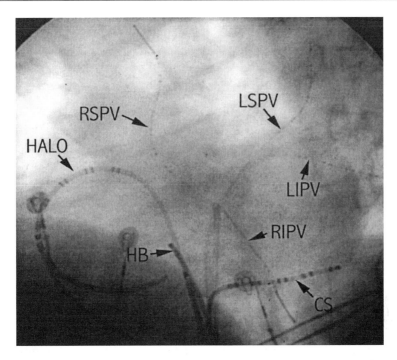

Fig. 2. Multielectrode mapping arrangement, designed to "regionalize" the SOO of AF (*see* text). Catheters were placed simultaneously into right atrial (Halo = multi-electrode catheter sampling areas ranging from septum to free wall; HB = His bundle or high septal region), coronary sinus (CS), and left atrial (multi-electrode catheters placed into each "main" pulmonary vein: RSPV = right superior vein, LSPV = left superior vein, RIPV = right inferior vein, LIPV = left inferior vein).

Extensive embryologic and electroanatomic data suggests why the posterior left atrial and pulmonary venous myocardium would be a major seat of AF origin (*10–12*). More recent clinical data certainly testifies to the unique nature of this tissue (*13,14*). A particularly intriguing observation has been the frequent observation of left ventricular compliance abnormalities, even in the absence of echocardiographic hypertrophy or hypertension history, among patients in whom AF initiated with pulmonary vein-based APDs. It is conceivable that left atrial hypertension resulting from the compliance abnormality causes remodeling of the posterior left atrium/pulmonary venous myocardium in a way which is proarrhythmic. If demonstrable, the details of such remodeling could have important therapeutic implications. However, it is important to recognize that we have barely scratched the surface. Critical issues in relating the current state of knowledge to the majority of patients with AF have yet to be addressed. For example, information regarding AF initiation in patients with significant structural heart disease is almost completely lacking. In addition, AF "onset mapping" is not intrinsically valid. It is possible that SOO which are recorded in the electrophysiology laboratory are irrelevant to the spontaneous ambulatory initiation of AF.

Nevertheless, the results of two relatively large single-center trials of focal ablation targeting SOO to suppress AF initiation have been published. Haissaguerre et al., in their latest report, have gathered 130 patients with paroxysmal AF (*15*). Among these patients, AF-onset mapping demonstrated 306 pulmonary-vein SOO. Catheter ablation of these foci has resuletd in antiarrhythmic drug-free suppression of AF (8-mo mean

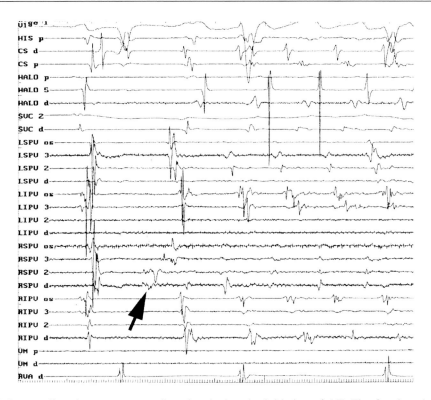

Fig. 3. Intracardiac electrogram recordings bracketing the initiation of AF. The first beat is sinus. The next beat is the AF-initiating APD: the arrow demonstrates its origin, deep and within the right superior pulmonary vein.

follow-up) in 67% of patients. Chen et al., in their latest report, have gathered 167 patients with AF. Among these patients, mapping demonstrated 247 SOO. Catheter ablation of these foci has resulted in antiarrhythmic drug-free suppression (13-mo mean follow-up) in approx 80% of patients. This group has been particularly effective in demonstrating non-pulmonary-vein SOO: in their experience, approx 22% of sites were in other locations, including the superior vena cava (SVC) and the ligament of Marshall, crista terminalis, coronary sinus (CS), and left atrial body *(16,16a,16b)*. This has been corroborated by others *(17)*. Smaller series of focal AF ablation in patients with paroxysmal AF have also been presented, with highly varied results. In our own experience with focal ablation in 33 patients (42 foci), antiarrhythmic drug-free AF suppression (7-mo mean follow-up) has been observed in 55% of patients. Varied outcomes from otherwise experienced operators reflect the nascent state of this art. Difficult-to-communicate issues, such as patient selection biases, electrogram interpretation, ablation-site selection and ablation energy titration habits are some of the likely factors underlying the current variability in procedural success. Some groups have begun to expand the clinical profiles of their ablation cohorts. Haissaguerre et al. recently reported a cohort of 15 patients with persistent AF who underwent focal ablation, resulting in antiarrhythmic drug-free AF suppression (mean follow-up 11 mo) in 60% *(18)*. Chen et al. have not had such a promising experience *(19)*.

It is important to note that focal AF ablation procedures are currently beset by vexing

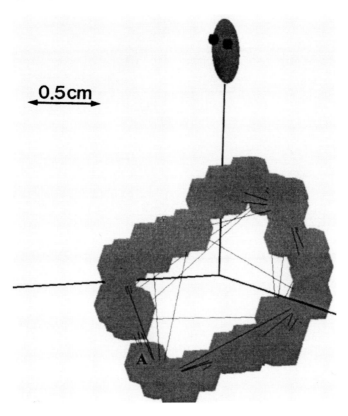

Fig. 4. Electroanatomical map (CARTO™), (Biosense/Webster Inc., Diamond Bar, CA, USA) of ablation lesions encircling a right superior pulmonary vein in a patient in whom AF was consistently triggered by atrial premature beats emanating from myocardium deep within this vein. Each circle (**A**) represents the site of an individual focal radiofrequency energy application. The summed effect of this series of lesions was "electrical isolation" of the vein. (*See* color plate 2 appearing in the insert following p. 208.)

logistical problems. For example, in many patients, once AF is started, it is difficult to resolve. This often leads to multiple cardioversions and limited onset mapping data, particularly when onset occurs within a few beats of cardioversion. Conversely, it is also common to observe patients with no/infrequent AF and sparse atrial ectopy. In many labs, selection of an ablation site is based on activation mapping, necessitating adequate ectopy. Patient behavior in the electrophysiology laboratory is largely unpredictable and ablation procedures are often abandoned. This limitation has led some groups to reduce their dependence on mapping. For example, we have gathered 15 patients in whom activation mapping could not be adequately performed. In each patient, available data suggested that AF initiation was caused by a focus/foci within a single pulmonary vein. This vein was "electrically isolated," utilizing sequential contiguous encircling focal ablation lesion applications at the venoatrial junction *(20)* (Fig. 4). This "anatomy-guided" procedure has resulted in antiarrhythmic drug-free suppression of AF (mean follow-up 8 mo) in 8 patients. Haissaguerre et al. have evolved to a technique which requires little or no atrial ectopy in designating "arrhythmogenic" pulmonary veins, with ablation performed in sinus rhythm *(21)*. Pappone et al. have

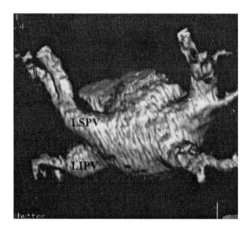 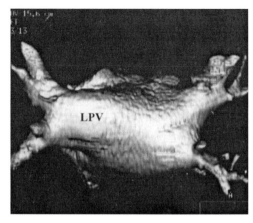

Fig 5. Three-dimensional CT reconstructions of the left atria and proximal pulmonary veins (poster-oanterior view) from two patients with AF; magnifications are identical. In the left figure, the left superior (LSPV) and inferior (LIPV) pulmonary veins join the body of the left atrium independently. In contrast, in the right figure, the left superior and inferior veins join into a common vein which then joins the left atrial body.

taken the most extreme approach, advocating empiric isolation of all four main pulmonary veins *(22)*.

Currently, focal ablation procedures are usually quite time-consuming, even in patients with in whom activation mapping can be adequately performed. This has raised safety concerns and has limited application. It is reasonable to strive for highly abbreviated procedures; this is certainly necessary from an economic perspective. In collaboration with the procedural problems described here, many have envisioned abandoning activation mapping altogether and proceeding with empiric pulmonary-vein ablation, accepting the potential for failure caused by non-pulmonary-vein trigger-ing foci. To this end, an aggressive device development effort is underway by several manufacturers. Each has conceptualized electrical isolation of veins utilizing a catheter designed to create circumferential ablation lesions adjacent to an atriovenous junction. Several prototypes have been tested in animal models *(23,24)*. These studies have emphasized the difficulties of such a venture. For example, Asirvatham et al. utilized intracardiac echocardiography to elucidate that, despite optimal fluoroscopic catheter deployment, contact of the ablation apparatus with the target area was incomplete, resulting in lesion failure *(23)*. Critical considerations for circumferential pulmonary-vein ablation include the marked interindividual variability of human atriovenous anat-omy (Fig. 5) and the distensibility of these areas *(24a,24b)*. The first human data summarizing a multicenter experience with a catheter designed specifically to isolate pulmonary veins was recently reported by Natale et al. *(25)*. In contrast to the conceptual-ized "single pass" efficacy of this device, vein isolation usually necessitated multiple lesion applications, and could not be achieved successfully in all veins *(25)*.

Assuming that AF is not inherently life-threatening, the optimum "value" of catheter ablative cure would be to provide relief from AF-attributable morbidity/symptomatology in a cost-effective manner. This presupposes a low procedural complication rate. Unfor-tunately, serious complications have been reported in patients undergoing catheter ablation in the left atrium, most importantly cardioembolism and pulmonary-vein stenosis. Cardioembolism is well reported in association with left heart ablation. Although direct data are difficult to find, the incidence is likely to be higher with procedures that require longer dwell times, more hardware, and more extensive ablation *(26–28)*. Cardioembolism has been reported after focal AF ablation *(29)*. One important factor may be ablative energy titration technique *(30)*. Given the variation in technique among investigators, it is difficult to determine the current magnitude of risk. Undoubtedly, this will remain a major obstacle for new catheter technologies. Stenosis has long been recognized as a sequela of operative trauma to the pulmonary veins. In the context of catheter ablation of AF, it was initially observed after deployment of linear lesions. In a study by Robbins et al., multiple vein stenoses had led to a syndrome of pulmonary hypertension *(31)*. Stenosis is now well-described in association with focal ablation *(29)*. Although human pathologic analyses are lacking, most data indicate that the mechanism of stenosis is heat-induced collagen contraction. Even single-vein stenosis can cause severe signs and symptoms. The risk of pulmonary-vein stenosis is currently unclear. Important considerations appear to include the number of lesions, ablative energy titration technique, and baseline vein lumen diameter. Most cases are apparent early after ablation; there seems to be no progressive or late-onset element *(31a)*.

In summary, a reliable ablative cure of AF by targeting initiation should be currently classified as experimental. Although ablation in a small subset of AF patients has provided proof of concept, and has emphasized the importance of the posterior left atrium and pulmonary veins, relevance to "common" AF has yet to be determined. At present, applicability is highly limited. Efficacy rates remain rather low, even in the most experienced hands. Variation in patient selection and mapping/ablation technique inhibit the establishment of core principles. However, despite the problems, there is an astonishing amount of catheter development coalescing around the concept of empiric ablation in the posterior left atrium/pulmonary veins. Ironically, it will be the fruit of this development, by providing anatomical ablation end points reliably achieved and defined, that will permit progress in defining whether initiation ablation works, and for which patients.

TRANSITION

Hypothetically, during the evolution from AF initiation to sustenance, an obligatory "transitional" condition occurs. The condition may involve a relatively uniform rhythm and/or a confined anatomical region.

The notion of a transitional rhythm is not new. For example, multiple studies have documented patients with both spontaneous paroxysmal supraventricular tachycardia (SVT) and AF, in whom the latter was believed to occur consistently during the former *(32,33)* (Fig. 6).

Mechanistically, AF occurring in the setting of ongoing SVT could be related to atrial electrophysiologic alterations induced by factors including rapid stimulation, pressure overload, or changes in autonomic tone *(34–36)*. Several studies have demonstrated a low incidence of AF recurrence in patients with apparent SVT-mediated AF who undergo SVT ablation *(37,38)*. However, this data is largely limited to those with Wolff-Parkinson-White syndrome (WPW); there is little data in patients with other types of SVT *(39)*. AF in WPW patients may involve more complex issues regarding atrial vulnerability independent of SVT *(40–45)*. Nevertheless, this has resulted in the

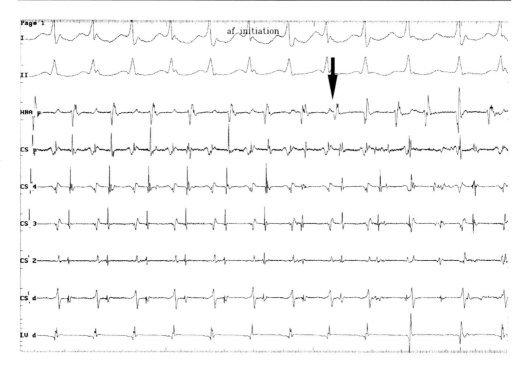

Fig. 6. Surface (leads I, II, top) and intracardiac (right atrial appendage: HRA; coronary sinus: CS; left ventricular lateral base: LV) electrograms during orthodromic AV reentrant tachycardia (ORT) utilizing a concealed left free-wall accessory pathway. Spontaneous degeneration of ORT to AF is observed (arrow).

unsubstantiated but common practice of electrophysiologic testing to exclude any SVT in patients with AF, particularly those who are young with no structural heart disease.

More recently, the potential role of type I atrial flutter as a transitional rhythm has been evaluated. It has been demonstrated in animal models that atrial flutter can trigger AF *(46)*. It has long been known that the spontaneous occurrence of atrial flutter is a marker for advanced atrial electrophysiologic pathology, and frequently coexists with AF *(47)*. However, data from several reports evaluating the incidence of AF after catheter ablation of atrial flutter strongly suggest that atrial flutter does *not* function as an obligatory transitional rhythm for AF (Table 1). In fact, in most cases, atrial flutter appears to transition from AF, occurring principally as a result of the anatomical features of the right atrium and persisting when other wavelets spontaneously extinguish *(55)*. This may help to explain the dominance of counterclockwise reentry in spontaneous atrial flutter (Fig. 7).

The examples of SVT and type I atrial flutter discussed here both insinuate the "degeneration" of an ongoing uniform atrial tachyarrhythmia to AF. There is very little data on the issue of transitional rhythms that appear early after APD initiation. In this regard, one type of atrial tachycardia to consider is so-called "repetitive firing," sometimes seen emanating from the same site as AF-initiating APDs (Fig. 8). Defining repetitive firing is problematic in clinical studies because of the scarcity of electrodes, which limits designation of the moment of degeneration to multiple wavelet reentry. The majority of repetitive firing appears to be (effectively) transient, either spontaneously

Table 1
Studies Evaluating the Incidence of Electrocardiographic AF Prior To and After
Successful Radiofrequency Catheter Ablation of Type I Atrial Flutter

| Author | N | AF Incidence | |
		Pre-ablation	Post-ablation
Movsowitz (48)	32	55%	44%
Philippon (49)	59	20%	26%
Nath (50)	22	27%	23%
Tai (51)	144	23%	24%
Anselme (52)	100	35%	36%
Paydak (53)	110	40%	25%
Frey (54)	17	41%	47%

terminating or cloaked by supervening multiple wavelet reentry. Continuous repetitive firing with varying dependent atrial activation appears to be rare (3). Repetitive firing may have more than one mechanism among patients, but reentry is almost certainly common. The scale of these reentrant circuits is unclear; this may have significant ramifications for catheter ablation. Because of its transience, repetitive firing has generally not been targeted for ablation.

However, it may be the successful suppression of such firing rather than actual eradication of a SOO that yields a "focal" ablative cure. Similarly, it may be our inability to understand repetitive firing circuits that leads to focal ablation failure despite the impression of precise targeting of the SOO.

Type II macroentrant atrial flutter is a rhythm that is commonly observed early after APD initiation of AF. We have encountered six patients in whom this rhythm served reproducibly in transition between the initiating APD and AF (Fig. 9). AFL was mapped to the right atrium in two patients and to the left atrium in four patients. Successful catheter ablation of the atrial flutter was achieved in each case. With more than 6 mo of follow-up in all patients, three have been free of atrial tachyarrhythmias. The remaining patients continue to have episodic AF.

The notion of a "transitional anatomical region" is substantially more theoretical than that of a transitional rhythm. Conceptually, there is an atrial region(s), and it is necessarily engaged early in the evolution beetween APD and AF that is critical to the transition process. Although this region may vary among individuals, this is not always the case. For example, previous reports have suggested that interatrial conduction can be an important factor in the sustenance of AF (56–59). In a canine model, Sparks et al. demonstrated a reduction in AF inducibility associated with attenuation of interatrial conduction by septal catheter ablation (60). Anecdotal experience has suggested that this concept may be useful in man. A second region of potential interest in this regard is the posterior left atrium. It is conceivable that inadvertent ablative eradication of such regions is partly responsible for successful outcomes utilizing focal/linear ablative techniques.

In summary, a reliable ablative cure for AF by targeting transition currently has little precedent. With the possible exception of WPW, there is little data confirming the utility of ablating paroxysmal SVT. Type I atrial flutter does not appear to be a

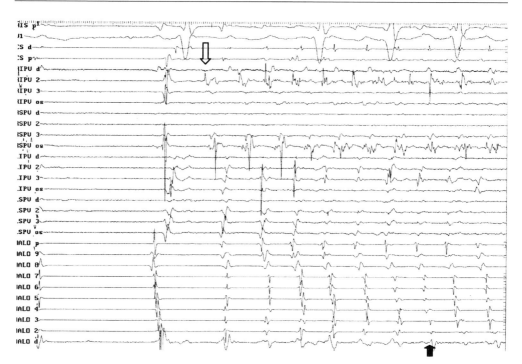

Fig. 7. Initiation of atrial flutter by a transient burst of tachycardia emanating from the right inferior pulmonary vein. Intracardiac electrodes are positioned in the high septal right atrium (His), coronary sinus proximal (CSp) and distal (CSd), right inferior pulmonary vein (RIPV), right superior pulmonary vein (RSPV), left inferior pulmonary vein (LIPV), left superior pulmonary vein (LSPV), and right atrium adjacent and parallel to the tricuspid annulus (Halo: distal = cavotricuspid isthmus; proximal = right atrial roof). The initial and subsequent tachycardia beats emanate from the right inferior pulmonary vein (hollow arrow). Initially, activation of the Halo catheter is early in both proximal and distal electrodes and later in the middle electrodes, suggesting the collision of separate right atrial wavefronts. After several beats, the Halo activation suddenly becomes counterclockwise without a significant change in activation cycle length (solid arrow). A few seconds later, the initiating pulmonary vein abruptly ceased to activate, right atrial counterclockwise activation continued, and subsequent cycle lengths were significantly longer. The rhythm at that point was atrial flutter. Note that because of the short cycle length of the atrial tachycardia burst, the surface ECG may give the impression of AF. These observations demonstrate a mechanism for spontaneous initiation of counterclockwise atrial flutter in which it is actually a "second" rhythm. In this patient, on many occasions the same initiation sequence would lead to AF (multiple wavelet reentry) rather than atrial flutter.

viable target. Although we have observed several cases in which macroreentrant type II atrial flutter appeared to be an obligatory transitional rhythm, despite consistent atrial flutter ablation success, recurrence of AF has been common, with follow-up short. The concept of transitional anatomical regions requires further evaluation.

SUSTENANCE

Like other percutaneous interventions in cardiovascular medicine, it was the development of a surgical procedure which ushered in the era of catheter ablation for AF sustenance. Utilizing the concepts of multiple wavelet reentry, Cox et al. hypothesized that if the atrium were sectioned in order to limit the region of contiguous conduction,

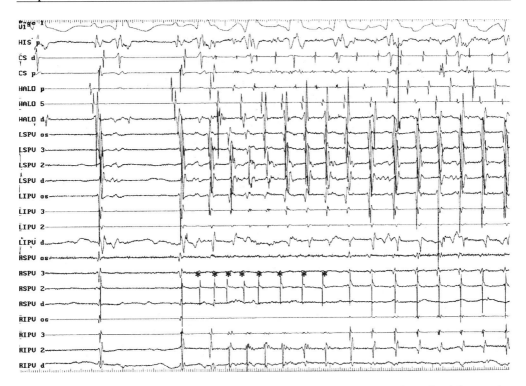

Fig. 8. Initiation of AF by a period of repetitive firing (asterisks) emanating from the right superior pulmonary vein. The firing is irregular at times. In this patient, the duration of firing would range from several beats to several seconds, either resolving with restitution of sinus rhythm or degenerating into atrial flutter or AF.

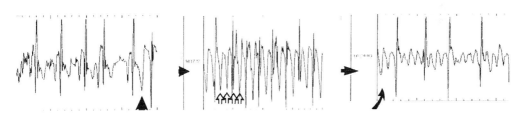

Fig. 9. Time-lapse recordings from a subcutaneous (SC) loop recorder (recordings similar to MCL 1) demonstrating a reliable electrocardiographic sequence culminating in AF. On the left, sinus rhythm is interrupted by an APD (arrowhead). This initiates a rapid, uniform atrial tachyarrhythmia (hollow arrows), demonstrated on the center panel. Within minutes, this rhythm would degenerate to "typical" AF, demonstrated in the right panel (curved arrow).

AF sustenance could not occur *(2)*. Utilizing a series of "linear" surgical incisions, which permitted atrioventricular conduction but severely limited contiguous conduction, these investigators developed and deployed the Maze procedure *(61,62)*. The high rates of long-term success reported by groups performing this procedure has served as clear proof of concept. In subsequent years, modified and less extensive surgical procedures also demonstrated high rates of efficacy. This led investigators to conceptualize that AF sustenance could be prevented without the severe limitation of contiguous conduction

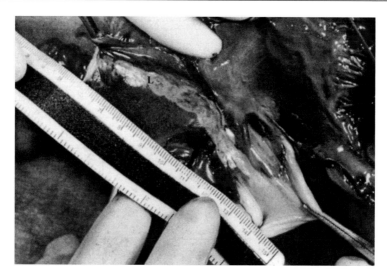

Fig. 10. Endocardial view of a 1-d-old lesion (**L**) deployed in the right atrium percutaneously utilizing radiofrequency energy. Unablated myocardium stains red. (*See* color plate 3 appearing in the insert following p. 208.)

(63,64). Together with the development of catheter and imaging technologies, these observations emboldened interventional electrophysiologists to embark on a program of mimicry of atrial incisions utilizing catheter ablation. Technically, anatomy-based transmural "linear" lesions, which function as complete conduction barriers, can be deployed *(65)* (Fig. 10). Histologically, these lesions are quite similar to surgical incisions *(66).* Unfortunately, the accumulated experience with linear catheter ablation to inhibit AF sustenance is comprised of several different catheter technologies. In most studies, there is no conclusive evidence that the conceptualized lesions were successfully deployed. Nonetheless, multiple trials evaluating the efficacy of linear ablation have been reported (Table 2). Results thus far are short-term, with serial results from single centers demonstrating a progressive failure rate *(80).* However, several important observations have been made. First, superior efficacy has been consistently demonstrated in procedures that incorporate left atrial ablation relative to those which do not *(80a).* Data from animal models have long suggested that AF sustenance is primarily a "left atrial problem." The encouraging results from surgical ablation procedures with lesions limited to the left atrium have reinforced this concept *(81–83).* Furthermore, several investigators have reported the phenomenon of post-ablation drug "sensitization"—successful AF suppression by an antiarrhythmic drug/dose which had previously failed to do so *(67,69,74).* In the case of right atrial ablation, the "partial success" group (AF suppression on a previously inefficacious antiarrhythmic drug) appears to be significantly larger than the "complete success" group (drug-free AF suppression). Third, several investigators have reported early post-ablation failures (no change from pre-ablation syndrome or exacerbation of syndrome) which improve with time *(69,74).* This phenomenon has also been observed early after surgical AF ablation, and may be the result of transient inflammation-mediated alterations in atrial electrophysiology, particularly contiguous to lesion zones *(84).*

In contrast to the evolution of focal ablation procedures described here, linear ablation

Table 2
Results of Linear Atrial Ablation Trials for Suppression of AF

Author	N	FU	AF	Atrium	Cure Complete	Partial
Haissaguerre (67)	45	11 ± 4	P	R	13%	20%
	10		P	L	40%	60%
Swartz (68)	29	24	C	R,L	79%	—
Schwartzman (69)	22	18 ± 7	P,C	R	14%	18%
Gaita (70)	23	12	P	R	9%	21%
Ernst (71)	13	NR	P,C	R,L	0%	—
	32	NR		R	11%	—
Garg (72)	12	21 ± 11	P,C	R	8%	58%
Calkins (73)	15	3 ± 2	P,C	R	21%	
Olgin (74)	20	NR	P,C	R	75%	
Pappone (75)	27	11 ± 3	P	R,L	44%	15%
Tondo (76)	26	17 ± 8	P	R	30%	31%
Natale (77)	18	22 ± 11	P	R	28%	22%
Haines (78)	23	6 ± 4	P,C	R,L	26%	22%
Man (79)	12	2	P	R	8%	42%

N = number of patients; FU = mean follow-up (± standard deviation, when reported); AF = clinical syndrome (P = paroxysmal, C = persistent or permanent); Atrium = chamber in which ablation was performed (R = right, L = left); Complete cure = free of AF and antiarrhythmic drug; partial cure = free of AF while taking an antiarrhythmic drug which was previously documented to be ineffective. Cure data straddling the 2 columns was not reported separately. NR = not reported.

has always been considered an essentially anatomical problem. There have been few attempts at utilizing electrophysiologic findings during ongoing AF to guide specific lesion types/locations (65,68). However, like focal ablation, the current art of linear ablation is plagued by several key problems. First, linear ablation is associated with unacceptably long procedure times. Currently, linear ablation is practiced using single (65,69,71,72,77,79) or multielectrode (70,73,74,76,78) catheters; this does not appear to have a major impact on procedure/fluoroscopy time. A major cause of long procedure times is inadequate imaging of the atrial endocardium. Smooth atrial endocardial areas are topographically complex; combined with their phenomenal resistance to stable ablation electrode purchase, imaging becomes critical. Several investigators have incorporated intracardiac echocardiography, the only currently available technology for real-time endocardial imaging, into lesion deployment techniques (65,69,74,86). Second, "completion" (linear lesion as complete barrier to conduction) of planned lesions often cannot be achieved (65). This appears to be particularly common in the left atrium (71). Third, lesion healing with associated recovery of translesion conduction has been a serious problem. This was first shown to be common with cavotricuspid isthmus ablation for atrial flutter (87). The incidence of recovery of conduction appears to increase with the longer, more complex lesions utilized for ablation of AF. Fourth, postlinear ablation recurrence of uniform atrial tachyarrhythmias is common, probably because of incomplete lesion deployment and lesion healing. This has resulted in the need for multiple ablation procedures in many patients. Finally, and most critically, current lesion paradigms are empiric. Most mimic some component of the surgical Maze procedure, but none has intrinsic validity. The marked variation in lesion paradigms has severely limited data comparison among centers, which has hampered the evolution of this technique.

As for focal ablation of AF, linear ablation has been associated with a significant number of procedural complications, including cardioembolism, pulmonary-vein stenosis, and pericarditis (26,28,31,71). Given the variability in techniques and catheter technologies, risk factors and magnitude assessments are difficult. Similar to Maze surgery, linear ablation can be associated with diminished atrial transport function, and the rate and degree of recovery from this procedure is now poorly characterized.

In summary, a reliable ablative cure of AF by targeting sustenance should be currently classified as experimental. Although the Maze procedure provided proof of concept, current catheter ablation procedures are far less extensive, which may render the comparison irrelevant. Some inroads have been made—particularly with "hybrid" treatment, in which antiarrhythmic drugs are combined with ablation. However, procedural complications have been significant, and long-term data is lacking. Future efforts must concentrate on the left atrium, and this will be dependent on new technology development. Notably, there is a growing literature regarding intra-operative linear ablation under direct vision using a catheter-type device (81–83). To date, most procedures have been performed on the left atrium in a dry surgical field in patients undergoing mitral valve repair/replacement. Although they have been short term, success rates have been impressive and ablation-attributable morbidity has been low. Direct-vision ablation eliminates problems with electrode-endocardial contact, power titration, and lesion assessment. If this experience continues to be favorable, it is likely that it will be extended to other groups, such as patients undergoing cardiac surgery in whom left atrial access would not otherwise be needed. In addition, there is significant ongoing development in the area of off-pump epicardial ablation (88). If perfected and combined with rapidly developing minimally invasive/thoracoscopic cardial surgical techniques, the surgical approach may become the approach of choice.

CONCLUSION

In my opinion, percutaneous catheter ablation for the cure of AF is a promising concept, although it now offers unclear viability. A reasonable cognitive framework (initiation, transition, sustenance) exists, but much development is needed. For example, clinical subsets must be discerned, based preferably on ambulatory indices such as AF pattern and cardiac structure/function. Technology which is both reliable and reproducible must be developed to rapidly deploy lesions.

REFERENCES

 1. Schwartzman D, Brown ML, Fitts SM. Electrocardiographic events preceding the onset of atrial fibrillation: insights gained using an implantable loop recorder. J Am Coll Cardiol 2000;35(2):130A.
 2. Janse MJ. Mechanisms of atrial fibrillation. In: Zipes DP, Jalife J, eds. Cardiac Electrophysiology: From Cell to Bedside. 3rd ed. Saunders, Philadelphia, PA: 2000;476–481.
 3. Scherf D. Studies on auricular tachycardia caused by aconitine administration. Proc Soc Exp Biol Med 1947;64:233–239.
3a. Lu TM, Tai CT, Hsieh MH, et al. Electrophysiologic characteristics in initiation of paroxysmal atrial fibrillation from a focal area. J Am Coll Cardiol 2001;37(6):1658–1664.
 4. Haissaguerre M, Gencel L, Fischer B. Successful catheter ablation of atrial fibrillation. J Cardiovasc Electrophysiol 1994;5:1045–1052.

5. Jais P, Haissaguerre M, Shah DC. A focal source of atrial fibrillation treated by discrete radiofrequency ablation. Circulation 1997;95:572–576.

6. Haissaguerre M, Jais P, Shah DC. Spontaneous initiation of atrial fibrillation by ectopic beats originating in the pulmonary veins. N Engl J Med 1998;339:659–666.

7. Chen S-A, Tai C-T, Yu W-C. Right atrial focal atrial fibrillation: electrophysiologic characteristics and radiofrequency catheter ablation. J Cardiovasc Electrophysiol 1999;10:328–335.

8. Hwang C, Wu T-J, Doshi RN. Vein of Marshall cannulation for the analysis of electrical activity in patients with focal atrial fibrillation. Circulation 2000;101:1503–1505.

9. Schwartzman D, Predis L. Simultaneous multielectrode microcatheter mapping of the pulmonary veins in patients with paroxysmal atrial fibrillation. (Abstracts) Pacing Clin Electrophysiol 1999;22:15–88.

10. Nathan H, Eliakim M. The junction between the left atrium and the pulmonary veins: an anatomic study of human hearts. Circulation 1996;34:412–422.

11. Cheung DW. Electrical activity of the pulmonary vein and its interaction with the right atrium in the guinea pig. J Physiol 1980;314:445–456.

12. Spach MS, Barr RC, Jewitt PH. Spread of excitation from the atrium into thoracic veins in human beings and dogs. Am J Cardiol 1972;30:844–854.

13. Chen S-A, Hsieh M-H, Tai C-T, et al. Initiation of atrial fibrillation by ectopic beats originating from the pulmonary veins: electrophysiologic characteristics, pharmacological responses, and effects of radiofrequency ablation. Circulation 1999;100:1879–1886.

14. Schwartzman D. Atrial premature depolarization concealed in two pulmonary veins. J Cardiovasc Electrophysiol 2000;11:931–934.

15. Haissaguerre M, Jais P, Shah DC, et al. Sites of recurrences after catheter ablation of pulmonary vein initiated atrial fibrillation. Pacing Clin Electrophysiol 2000;23:583.

16. Chen S-A, Tsai C-F, Tai C-T, et al. Predictors of recurrence after focal ablation of the initiating beats in patients with paroxysmal atrial fibrillation: risk prediction, endpoint, and clinical course. Pacing Clin Electrophysiol 2000;23:651.

16a. Tai CT, Hsieh MH, Tsai CF, et al. Differentiating the ligament of Marshall from the pulmonary vein musculature potentials in patients with paroxysmal atrial fibrillation: electrophysiological characteristics and results of radiofrequency ablation. Pacing Clin Electrophysiol 2000;23:1493–1501.

16b. Tsai CF, Tai CT, Hsieh MH, et al. Initiation of atrial fibrillation by ectopic beats originating from the superior vena cava: electrophysiological characteristics and results of radiofrequency ablation. J Cardiovasc Electrophysiol 2000;11:744–749.

17. Vergara I, Martin D, Bahnson T, et al. Clinical predictors of successful focal atrial fibrillation ablation. Pacing Clin Electrophysiol 1999;22:772.

18. Haissaguerre M, Jais P, Shah DC. Catheter ablation of chronic atrial fibrillation targeting the reinitiating triggers. J Cardiovasc Electrophysiol 2000;11:2–10.

19. Chen S-A, Tai C-T, Hsieh M-H, et al. Focal ablation of ectopic foci has limited efficacy in patients with persistent atrial fibrillation. Pacing Clin Electrophysiol 2000;23:694.

20. Schwartzman D. Circumferential radiofrequency ablation of pulmonary vein orifices: feasibility of a new technique. Pacing Clin Electrophysiol 1999;22:711.

21. Haissaguerre M, Shah DC, Jais P. Circular multipolar pulmonary vein catheter for mapping guided minimal ablation for atrial fibrillation. Pacing Clin Electrophysiol 2000;23:574.

22. Pappone C, Rosanio S, Oreto G, et al. Circumferential radiofrequency ablation of pulmonary vein ostia: a new anatomic approach for curing atrial fibrillation. Circulation 2000;102(21):2562–2564.

23. Asirvatham S, Johnson SB, Packer DL. Utility of intracardiac ultrasound (ICUS) in guiding circumferential pulmonary venous ablation with a tandem balloon catheter. Pacing Clin Electrophysiol 1999;22(4):822.

24. Wilber DJ, Arruda M, Wang ZG, et al. Circumferential ablation of pulmonary vein ostia with an ultrasound ablation catheter: acute and chronic studies in a canine model. Circulation 1999;100(18):I–373.

24a. Lin WS, Prakash VS, Tai CT, et al. Pulmonary vein morphology in patients with paroxysmal atrial fibrillation initiated by ectopic beats originating from the pulmonary veins: implications for catheter ablation. Circulation 2000;101(11):1274–1281.

24b. Tsao HM, Yu WC, Cheng HC, et al. Pulmonary vein dilation in patients with atrial fibrillation: detection by magnetic resonance imaging. J Cardiovasc Electrophysiol 2001;12(7):809–813.

25. Natale A, Pisano E, Shewchick, et al. First human experience with pulmonary vein isolation using

a through-the-balloon circumferential ultrasound ablation system for recurrent atrial fibrillation. Circulation 2000;102(16):1879–1882.

26. Mitchell M, McRury I, Haines D. Linear atrial ablation in a canine model of chronic atrial fibrillation: morphological and electrophysiologic observations. Circulation 1998;1176–1185.

27. Ernst S, Schluter M, Ouyang F, et al. Modification of the substrate for maintenance of idiopathic human atrial fibrillation. Circulation 1999;100:2085–2092.

28. Swartz JF, Gencel L, Fischer B, et al. A catheter-based curative approach to atrial fibrillation in humans. Circulation 1994;90:I–335.

29. Jais P, Haissaguerre M, Shah DC, et al. Complications of radiofrequency catheter ablation in the pulmonary veins in 200 consecutive patients. Pacing Clin Electrophysiol 2000;23:627.

30. Schwartzman D, Michele JJ, Trankiem CT, et al. Radiofrequency power titration for atrial ablation: prospective comparison of thermometry versus electrogram amplitude reduction. Pacing Clin Electrophysiol 1998;21(4):849.

31. Robbins IM, Colvin EV, Doyle TP, et al. Pulmonary vein stenosis after catheter ablation of atrial fibrillation. Circulation 1998;98:1769–1775.

31a. Yu WC, Hsu TL, Tai CT, et al. Acquired pulmonary vein stenosis after radiofrequency catheter ablation of paroxysmal atrial fibrillation. J Cardiovasc Electrophysiol 2001;12(8):887–892.

32. Sung RJ, Castellanos A, Mallon SM, et al. Mechanism of spontaneous alteration between reciprocating tachycardia and atrial flutter-fibrillation in the Wolff-Parkinson-White syndrome. Circulation 1977;56:406–416.

33. Roark SF, McCarthy EA, Lee KL, et al. Observations on the occurrence of atrial fibrillation in paroxysmal supraventricular tachycardia. Am J Cardiol 1986;57:571–575.

34. Wyndham CRC, Amt-y-Leon F, Wu D, et al. Effect of cycle length on atrial vulnerability. Circulation 1977;55:260–267.

35. Calkins H, El-Atassi R, Kalbfleisch S, et al. Effect of an acute increase in atrial pressure on atrial refractoriness in humans. Pacing Clin Electrophysiol 1992;15:1674–1680.

36. Alessi R, Nusynowitz M, Abildskov JA, et al. Nonuniform distribution of vagal effects on the atrial refractory period. Am J Physiol 1958;194:406–410.

37. Sharma AD, Klein GJ, Guiraudon G, et al. Atrial fibrillation in patients with Wolff-Parkinson-White syndrome: incidence after surgical ablation of the accessory pathway. Circulation 1985;72 (1):161–169.

38. Haissaguerre M, Fischer B, Labbe T, et al. Frequency of recurrent atrial fibrillation after catheter ablation of overt accessory pathways. Am J Cardiol 1992;69:493–497.

39. Weiss R, Knight BP, Bahu M. Long-term followup after radiofrequency ablation of paroxysmal supraventricular tachycardia in patients with tachycardia-induced fibrillation. Am J Cardiol 1997;80 (12):1609–1610.

40. Konoe A, Fukatani M, Tanigawa M, et al. Electrophysiologic abnormalities of the atrial muscle in patients with manifest Wolff-Parkinson-White syndrome associated with paroxysmal atrial fibrillation. Pacing Clin Electrophysiol 1992;15(7):1040–1052.

41. Peters RW, Gonzalez R, Scheinman MM. Atrial and ventricular vulnerability in a patient with the Wolff-Parkinson-White syndrome. Pacing Clin Electrophysiol 1981;4(1):17–22.

42. Wathen M, Natale A, Wolfe K, et al. Initiation of atrial fibrillation in the Wolff-Parkinson-White syndrome: the importance of the accessory pathway. Am Heart J 1993;125(3):753–759.

43. Fujimura O, Klein GJ, Yee R, et al. Mode of onset of atrial fibrillation in the Wolff-Parkinson-White syndrome: how important is the accessory pathway? J Am Coll Cardiol 1990;15(5):1082–1086.

44. Iesaka Y, Yamane T, Takahashi A, et al. Retrograde multiple and multifiber accessory pathway conduction in the Wolff-Parkinson-White syndrome: potential precipitating factor of atrial fibrillation. J Cardiovasc Electrophysiol 1998;9(2):141–151.

45. Muraoka Y, Karakawa S, Yamagata T, et al. Dependency on atrial electrophysiologic properties of appearance of paroxysmal atrial fibrillation in patients with Wolff-Parkinson-White syndrome: evidence from atrial vulnerability before and after radiofrequency catheter ablation and surgical cryoablation. Pacing Clin Electrophysiol 1998;21(2):438–446.

46. Ortiz J, Niwano S, Abe H, et al. Mapping the conversion of atrial flutter to atrial fibrillation and atrial fibrillation to atrial flutter: insights into mechanisms. Circ Res 1994;74:882–894.

47. Watson RM, Josephson ME. Atrial flutter I: electrophysiologic substrates and modes of initiation and termination. Am J Cardiol 1980;45:732–740.

48. Movsowitz C, Callans DJ, Schwartzman D, et al. The results of atrial flutter ablation in patients with and without a history of atrial fibrillation. Am J Cardiol 1996;78:93–96.

49. Philippon F, Plumb VJ, Epstein A, et al. The risk of atrial fibrillation following radiofrequency catheter ablation of atrial flutter. Circulation 1995;92:430–435.

50. Nath S, Mounsey P, Haines DE, et al. Predictors of acute and long-term success after radiofrequency catheter ablation of type I atrial flutter. Am J Cardiol 1995;75:604–606.

51. Tai CT, Chen SA, Chiang CE, et al. Long-term outcome of radiofrequency catheter ablation for typical atrial flutter: risk prediction of recurrent arrhythmias. J Cardiovasc Electrophysiol 1998;9:115–121.

52. Anselme F, Saoudi N, Poty H, et al. Radiofrequency catheter ablation of common atrial flutter: significance of palpitation and quality-of-life evaluation in patients with proven isthmus block. Circulation 1999;99:534–540.

53. Paydak LI, Kall JG, Burke MC, et al. Atrial fibrillation after radiofrequency ablation of type I atrial flutter: time to onset, determinants, and clinical course. Circulation 1998;98:315–322.

54. Frey B, Kreiner G, Binder T, et al. Relation between left atrial size and secondary atrial arrhythmias after successful catheter ablation of common atrial flutter. Pacing Clin Electrophysiol 1997;20:2936–2942.

55. Roithinger F, Karch MR, Steiner PR, et al. Relationship between atrial fibrillation and typical atrial flutter in humans: Activation sequence changes during spontaneous conversion. Circulation 1997;96:3484–3491.

56. Kumagai K, Khrestian C, Waldo AL. Simultaneous multisite mapping studies during induced atrial fibrillation in the sterile pericarditis model. Circulation 1997;95:511–521.

57. Allessie MA, Lammers WJEP, Bonke FIM, Hollen J. Experimental evaluation of Moe's multiple wavelet hypothesis of atrial fibrillation. In: Zipes DP, Jalife J, eds. Cardiac Electrophysiology and Arrhythmias. Grune and Stratton, Orlando, Fl, 1985, pp. 265–275.

58. Allessie M, Lammers W, Smeets J, Bonke F, Hollen J. Total mapping of atrial excitation during acetylcholine-induced atrial flutter and fibrillation in the isolated canine heart. In: Kulbertus HE, Olsson SB, Schlepper M, eds. Atrial Fibrillation. Molndal, Sweden, Lindgren and Soner, 1982.

59. Skanes AC, Mandapati R, Berenfeld O, Davidenko JM, Jalife J. Spatiotemporal periodicity during atrial fibrillation in the isolated sheep heart. Circulation 1998;98(12):1236–1248.

60. Sparks PB, Goseki Y, Gerstenfeld EP, et al. Ablation of the connections between the left and right atrium guided by electroanatomic mapping: effects on perpetuation of atrial fibrillation. Pacing Clin Electrophysiol 2000;23:693.

61. Cox JL, Schuessler RB, D'Agostino HJ Jr., et al. The surgical treatment of atrial fibrillation. III. Development of a definitive surgical procedure. J Thorac Cardiovasc Surg 1991;101:569–583.

62. Cox JL, Schuessler RB, Lappas DG, et al. An 8½-year clinical experience with surgery for atrial fibrillation. Ann Surg 1996;224:267–275.

63. Sueda T, Nagata H, Orihashi K, et al. Efficacy of a simple left atrial procedure for chronic atrial fibrillation in mitral valve operations. Ann Thorac Surg 1997;63:1070–1075.

64. Shyu K-G, Cheng J-J, Chen J-J, et al. Recovery of atrial function after atrial compartment operation for chronic atrial fibrillation in mitral valve disease. J Am Coll Cardiol 1994;24:392–398.

65. Schwartzman D, Kuck KH. Anatomy-guided linear atrial lesions for radiofrequency catheter ablation of atrial fibrillation. Pacing Clin Electrophysiol 1998;21:1959–1978.

66. Schwartzman D, Fischer WD, Spencer EP, Parishkaya M, Devine W. Linear radiofrequency atrial lesions deployed using an irrigated electrode: electrical and histologic evolution. J Intervent Cardiac Electrophysiol 2001;5(1):17–26.

67. Haissaguerre M, Jais P, Shah DC, et al. Right and left atrial radiofrequency catheter therapy of paroxysmal atrial fibrillation. J Cardiovasc Electrophysiol 1996;7:1132–1144.

68. Swartz JF, Gencel L, Fischer B. A catheter-based curative approach to atrial fibrillation in humans. Circulation 1994;90:I-335.

69. Schwartzman D, Wackowski C, Scharfenberg C. Outcome of right atrial linear radiofrequency ablation for suppression of atrial fibrillation. Pacing Clin Electrophysiol 1999;22:904.

70. Gaita F, Riccardi R, Scaglione M, et al. Catheter ablation of paroxysmal atrial fibrillation: comparison of outcomes between right atrial linear and pulmonary veins ablation. Pacing Clin Electrophysiol 2000;23:674.

71. Ernst S, Schluter M, Ouyang F, et al. Modification of the substrate for maintenance of idiopathic human atrial fibrillation: efficacy of radiofrequency ablation using nonfluoroscopic catheter guidance. Circulation 1999;100:2085–2092.

72. Garg A, Finneran W, Mollerus M, et al. Right atrial compartmentalization using radiofrequency catheter ablation for management of patients with refractory atrial fibrillation. J Cardiovasc Electrophysiol 1999;10:763–771.

73. Calkins H, Hall J, Ellenbogen K, et al. A new system for catheter ablation of atrial fibrillation. Am J Cardiol 1999;83:227D–236D.

74. Olgin J, Strickberger SA, Lesh M, et al. Right atrial ablation of lone atrial fibrillation with multielectrode coil catheters. Pacing Clin Electrophysiol 1999;22:904.

75. Pappone C, Oreto G, Lamberti F, et al. Catheter ablation of atrial fibrillation using a 3D mapping system. Circulation 1999;100(11):1203–1208.

76. Tondo C, Riva S, Carbucicchio C, et al. Long term clinical outcome of right atrial ablation for paroxysmal atrial fibrillation. Pacing Clin Electrophysiol 2000;23:672.

77. Natale A, Leonelli F, Beheiry S, et al. Catheter ablation approach on the right side only for paroxysmal atrial fibrillation therapy: long-term results. Pacing Clin Electrophysiol 2000;23(2):224–233.

78. Haines DE, Hummel JD, Kalbfleisch SJ, et al. Bi-atrial linear ablation with the multiple electrode catheter ablation (MECA) system in patients with atrial fibrillation. Pacing Clin Electrophysiol 2000;23:567.

79. Man KC, Daoud E, Knight BP, et al. Right atrial radiofrequency catheter ablation of atrial fibrillation. J Am Coll Cardiol 1996;27:768.

80. Jais P, Shah DC, Takahashi A, et al. Long-term follow-up after right atrial radiofrequency catheter treatment of paroxysmal atrial fibrillation. Pacing Clin Electrophysiol 1998;21:2533–2538.

80a. Ernst S, Ouyang F, Schneider B, Kuek KH. Prevention of atrial fibrillation by complete compartmentalization of the left atrium using a catheter technique. J Cardiovasc Electrophysiol 2000;11(6):686–690.

81. Kottkamp H, Hindricks G, Hammel D, et al. Intraoperative radiofrequency ablation of chronic atrial fibrillation: a left atrial curative approach by elimination of anatomic "anchor" reentrant circuits. J Cardiovasc Electrophysiol 1999;10:772–780.

82. Melo JQ, Adragao P, Neves J, et al. Surgery for atrial fibrillation using intraoperative radiofrequency ablation. Rev Port Cardiol 1998;17:377–379.

83. Patwardhan AM, Dave HH, Tamhane AA, et al. Intraoperative radiofrequency micropolar coagulation to replace incisions of maze III procedure for correcting atrial fibrillation in patients with rheumatic valvular disease. Eur J Cardio-Thorac Surg 1997;12:627–633.

84. Ren JF, Schwartzman D, Michele JJ, Brode SE, Trankiem CT, Li KS, et al. Intracardiac echocardiographic quantitation of atrial wall thickness changes associated with radiofrequency ablation. J Am Coll Cardiol 1998;31:259A.

85. Gaita F, Riccardi R, Calo L, et al. Atrial mapping and radiofrequency catheter ablation in patients with idiopathic atrial fibrillation: electrophysiologic findings and ablation results. Circulation 1998;2136–2145.

86. Brode SE, Schwartzman D, Ren J-F, et al. A new non-fluoroscopic method for guiding the creation of linear right atrial radiofrequency lesions with standard ablation electrode. Pacing Clin Electrophysiol 1997;20(4):1203.

87. Schwartzman D, Callans DJ, Gottlieb CD, Dillon SM, Movsowitz C, Marchlinski FE. Conduction block in the inferior vena caval-triscupid valve isthmus: an alternative endpoint for radiofrequency catheter ablation of atrial flutter. J Am Coll Cardiol 1996;28(6):1519–1531.

88. Williams M, Sanchez J, Barbone A, et al. Feasibility of epicardial radiofrequency pulmonary vein isolation for thoracoscopic treatment of atrial fibrillation. Pacing Clin Electrophysiol 2000;23:600.

9 The Management of Atrial Flutter

Robert W. Rho, MD,
and David J. Callans, MD

CONTENTS

HISTORICAL PERSPECTIVES

Atrial flutter was first described in 1911 by Jolly and Ritchie *(1)*, who differentiated this arrhythmia from atrial fibrillation (AF) and reported the typical saw-tooth-shaped atrial waves in leads II and III. Early insight into atrial flutter was facilitated by Lewis, who defined the electrocardiographic findings and through a series of animal experiments concluded that the arrhythmia resulted from circus movement around one or both caval orifices *(2–4)*.

After five decades of debate over the mechanism of atrial flutter between proponents of a single-focus theory and those favoring reentry *(5)*, it is now clear that atrial flutter arises from a single macroreentry circuit confined to the right atrium. This theory has been supported by animal studies and confirmed over the last two decades in humans via electrophysiologic studies utilizing detailed multiple electrode pace mapping and entrainment mapping techniques *(6–17)*. In typical atrial flutter, the anatomic barriers within the right atrium have mostly been defined *(18–20)*. The circuit depends on an area of slow conduction within the inferior, medial right atrium between the inferior vena cava (IVC) and the tricuspid valve *(16,21–24)*. This anatomic zone of slow conduction is the target of modern ablation techniques.

INCIDENCE

Atrial flutter is a relatively rare arrhythmia in comparison to AF. Both arrhythmias share a very similar clinical profile, and often coexist within the same individual.

From: *Contemporary Cardiology: Management of Cardiac Arrhythmias*
Edited by: L. I. Ganz © Humana Press Inc., Totowa, NJ

Because of their similarities, they are often combined together in studies reporting incidence and treatment efficacy. Therefore, there is insufficient independent data on the incidence of atrial flutter and its response to pharmacologic therapy. In one retrospective analysis of ICD-9 (i.e., billing) codes for atrial flutter in 54,000 patients in the Marshfield Epidemiologic Study Area, there was an annual incidence rate of 0.9 per 1000 patients. The annual incidence rate was 7.3 per 1000 patients greater than 80 yr of age. It is estimated that there are approx 200,000 new cases of atrial flutter in the United States per year *(25)*.

Atrial flutter is commonly associated with AF, and may often coexist in some patients, occasionally simultaneously, manifesting as "flutter-fibrillation." Atrial flutter often complicates the postoperative management of patients who have undergone cardiac surgery. It has an association with chronic obstructive pulmonary disease (COPD), thyrotoxicosis, structural heart disease including mitral or tricuspid valve disease, atrial enlargement of any etiology, and surgical correction of congenital heart disease *(26–29)*.

A REVIEW OF RIGHT ATRIAL ANATOMY

Because atrial flutter is usually confined to the right atrium, an appreciation of the anatomy of the endocardial surface of the right atrium is essential. The interior surface of the right atrium can be divided into three regions: a smooth-walled venous component derived from the embryonic sinus venosus; a trabeculated atrium proper; and the right atrial appendage *(33)*.

The crista terminalis is a ridge on the internal surface of the right atrium which is located lateral to the superior vena cava (SVC) and IVC. It separates the venous component from the trabeculated atrium. The venous component of the right atrium receives the superior and inferior vena cavae posterior to the crista terminalis as well as the coronary sinus (CS).

Located anterior and medial to the orifice of the IVC is the Eustachian valve (EV). The EV, if present, is the remnant of an embryonic baffle that shunted blood from the IVC (oxygenated from the placenta) into the left atrium via the foramen ovale. The lateral portion of the EV continuous with the inferior portion of the crista terminalis. The Eustachian ridge continues inferiorly and anteriorly to the atrial septum between the orifice of the IVC and tricuspid annulus. The CS runs in the left atrioventricular groove, and its ostium is in the interior medial right atrium, posterior to the tricuspid annulus *(33)* (*see* Fig. 1).

The macroreentrant circuit of typical atrial flutter is dependent on an isthmus or zone of slow conduction, which lies between the IVC and the tricuspid annulus. The posterior barrier of the circuit is the crista terminalis, EV, and Eustachian ridge. The anterior barrier is the tricuspid annulus. In counterclockwise typical atrial flutter, the circuit moves through the isthmus of slow conduction, up the intra-atrial septum, over the superior vena cavae, down the lateral wall, and through the isthmus, thus completing the loop.

In clockwise typical atrial flutter, the circuit is bound by the same barriers and is also dependent on the isthmus of slow conduction. The direction of rotation is up the lateral wall, over the SVC, down the intra-atrial septum, through the isthmus, and up the lateral wall, thus continuing the loop. In both counterclockwise and clockwise

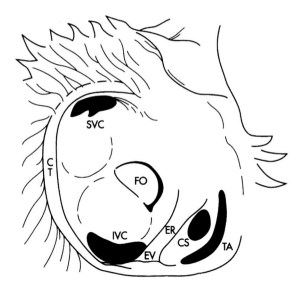

Fig. 1. Anatomic landmarks in the right atrium. Superior vena cava (SVC); crista terminalis (CT); inferior vena cava (IVC); fossa ovalis (FO); Eustachian valve (EV); Eustachian ridge (ER); coronary sinus (CS); tricuspid annulus (TA). The venous orifices (vena cavae and coronary sinus) and the crista terminalis are believed to act as central barriers to prevent "short circuiting" of the atrial flutter circuit. (Reproduced with permission from Marriot JL, Conover MB: Advanced Concepts in Arrhythmias. 3rd ed. Mosby, St. Louis, MO, 1998, p. 111.)

typical atrial flutter, the isthmus between the IVC and tricuspid annulus is the vulnerable segment of the circuit, and is the target for successful radiofrequency ablation of atrial flutter.

CLASSIFICATION OF ATRIAL FLUTTER

Macroreentrant circuits manifesting as atrial flutter may propagate around anatomic, surgical, or functional barriers. Atrial flutter is therefore a general term used to define a heterogeneous group of macroreentrant supraventricular tachyarrhythmias that may exist in either atrium.

Recognizing the many subtypes of atrial flutter and the need for a more specific system of nomenclature to facilitate sharing of new insights by investigators into the various forms of macroreentrant tachycardias, electrophysiologists proposed this new classification schema, based on electrophysiologic criteria *(30)*:

1. Typical atrial flutter (Type 1; or isthmus-dependent) reentry depends on a zone of slow conduction in the narrow isthmus confined by the inferior vena cavae, Eustachian ridge, CS, and tricuspid annulus. It is usually counterclockwise (also known as "common" or "usual" atrial flutter [*see* Fig. 2A]) but may less frequently be clockwise ("atypical atrial flutter" distinguished from "true atypical atrial flutter." Counterclockwise typical atrial flutter is the most common type of atrial flutter seen clinically. It has an atrial rate of approx 300 (240–350) cycles per min, and has negative flutter waves in the inferior leads. Clockwise typical atrial flutter also has a flutter rate of approx 300 cycles per min, but the flutter waves are usually positive in the inferior leads (*see* Fig. 2b).

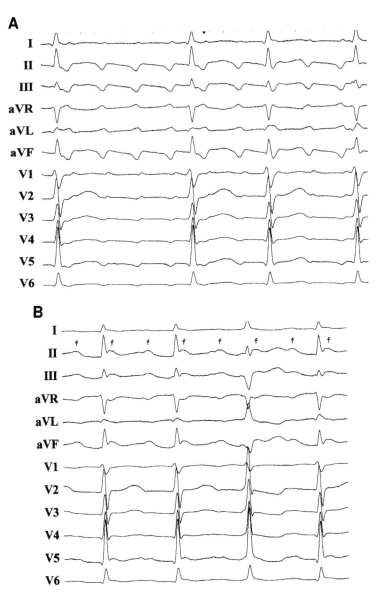

Fig. 2. Surface electrocardiograms demonstrating both clockwise and counterclockwise typical atrial flutter in the same patient. Paper speed 100 mm/s. (**A**) Counterclockwise atrial flutter with 4:1 and 2:1 conduction. (**B**) Clockwise atrial flutter with 2:1 conduction. Note the positive flutter (f) waves in aVF.

2. True atypical atrial flutter (also called Type II, "rare," or "uncommon") is a rare type of atrial flutter that describes a heterogeneous group of single macroreentrant atrial tachycardias. This includes leading circle reentry or reentry around a variety of naturally occurring anatomic boundaries. The atrial rate in true atypical atrial flutter is usually more rapid (340–440 cycles per minute) than that of typical atrial flutter, and the direction of rotation may be clockwise or counterclockwise. (*see* Fig. 3).

3. Incisional reentrant atrial tachycardia is macroreentry around a surgical incision. It occurs frequently in patients who have undergone surgical repair of congenital heart

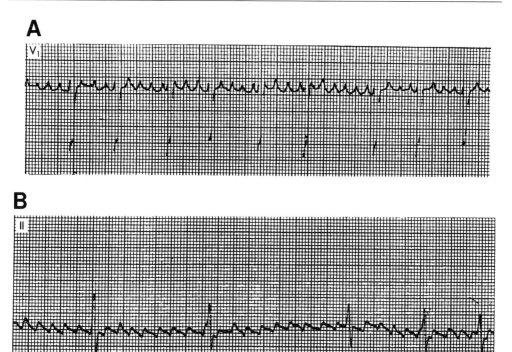

Fig. 3. True atypical atrial flutter. **(A)** The atrial rate is 428 BPM with variable AV conduction. **(B)** The atrial rate is 345 BPM with high-grade AV block. (Reproduced with permission from Marriot JL, Conover MB. Advanced Concepts in Arrhythmias. 3rd ed. Mosby, St. Louis, MO, 1998, p. 123.)

disease (Mustard, Senning, Fontan, and ASD repairs). Bi-atrial anastamosis for orthotopic heart transplantation provides an ideal substrate for reentry, as the incision forms the posterior barrier to conduction and the atrium is usually enlarged to accommodate the arrhythmia circuit.

ELECTROCARDIOGRAPHIC FEATURES

The term "atrial flutter" refers to a heterogeneous group of macro-reentrant arrhythmias including isthmus-dependent (typical) reentry around the tricuspid annulus, reentry around a surgical incision that is not necessarily isthmus-dependent, functional reentry (leading circle reentry), or reentry involving a combination of these conduction barriers *(30)*.

The diagnosis of atrial flutter is usually made by the surface electrocardiogram (ECG). The findings in the atrium are fundamentally those of the waveforms described by Lewis: rapid rate—usually 300 beats per minute (BPM) in typical atrial flutter, high degree of regularity, no isoelectric period but instead contiguous auricular complexes, and uniformity in outline *(2)*. In counterclockwise typical atrial flutter (the most common clinically), the flutter waves are negative in leads II, III, and aVF (*see* Fig. 2A). In clockwise typical atrial flutter (also referred to as atypical atrial flutter), the rates are usually the same (300 BPM), but the flutter waves are positive in leads II, III, and aVF (*see* Fig. 2B). In true atypical atrial flutter, the atrial rates are usually more rapid

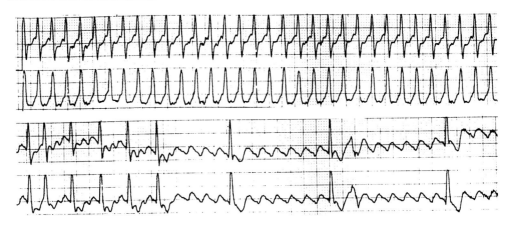

Fig. 4. Atrial flutter with 1:1 ventricular conduction. Two lead telemetry strips recorded during atrial flutter with 1:1 conduction (top two strips) and after adenosine, with transient high level AV-nodal block (bottom two strips). The key to the diagnosis of 1:1 atrial flutter, is that the interval between QRS complexes in the top tracing is equivalent to the atrial cycle length in the bottom two tracings.

(greater than 350 BPM) and the flutter waves in leads II, III, and aVF are usually positive (*see* Fig. 3).

The ventricular rate in atrial flutter depends on the AV conduction ratio and is usually 140–160 BPM because of 2:1 atrioventricular (AV) conduction. Atrial flutter should be considered in any supraventricular tachycardia (SVT) with rates near 150 BPM. The conduction ratio is usually a multiple of the atrial rate, and may be 2:1, 4:1, 6:1, etc. Higher conduction ratios may be seen in patients with AV nodal disease or in the presence of drugs slowing AV conduction (such as digitalis, verapamil, or beta-blockers). Importantly, 1:1 conduction is usually poorly tolerated hemodynamically, and if prolonged, may degenerate into ventricular fibrillation (VF). One-to-one conduction during atrial flutter may be seen in patients with accessory pathways and in the presence of hyperadrenergic states (such as critical care, postsurgical, and intravenous [iv] inotopes). Patients taking class I agents without adequate protection from medications to slow AV conduction are at risk for rapid ventricular conduction because the atrial rate may be slowed sufficiently to allow 1:1 conduction *(27,28)* (*see* Fig. 4). Patients started on a class I antiarrhythmic should always be treated with a beta-blocker, verapamil, or diltiazem to slow AV conduction enough to prevent this serious complication.

The ventricular rhythm may be regular if there is a fixed AV conduction ratio, or irregular if there is variable AV conduction. Grouped beating may be observed in the presence of Wenckebach periodicity within the AV node.

Vagal stimulation (i.e., carotid sinus massage, Valsalva maneuver) or iv adenosine may temporarily slow the ventricular rate to reveal the typical saw-toothed atrial pattern. Atrial flutter usually does not "break" with these interventions, whereas AV-node reentry or AV-reciprocating tachycardia usually converts to sinus rhythm.

Coarse AF may look organized in lead V1, and can be mistaken for atrial flutter (*see* Fig. 5). The distinction between AF and atrial flutter is helped by the lack of organized and regular flutter waves in the *inferior* leads and the irregular ventricular rates in AF.

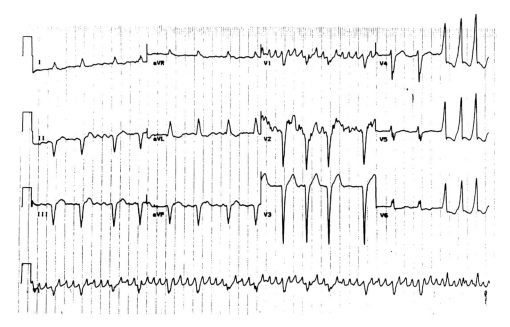

Fig. 5. Coarse AF. Note the organized undulations in lead V1, which can be mistaken for flutter waves. The variability in the cycle length of the "pseudo-flutter waves," the irregular ventricular rhythm, and the lack of organized flutter waves in the inferior leads are evidence that this is AF.

MECHANISM OF ATRIAL FLUTTER

Typical Atrial Flutter

Detailed atrial mapping and entrainment mapping studies in humans have confirmed that atrial flutter is caused by a macroreentrant circuit localized in the right atrium *(14,15,17,19)*. The circuit boundaries are the tricuspid annulus (anteriorly) and the crista terminalis, EV, and Eustachian ridge and venous orifices (posteriorly) *(18–20)*. There is a zone of slow conduction in the narrow isthmus of tissue between the inferior vena cava (IVC) and the tricuspid annulus *(16,21–24)*. A critical element in the propagation of a reentry circuit is the presence of a fully excitable gap preceding the depolarization wavefront. The reentry circuit in typical atrial flutter contains a fully excitable gap between the depolarization wavefront and the tail of repolarization *(34–39)*. The excitable gap comprises up to 25% of the cycle length of the reentry circuit *(34,39)*.

True Atypical Atrial Flutter

As mentioned previously, true atypical atrial flutter usually has a faster rate than typical atrial flutter, and may not have the same flutter-wave morphology on the surface electrocardiogram (ECG). The initial definition of atypical atrial flutter also included its usual lack of response (either termination or degeneration into AF) to atrial overdrive pacing *(40)*. A more mechanistic and particularly anatomic definition has thus far been lacking, probably because atypical flutter is a descriptive term referring to a heterogeneous group of reentrant arrhythmias revolving around functional and/or ana-tomic barriers. Kalman et al. *(41)* described a cohort of 20 patients with "true atypical atrial flutter" (distinguished from clockwise typical flutter and incisional flutter). These patients had a heterogeneous group of surface ECG morphologies and atrial cycle lengths of 192 ± 24 ms (range 152–265 ms). Detailed localization of the atypical flutter circuit was not performed in this study. Natale et al. *(42)* described a form of atypical atrial flutter than used the pulmonary veins as a central barrier. In 13 of 13 patients, radiofrequency ablation to produce a line of block from the mitral annulus to the pulmonary veins eliminated the tachycardia, although the recurrence rate was high. Cheng et al. *(43)* described a form of atypical flutter that was isthmus-dependent; the circuit traversed the isthmus but "short-circuited" across the crista terminalis instead of the roof of the right atrium as in typical atrial flutter. Finally, Kall et al. *(44)* described a form of "true atypical atrial flutter" that used a right atrial free-wall circuit with a central barrier that was incompletely characterized in six patients. Detailed mapping allowed linear ablation that prevented atypical flutter recurrence. In summary, atypical atrial flutter is a term that describes a range of different reentrant circuits, with various potential mechanisms and anatomic locations. This arrhythmia is unusual, but probably represents a fair proportion of the failed attempts at isthmus ablation for presumed typical atrial flutter.

Incisional Atrial Flutter

Incisional atrial flutter frequently occurs in patients who have had surgically corrected congenital heart disease such as ASD repair, Fontan Mustard, or Senning procedure. The reentry circuit is variable, depending on the incision and its relation to other anatomic structures. Multiple reentry circuits may exist within the same patient. The circuit may rotate around the incision itself or may rotate around the incision and other anatomic structures. Because there is a fixed incisional and/or anatomic barrier, this type of atrial flutter has an excitable gap and can therefore be entrained. Through detailed activation and entrainment mapping, Kalmar et al. identified incisional reentry in 18 patients with 26 intra-atrial reentrant tachycardias complicating surgery for congenital heart disease. In this series, nine patients had an ASD repair, four patients had a Fontan repair, two patients had a Mustard repair, two patients had a Senning repair, and one patient had a Rastelli procedure. Using detailed atrial activation and entrainment mapping to identify a unique narrow isthmus bound by anatomic/incisional barriers to conduction, radiofrequency ablation across this isthmus achieved acute success in 15 of 18 (83%) of patients. At a mean follow-up of 17 mo, 9 of 18 (50%) patients were symptom-free and required no medical therapy *(45)*.

TREATMENT OF ATRIAL FLUTTER

The goals of treatment in atrial flutter are to control ventricular rate, convert to and maintain sinus rhythm, and prevent thromboembolic complications in patients with prolonged episodes of atrial flutter.

Drugs used for ventricular rate control in atrial flutter include digitalis, verapamil, diltiazem, and beta-blockers. The efficacy of these drugs in preventing 1:1 conduction in atrial flutter is assumed, but has not been proven. Digitalis is a poor single choice for rate control, because circulating catecholamines from daily stressors may easily overwhelm its vagotonic effects on the AV node. Given the typical even-integral (i.e.,

2:1, 4:1, 8:1) ventricular response to atrial flutter, rate control without corresponding bradycardia during sinus rhythm is often difficult to achieve.

The therapeutic options for cardioversion of atrial flutter include electrical or direct current (DC) cardioversion, antiarrhythmic agents (class I and III antiarrhythmics), overdrive pacing, and radiofrequency ablation. Notably, any attempt at acute cardioversion (independent of whether electrical, chemical, pacing or ablative techniques are used) necessitates careful consideration of the risk of thromboembolism.

DC Cardioversion

Direct current (DC) cardioversion was first introduced as a treatment for atrial tachyarrhythmias in 1962 *(46)*. DC cardioversion for atrial flutter is initially successful in 93–100% of patients *(47–51)*. In patients with chronic atrial flutter, recurrence rates are high *(52)*. Traditionally, an initial shock of 50 J has been recommended for atrial flutter, yet more recent evidence reveals a higher rate of first-shock cardioversion, fewer total shocks, and less AF complicating cardioversion when 100 J or higher is used as the initial shock *(47,53)*.

Patients undergoing direct current cardioversion should have an empty stomach, and therefore should not eat for 8 h prior to the procedure. External cardioversion is performed with general anesthesia, typically with a short-acting agent such as propofol. Once the patient is adequately sedated, a synchronized shock at an initial energy of 100 J is successful 85% of the time *(53)*. If the initial shock is unsuccessful, 200-J and 300-J shocks should follow until the patient is in sinus rhythm. In patients refractory to DC cardioversion, the use of a biphasic external defibrillator may be successful. Intracardiac cardioversion is also an option.

Pharmacologic Treatment of Atrial Flutter

ACUTE CARDIOVERSION

Anti-arrhythmic agents used for cardioversion of atrial flutter include class I and class III drugs. Class I agents block sodium channels and slow conduction within the atrium. Theoretically, sufficient slowing of conduction across the isthmus of slow conduction in typical atrial flutter should result in localized conduction block (depressed excitability) and termination of the arrhythmia. Class III agents block potassium channels and prolong refractoriness. In theory, prolonging the refractory period should narrow the excitable gap and/or force the activation pathway to expand beyond the dimensions of the available atrial tissue.

Most of the clinical evidence about antiarrhythmic drug therapy in atrial flutter comes from studies in which atrial flutter is combined with AF *(54)*. Furthermore, most of these studies lack a placebo group for comparison, and therefore the incidence of spontaneous cardioversion was not determined. Studies in which drug effects on atrial flutter have been separated from AF include only a small number of patients. In turn, there is a tremendous lack of information on antiarrhythmic drug efficacy in atrial flutter itself. Cardioversion rates in these studies are disappointing and are in general reported to be less than 40% *(55,56)*.

Ibutilide appears to be more effective than other antiarrhythmic agents in acute cardioversion of atrial flutter. Vos et al. in a double-blind, randomized study of ibutilide vs *dl*-sotalol (251 patients with AF and 57 patients with atrial flutter), reported successful cardioversion in 70% of patients with atrial flutter treated with ibutilide (2 mg iv). Only 19% of patients treated with sotalol converted to sinus rhythm. Of the 109 patients treated with 2 mg of iv ibutilide, 8 patients (7.3%) had nonsustained polymorphic ventricular tachycardia (PVT), one patient had nonsustained monomorphic VT, and 1 patient had sustained PVT requiring electrical cardioversion. All proarrhythmic events occurred within 30 min of the infusion of ibutilide (57). Stambler et al. reported a comparison of ibutilide, procainamide, and placebo given for attempted cardioversion in 89 patients with atrial flutter. Ibutilide converted 29 of 45 (64%) patients, procainamide converted 0 of 33 patients, and 0 of 11 patients who received placebo converted to sinus rhythm. Nonsustained PVT was observed in 4% of patients who received ibutilide for atrial flutter (58).

The incidence of pro-arrhythmia in these two trials is consistent with other published data. The overall incidence of PVT in a report of 586 patients who received ibutilide in clinical trials was 4.4%. The incidence of sustained PVT was 1.7% (59). Although ibutilide appears to be efficacious in the acute termination of atrial flutter, there is a significant risk of proarrhythmia, and patients should be closely monitored until resolution of drug-induced QT prolongation (minimum of 60 min after the iv infusion is complete).

Chronic Maintenance of Sinus Rhythm

Data on the efficacy of long-term maintenance of sinus rhythm with pharmacologic therapy of atrial flutter is lacking, again because of the inclusion of patients with AF in most trials. A potential danger with antiarrhythmic therapy is that it may cause sufficient slowing of the flutter rate to allow the AV node to conduct 1:1 in the absence of sufficient AV-nodal blocking agents. This may result in hemodynamic instability, myocardial ischemia, or sudden death. It is important that patients treated with antiarrhythmic therapy (for AF or atrial flutter) are placed on medications that will sufficiently slow AV conduction, such as beta-blockers or calcium-channel blockers.

Treatment of Atrial Flutter with Atrial Pacing

When atrial pacing is readily available (as in the presence of a DDD pacemaker or an atrial lead inserted after cardiac surgery), rapid atrial pacing may be utilized to terminate atrial flutter. This procedure is performed by pacing at a slightly faster rate than the flutter rate. When an atrial lead is available, this method is attractive because it causes little discomfort to the patient and does not require anesthesia.

Clinical trials of antitachycardia pacing for atrial flutter have yielded modest results for pacing alone (60–66). Atrial pacing may be complicated by the induction of AF, which may occur in up to 70% of patients after rapid pacing of atrial flutter (62,63,65). Improvement in pace termination rates with significant reduction in the induction of AF can be achieved with the addition of class IA (procainamide, disopyramide) agents prior to atrial overdrive pacing. The efficacy of combination therapy is reported to be 70–100% (61–63,66,67). Class IA agents prolong the cycle length to a greater extent than the effective refractory period, and significantly increase the excitable gap in atrial flutter (66). These agents appear to exert their effect by decreasing the conduction velocity and widening the excitable gap, and therefore facilitating the penetration of the pacing stimulus into the atrial flutter circuit.

Ibutilide, a class III agent, appears as efficacious as procainamide in aiding the success of overdrive pacing for atrial flutter. Stambler et al. *(67)* reported conversion of atrial flutter in 2 of 11 (18%) patients with pacing alone, 13 of 15 (87%) patients who received iv ibutilide and overdrive pacing, and 29 of 33 (88%) patients who received iv procainamide and overdrive pacing.

Treatment of Atrial Flutter with Radiofrequency Ablation

Radiofrequency catheter ablation has revolutionized the treatment of supraventricular tachyarrhythmias. Understanding the anatomic barriers that confine the macroentry circuit of typical atrial flutter has allowed electrophysiologists to focus treatment on the narrow isthmus between the IVC and tricuspid annulus *(23,68,69)* *(see* Fig. 6). A linear lesion is applied with radiofrequency energy within the isthmus to the end point of bidirectional conduction block, demonstrated with pacing and multi-electrode catheter recordings *(see* Fig. 7). The acute success rate is greater than 95% *(23,68,70–72)* and when bidirectional block is demonstrated within the isthmus, the recurrence rate is 6–9% *(71,73)*. The procedure is performed anatomically, and can therefore be performed with the patient in sinus rhythm *(72,75)*. Radiofrequency ablation of atrial flutter is safe, with relatively few reported complications, and is effective. Success rates in excess of 95% have been reported; recurrence rates are less than 10% with current techniques.

Natale et al. prospectively studied outcomes of patients with atrial flutter who were randomly assigned to initial antiarrhythmic therapy vs primary radiofrequency ablation *(74)*. Of 61 patients, 30 were assigned to drug therapy and 31 were assigned to radiofrequency ablation therapy. After a mean follow-up of 21 ± 11 mo, only 11 of 30 (36%) patients treated with antiarrhythmics were in sinus rhythm, vs 25 of 31 (80%) who received radiofrequency ablation ($p < 0.01$). Furthermore, 63% of patients who were treated with antiarrhythmics required one or more hospitalizations after initiation of therapy vs 22% of patients post-radiofrequency ablation. Importantly, a quality-of-life and symptom questionnaire (Endicott Quality of Life Enjoyment and Satisfaction Questionnaire) was administered at the beginning of the study and 6 and 12 mo thereafter. Sense of well-being and function in daily life improved significantly after ablation (2.0 ± 3 pre radiofrequency vs 3.8 ± 0.5 post-radiofrequency, $p < 0.01$); 2.3 ± 0.4 pre-radiofrequency vs 3.6 ± 0.6 post-radiofrequency, $p < 0.01$ respectively). These parameters did not change significantly in patients treated with drugs *(74)*. Interestingly, 53% patients treated with antiarrhythmic medication in this study developed AF vs 29% of patients who were treated with radiofrequency ablation ($p < 0.05$). This finding casts further doubts into the efficacy of antiarrhythmic therapy.

AF following radiofrequency ablation for typical atrial flutter occurs in approx 25% of patients. Philippon et al. reported an incidence of 26.4% (14 patients) in 53 consecutive patients during a mean follow-up of 13 mo after radiofrequency ablation *(76)*. Paydak reported a rate of 25% (28 patients) in 110 consecutive patients treated with ablation during a mean follow-up of 20 mo *(77)*. Patients with structural heart disease and a history of AF are at greatest risk *(76,77)*. In the absence of structural heart disease, patients with this complication can be treated safely with class I antiarrhythmic drugs *(see* section on Hybrid therapy). Patients with AF and structural heart disease should be treated on an individual basis with either anticoagulation and rate control or anti-arrhythmic therapy (such as amiodarone or dofetilide).

The efficacy of radiofrequency ablation in true atypical atrial flutter is not as well defined. Experience with ablation of true atypical atrial flutter with fixed anatomic

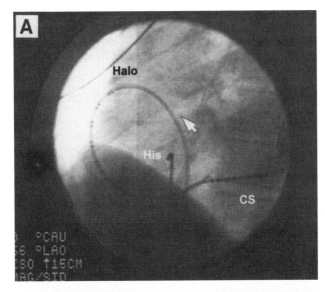

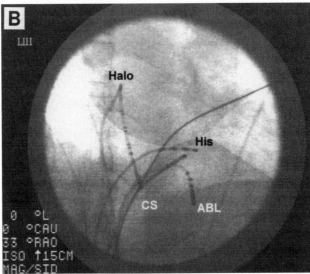

Fig. 6. Fluoroscopic images of catheters within the right atrium. **(A)** Left anterior oblique 30° projection. The halo catheter encircles the tricuspid annulus and has 10 bipolar electrodes (from distal to proximal, labeled T1–T10). The His catheter sits immediately on the atrial side of the tricuspid annulus over the bundle of His. The coronary sinus (CS) catheter is placed within the coronary sinus. In counterclockwise typical atrial flutter, activation around the Halo follows the direction of the arrow. **(B)** Right anterior oblique 60° projection of the same catheters, now including the ablation (ABL) catheter. During ablation of typical atrial flutter, a lesion is created in the isthmus between the tricuspid annulus and the IVC. This is usually between the CS catheter and T1 on the Halo catheter.

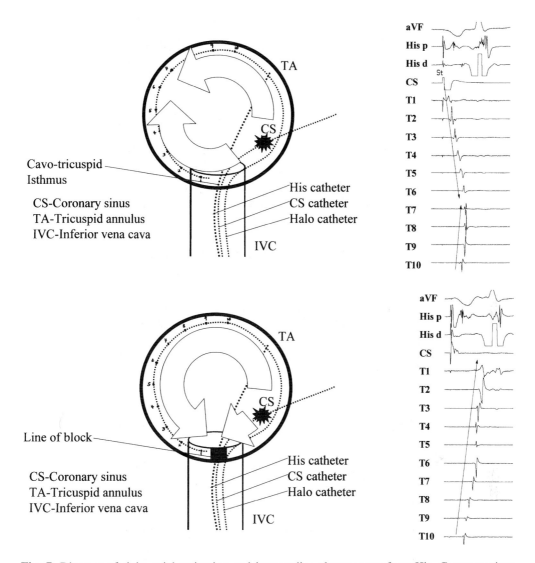

Fig. 7. Diagram of right atrial activation and intracardiac electrograms from His, Coronary sinus ostium (CS), Halo catheter electrodes. **(A)** Activation sequence prior to ablation of typical atrial flutter. Schematic diagram (left) represents position of electrodes in relation to anatomic structures within the right atrium. The critical isthmus lies between the inferior vena cava (IVC) and the tricuspid annulus (TA). Pacing from the CS os starts a wavefront that conducts in both directions through the atrium, the impulse proceeds "colliding" at approx T7. This is seen clearly in the intracardiac electrograms on the right. **(B)** Activation sequence after successful ablation of isthmus. The paced impulse blocks at the site of the lesion, but proceeds superiorly on the atrial septum (CS to His), across the roof of the atrium, and then inferiorly on the atrial free wall (T10 to T1). The T1 electrode is now the latest electrode site activated, despite its proximity to the CS pacing site. Bidirectional block is demonstrated by a similar discontinuous conduction pattern during pacing from the low lateral right atrium (T3 position). When this site is paced, the CS os electrode site should be the latest in the sequence with successful ablation.

substrates is limited. Because of the variable anatomic location, detailed mapping and a case-specific approach are necessary.

Ablation of incisional atrial flutter may be achieved by creating a lesion in a critical isthmus of conduction bounded by anatomic barriers. This isthmus can be localized by entrainment mapping. Once the critical isthmus is localized, a line of block is created from the incision to an anatomic barrier (such as the tricuspid annulus, atrial septal patch, IVC, or SVC) *(77a)*. Kalman et al. reported an acute success rate of 83% (15 of 18 patients). During a mean follow-up of 17 mo, clinical improvement was observed in 73% (13 of 18 patients), and 50% (9 of 18 patients) remained asymptomatic without recurrence of atrial flutter *(45)*.

In refractory cases of incisional atrial flutter with a rapid ventricular rate, radio-frequency ablation of the His bundle with the implantation of a single-chamber ventricular pacing (VVIR)-pacemaker may be an alternative option *(78–81)*.

Typical atrial flutter is the most common subtype of atrial flutter seen clinically. Atrial flutter ablation in typical atrial flutter is curative and safe. Atrial flutter ablation results in a lower incidence of AF than pharmacologic treatment, improves quality of life, and may allow cessation of warfarin.

Treatment of Atrial Flutter After Cardiac and Thoracic Surgery

Atrial arrhythmias are common after cardiothoracic surgery. Right atrial enlargement from hemodynamic factors, pericardial irritation, and withdrawal from chronic beta-blocker therapy contribute to promote the occurrence of atrial tachyarrhythmias. The incidence of atrial arrhythmias after cardiac surgery is approximately 30%, with atrial flutter representing up to one-third of these cases *(82)*. The initial management of postoperative atrial flutter is similar to the management of postoperative AF. If the patient is hemodynamically unstable, DC cardioversion or anti-tachycardia pacing is indicated. If the patient is stable, ventricular rate control with a beta-blocker is preferred unless contraindicated. Most patients will spontaneously convert to sinus rhythm without antiarrhythmic therapy. In patients with late (> 3 d postoperative) onset or recurrent atrial flutter after the initiation of beta-blocker therapy, a reasonable approach is treatment with antiarrhythmic drugs (usually procainamide or amiodarone) and warfarin for 4–6 wk. Catheter ablation is not indicated in the acute postoperative setting, because of the usually transient nature of atrial flutter in this setting.

Prevention of Thromboembolic Complications in Atrial Flutter

Until recently, patients with atrial flutter had not been treated with anticoagulation. Several transesophageal echocardiographic studies have demonstrated a significant prevalence of left atrial thrombus and spontaneous echo contrast in patients referred for cardioversion or ablation of atrial flutter *(83–85)*. Recent studies have demonstrated a risk of thromboembolic complications in patients with atrial flutter. Seidl et al. reported a 7% thromboembolic event-rate flutter over a mean follow-up of 26 mo in a prospective study of 191 consecutive patients referred for treatment of atrial flutter *(86)*. Wood et al. found an embolic rate of 14% over a period of 4.5 yr in 86 patients referred for radiofrequency ablation for atrial flutter *(87)*. Lanzarotti et al. retrospectively reviewed thromboembolic events in 100 patients who underwent direct current cardioversion for atrial flutter, and reported a 6% event rate *(88)*. The preliminary evidence for thromboembolic risk in atrial flutter demonstrates a significant risk rate, approaching the risk seen in AF.

With anticoagulation therapy, there is a fine balance between decreasing the risk of thromboembolic events and the increased risk of bleeding. Bleeding complications from anticoagulation therapy can be estimated from the six major trials examining the effectiveness of anticoagulation in the prevention of stroke in patients with atrial AF (AFASAK, SPAF, BAATAF, CAFA, SPINAF, and SPAFII) *(89–94)*. The target INR in these trials varied, with a range between 1.4 and 4.5. The annual incidence of stroke in these trials was approx 4.5% (range 3.0–7.4%). With warfarin therapy, the incidence of stroke was reduced to a mean of 1.4%. The risk of major bleeding in these studies was extremely low, with an incidence of approx 1.3% per yr in the warfarin groups.

Further insights into the risk of bleeding during anticoagulation therapy can be derived from recent studies of anticoagulation for myocardial infarction (MI). In the ASPECT trial, patients were randomized to anticoagulant treatment following an acute MI with a target International Normalized Ratio (INR) of 2.8 to 4.8 *(95)*. Major bleeding in this trial was reported at a rate of 1.5 per 100-patient years of follow-up. The risk of major bleeding increased dramatically as the INR increased over 4.0. The risk of thromboembolic events increased at an INR <2.0.

Based on the available data, patients with atrial flutter of greater than 48 h duration should be anticoagulated with warfarin (target INR 2.0–3.0). A transesophageal echocardiogram should be obtained if cardioversion or ablation is planned prior to at least 3 wk of adequate anticoagulation. Anticoagulation should be continued for 4 wk after cardioversion or radiofrequency ablation of atrial flutter. Long-term anticoagulation is recommended for paroxysmal or chronic atrial flutter, except in patients less than 65 yr of age with "lone" or idiopathic atrial flutter. In these patients, the risk of thromboembolic complications is extremely low, and aspirin therapy is typically recommended *(96)*.

Hybrid Therapy for Atrial Fibrillation

Atrial flutter often coexists with AF within the same individual. It has been observed that up to 11% of patients with lone AF treated with antiarrhythmics will develop persistent atrial flutter. Schumacher et al. studied 187 patients with paroxysmal AF who were treated with class (IC) antiarrhythmic agents (96 patients received flecainide, 91 patients received propafenone) *(97)*. Twenty-four patients (12.8%) developed atrial flutter during treatment. Twenty of the 24 patients (10.7%) were found to have typical atrial flutter by electrophysiologic studies. These 20 patients underwent radiofrequency ablation, which was acutely successful in 19 of 20 patients. These patients were followed by ambulatory Holter monitoring and serial questionnaires for a mean follow-up period of 11 ± 4 mo. The incidence of AF episodes were significantly lower in patients with combined therapy (2.7 ± 3.6 per yr) vs patients treated with drugs alone (7.8 ± 9.2 per yr, $p < 0.05$). During the follow-up period, 7 patients remained symptom-free with no evidence of atrial tachyarrhythmias, and 8 patients had paroxysmal AF but at a significant lower frequency than before combined therapy (2.3 ± 1.6 per yr vs 11.5 ± 1.50 per yr, $p < 0.001$). In the remaining four patients, no benefit was found *(97)*. Huang et al. reported 13 patients who developed atrial flutter when treated for AF with antiarrhythmic agents. Nine of these patients had typical atrial flutter and underwent successful radiofrequency ablation. These nine patients were followed by clinic visits, record review, and telephone interviews and during a mean follow-up of 14.3 ± 6.9 mo, 88.9% remained in sinus rhythm *(98)*. Tai et al. reported atrial flutter in 15 of 136 (11%) patients treated for AF with amiodarone (*n* = 96) or propafenone (*n* = 40). Atrial flutter occurred in equal frequency in patients treated with amiodarone vs propafenone. Eleven of these 15 patients had counterclockwise typical atrial flutter and four had clockwise typical atrial flutter. All 15 patients underwent successful radiofrequency ablation. During a mean follow-up period of 12.3 ± 4.2 mo, 14 (93%) remained in sinus rhythm *(99)*.

Hybrid pharmacologic and ablative therapy may be a safe and effective means of maintaining sinus rhythm in a subset of patients who develop atrial flutter during antiarrhythmic treatment for AF.

CONCLUSION

There is compelling evidence that patients with atrial flutter should be offered radiofrequency ablation as a "first-line" therapy for this arrhythmia. Radiofrequency ablation is highly successful, safe, and for most patients, a curative treatment for atrial flutter. Furthermore, patients successfully treated with radiofrequency ablation may be taken off warfarin therapy approx 4 wk after the procedure. In patients who are unable to or choose not to undergo radiofrequency ablation, DC cardioversion, overdrive pacing with the aide of procainamide or disopyramide, or iv antiarrhythmic drug infusion may be attempted when appropriate for acute cardioversion.

Acute cardioversion and maintenance of sinus rhythm with pharmcological treatment of atrial flutter is disappointing, and is associated with the risk of proarrhythmia, side effects, drug toxicities, and a significant risk of tachyarrhythmia resulting from 1:1 conduction through the AV node.

Unless contraindicated, patients with chronic or paroxysmal atrial flutter should generally be anticoagulated with warfarin.

REFERENCES

1. Jolly WA, Ritchie WT. Auricular flutter and fibrillation. Heart 1911;2:177–221.
2. Lewis T. Observations upon flutter and fibrillation. I. The regularity of clinical auricular flutter. Heart 1920;7:127–130.
3. Lewis T, Feil HS, Stroud WD. Observations upon flutter and fibrillation. II. The nature of auricular flutter. Heart 1920;7:191–245.
4. Lewis T, Drury AN, Iliescu CC. A demonstration of circus movement in clinical flutter of the auricles. Heart 1921;8:341–357.
5. Mary-Rabine L, Mahaux V, Waleffe A, Kulbertus H. Atrial flutter: historical background. J Cardiovasc Electrophysiol 1997;8:353–358.
6. Puech P, Latour H, Grolleau R. Le flutter et ses limites. Arch Mal Coeur 1970;61:116–144.
7. Rosenblueth A, Garcia-Ramos J. Studies on flutter and fibrillation. II. The influence of artificial obstacles on experimental auricular flutter. Am Heart J 1947;33:677–684.
8. Frame LH, Page RI, Hoffman BF. Atrial reentry around an anatomic barrier with a partially refractory excitable gap: a canine model of atrial flutter. Circ Res 1986;58:495–511.
9. Frame L, Page R, Boyden P, et al. Circus movement in the canine atrium around the tricuspid ring during experimental atrial flutter and during reentry in vitro. Circulation 1987;76:1155–1175.
10. Boineau JP, Schuessler RB, Mooney CR, et al. Natural and evoked atrial flutter due to circus movement in dogs. Am J Cardiol 1980;45:1167–1181.
11. Allessie MA, Lammers WJEP, Bonke FIM, et al. Intra-atrial reentry as a mechanism for atrial flutter induced by actylcholine and rapid pacing in the dog. Circulation 1984;70:123–135.
12. Boyden PA. Activation sequence during atrial flutter in dogs with surgically induced right atrial enlargement. I. Observations during sustained rhythms. Circ Res 1988;62:596–608.

13. Feld GK, Shahandeh RF. Activation patterns in experienced canine atrial flutter produced by right atrial crush injury. J Am Coll Cardiol 1992;20:441–451.

14. Klein GJ, Guiraudon GM, Sharma AD, et al. Demonstration of macroreentry and feasibility of operative therapy in the common type of atrial flutter. Am J Cardiol 1986;57:587–591.

15. Cosio FG, Lopez-Gil M, Goicolea A, et al. Electrophysiologic studies in atrial flutter. Clin Cardiol 1992;15:667–673.

16. Cosio FG, Arribas F, Palacios J, et al. Fragmented electrograms and continuous electrical activity in atrial flutter. Am J Cardiol 1986;57:1309–1314.

17. Waldo AL, Mclean WAH, Karp RB, et al. Entrainment and interruption of atrial flutter with atrial pacing: studies in man following open heart surgery. Circulation 1977;56:737–745.

18. Nakagawa H, Lazzara R, Khastgir T, et al. Role of the tricuspid annulus and the eustachian valve/ridge on atrial flutter. Circulation 1996;94(3):407–424.

19. Olgin JE, Kalman JM, Fitzpatrick AP, et al. Role of right atrial endocardial structures as barriers to conduction during human type I atrial flutter. Circulation 1995;92(7):1839–1848.

20. Kalman JM, Olgin JE, Saxon LA, et al. Activation and entrainment mapping defines the tricuspid annulus as the anterior barrier in typical atrial flutter. Circulation 1996;94(3):398–406.

21. Olshansky B, Okumura K, Hess PG, Waldo AL. Demonstration of an area of slow conduction in human atrial flutter. J Am Coll Cardiol 1990;16:1639–1648.

22. Olshanski B, Okumura K, Henthorn RW, Waldo AL. Characterization of double potentials in human atrial flutter: studies during transient entrainment. J Am Coll Cardiol 1990;15:833–841.

23. Feld GK, Fleck RP, Chen PS, et al. Radiofrequency catheter ablation of human type I atrial flutter: identification of a critical zone in the reentrant circuit by endocardial mapping techniques. Circulation 1992;86:1233–1240.

24. Cosio FG, Arribas F, Barbero JM, et al. Validation of double spike electrograms as markers of conduction delay or block in atrial flutter. Am J Cardiol 1988;61:755–780.

25. Uribe W, Vidaillet H, Granada J, et al. Incidence and cause of death among patients with atrial flutter in the general population. Circulation 1996;94(Suppl 8):2269.

26. Garson A Jr, Bink-Boelkens M, Hesslein PS, et al. Atrial flutter in the young: a collaborative study of 380 cases. J Am Coll Cardiol 1990;6:871–878.

27. Waldo AL. Clinical evaluation in therapy of patients with atrial fibrillation or flutter. Cardiol Clin *Supraventricular Tachycardia* 1990;8:479.

28. VanHare GF, Lesh MD, Ross BA, et al. Mapping and radiofrequency ablation of intraatrial reentrant tachycardia after the Senning or Mustard procedure for transposition of the great arteries. Am J Cardiol 1996;77:985–991.

29. Boyden PA, Hoffman BF. The effects on atrial electrophysiology and structure of surgically induced right atrial enlargement in dogs. Circ Res 1981;49:1319–1331.

30. Lesh MD, Kalman JM. To fumble flutter or tackle "tach"? Toward updated classifiers for atrial tachyarrhythmias. J Cardiovasc Electrophysiol 1996;7:460–466.

31. London F, Howell M. Atrial flutter: 1 to 1 conduction during treatment with quinidine and digitalis. Am Heart J 1954;48:152–156.

32. Robertson CE, Miller HC. Extreme tachycardia complicating the use of disopyramide in atrial flutter. Br Heart J 1980;44:602–603.

33. Williams PL. Gray's anatomy—The anatomical basis of medicine and surgery. 38th ed. Churchill Livingstone, 1995.

34. Inoue H, Matsuo H, Takayanagi et al. Clinical and experimental studies of the effects of atrial extrastimulation and rapid pacing on atrial flutter cycle: evidence of macro-reentry with an excitable gap. Am J Cardiol 1981;48:623–630.

35. Disertori M, Inama G, Vergara G, et al. Evidence of a reentry circuit in the common type of atrial flutter in man. Circulation 1983;67:434–440.

36. Della Bella P, Marenzi G, Tondo C, et al. Usefulness of excitable gap and pattern of resetting in atrial flutter for determining reentry circuit location. Am J Cardiol 1991;68:492–497.

37. Arenal A, Almendral J, San Roman D, Delcan JL, Josephson ME. Frequency and implications of resetting and entrainment with right atrial stimulation in atrial flutter. Am J Cardiol 1992;70:1292–1298.

38. Stambler BS, Wood MA, Ellenbogen KA. Pharmacologic alterations in human type I atrial flutter cycle length and monophasic action potential duration: evidence of a fully excitable gap in the reentrant circuit. J Am Coll Cardiol 1996;27:453–461.

39. Callans DJ, Schwartzman D, Gottlieb CD, et al. Characterization of the excitable gap in human type I atrial flutter. J Am Coll Cardiol 1997;30:1793–1801.

40. Wells JL, MacLean WAH, James TN, et al. Characterization of atrial flutter: studies in man after open heart surgery using fixed atrial electrodes. Circulation 1979;60:665–673.

41. Kalman JM, Olgin JE, Saxon LA, et al. Electrocardiographic and electrophysiologic characterization of atypical atrial flutter in man: using activation mapping and implications of catheter ablation. J Cardiovasc Electrophysiol 1997;8:121–144.

42. Natale A, Richey M, Tomassoni GF, et al. Clinical characteristics and ablation of left sided atrial flutter. J Am Coll Cardiol 1999;33 (Suppl 2) a):116A.

43. Cheng J, Cabeen WR, Scheinman MM. Right atrial flutter due to lower loop reentry: mechanism and anatomic substrates. Circulation 1999;99(13);1700–1705.

44. Kall JG, Rubenstein DS, Kopp DE, et al. Atypical atrial flutter originating in the right atrial free wall. Circulation 2000;101:270–281.

45. Kalman JM, Van Hare GF, Olgin JE, et al. Ablation of 'incisional' reentrant atrial tachycardia complicating surgery for congenital heart disease: use of entrainment to define a critical isthmus of conduction. Circulation 1996;93:502–512.

46. Lown B, Amana Bingham R, Neuman J. A new method for terminating cardiac arrhythmias. JAMA 1962;182:548–551.

47. Castellanos A, Lemberg L, Gosselin A., et al. Evaluation of countershock treatment of atrial flutter. Arch Int Med 1965;115:426–433.

48. Frith ZG, Aberg H. Direct current cardioversion of atrial flutter. Acta Med Scand 1970;271–274.

49. Morris JJ, Kong Y, North WC, McIntosh HD. Experience with cardioversion of atrial fibrillation and atrial flutter. Am J Cardiol 1964;14:94–100.

50. VanGelder H, Crijns HJ, VanGilst WH, et al. Prediction of uneventful cardioversion and maintenance of sinus rhythm from direct current cardioversion of chronic atrial fibrillation and atrial flutter. Am J Cardiol 1991;68:41–46.

51. Chalasani P, Cambre S, Silverman ME. Direct current cardioversion of atrial flutter. Am J Cardiol 1996;77(8):658–660.

52. Crijns HJ, VanGelder IC, Tieleman RG, et al. Long term outcome of electrical cardioversion in patients with chronic atrial flutter. Heart 1997;77:56–61.

53. Pinski SL, Sgarbossa EB, Ching E, et al. A comparison of 50 J versus 100 J shocks for direct current cardioversion of atrial flutter. Am Heart J 1999;137(3):439–432.

54. Campbell RWF. Pharmacologic therapy of atrial flutter. J Cardiovasc Electrophysiol 1996;7:1008–1012.

55. Bianconi L, Boccadamo R, Pappalardo A, et al. Effectiveness of intravenous propafenone for conversion of atrial fibrillation and flutter of recent onset. Am J Cardiol 1989;64:335–338.

56. Suttorp MJ, Kingma JH, Lie-A-Huen L, et al. Intravenous flecainide versus verapamil for conversion of paroxysmal atrial fibrillation or flutter to sinus rhythm. Am J Cardiol 1989;63:693–696.

57. Vos MA, Golitsyn SR, Stangl K, et al. Superiority of ibutilide (a new class III agent) over DL-sotalol in converting atrial flutter and atrial fibrillation. Heart 1998;79(6):568–575.

58. Stambler BS, Wood MA, Ellenbogen KA. Antiarrhythmic actions of intravenous ibutilide compared with procainamide during human atrial flutter and fibrillation: electrophysiological determinants of enhanced conversion efficacy. Circulation 1997;96(12):4298–4306.

59. Foster RH, Wilde MI, Markham A. Ibutilide: a review of its pharmacological properties and clinical potential in the acute management of atrial flutter and fibrillation. Drugs 1997;54(2):312–330.

60. Haft JI, Kosowsky BD, Lau SH, et al. Termination of atrial flutter by rapid electrical stimulation of the atrium. Am J Cardiol 1967;20:239–244.

61. Camm J, Ward D, Spurrell R. Response of atrial flutter to overdrive atrial pacing and intravenous disopyramide phosphate, singly and in combination. Br Heart J 1980;44:240–247.

62. Olshansky B, Okumura K, Hess PG, Henthorn RW, Waldo AL. Use of procainamide with rapid atrial pacing for successful conversion of atrial flutter to sinus rhythm. J Am Coll Cardiol 1988;11:359–364.

63. Della Bella P, Tondo C, Marenzi G, et al. Facilitating influence of disopyramide on atrial flutter termination by overdrive pacing. Am J Cardiol 1988;61:1046–1049.

64. Rosen KM, Sinno MZ, Gunnar RW, Rahimtoola SH. Failure of rapid atrial pacing in the conversion of atrial flutter. Am J Cardiol 1970;26:262–269.

65. Fujimoto T, Inoue T, Hidemi O, et al. The effects of class IA antiarrhythmic drug on the common type of atrial flutter in combination with pacing therapy. Jpn Circ J 1989;53:237–244.

66. Della Bella P, Marenzi G, Tondo C, Doni F, et al. Effects of disopyramide on cycle length, effective refractory period and excitable gap of atrial flutter, and relation to arrhythmia termination by overdrive pacing. Am J Cardiol 1989;63:812–816.

67. Stambler BS, Wood MA, Ellenbogen KA. Comparative efficacy of intravenous ibutalide versus procainamide for enhancing termination of atrial flutter by atrial overdrive pacing. Am J Cardiol 1996;77(11):960–966.

68. Cosio FG, Lopez-Gil M, Goicolea A, et al. Radiofrequency ablation of the inferior vena cava-tricuspid valve isthmus in common atrial flutter. Am J Cardiol 1993;71:705–709.

69. Saoudi N, Atallah G, Kirkorian G, Touboul P. Catheter ablation of the atrial myocardium in human type I atrial flutter. Circulation 81:762–771.

70. Fischer B, Jais P, Shah D, et al. Radiofrequency catheter ablation of common atrial flutter in 200 patients. J Cardiovasc Electrophysiol 1996;7:1225–1233.

71. Tai CT, Chen SA, Chiang CE, et al. Long-term outcome of radiofrequency catheter ablation for typical atrial flutter: risk prediction of recurrent arrhythmias. J Cardiovasc Electrophysiol 1998;9:115–121.

72. Poty H, Saoudi N, Anair M, et al. Radiofrequency catheter ablation of atrial flutter: further insights into the various types of isthmus block: application to ablation during sinus rhythm. Circulation 1996;94:3204–3213.

73. Schumacher B, Pfeiffer D, Tebbenjohanns J, et al. Acute and long-term effects of consecutive radiofrequency applications on conduction properties of the subeustachian isthmus in type I atrial flutter. J Cardiovasc Electrophysiol 1998;9:152–163.

74. Natale A, Leonelli F, Newby K, et al. Prospective randomized comparison of antiarrhythmic therapy versus first line radiofrequency ablation in patients with atrial flutter. J Am Coll Cardiol 2000;35:1898–1904.

75. Kirkorian G, Moncada E, Chevalier P, et al. Radiofrequency ablation of atrial flutter: efficacy of an anatomically guided approach. Circulation 1994;90:2804–2814.

76. Philippon F, Plumb VJ, Epstein AE. The risk of atrial fibrillation following radiofrequency catheter ablation of atrial flutter. Circulation 1995;92:430–435.

77. Paydak H, Kall JG, Burke MC. Atrial fibrillation after radiofrequency ablation of type I atrial flutter: time to onset, determinants, and clinical course. Circulation 1998;98:315–322.

77a. Delacretaz E, Ganz LI, Soejima K, Friedman PL, Walsh EP, Triedman LJ, Landzberg MJ, Stevenson WG. Multi atrial maco-re-entry circuits in adults with repaired congenital heart disease: entrainment mapping combined with three-dimensional electroanatomic mapping. J Am Coll Cardiol 2001; 37(6):1665–1676.

78. Vaksmann G, Lacroix D, Klug D. Radiofrequency ablation of the His bundle for malignant atrial flutter after Mustard procedure for transposition of the great arteries. Am J Cardiol 1996;77(8):669–670.

79. Russell MW, Dorostkar PC, Dick M II, et al. Catheter interruption of the atrioventricular conduction using radiofrequency energy in a patient with transposition of the great arteries. PACE 1995;18:113–116.

80. Greene CA, Case CL, Gillette PC. Successful catheter fulguration of the His bundle in a postoperative Mustard patient after unsuccessful fulguration of ectopic atrial foci. PACE 1991;14:1593–1597.

81. Urcelay G, Dick M II, Bove EL, et al. Intraoperative mapping and radiofrequency ablation of the His bundle in a patient with complex congenital heart disease and intractable atrial arrhythmias following the Fontan operation. PACE 1993;16:1437–1440.

82. Waldo AL, MacLean WAH. Diagnosis and treatment of arrhythmias following open heart surgery: emphasis on the use of epicardial wire electrodes. Futura Publishing, New York, NY, 1980.

83. Irani WN, Grayburn PA, Afridi I. Prevalence of thrombus, spontaneous echo contrast, and atrial stunning in patients undergoing cardioversion of atrial flutter: a prospective study using transesophageal echocardiography. Circulation 1997;95:962–966.

84. Santiago D, Warshofsky M, Li-Mandri G, et al. Left atrial appendage function and thrombus formation in atrial fibrillation-flutter: a transesophageal echocardiographic study. J Am Coll Cardiol 1994;24:159–164.

85. Feltes TF, Friedman RA. Transesophageal echocardiographic detection of atrial thrombi in patients with non-atrial fibrillation atrial tachycardias and congenital heart disease. J Am Coll Cardiol 1994;24:1365–1370.

86. Siedl K, Hauer B, Schwick N, et al. Rick of thromboembolic events in patients with atrial flutter. Am J Cardiol 1998;82:580–583.

87. Wood KA, Eisenberg SJ, Kalman JM, et al. Risk of thromboembolism in chronic atrial flutter. Am J Cardiol 1997;79:1043–1047.

88. Lanzarotti C, Olshanski B. Thromboembolic risk of chronic atrial flutter: is the risk underestimated? J Am Coll Cardiol 1997;30:1506–1511.

89. Petersen P, Boysen G, Godtfredsen J, et al. Placebo-controlled, randomized trial of warfarin and aspirin for prevention of thromboembolic complications in chronic atrial fibrillation: the Copenhagen AFASAK study. Lancet 1989;1:175–178.

90. Stroke Prevention in Atrial Fibrillation Investigators. Stroke Prevention in Atrial Fibrillation Study: final results. Circulation 1991;84:527–539.

91. The Boston Area Anticoagulation Trial for Atrial Fibrillation Investigators. The effect of low-dose warfarin on the risk of stroke in patients with nonrheumatic atrial fibrillation. N Engl J Med 1990; 323:1505–1511.

92. Connolly SJ, Laupacis A, Gent M, et al. Canadian Atrial Fibrillation Anticoagulation (CAFA) study. J Am Coll Cardiol 1991;18:349–355.

93. Ezekowitz MD, Bridgers SL, James KE, et al. Warfarin in the prevention of stroke associated with nonrheumatic atrial fibrillation. N Engl J Med 1992;327:1406–1412.

94. Stroke Prevention in Atrial Fibrillation Investigators: Warfarin versus aspirin for prevention of thrombo-embolism in atrial fibrillation: Stroke Prevention in Atrial Fibrillation II study. Lancet 1994;343:687–691.

95. Anticoagulants in the Secondary Prevention of Events in Coronary Thrombosis (ASPECT) Research Group: effect of long-term oral anticoagulant treatment on mortality and cardiovascular morbidity after myocardial infarction. Lancet 1994;343:499–503.

96. Albers GW, Dalen JE, Laupacis A, Manning WJ, Petersen P, Singer DE. Antithrombotic therapy in atrial fibrillation. Chest 2001;119:194S–206S.

97. Schumacher B, Jung W, Lewalter T, et al. Radiofrequency ablation of atrial flutter due to administration of class 1C antiarrhythmic drugs for atrial fibrillation. Am J Cardiol 1999;83:710–713.

98. Huang DT, Monahan KM, Zimetbaum P, et al. Hybrid pharmacologic and ablative therapy: a novel and effective approach for the management of atrial fibrillation. J Cardiovasc Electrophysiol 1998; 98:315–322.

99. Tai CT, Chiang CE, Lee SH, et al. Persistent atrial flutter in patients treated for atrial fibrillation with amiodarone and propafenone: electrophysiologic characteristics, radiofrequency catheter ablation and risk prediction. J Cardiovasc Electrophysiol 1999;10:1180–1187.

10 Evaluation and Management of Syncope

Blair P. Grubb, MD, and Daniel Kosinski, MD

CONTENTS

INTRODUCTION

Syncope, defined as the transient loss of consciousness and postural tone with spontaneous recovery, has fascinated, challenged, and often frustrated physicians for millennia. Indeed, the first clinical description of syncope comes from Hippocrates (the "father of medicine"), and it is from the Greek that the medical term for fainting is taken (syncopen—"to cut short"). Both a sign and a symptom, syncope can result from a bewildering array of quite varied disorders ranging from the benign and self-limited, to an indication of a serious chronic disease or a potentially fatal disorder. Perhaps no other condition so challenges the diagnostic acumen of the practitioner. This chapter reviews the epidemiology of syncope, outlines a practical approach to the evaluation of syncope, and briefly outlines the major causes of syncope, focusing on autonomic disturbances.

EPIDEMIOLOGY

Syncope is a common complaint that almost every practitioner will encounter (or experience). Data obtained from 26 yr of surveillance by the Framingham Study suggest that 3.0% of all men and 3.5% of all women experience syncope (1). The incidence in the elderly (those older than 65 yr) is as high as 5.6%, but many investigators feel

From: *Contemporary Cardiology: Management of Cardiac Arrhythmias*
Edited by: L. I. Ganz © Humana Press Inc., Totowa, NJ

that these estimates probably fall short of the true prevalence *(2)*. Over one million people each year undergo evaluation and treatment for recurrent syncope, and at the same time many others who have suffered from syncope do not seek out medical attention.

Each year in the United States alone, syncope accounts for 6% of all hospital admissions and 3–5% of all emergency room visits *(2,3)*. Syncope provokes an extreme sense of anxiety among both physicians and patients for, as Hippocrates noted, "those who suffer from recurrent fainting often die suddenly" *(4)*. In a number of cardiovascular conditions syncope may be the only warning that occurs before an episode of sudden death. Even if the case of syncope is benign, sudden unpredictable episodes of loss of consciousness may result in serious injury *(2)*. Syncope is more common in the elderly (especially those over 75 yr of age), and the elderly now constitute an ever-increasing proportion of the world's population *(5)*. Falls are now the fourth leading cause of death in the elderly, and at least half of these are believed to occur because of syncope *(6)*. In addition, recurrent syncope places a tremendous psychological burden on both patients and their families, and often significantly limits their social, educational, and employment opportunities *(7)*. Indeed, recurrent syncope can produce a degree of functional impairment similar to chronic debilitating diseases such as rheumatoid arthritis *(8)*.

The cost of evaluating and treating syncope is quite high, especially if done in a haphazard and undirected fashion. A recent study showed that the average undirected syncope evaluation presently used by many physicians costs up to $16,000 per patient *(9)*. This would place the cost of syncope evaluation in the United States alone at over one billion dollars per year *(2)*. However, this figure does not take into account the costs associated with lost time from work by both patients and family members and the resultant loss in productivity to the economy.

POTENTIAL CAUSES

The cause of syncope is rarely completely obvious, and those individuals at the highest risk of sudden death may be the hardest to detect. In reality, almost every case of syncope is of unknown origin. Unless one is fortunate enough to have recorded a spontaneous episode, establishing a causal relationship between any abnormality detected during testing and the cause of a particular episode is tenuous. All too often, practitioners base their diagnoses on incorrect assumptions and flawed methodology. Thus, even when the evaluation is properly carried out by skilled clinicians, the diagnosis often requires a "leap of faith" that the suspected cause is the actual mechanism of the patient's syncope. The physician must learn to cope with a degree of uncertainty in dealing with these patients, and must have the inner strength to dismiss a diagnosis and consider other diagnoses when things do not go as predicted. The best clinicians are honest with themselves and their patients, and are humble, uncertain, and open to revision.

Virtually any condition that results in a significant reduction in cerebral blood flow, particularly to the area of the brain known as the reticular activating system, may result in a transient loss of consciousness *(see* Tables 1,2). Most investigators divide the causes of syncope into three broad groupings: cardiovascular, noncardiovascular, and syncope of unknown origin *(see* Table 1). Each category is associated with a very different prognosis *(14)*. For example, in patients with cardiovascular syncope, mortality

Table 1
Various Causes and Types of Syncope

Cardiovascular
    Arrhythmias
        Atrioventricular block with bradycardia
        Sinus bradycardia
        Ventricular tachycardia
    Nonarrhythmic
        Hypertrophic cardiomyopathy
        Aortic stenosis
Non-cardiovascular
    Reflex mechanisms
        Neurocardiogenic
        Micturition
        Defecation
        Cough
        Deglutition
        Post prandial
        Carotid sinus hypersensitivity
    Orthostatic hypotension
        Dysautonomia
        Fluid depletion
        Bed rest, debilitation
        Drugs
    Psychogenic
        Conversion reactions
        Hysteria
        Panic/anxiety disorder
Conditions that can be mistaken for syncope
    Epileptic seizures
    Hypoglycemia
    Stroke
    Drug-induced (alcohol, narcotics)
Syncope of unknown origin

rates are as high as 20–30% over a period of 1–2 yr. For noncardiac causes, the mortality tends to be comparatively low, averaging 1–6% over 1–2 yr. Among patients with recurrent syncope for whom a very thorough evaluation yields no diagnosis, mortality rates are also comparatively low. At one point in time, a large number of patients (40–50%) were given the diagnosis of syncope of unknown origin. However, the development of better diagnostic modalities such as tilt table testing and implantable loop recorders (ILRs) have reduced the percentage of patients in this group to approx 10–15% *(11)*.

THE EVALUATION OF SYNCOPE

The cornerstone of the syncope evaluation is a comprehensive history and detailed physical examination *(2,11)*. The history should include any information on current or previous cardiovascular conditions, current medications, comorbid conditions, and a

Table 2
Causes of Syncope by Age

Young patients (< 35 yr)
   Neurocardiogenic
   Psychiatric
   Situational
   Epileptic seizures*
   Long QT Syndrome*
   Hypertrophic cardiomyopathy*
   Supraventricular tachycardia*
Mid-life (35–65 yr)
   Neurocardiogenic
   Cardiac arrhythmias
Older patient
   Cardiac: Hemodynamic
             Arrhythmic
   Dysautonomic (orthostatic hypotension)
   Drug-induced
   Multifactorial
   Reflex syncope: carotid sinus hypersensitivity
                 micturition/defecation
                 neurocardiogenic

*Important but less common causes.

thorough family history. The family history should include any history of syncope, seizure disorders, congenital heart disease, premature atherosclerosis, arrhythmias, unexplained death, or Sudden Infant Death Syndrome. Information should be obtained as to the clinical nature of the syncopal episodes. Such information should include the frequency of episodes, relationship to body position and exertion, prodromal symptoms, the presence or absence of any convulsive activity, and the presence or absence of a postictal state. It should be kept in mind, however, that convulsive activity may accompany any condition where cerebral hypoperfusion occurs; true seizure disorders rarely present as syncope. Any observations from witnesses may be useful.

The physician should keep in mind that various psychologic factors may play a significant role in the patient's condition. In all chronic disorders there is often a common and complex interplay between the physical and mental, leading to a "physiology of illness" (7). In some patients, syncope may be purely psychogenic in nature (12).

It is imperative that the physician should explore the potential for drug use as a cause of syncope. Illicit use of recreational drugs, such as cocaine, heroin, methylamphetamine, and alcohol may result in syncope because of heart rhythm or blood pressure disturbances (2). A number of therapeutic agents may also produce syncope, either by provocation or exacerbation of arrhythmias or by the volume depleting or vascular relaxing effects of antihypertensives.

The physical exam may be extremely helpful in ascertaining an etiology for syncope. Patients must be checked for the presence or absence of orthostasis. Such a maneuver may provide a diagnosis. Carotid sinus massage should be performed if no evidence for carotid occlusive disease is suspected. The remainder of the cardiac examination

Table 3
Diagnostic Evaluation of Syncope

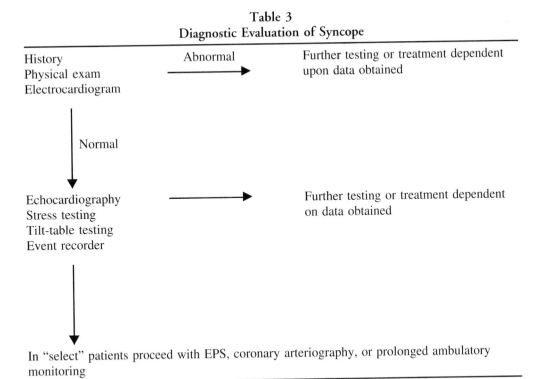

History
Physical exam
Electrocardiogram

                Abnormal   Further testing or treatment dependent
                                                upon data obtained

        Normal

Echocardiography   Further testing or treatment dependent
Stress testing   on data obtained
Tilt-table testing
Event recorder

In "select" patients proceed with EPS, coronary arteriography, or prolonged ambulatory
monitoring

should focus on identifying significant abnormalities, such as congenital or valvular
heart disease, that could potentially be a cause for syncope.

In addition to potentially suggesting a cause for syncope, the history and physical
exam may also allow risk stratification to be performed. Although the 1-yr mortality
rate for patients with cardiovascular syncope has been identified as approx 30%, this
varies depending upon the etiology *(10)*. Patients without primary electrical abnormalities or structural heart disease generally have a better prognosis than patients with
structural heart disease or a conduction system abnormality. In addition, the results of
the history and physical examination are utilized to direct further evaluation. It is critical
to attempt to identify individuals in whom structural heart disease of any sort is present
(*see* Table 3).

A note of special interest shall be made in the evaluation of the patient with a
single syncopal episode. It is sometimes incorrectly assumed that a single episode of
unexplained syncope is not of significant magnitude to warrant a thorough evaluation.
This notion can prove to be very dangerous. Syncope of uncertain etiology can be
caused by a wide array of causes, and the prognosis after a single episode of syncope
is variable in relation to the underlying cause. A single syncopal episode may be the
only warning of a potentially life-threatening disorder.

One common question is whether to hospitalize a patient after an episode of syncope.
A patient with known cardiovascular disease, in whom there is a high suspicion of
conditions such as ventricular tachycardia (VT) may benefit from hospitalization. In
this subpopulation, hospitalization could prevent recurrent symptoms, injury, and even
death. However, most patients with syncope do not seem to benefit from hospitalization,

Table 4
Patients with Syncope Who Should be Considered for Hospitalization

1. The elderly.
2. Patients with suspected or proven structural heart disease.
3. A potential arrhythmic cause of syncope (i.e., Long QT syndrome).
4. Severe orthostatic hypotension.
5. Unexplained syncope that has led to significant injury.
6. Concomitant conditions that require treatment.
7. Syncope associated with new neurologic findings, including weakness or hemiparesis).

and in some the social and economic impact may actually be detrimental. Before hospitalizing a patient with syncope, you must have a clear idea of what diagnostic and therapeutic goals you would like to achieve.

Studies on the effects of hospitalization for syncope have revealed an average length of stay of 6–7 d, usually with no observable benefit (2). In one study of 161 patients with syncope, 78% were hospitalized with an average stay of 6.8 d (13). Of these patients, a cause was identified in only 17%; the cause was cardiac in 7%. The cost of hospitalization can be quite expensive. Mozes et al. reported that the average syncope admission costs up to $38,565 per patient (14). A list of potential syncope patients who might be considered for admission is found in Table 4.

Electrocardiography

Our opinion is that a baseline 12-lead scalar electrocardiogram (ECG) should be part of the evaluation in all patients with syncope. Although the yield of such testing is not entirely certain, valuable information can be obtained. In younger patients the clinician should evaluate for evidence of pre-excitation, long QT, accelerated AV conduction or conduction block, right ventricular dysplasia, or hypertrophic cardiomyopathy. In older individuals, evidence for coronary artery disease (CAD) (Q waves), conduction block or bundle-branch block, and hypertensive heart disease are among the abnormalities to look for. Although abnormalities noted may not assign a cause to syncope, they may serve to risk-stratify the patient and direct further evaluation. An example would be that in the evaluation of syncope in a 50-yr-old male patient, the presence of Q waves would direct evaluation towards ischemic heart disease. If the ECG is nonrevealing, further noninvasive evaluation is warranted.

Echocardiography

Echocardiography may be very useful as a next step of evaluation. Certainly abnormalities such as HOCM or other structural heart disease would be detected by echocardiography. However, the issue is whether or not routine echocardiography can be recommended.

The majority of data involving screening echocardiography has been drawn from athletes and not persons with prior syncope (15–18). These data suggest a very low yield in identifying significant abnormalities. Murray et al. reported that 10% of the athletes screened had findings that merited medical follow-up (15). However, the majority of these athletes (11 of 13) with abnormalities had only mitral-valve prolapse.

Recchia and Brazilai examined the value of echocardiography in 128 patients with syncope admitted over an 8-mo period *(19)*. Echocardiography was performed in 64% of these patients. In the patients for whom echocardiography was performed, the majority were normal. The authors found, however, that in patients with a normal ECG and no clinical markers for cardiovascular disease, 100% of the echocardiograms were normal. In patients with a clinical or electrocardiographic indicator of cardiovascular disease, 34% had abnormal echocardiograms. The authors concluded that in the absence of a clinical or electrocardiographic predictor of cardiovascular disease, the yield of echo-cardiography was exceptionally low. This conclusion should be somewhat tempered, because 36% of the patients did not have echocardiography; this may have affected the results *(19)*. Also, the study was a retroprospective evaluation. At this point, although the yield of an echocardiogram is likely to be low with a lack of substantial perspective data, there should be sufficient latitude granted to clinical judgment in this area.

Exercise Stress Testing

Certainly in individuals for whom an ischemic etiology is suspected, exercise testing may be appropriate. However, exercise testing is useful in other subsets of patients as well, and should be considered in individuals for whom syncope occurred during exercise or exertion.

It is now appreciated that in younger patients with structurally normal hearts, exercise-induced neurocardiogenic syncope is a legitimate entity *(1,5,20–24)*. These patients have the features of neurally mediated syncope present on both exercise and head-upright tilt testing. Sakaguchi et al. found neurocardiogenic syncope to be the leading cause of syncope in patients with syncope associated with exercise *(20)*.

Exercise-related syncope may be caused by other nonarrhythmic, nonischemic etiolo-gies. Both post-exercise asystole *(22,25,26)* and post-exercise postural hypotension are capable of provoking syncope.

It is also possible to have nonischemic exercise-induced arrhythmia *(28–33)*. In some patients, electrophysiology study may be negative, and exercise may be the only method to provoke arrhythmia.

Ischemic-induced exercise-related syncope may be the result of a permanent substrate or to a transient ischemia itself *(33)*. Although this condition is generally believed to occur in the older population, other age groups may be affected. In a study of sports-related sudden death in individuals with a mean age of 32 yr, 26% were believed to be caused by atherosclerotic heart disease *(34)*. Younger patients without atheroscle-rotic heart disease may also experience transient ischemia from conditions such as anomalous coronary artery distribution *(35,36)*, and hypoplastic *(37)* or tunnel coronary arteries *(35)*.

Head-Upright Tilt Testing

In patients with cardiovascular syncope and no structural heart disease or ischemic heart disease, neurocardiogenic syncope is the most common etiology *(38)*. This has been demonstrated in adults and children *(38–40)*. Much controversy has been generated over the appropriate angle of tilt and duration of tilt. A recent American College of Cardiology (ACC) consensus document recommended an angle of 60–80 degrees with a duration of 30–45 min for the baseline tilt test *(41)*. These parameters appear to provide a reasonable sensitivity. False-positive rates are generally less than 10% *(43)*. Practices regarding pharmacologic provocation vary widely; a number of pharmacologic agents have been used, including isoproterenol, epinephrine, edrophonium, and nitroglycerine.

The use of isoproterenol provocation has also come under attack as being nonspecific; however, this is dependent upon the dosing protocol (43,44). Most experts would agree on a protocol of low-dose isoproterenol infusion. In a recent trial, Natale et al. evaluated 150 control patients in the baseline state, at various isoproterenol doses (47). They found that in the baseline state, a tilt angle of 60–70 degrees provided an excellent specificity. Testing at an 80-degree angle for greater than 10 min was less specific. The addition of a low-dose isoproterenol protocol reduced the specificity minimally (from 92–88%). Higher doses of isoproterenol (3–5 µg/min) substantially affected specificity.

Our current practice is to perform a baseline test at an angle of 70 degrees for 30 min. If necessary, a subsequent isoproterenol test is done in a low-dose protocol. We titrate an isoproterenol dose to increase heart rate by 25–30% over the baseline supine rate and then perform tilt testing at a 70-degree angle for 10 min.

Several investigators have explored the potential of other provocative agents during tilt-table testing, primarily nitroglycerin and adenosine (41). Similar sensitivities have been obtained with these agents, although it may be that a positive test with one of these agents and not another may identify different subgroups of neurocardiogenic syncope (42). Further studies will be necessary to better define the utility of each of these various agents.

Electrophysiology Study

The utility of electrophysiology study (EPS) in patients with syncope is largely dependent upon the patient's underlying cardiac substrate. A thorough history, physical exam, and noninvasive testing are likely to identify patients in whom a tachyarrhythmia or bradyarrhythmia is known or suspected to be the causative agent of syncope. Such individuals would include these with ischemic heart disease, other structural heart disease such as cardiomyopathy, or those with known or suspected conduction system abnormalities. Guidelines were established as to the appropriateness of EPS in such patients (43). A class I indication is given to EPS in patients with structural heart disease and syncope that remains unexplained after appropriate initial evaluation. More controversial is the role of EPS in patients with unexplained syncope without structural heart disease.

In general terms, the diagnostic yield of EPS is low in patients with syncope and no structural heart disease (44). In one review (45), the role of electrophysiology testing in syncope of unknown origin was examined in four studies totaling 327 patients. EPS provided a diagnosis for syncope in 71% of patients with structural heart disease and 36% of patients without heart disease (46–49). One study examined nine major series dealing with electrophysiology only in patients with syncope. A diagnostic abnormality was found in 59% of the combined total of 647 patients (50).

Current guidelines provide a class II indication for EPS in patients with recurrent syncope without structural heart disease and with a negative head-up tilt test (43). In patients with no structural heart disease, neurocardiogenic syncope is the more likely etiology (51). In a study evaluating unexplained syncope, patients underwent EPS, and if this was negative, then underwent head-up tilt testing (52). A diagnosis was established in 74% of the patients. In patients with abnormal EPS, structural heart disease was present in 76% of these patients. In contrast, in the group of patients with a negative EPS and a subsequent positive tilt test, only 6% had structural heart disease.

Noninvasive Monitoring

Several reports have described the utility of Holter monitoring for the evaluation of syncope. The predominant use is in substantiating or excluding a dysrhythmia as the etiology of the event(s) *(53–63)*. Many of the studies were summarized in a 1990 review of DiMarco and Philbrick *(53)*. The trials were retrospective studies *(54–60)*, and attempted to correlate symptoms with arrhythmias. Correlation between symptoms and simultaneous ECG findings could only be made on 22% of patients; the remaining 78% had nondiagnostic studies.

Interestingly, between 4% and 30% of patients who were asymptomatic during these recordings had significant arrhythmias. DiMarco and Philbrick concluded that ambulatory Holter monitoring has a relatively low yield unless symptoms are frequent an/or the period of monitoring is prolonged *(53)*.

More recently Pasyk and Srediniawa *(61)* evaluated 32 patients with syncope utilizing 72-h Holter monitoring. Syncope occurred in 16 of 32 patients. Cardiac arrhythmias were the cause of syncope in 14 of these 16 patients. Therefore, a 72-h monitoring period appeared to provide a reasonable diagnostic yield. Racco et al. *(62)* prospectively evaluated 134 patients with syncope. Although 102 of 134 patients showed some rhythm disturbance, continuous ECG recording provided a decisive diagnosis in only six patients. They concluded that continuous ECG recording was of limited value in the evaluation of syncope. However, they believed that because of its moderate cost and noninvasive nature, it may prove worthwhile in certain cases.

Beauregard et al. examined the combined use of 24-h electrocardiographic and electroencephalographic monitoring in 45 patients with syncope *(63)*. Isolated cardiac rhythm abnormalities were seen in 21 patients, and none of these were symptomatic. Isolated EEG abnormalities were observed in 11 patients. Simultaneous ECG and EEG abnormalities were seen in four patients. In two of these four patients, an unsuspected etiology for syncope was noted.

In 1986 Braun et al. reported the utility of memory-loop event recording in 100 patients, and 74 of these patients had either presyncope or syncope *(64)*. Sixty-nine patients made recordings, and 56 patients made recordings believed to be diagnostic. We are not aware of prospective direct comparison of loop-event recorders vs Holter monitoring in the evaluation of syncope. However, in a 1996 publication, Kinlay et al. found the cardiac-event recorder superior to 48-h Holter monitoring in patients with palpitations *(65)*. In this study, patients with syncope were excluded.

Our own beliefs regarding Holter monitoring are similar to those of DiMarco and Philbrick *(53)*: unless patients are having frequent episodes and/or the monitoring period is prolonged, the diagnostic yield in syncope is likely to be low. We generally employ loop-event recording more frequently than Holter monitoring.

Another interesting monitoring device is an implantable long-term subcutaneous (SC) monitoring device. Krahn et al. evaluated such a device in 16 patients with syncope for whom ambulatory monitoring, EPS, and tilt-table testing were all nondiagnostic *(66)*. In a monitoring period of 4 ± 4 mo, 15 of 16 patients had syncope and a diagnosis was established for all 15 patients. Nine of these 15 patients had an arrhythmic cause of syncope; 7 of these 9 were bradyarrhythmias, and 2 of 9 had tachyarrhythmias. This device may be of benefit in selected patients with very rare episodes.

Several studies have evaluated the usefulness of signal-average electrocardiography in identifying patients with syncope for whom EPS may be appropriate (67–70). These studies examined the relationship between late potentials and the risk of VT. These studies were summarized by Kjellgren and Gomes in a 1993 review (71). They concluded that late potentials appeared to offer a good sensitivity and specificity in identifying individuals in whom VT was inducible on EPS. However, they cautioned that the utility is variable depending on the underlying substrate. More recently, Morillo et al. evaluated the usefulness of Signal-averaged electrocardiogram (SAECG) head-up tilt-table testing and EPS in 70 patients with recurrent unexplained syncope (72). Overall, a cause for syncope was found in 77% of these patients. A positive SAECG was more likely to be found in patients with a prior myocardial infarction (MI) and lower ejection fraction than patients with a negative SAECG. The patients with a positive ECG were also much more likely to have inducible VT on EPS. They conclude a positive SAECG along with a previous MI and ejection fraction less than 40% were highly predictive of inducible VT.

SPECIFIC CAUSES OF SYNCOPE

The following sections review some of the various disorders that may result in syncope. Many of these disorders (such as VT and heart block) are dealt with in greater detail elsewhere in this book and will not be reviewed here. Conditions that are not covered in other sections will be discussed in more detail.

Noncardiac Causes of Syncope

Noncardiac causes predominate in patients suffering from recurrent unexplained syncope. Of these, the majority appear to occur because of transient alterations in autonomic nervous system (ANS) tone that lead to periods of hypotension and ultimately, loss of consciousness. Until recently, these syndromes of autonomic dysfunction associated with orthostatic intolerance were poorly understood. However, over the last decade there has been a virtual explosion of information on these disorders. Recently these disorders have been subdivided into various syndromes which—although similar—are nonetheless fairly distinct entities. Each seems to result from an inability of the ANS to compensate for positional change. The following is a brief review of the mechanisms by which the body maintains postural normotension, as well as some basic aspects of autonomic structure and function.

The human nervous system has two basic components: the central nervous system (CNS), made up of the brain and the spinal cord (73), and the peripheral nervous system, which is comprised of groups of neurons known as ganglia and of peripheral nerves that lie outside the brain and spinal cord. Although anatomically separate, the two systems are functionally interconnected. The peripheral nervous system is further divided into somatic and autonomic divisions. The somatic division is principally involved with sensory information about the environment outside the body as well as muscle and limb position. The autonomic division (usually called the autonomic nervous system or ANS) is the motor system for the viscera, the smooth muscles of the body (especially those of the vasculature), and the exocrine glands. It is composed of three distinct parts: the sympathetic, parasympathetic, and enteric nervous systems. The sympathetic nervous system helps control the reaction of the body to stress, and the parasympathetic system works to conserve the body's resources and to restore equilibrium to the resting state. The enteric system controls the function of the gut. The organ systems governed by the ANS are, for the most part, independent of volitional control (although they are sometimes affected by volitional or emotional inputs) and include the cardiorespiratory organs and the gastrointestinal and genitourinary tracts. The ANS is vital to the maintenance of internal homeostasis, and achieves this through mechanisms that regulate blood pressure, fluid and electrolyte balance, and body temperature.

Although representative of one of the defining aspects of the evolution of Homo sapiens, the adoption of upright posture presented a novel challenge to a blood-pressure control system that developed to meet the requirements of an animal in the dorsal position. Indeed, the organ that defines our humanity—the brain—was placed in a somewhat precarious position with regard to vascular perfusion and oxygenation. It is the ANS that governs both the short- and medium-term blood-pressure responses to positional change *(74)*. Normally, approx 25% of the circulating blood volume is in the thorax. Immediately following the assumption of upright posture, gravity produces a downward displacement of approx 500 cc of blood to the abdomen and lower extremities. Approximately 50% of this amount is redistributed within seconds after standing, and almost one-quarter of total blood volume may be involved in the process. The process causes a decrease in venous return to the heart and cardiac filling pressures, and stroke volume may fall by 40%. The reference point for determination of these changes is known as the venous hydrostatic indifference point (HIP), and represents the part of the vascular system where pressure is independent of posture. In humans, the venous HIP is near the level of the diaphragm, and the arterial HIP is at the left ventricle. The venous HIP is somewhat dynamic in that it can be altered by changes in venous compliance brought on by muscular activity *(74)*. After standing, the normal subject achieves orthostatic stabilization in 1 min or less. It should be noted that the exact circulatory responses brought on by standing (an active process) are somewhat different than those brought on by head-up tilt (a passive process). In the moments following the assumption of upright posture, a slow decline in arterial pressure and cardiac filling occurs. This causes activation of the high-pressure receptors of the carotid sinus and aortic arch, as well as the low-pressure receptors of the heart and lungs. The mechanoreceptors within the heart are linked by unmyelinated vagal afferents in both the atria and ventricles *(73–76)*. These fibers have been found to cause continuous inhibitory actions on the cardiovascular areas of the medulla (the nucleus tractus solitarii) *(73)*. The fall in venous return that results from upright posture produces less stretch on these receptors, causing discharge rates to decrease. This change in input to the brain stem causes an increase in sympathetic outflow resulting in systemic vasoconstriction. At the same time, the fall in arterial pressure during upright position actuates the high-pressure receptors in the carotid sinus which stimulates an increase in heart rate. These early steady-state adaptations to upright posture therefore result in a 10–15 beat-per-minute (BPM) increase in heart rate, a diastolic pressure increase of 10 mmHg, and little or no change in systolic blood pressure. Once these adjustments are complete, as compared to the supine state, in the upright stance the thoracic blood volume and total cardiac output are 30% less and the mean heart rate is 10–15 BPM higher. More detailed descriptions of this process are available to the interested reader *(74)*.

As a person continues to stand, activation of neurohumoral responses occurs, and the amount is dependent on the subject's volume status. As a rule, the lower the volume, the higher the degree of the renin-angiotensin-aldosterone system activation *(74)*. The inability of any of these processes to function adequately (or in a coordinated manner) can potentially result in a failure in the normal responses to sudden shifts in posture (or their maintenance) with resultant hypotension, which may be sufficiently high to cause cerebral hypoperfusion, hypoxia, and loss of consciousness.

DISORDERS OF ORTHOSTATIC CONTROL

Studies conducted in the last decades of the 20th century have significantly contributed to our understanding of autonomically mediated disorders of orthostatic control. Although they are similar in many respects, many of these disorders have distinct characteristics. In order to make sense of the apparent chaos of nature, mankind has always attempted to classify it in a coherent manner. Therefore, any mode of classification is somewhat arbitrary and open to modification. The current system of classification is outlined in Fig. 1. Some investigators have divided autonomic disorders into primary or secondary forms. The primary forms of these disorders tend to be idiopathic in nature, and are further subdivided into acute and chronic forms. The secondary forms usually occur in conjunction with a particular disease or are known to occur because of a known biochemical abnormality (*see* Table 5).

There are currently four major subtypes of orthostatic control disorders, which include Reflex Syncope, Pure Autonomic Failure, Multiple System Atrophy, and the Postural Orthostatic Tachycardia Syndrome (POTS) (*see* Fig. 1).

Reflex Syncope

Physicians tend to be most familiar with this form of syncope, and thus our discussion of it will be limited *(75)*. First described by both Gower and Sir Thomas Lewis as vasovagal syncope, it is better known today as either neurocardiogenic or neurally mediated syncope. Although diverse in presentation, it occurs most frequently in younger people, and is characterized by a distinct prodrome of variable duration followed by an abrupt loss of consciousness. Recovery is rapid and is usually not accompanied by a postictal state. These episodes are believed to represent a "hypersensitive" autonomic system that over-responds to various stimuli. Most commonly this is prolonged orthostatic stress; venous pooling causes venous return to the right ventricle to fall so precipitously that an increase in inotropy causes activation of mechanoreceptors that would normally fire only during stretch *(76)*. This sudden surge in neural traffic to the brain stem mimics the conditions seen in hypertension, thus provoking an apparently "paradoxic" sympathetic withdrawal with resultant parasympathetic predominance. Hypotension, bradycardia, and syncope ensue. It is important to remember that other stimuli such as strong emotion or epileptic discharge can provoke identical responses, thus suggesting that these individuals have an inherent increase in sensitivity to such stimuli. During head-upright tilt-table testing, these individuals have a sudden profound

Table 5
Autonomic Disorders Associated with
Orthostatic Intolerance

I. Primary autonomic disorders
  A. Acute pandysautonomia
  B. Pure autonomic failure
  C. Multiple system atrophy
    1. Parkinsonian
    2. Pyramidal/cerebellar
    3. Mixed
  D. Reflex syncopes
    1. Neurocardiogenic syncope
    2. Carotid sinus hypersensitivity
II. Secondary autonomic failure
  A. Central origin
    1. Cerebral cancer
    2. Multiple sclerosis
    3. Age-related
    4. Syringobulbia
  B. Peripheral forms
    1. Afferent
      a. Guillian-Barré syndrome
      b. Tabes dorsalis
      c. Holmes-Adie syndrome
    2. Efferent
      a. Diabetes mellitus
      b. Nerve growth-factor deficiency
      c. Dopamine beta-hydroxylase deficiency
    3. Afferent/Efferent
III. Familial dysautonomia
IV. Spinal origin
    a. Transverse myelitis
    b. Syringomyelia
    c. Spinal tumors
V. Other causes
    a. Renal failure
    b. Paraneoplastic syndromes
    c. Autoimmune/collagen vascular disease
    d. Human immunodeficiency virus infection
    e. Amyloidosis

fall in blood pressure, that is closely followed by a fall in heart rate (sometimes to the point of asystole).

Sutton has made the insightful observation that the responses seen during neurocardiogenic syncope and carotid sinus hypersensitivity are quite similar, and may be different aspects of the same disorder *(77)*. Indeed, in such a predisposed individual, rapid mechanoreceptor activation from any site (blood, bladder, or cough) could elicit similar responses, producing the conditions variously described as micturition, defecation,

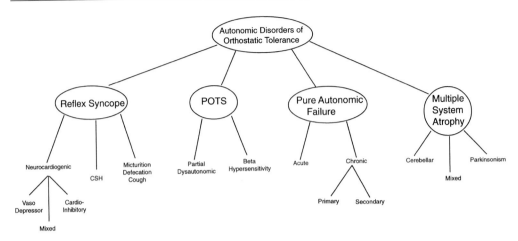

Fig. 1. Autonomic Disorders of Orthostatic Tolerance.

deglutition syncope. More detailed descriptions of these disorders can be found else-where *(78)*. What seems to distinguish these disorders from the remainder of those discussed here is that between episodes these patients are quite normal and report few other symptoms, if any. Indeed, their autonomic systems appear to function normally despite their "hypersensitive" nature, as opposed to other conditions where the auto-nomic system seems to "fail."

Primary Disorders of Autonomic Failure

Chronic Disorders

The physician is more likely to encounter the chronic forms of autonomic failure than their acute counterparts. The first report of chronic autonomic failure was the groundbreaking report by Bradbury and Eggleston in 1925, in which they labeled the condition "idiopathic orthostatic hypotension" because of the apparent lack of other neurologic features *(79)*. Since then, it has become quite apparent that in these patients there exists a generalized state of autonomic dysfunction manifested by orthostatic hypotension and syncope, as well as disturbances in bowel, and bladder and thermoregu-latory, sudomotor (sweating), and sexual function. The American Autonomic Society has named this disorder Pure Autonomic Failure (or PAF) *(80)*. Although the cause of PAF remains unknown, several investigators have postulated that there is a degenera-tion of the peripheral post-ganglionic autonomic neurons. This condition is more com-monly seen in older adults but it can occur in almost any age group (including children).

Another type of autonomic failure was reported in 1960 in a landmark study by Shy and Drager *(81)*. In contrast to PAF, this more severe condition is manifested by severe orthostatic hypotension, progressive urinary and rectal incontinence, loss of sweating, iris atrophy, external ocular palsy, impotence, rigidity, and tremors. Both muscle fascicu-lations and distal muscle wasting may be seen late in the disorder. In order to better identify this complex multi-system disorder, the American Autonomic Society has named this disease Multiple System Atrophy (MSA) and has divided it into three major subtypes *(82)*. The first group of patients demonstrate tremors that are strikingly similar to Parkinson's disease (some authors prefer to refer to this group as having striatonigral

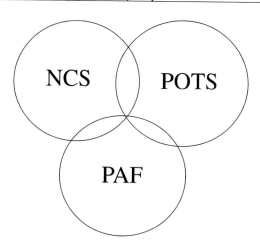

Fig. 2. Overlap of Autonomic Disorders.

degeneration). A second group of these patients display mainly cerebellar and/or pyrami-
dal symptoms (some investigators have termed this the olivopontocerebellar atrophy/
degeneration form). A third group displays aspects of both these types. An autopsy
study recently found that 7–22% of people believed to have Parkinson's disease actually
had neuropathologic findings diagnostic for MSA. Although the vast majority of MSA
patients do not present until somewhere between the 5th and 7th decade of life, some
individuals begin to experience symptoms in their late thirties (82).

Recently, a considerable amount of attention has been focused on a milder form of
chronic autonomic failure referred to as the Postural Orthostatic Tachycardia Syndrome
(POTS) (83). The hallmark of the syndrome is a persistent sinus tachycardia that occurs
while upright (which sometimes reaches rates of 160 BPM or more). Patients have
associated symptoms of severe fatigue, near-syncope, exercise intolerance, and light-
headedneses or dizziness. Many also complain of always being cold, and are also unable
to tolerate extreme heat. During head-upright tilt, these patients will display a sudden
increase in heart rate of greater than 30 BPM within the first 5 min, or achieve a
maximum heart rate of 120 BPM associated with only mildly reduced blood pressures.

The mechanism that causes this condition appears to be a failure of the peripheral
vasculature to appropriately vasoconstrict under orthostatic stress, which is then compensated for by an excessive increase in heart rate. Several authors believe that POTS
represents the earliest sign of autonomic dysfunction, and some of these patients have
later progressed into PAF. It is important to recognize this disorder, as we have seen
several patients with POTS who had been misdiagnosed as having an inappropriate
sinus tachycardia (IST) and who had undergone radiofrequency modification of the
sinus atrial mode (at other centers). After the apparently successful elimination of their
"sinus tachycardia," they were left with profound orthostatic hypotension. Moreover,
these patients may be misdiagnosed as suffering from Chronic Fatigue Syndrome.
Several recent reports have suggested that there may be considerable overlap between
these two disorders (84). In addition, there appears to be overlap among POTS, neurocardiogenic syncope, and PAF (see Fig. 2).

Most investigators believe that there are two distinct forms of POTS, a principally peripheral form referred to as the peripheral dysautonomic form, and a centrally mediated type referred to as the beta hypersensitivity form.

ACUTE AUTONOMIC DYSFUNCTION

Although these syndromes are rare, the acute autonomic neuropathesis that produce hypotension and syncope are frequently dramatic in presentation (85). These disorders are usually acute, and demonstrate severe and widespread failure of both the sympathetic and parasympathetic systems while leaving the somatic fibers unaffected. Many of these patients tend to be young and in good health prior to the illness. The development of the illness is surprisingly rapid and patients can frequently relate to the exact day that symptoms first began. One interesting observation has been that a large number of these individuals report having had a febrile illness (presumed to be viral) prior to the onset of symptoms, giving rise to the notion that there may be an autoimmune component to the disorder.

Severe disruption of the sympathetic nervous system often causes orthostatic hypotension of such a degree that the patient cannot even sit upright in bed without fainting. Patients often totally lose their ability to sweat, and suffer bowel and bladder dysfunction. These patients frequently complain of bloating, nausea, vomiting, and abdominal pain. Constipation is frequent, and sometimes alternates with diarrhea. One fascinating finding is that the heart rate will often be at a fixed rate of 40–50 BPM associated with complete chronotropic incompetence. The pupils are often dilated and poorly reactive to light. Patients may experience several syncopal episodes daily. The long-term prognosis of these patients is quite variable—some experience complete recoveries, and others suffer a chronic debilitating course. Patients are often left with significant residual effects.

Secondary Causes of Autonomic Dysfunction

A wide variety of disorders may cause varying degrees of autonomic disturbance. A list of some of these disorders is found in Table 5. It is important for the physician to be able to recognize when autonomic dysfunction is part of a greater disorder. In occasional patients, several conditions may coexist that produce synergistic detrimental effects on autonomic function. During the last decade, a number of enzymatic abnormalities have been identified that can result in autonomic disruption. Principal among these is isolated dopamine beta hydroxylase (DBH) deficiency syndrome, a condition which is now easily treated by replacement therapy. Other deficiency syndromes involving nerve-growth factor, monamine oxidase, aromatic L-amino decarboxylase, and some sensory neuropeptides may all result in autonomic failure and hypotension. Diffuse systemic illnesses such as renal failure, cancer, or the acquired immune deficiency syndrome (AIDS) may all cause hypotension and syncope. Studies have also demonstrated a link between orthostatic hypotension and Alzheimer's disease (86).

Perhaps one of the most important things to remember are the vast number of pharmacologic agents that may either cause or worsen orthostatic hypotension (see Table 6). Chief among these are the peripherally acting vasodilatory agents such as the angiotensin-converting enzyme (ACE) inhibitors; prazosin, hydralazine, and guanethidine. Beta-blocking agents may also worsen syncope in some patients. Lately we have observed an increased frequency of dysautonomic syncope in patients suffering from congestive heart failure (CHF). In this group, the combination of a low cardiac output and volume depletion caused by diuretics and vasodilator therapy serve to interfere with the body's aforementioned mechanisms for adapting to upright posture. Centrally acting agents, such as the tricyclic antidepressants reserpine and methyldopa, may also exacerbate otherwise mild hypotension.

CLINICAL FEATURES

The principal feature shared by all of these conditions is that normal cardiovascular regulation is disturbed, resulting in postural hypotension. Although orthostatic hypotension was once defined as a drop of greater than 20 mm/Hg in systolic blood pressure over a 3-min period after standing upright, a smaller drop in blood pressure associated with symptoms can be just as important. A large percentage of these patients will display a slow, steady fall in blood pressure over a longer time period (approx. 10–15 min) that can be quite symptomatic. Whether the patient experiences symptoms is as much dependent on the rate of fall in pressure as it is upon the absolute degree of change. The loss of consciousness in the dysautonomic tends to be slow and gradual, usually when the patient is walking or standing. However, many older patients do not seem to perceive this decline in pressure—they report little or no prodrome prior to syncope, and will describe these episodes as "drop attacks." Those who do experience prodromes will describe a wide variety of symptoms such as dizziness, blurring of vision, "seeing stars," and tunnel vision. A feature that distinguishes neurocardiogenic from dysautonomic syncope is that in the latter, bradycardia and diaphoresis rarely occur during an episode. Dysautonomic syncope tends to be more common in the early morning hours. Any factor that enhances peripheral venous pooling, such as extreme heat, fatigue, or alcohol ingestion, will exacerbate hypotension. As time goes on, some patients may develop a relatively fixed heart rate that shows little response to either postural change or exercise. In addition, some patients will develop a syndrome of supine hypertension that alternates with upright hypotension, presumably caused by a failure to vasodilate when prone. Patient suffering from this combination of supine hypertension and upright hypotension can quite be difficult to treat. Sometimes distinguishing between these disorders can be difficult, as there may be a considerable degree of overlap between them (a situation not dissimilar to that seen with the various forms of chronic obstructive lung disease) (see Fig. 2).

EVALUATION OF PATIENTS

The cornerstone of evaluation is a detailed history and physical examination. When do syncopal or near-syncopal episodes occur, and when did they begin? How often do they occur? Is there a pattern to the events or any known precipitating factors? What are episodes like for the patient, and how do they appear to bystanders? What other organ systems are involved? Other than syncope, what symptom bothers the patient most? A careful and concise history and physical exam (which must include a concise neurologic examination) will have a far greater diagnostic yield than the routine ordering of multiple tests. Laboratory examinations should be obtained in a careful and directed manner, based upon history and physical findings, to confirm one's clinical impressions.

It is far beyond the scope of this chapter to review every autonomic disorder and the various tests used in evaluation. The interested reader is directed to several excellent texts on the subject (80,87–90). It is important to note that any drugs the patient is taking that could produce hypotension should be identified (see Table 6). This includes not only pharmaceuticals, but over-the-counter medications and herbal remedies as well. Sadly, in the modern era, when a young person presents with symptoms of autonomic dysfunction, the potential use of illicit drugs or alcohol should be considered. In women, symptoms may vary with the menstrual cycle, or an otherwise mild tendency toward autonomic dysfunction may be exacerbated by the onset of menopause.

Since the autonomic areas of the brain are not accessible to direct measurement, one must measure the responses of various organ systems to various physiologic or pharmacologic challenges. In addition, recent advances have allowed for the determination of serum urine and cerebrospinal fluid levels of some autonomic neuromodulators and neurotransmitters. Foremost, however, is the determination of the blood pressure and heart rate response to positional change, with measurements taken while supine, sitting, and standing. The exact change in pressure considered to be significant is still under discussion, but is usually believed to be 20–30 mm/Hg systolic and 10–15 mm/Hg diastolic. Remember that standing blood pressure should be measured with the arm extended horizontally (to avoid the possible hydrostatic effects of the fluid column of the arm). Since the body's responses to active standing differ from those of passive tilting, we also frequently perform tilt-table testing on these patients (91). A number of other autonomic tests are also available, and are quite useful in selected patients (87–90).

We have found it useful to distinguish between these broad response patterns as outlined in Fig. 3. The first of these is the classic neurocardiogenic (or vasovagal) response. This is characterized by a sudden fall in blood pressure often followed by a fall in heart rate. The second pattern is referred to as dysautonomic and demonstrates a gradual but progressive decline in blood pressure to hypotensive levels leading to loss of consciousness. The third pattern is characteristic of POTS (83). Initially, we defined this group as exhibiting an increase of at least 30 BPM (or a maximum of 120 BPM) within the first 10 min of passive upright tilt, which is usually not associated with profound hypotension. Recently, we have realized that there are probably subgroups within the POTS population, and we are working to better categorize these.

POTENTIAL TREATMENTS

A complete discussion of the treatment options available is beyond the scope of this chapter; however, some basic principals are briefly outlined (75). One of the physician's most important tasks is to identify whether hypotensive syncope is primary or secondary in nature, and to determine if there are any potentially reversible causes (such as drugs, anemia, or volume depletion) (see Table 6).

It is equally important to educate the patient and their family about the nature of the problem. Teaching the patient to avoid aggravating factors (such as extreme heat, dehydration, and alcohol consumption), as well as recognizing any prodromal symptoms and assuming a recumbent position at their onset, are extremely helpful measures.

Nonpharmacologic therapies that are useful include sleeping with the head of the bed upright (approx 6–12 inches), and elastic support hose (at least 30–40 mm/Hg ankle counter-pressure). Biofeedback has also proven useful in selected patients.

Pharmacotherapy should be used cautiously, and should be tailored to fit the needs of the patient based on the type of autonomic disorder being treated, as well as coexisting symptoms and conditions. It should also be remembered that virtually any drug used in treatment can occasionally worsen symptoms (a "prosyncopal" effect).

In neurocardiogenic syncope, a number of reports have found that beta-blocker

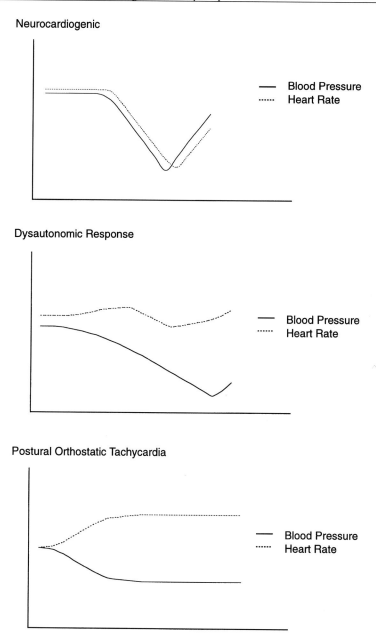

Fig. 3. Response Patterns During Tilt-Table Testing.

therapy is effective, presumably because its negative inotropic effects lessen the degree of cardiac mechanoreceptor activation associated with abrupt falls in venous return *(92)*. The increase in peripheral vascular resistance that accompanies unopposed beta blockade may also contribute to its therapeutic effects. We have not found beta blockade as useful in other forms of reflex syncope, and it may be detrimental in the dysautonomic syndromes. A useful agent in patients with dysautonomic syncope (and in younger patients with neurocardiogenic syncope) is the mineral corticoid agent fludrocortisone *(93)*. It results in fluid and sodium retention, and also appears to raise pressure via an

Table 6
Pharmacologic Agents That May Cause
or Worsen Orthostatic Intolerance

Angiotensin-converting enzyme inhibitors
Alpha-receptor blockers
Calcium-channel blockers
Beta-blockers
Phenothiazines
Tricyclic antidepressants
Bromocriptine
Ethanol
Opiates
Diuretics
Hydralazine
Ganglionic blocking agents

indirect vasoconstrictive effect resulting from sensitization of peripheral alpha receptors. Since the drug may cause hypokalemia and hypomagnesemia, serum potassium and magnesium levels must be periodically monitored.

Since failure to properly vasoconstrict the peripheral vessels is common to all of these disorders, vasoconstrictive substances can be employed. Initially, we employed the amphetamine-like agent, methylphenidate, with excellent results (94). However, the fact that it is a controlled substance with potent CNS-stimulating activity tended to limit our use of the drug. An excellent alternative is the new peripherally acting alpha agonist, midodrine. It has virtually no CNS effects or cardiac stimulation, and provides identical degrees of peripheral alpha-receptor stimulation. Several studies have demonstrated the efficacy of midodrine in both neurocardiogenic and dysautonomic disorders (95–97).

It has been found that the alpha-2-receptor blocking agent, clonidine, can actually elevate blood pressure in dysautonomic patients for whom hypotension is secondary to a severe post-ganglionic sympathetic lesion (98). In patients with severe autonomic failure, the post-junctional vascular alpha-2 receptors that are plentiful in the venous system are actually hypersensitive. Although, in normal individuals, clonidine acts on the CNS to lessen sympathetic output and blood pressure, in autonomic failure, some patients exhibit little or no sympathetic output, thus permitting its peripheral actions to become manifest.

Interestingly, a number of patients with autonomic failure will be anemic. A brilliant study by Hoeldtke and Streeten demonstrated that subcutaneous injections of erythropoietin while raising blood count will also produce dramatic increases in blood pressure (99). This pressure effect seems to occur independent of the red cell effect (100).

A series of both animal and human studies have demonstrated that the neurotransmitter serotonin (5-hydroxytryptamine) plays an essential role in the central regulation of blood pressure and heart rate. It has been postulated that some patients with autonomic disorders may have disturbances in central serotonin production or regulation (101). The observation that serotonin reuptake inhibitors can be effective in both the treatment of neurocardiogenic syncope and orthostatic hypotension supports this concept (102,103).

The exact role of pacemaker therapy in the treatment of these disorders remains controversial, and is beyond the scope of this discussion. However, a number of investigators have found that in selected patients pacemaker therapy can be effective in reducing symptoms and may sometimes eliminate syncope altogether *(104)*. The recent North American Vasovagal Pacemaker Study demonstrated that pacing using a rate-drop hysteresis algorithm was effective in preventing syncope *(105)*. More recently, the VASIS trial, using DDI pacing with simple rate hysteresis, yielded similar results *(106)*.

It should be considered that in dysautonomic disorders (as opposed to the reflex syncopes), hypotensive syncope is only one aspect of a broader constellation of symptoms relating to autonomic failure. The physician should therefore not give the patient unrealistic expectations as to what symptoms can and cannot be eliminated. Both physician and patient should remain aware that these disorders can be progressive in nature, and that therapies may need to be altered over time.

SUMMARY

Syncope is caused by a very wide range of quite varied clinical disorders. A careful history and physical examination, in conjunction with appropriately selected laboratory tests, often enables the cause to be determined.

REFERENCES

1. Savage DD, Carwin L, McGee DL, Kennel WB, Wolf PA. Epidemiologic features of isolated syncope. The Framingham Study. Stroke 1985;16:626–629.
2. Olshansky B. Syncope: An overview and approach to management. In: Grubb BP, Olshansky B, eds. Syncope: Mechanisms and Management. Futura Publishing Co. Inc., Armonk, NY, 1998, pp. 15–71.
3. Day SC, Cook EF, Funkenstein H, Goldman L. Evaluation and outcome of emergency room patients with transient loss of consciousness. Am J Med 1982;73:15–23.
4. Olshansky B. Is syncope the same thing as sudden death except that you wake up? J Cardiovasc Electrophysiol 1997;8:1098–1101.
5. Lipsitz LA. Syncope in the elderly. Ann Int Med 1998;99:92–104.
6. Campbell AJ, Teinken J, Allen BC. Falls in old age: a study of frequency and related clinical factors. Age Aging 1981;10:264–270.
7. Linzer M, Gold DT, Pontinen M. Recurrent syncope as a chronic disease. J Gen Intern Med 1994; 9:181–186.
8. Linzer M, Pontinen M, Gold DT, Benarroch E. Impairment of physical and psychological function in recurrent syncope. J Clin Epidemiol 1991;44:1037–1043.
9. Calkins H, Byrne M, El-Atassi R, et al. The economic burden of unrecognized vasodepressor syncope. Am J Med 1993;35:473–479.
10. Kapoor WN, Karpf M, Wieand S, Peterson JR, Levey GS. A prospective evaluation and follow-up of patients with syncope. N Engl J Med 1983;309:197–204.
11. Kapoor WN. An overview of the evaluation and management of syncope. In: Grubb BP, Olshansky B, eds. Syncope: Mechanisms and Management. Futura Publishing Co., Inc., Armonk, NY, 1998, pp. 1–14.
12. Kapoor WN, Schulberg HC. Psychiatric disorders in patients with syncope. In: Grubb BP, Olshansky B (eds). Syncope: Mechanisms and Management. Futura Publishing Co., Inc., Armonk, NY, 1998, pp. 253–264.
13. Ferrick KJ, Pacio G, Fisher JD. Limited yield of acute hospitalization for evaluation of syncope. PACE 1997;20:1132.
14. Mozoo B, Confino-Cohen R, Halkin H. Cost-effectiveness of in-hospital evaluation of patients with syncope. Isr J Med Sci 1988;24:302–306.

15. Murray P, Cantwell J, Health D, Shoop J. The role of limited echocardiography in screening athletes. Am J Cardiol 1995;76:849–850.

16. Maron BJ, Bodison SA, Wesley YE, Tucker E, Green KJ. Results of screening a large group of intercollegiate competitive athletes for cardiovascular disease. J Am Coll Cardiol 1987;1214–1221.

17. Lewis JF, Maron BJ, Diggs JA, Spencer JE, Mehrotra PP, Curry CL. Pre-participation echocardiographic screening for cardiovascular disease in a large predominantly black population of college athletes. Am J Cardiol 1989;64:1029–1033.

18. Weidenbener CJ, Krauss MD, Waller BF, Taliercio CP. Incorporation of screening echocardiograhy in the pre-participation exam. Clin J Sports Med 1995;86–89.

19. Recchia D, Barzila I. Clinical predictors of a normal echocardiogram in patients with syncope. Abstract. Circulation 1994;90(4) Part 2:1–384.

20. Sakaguchi S, Schultz J, Remole S, Adler S, Lurie K, Benditt D. Syncope associated with exercise, a manifestation of neurally-mediated syncope. Am J Cardiol 1995;75:476–481.

21. Calkins H, Seifert M, Morady F. Clinical presentation and long term followup of athletes with exercise-induced vasodepressor syncope. Am Heart J 1995;129:1159–1164.

22. Tse H, Lau C. Exercise-associated asystole in persons without structural heart disease. Chest 1995; 107(2):572–576.

23. Sneddon J, Scalia G, Ward D, McKenna W, Camm AJ, Grenneaux M. Exercise-induced vasodepressor syncope. Br Heart J 1994;71:554–557.

24. Kosinski D, Grubb BP, Kip K, Hahn H. Exercise-induced neurocardiogenic syncope: case report. Am Heart J 1996;132:451–452.

25. Osswald S, Brooks P, O'Nunain S, Corwin J, Roelke M, Radvany P, et al. Asystole after exercise in healthy persons. Ann Int Med 1994;120:1008–1011.

26. Fleg JL, Asante AV. Asystole following treadmill exercise in a man without organic heart disease. Arch Int Med 1983;143:1821–1822.

27. Holtzhausen LM, Noakes T. The prevalence and significance of post exercise hypotension in ultra marathon runners. Med Sci Sports and Ex 1995;27(12):1595–1601.

28. Palileo EJ, Ashley WW, Sriryn S. Exercise provocable/right ventricular outflow tachycardia. Am Heart J 1982;104:185–193.

29. Woelfei A, Foster JR, Simpson RJ. Reproducibility and treatment of exercise-induced ventricular tachycardia. Am J Cardiol 1994;53:751–756.

30. Wu D, Kou HC, Hung JS. Exercise-triggered paroxysmal ventricular tachycardia: a repetitive rhythmic activity possibly related to after depolarization. Am Intern Med 1981;95:410–414.

31. Levy M, Villain E, Phillipe F, Kachaner J. Catecholamine-induced ventricular tachycardia: a cause of severe syncope during adolescence. De Daitrie 1993;48(7–8):533–535.

32. Eisenberg S, Scheinman M, Oullet N, Finkbeiner W, Griffin J, Eldar M, et al. Sudden cardiac death and polymorphic ventricular tachycardia in patients with normal QT intervals and normal cardiac systolic function. Am J Cardiol 1995;75:687–692.

33. Coumel P, Leenhardt A, Haddad G. Exercise ECG: prognostic implication of exercise-induced arrhythmias. PACE 1994;17:417–427.

34. Burke A, Farb A, Virmani R, Goodlin J, Smialek J. Sports related and non-sports related sudden cardiac death in young adults. Am Heart J 1991;121(2):568–575.

35. Burke A, Farb A, Virmani R. Causes of sudden death in athletes. Cardiol Clin 1992;10(2):303–315.

36. Liberthson RR, Zaman L, Weyman A, Kiger R, Dinsmore R, Leinbach R, et al. Aberrant origin of the left coronary artery from the proximal right coronary artery: diagnostic features and pre-post operative cause. Clin Cardiol 1982;5:377–381.

37. McClellan JT, Jokl E. Congenital anomalies of coronary arteries as a cause of sudden death associated with physical exertion. Med Sport 1971;5:91.

38. Kosinski D, Grubb BP. Neurally-mediated syncope with an update on indications and usefulness of head upright tilt table testing and pharmacologic therapy. Curr Opin Cardiol 1994;9:53–54.

39. Samoil D, Grubb BP. Head upright tilt table testing for recurrent, unexplained syncope. Clin Cardiol 1993;16:763–766.

40. Streiper M, Auld D, Hulse H, Campbell R. Evaluation of recurrent pediatric syncope: role of tilt table test. Pediatrics 1994;93:660–662.

41. Benditt D, Ferguson D, Grubb BP, et al. Tilt table testing for assessing syncope and its treatment: an American College of Cardiology consensus document. J Am Coll Cardiol 1996;28:263–275.

42. Menozzi C, Brignole M, Gaggioli A, et al. Adenosine sensitive syncope in Raviele A. Cardiac Arrhythmias 1999; Springer Verlag, Milan, Italy, 2000; pp. 423–429.

43. Zipes, et al. Guidelines for intracardiac electrophysiological and catheter ablation procedures. J Am Coll Cardiol 1995;26(2):555–573.

44. Galmhusein J, Naccarelli G, Ko P, et al. Value and limitations of clinical electrophysiologic study in assessment of patients with unexplained syncope. Am J Med 1982;73:700–706.

45. Benditt D, Remole S, Milstein S, Balin S. Syncope: causes, clinical evaluation, and current therapy. Ann Rev Med 1992;43:283–300.

46. Morady F, Shen E, Schwartz A, Hess D, Bhandari A. Long-term followup of patients with recurrent syncope evaluated by electrophysiologic testing. J Am Coll Cardiol 1983;2:1053–1059.

47. Akhtar M, Shenasa S, Denker S, et al. Role of electrophysiologic studies in patients with unexplained recurrent syncope. PACE 1983;6:192–201.

48. Teichman S, Felder S, Majas J, et al. The value of electrophysiologic studies in syncope of undetermined origin: report of 150 cases. Am Heart J 1985;110:469–479.

49. Crozer I, Kram H. Electrophysiologic evaluation and natural history of unexplained syncope. Aust NZ J Med 1986;16:587.

50. Camm AJ, Lau CP. Syncope of undetermined origin: diagnosis and management. Prog Cardiol 1988; 139–156.

51. Almquist A, Goldenberg IF, Milstein S., et al. Provocation of bradycardia and hypotension by isoproterenol and upright posture in patients with unexplained syncope. N Engl J Med 1989;320:346–351.

52. Sra J, Anderson A, Sheikh H, et al. Unexplained syncope evaluation by electrophysiologic study and head-up tilt testing. Ann Int Med 1991;114:1013–1019.

53. DiMarco J, Philbrick J. Use of ambulatory electrocardiographic monitoring. An Int Med 1990; 113(1):53–68.

54. Zeldus SM, Leune BJ, Michelson EL, Morganroth J. Cardiovascular complaints: correlation with cardiac arrhythmias on 24-hour electrocardiographic monitoring. Chest 1980;78:456–461.

55. Clark P, Glasser SP, Sporo E. Arrhythmias detected by ambulatory monitoring: lack of correlation with symptoms of dizziness and syncope. Chest 1980;77:722–725.

56. Jonas S, Klein I, Dimant J. Importance of Holter monitoring in patients with periodic cerebral symptoms. Amn Neurol 1977;1:470–474.

57. Kala R, Vittasalo M, Toivonen L, Eisalo A. Ambulatory ECG recording in patients with dizziness or syncope. ACTA Med Scand 1982;688 (Supp):13–19.

58. Gilton TC, Heitzman MR. Diagnostic efficacy of 24-hour electrocardiographic monitoring for syncope. Am J Cardiol 1984;53:1013–1017.

59. Boudoulas H, Schaal SF, Lewis RP, Robinson JL. Superiority of 24-hour outpatient monitoring over multi-stage exercise testing for the evaluation of syncope. J Electrocardiol 1979;12:103–108.

60. Diamond TH, Smith R, Myburgh D. Holter monitoring—a necessity for the evaluation of palpitations. S Afr Med J 1983;63:5–7.

61. Pasyk S, Sredniawa B. Holter monitoring in the diagnosis of syncope. Pulske Tygodnik Lekarski 1993;48(16–17):377–379.

62. Racco F, Sconocchini C, Reginelli R, Brizzi G, Alessi C, Rosario S, et al. Value of cardiac electrocardiographic monitoring of patients with syncope: results of a prospective study. Minerva Cardioangiol 1993;41(11):523–527.

63. Beauregard L, Fabiszewski R, Black CH, Lightfoot B, Schraeder PL, Toly T, et al. Combined ambulatory electroencephalographic and electrocardiographic monitoring for evaluation of syncope. Am J Cardiol 1991;68(10):1067–1072.

64. Braun A, Dawkins K, Davies J. Detection of arrhythmias: use of a patient-activated ambulatory electrocardiogram device with a solid state memory loop. Br Heart J 1987;58:251–253.

65. Kinlay S, Leitch J, Neil A, Chapman B, Hardy D, Fletcher P. Cardiac event recorders yield more diagnoses and are more cost effective than 48-hour Holter monitoring in patients with palpitations. Ann Int Med 1996;124(1):16–20.

66. Krahn A, Klein G, Norris C, Yee R. The etiology of syncope in patients with negative tilt table testing and electrophysiologic testing. Circulation 1995;42(7):1819–1824.

67. Kuchar DL, Thorburn CW, Sannuel NL. Signal averaged electrocardiogram for evaluation of recurrent syncope. Am J Cardiol 1986;58:949–953.

68. Gang ES, Peter T, Rosenthal ME. Detection of late potentials in the surface electrocardiogram in unexplained syncope. Am J Cardiol 1986;58:1014–1020.

69. Winters SL, Stewart D, Gome J. Signal averaging of the surface QRS complex predicts inducibility of ventricular tachycardia in patients with syncope of unknown etiology: a prospective study. J Am Coll Cardiol 1988;12:1481–1487.

70. Buxton A. Late potentials and syncope. In: El-Sherif N, Turitto G, eds. High Resolution Echocardiography. Futura Publishing Co., Inc., Mount Kisko, NY, 1992, pp. 521–532.

71. Kjellgren D, Gomes J. Current usefulness of the signal averaged electrocardiogram. Curr Prob & Cardiol 1993;18(6):396–398.

72. Morillo C, Zandri S, Klein G, Yee R. Usefulness of signal averaged ECG, head-up tilt and electrophysiologic study in patients with unexplained syncope. J Am Coll Cardiol 1995;21:92.

73. Benarroch E. The central autonomic network: functional organization, dysfunction and perspective. Mayo Clinic Proc 1993;68:988–1001.

74. Wieling W, Lieshout J. Maintenance of postural normotension in humans. In: Low P., ed. Clinical Autonomic Disorders. Little Brown Co., 1993, pp. 69–73.

75. Grubb BP. Neurocardiogenic syncope. In: Grubb BP, Olshansky B, eds. Syncope: Mechanisms and Management. Futura Publishing, Armonk, NY, 1998, in press.

76. Kosinski D, Grubb BP, Temesy-Armos P. Pathophysiological aspects of neurocardiogenic syncope. PACE 1995;18:716–721.

77. Sutton R, Petersen M. The clinical spectrum of neurocardiogenic syncope. J Cardiovasc Electrophysiol 1995;6:569–576.

78. Kosinski D. Miscellaneous causes of syncope. In: Grubb BP, Olshansky B, eds. Syncope: Mechanisms and Management. Futura Publishing, Armonk, NY, 1998, in press.

79. Bradbury S, Eggleston C. Postural hypotension: a report of three cases. Jam Heart J 1925;1:73–86.

80. Robertson D, Polinsky R, eds. A Primer on the Autonomic Nervous System. Academic Press, San Diego, CA, 1996.

81. Shy GM, Drager GA. A neurologic syndrome associated with orthostatic hypotension. Arch Neurol 1960;3:511–527.

82. Mathias CJ. The classification and nomenclature of autonomic disorders: ending chaos, restoring conflict, and hopefully achieving clarity. Clin Auton Res 1995;5:307–310.

83. Grubb BP, Kosinski D, Boehm K, Kip K. The postural orthostatic tachycardia syndrome: a neurocardiogenic variant identified during head up tilt table testing. PACE 1997;20:2205–2212.

84. Bou-Holaigh I, Rowe P, Kan J, Calkins H. The relationship between neurally mediated hypotension and chronic fatigue syndrome. JAMA 1995;274:961–967.

85. Grubb BP, Kosinski D. Acute pandysautonomic syncope. Eur J of Cardiac Pacing and Electrophysiol 1997;7:10–14.

86. Passant V, Warkentin S, Karlson, et al. Orthostatic hypotension in organic dementia: relationship between blood pressure, cortical blood flow, and symptoms. Clin Auton Res 1996;6:29–36.

87. Bannister R, Mathias C, eds. Autonomic Failure: A Textbook of Clinical Disorders of the Autonomic Nervous System. Oxford Medical Publications, Oxford, 1992.

88. Low P, ed. Clinical Autonomic Disorders. Little Brown Co., Boston, 1993.

89. Grubb BP, Olshansky B, eds. Syncope: Mechanisms and Management. Futura Publishing, Armonk, NY, 1997.

90. Robertson D, Biaggioni I, eds. Disorders of the Autonomic Nervous System. Harwood Academic Publishers, London, 1995.

91. Grubb BP, Kosinski D. Tilt table testing: Concepts and limitations. PACE 1997;20 (Part II):781–787.

92. Mahanonda N, Bhuripanyo K, Kangkagate C, et al. Randomized double blind placebo-controlled trial of oral atenolol in patients with unexplained syncope and positive upright tilt test results. Am Heart J 1995;18:655–662.

93. Scott WA, Pongiglione G, Bromberg BL, et al. Randomized comparison of atenolol and fludrocortisone acetate in the treatment of pediatric neurally-mediated syncope. Am J Cardiol 1995;76:400–402.

94. Grubb BP, Kosinski D, Mouhaffel A, Pothoulakis A. The use of methylphenidate in the treatment of refractory neurocardiogenic syncope. PACE 1996;19:836–840.

95. Low P, Gilden J, Freeman R, et al. Efficacy of midodrine vs placebo in neurocardiogenic orthostatic hypotension. JAMA 1997;277:1046–1051.

96. Sra J, Maglio C, Biehl M, et al. Efficacy of midodrine hydrochloride in neurocardiogenic syncope refractory to standard therapy. J Cardiovasc Electrophysiol 1997;8:42–46.

97. Ward CR, Gray JC, Gilroy JJ, Kenny RA. Midodrine: a role in the management of neurocardiogenic syncope. Heart 1998;79:45–49.

98. Robertson D, Davis TL. Recent advances in the treatment of orthostatic hypotension. Neurology 1995;5:526–532.

99. Hoeldtke RD, Streeton DH. Treatment of orthostatic hypotension with erythropoietin. N Engl J Med 1993;329:611–615.

100. Grubb BP, Lachant N, Kosinski D. Erythropoietin as a therapy for severe refractory orthostatic hypotension. Clin Auton Res 1994;4:212.

101. Grubb BP, Kosinski D. Serotonin and syncope: an emerging connection? Eur J Cardiac Pacing Electrophysiol 1996;5:306–314.

102. Girolamo ED, Iorio CD, Sabatini P, et al. Effects of paroxetine hydrochloride, a selective serotonin reuptake inhibitor on refractory neurocardiogenic syncope: a randomized double blind placebo-controlled study. J Am Coll Cardiol 1999;33:1227–1230.

103. Grubb BP, Samoil D, Kosinski D, et al. Fluoxetine hydrochloride for the treatment of severe refractory orthostatic hypotension. PACE 1993;16:801–805.

104. Benditt D, Petersen ME, Luriek, et al. Cardiac pacing for prevention of recurrent vasovagal syncope. Ann Int Med 1995;122:204–209.

105. Connolly SJ, Sheldon RS, Roberts RS, Gent M. The North American vasovagal pacemaker study: a randomized trial of permanent cardiac pacing for prevention of vasovagal syncope. J Am Coll Cardiol 1999;33:16–20.

106. Sutton R, Brignole M, Menozzi C, et al. Dual chamber pacing in the treatment of neurally mediated tilt positive cardioinhibitory syncope: pacemaker versus no therapy: a multicenter randomized study. Circulation 2000;102:294–299.

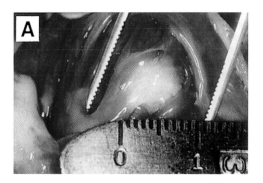 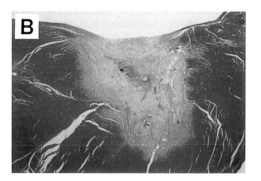

Color Plate 1, Fig. 1. (*See* discussion in Chapter 4, p. 52). **(A)** Endocardial radiofrequency ablation lesion demonstrating a round shape with sharp borders. **(B)** Histologic section of lesion in A, demonstrating hemispheric shape and extensive fibrosis. (From Jumrussirikul P, et al. Prospective comparison of temperature guided microwave and radiofrequency catheter ablation in the swine heart. PACE 1998;21[7]:1364–1374. Reproduced with permission.)

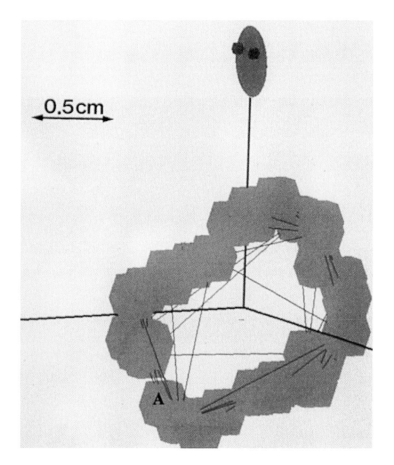

Color Plate 2, Fig. 4. (*See* discussion in Chapter 8, p. 149). Electroanatomical map (CARTO™), (Biosense/Webster Inc., Diamond Bar, CA, USA) of ablation lesions encircling a right superior pulmonary vein in a patient in whom AF was consistently triggered by atrial premature beats emanating from myocardium deep within this vein. Each circle **(A)** represents the site of an individual focal radiofrequency energy application. The summed effect of this series of lesions was "electrical isolation" of the vein.

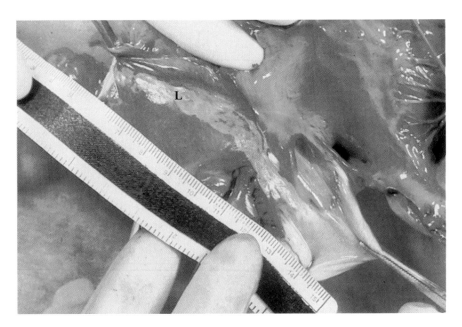

Color Plate 3, Fig. 10. (*See* discussion in Chapter 8, p. 156). Endocardial view of a 1-d-old lesion **(L)** deployed in the right atrium percutaneously utilizing radiofrequency energy. Unablated myocardium stains red.

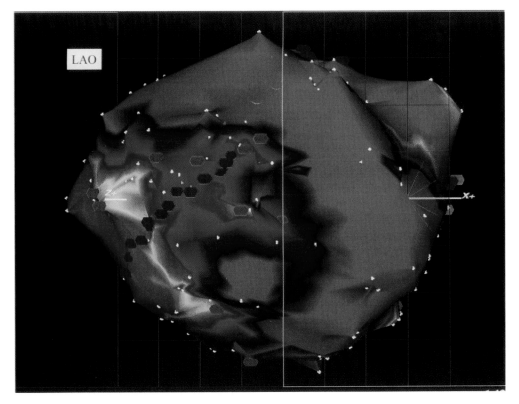

Color Plate 4, Fig. 7. (*See* discussion in Chapter 12, p. 250). Electro-anatomic map of the left ventricle in a patient with infarct-related VT, left anterior oblique (LAO) view. Radiofrequency lesions are depicted by dark red dots. Lesions are delivered in a line connecting densely scarred myocardium (red) to normal myocardium (purple).

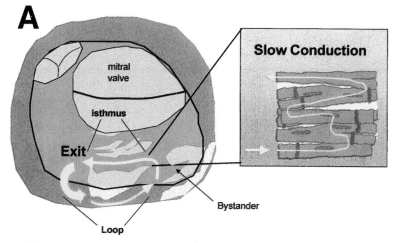

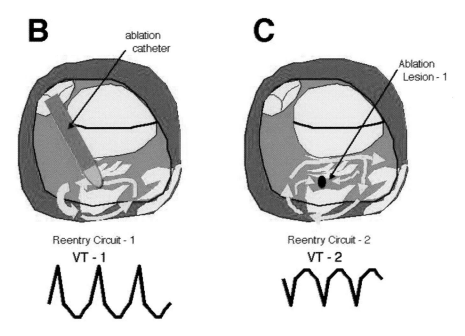

Color Plate 5, Fig. 4 A–C. (*See* discussion in Chapter 17, p. 367). Mechanism of reentry associated with ventricular scar is illustrated. The schematics show a view of the left ventricle from the apex looking into the ventricle towards the mitral and aortic valves. A region of heterogeneous scar is present in the inferior wall. In (**A**), the reentry wavefront circulates counterclockwise around and through the scar. Regions of dense scar create an isthmus in the circuit. The QRS onset occurs when the wavefront emerges from the isthmus at the Exit. It then circulates around the border of the scar, returning to the isthmus. Slow conduction through some regions in the scar is caused by discontinuities between myocyte bundles, as illustrated in the magnified image at the right. A wavefront that enters the bottom left myocyte bundles takes a circuitous course to emerge at the superior left bundle. In (**B**), an ablation catheter has been introduced through the aortic valve and positioned in the reentry circuit isthmus. In (**C**), following ablation of the isthmus for VT-1, a second VT is still possible because of reentry through an isthmus beneath the mitral valve. This circuit revolves in the opposite direction from the first circuit; the resulting VT has a different QRS morphology.

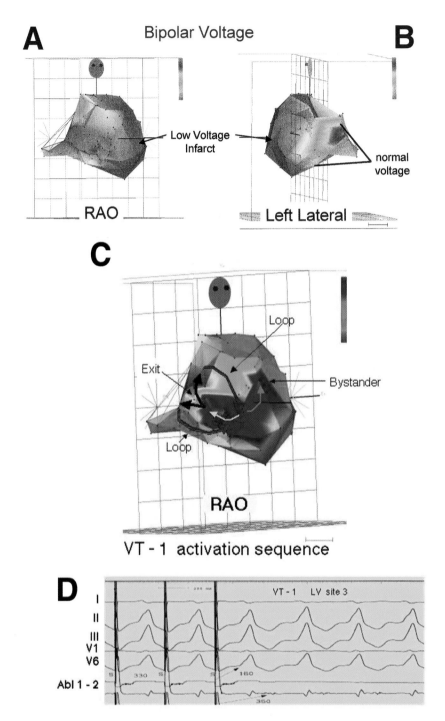

Color Plate 6, Fig. 5 A–C. (*See* full caption and discussion in Chapter 17, p. 369). Findings during catheter mapping in a patient with recurrent VT late after anterior-wall MI are shown. In (**A**) and (**B**) are shown the right anterior oblique (RAO) and left lateral views, respectively. Electrocardiogram voltage is designated by colors with the lowest voltage shown in red, progressing to greater voltage regions of yellow, green, blue, and purple. In (**C**), the activation sequence of induced VT is shown in the RAO view of the left vintricle. The colors now indicate the activation sequence, with red being the earliest activation (identifying the reentry circuit exit), progressing to yellow, green, blue, and purple. (**D**) Shows the effect of pacing during tachycardia (entrainment) in the central common pathway isthmus.

11

Bradyarrhythmias and Indications for Pacing

Current and Emerging

Robert W. Peters, MD,
and Michael R. Gold, MD, PhD

CONTENTS

INTRODUCTION

More than 100,000 permanent pacemakers are implanted in patients in the United States each year. From the most basic fixed-rate ventricular pacemakers that first became commercially available over 40 years ago, pacing systems have evolved dramatically in design and sophistication; current systems are both remarkably durable and reliable. This improvement in performance has been accompanied by an almost equally dramatic

From: *Contemporary Cardiology: Management of Cardiac Arrhythmias*
Edited by: L. I. Ganz © Humana Press Inc., Totowa, NJ

increase in complexity, so that patients with permanent pacemakers typically require follow-up in clinics staffed by specially trained individuals. In this chapter, we discuss in some detail the current and emerging indications for temporary and permanent pacing. In addition, we review some of the basic concepts and recent advances in pacing techniques and technology that are applicable to the various subsets of patients who require pacemakers.

DEMOGRAPHICS

With improvements in technology, the indications for pacing have been gradually expanding. In general, patients who develop symptoms and/or signs of hypoperfusion of critical organs or organ systems because of bradycardia, or an inadequate increase in heart rate during exertion or some other stress, may benefit from pacing. Many of these patients have evidence of intrinsic conduction-system disease as well as significant organic heart disease, although often the relationship between the etiology of the heart disease and conduction abnormalities is unclear. For example, most patients who require pacemakers for symptomatic atrioventricular conduction disease have underlying coronary-artery disease (CAD). In many cases, however, heart block did not develop in the setting of acute myocardial infarction (MI), and post-mortem examination of the conduction system shows nonspecific degeneration, rather than ischemic necrosis. Recently, there has been a growing interest in the use of pacing techniques in patients who are not necessarily bradycardic—such as congestive heart failure (CHF), or hypertrophic cardiomyopathy. Although the indications for pacing in these areas are still evolving, the clinical characteristics of the targeted patients may be markedly different from those of traditional pacemaker populations. Currently, it is estimated that greater than 85% of the more than one million individuals in the United States with permanent pacemakers are older than 65 yr of age (2). Almost one-half of these devices have been implanted because of some type of sinus-node dysfunction (3). The majority of implanted pacemakers are dual-chamber devices, and most have rate-responsive capabilities (2). It is anticipated that these statistics may become considerably different as the indications for permanent pacing continue to grow and evolve.

DEVELOPMENTS IN PACING TECHNOLOGY

Pacing occurs when a stimulus creates an electrical field at the interface between the pacing catheter and the adjacent myocardium. A wave of depolarization is created, which spreads across the heart and leads to myocardial contraction by means of excitation-contraction coupling. The earliest pacemakers were relatively primitive devices that produced pacing stimuli at regular intervals (at a rate that was preset by the manufacturer), but were not able to detect the heart's intrinsic rhythm. These "fixed-rate" pacemakers were soon supplanted by "demand" pacing units, equipped with circuitry to "sense" the local electrogram associated with intrinsic QRS complexes. As technology was further refined, dual-chamber pacing, rate-responsiveness, and programmability were added to the armamentarium. The current generation of permanent pacemakers is powered by lithium batteries that may last as long as 12 yr. Traditionally, the amplitude (voltage) has been programmed to twice the threshold level to ensure an adequate safety margin at the expense of battery longevity. New design elements incorporate a feature that automatically tests capture threshold on a regular basis so that a lower voltage can be used, improving battery longevity. Many pacemaker models are equipped with multiple sensors (to detect body movement or minute ventilation), which allow fine-tuning of rate-responsiveness and mimic the response of a normal sinus node), mode-switching (which automatically inactivates atrial tracking when a supraventricular tachyarrhythmia is detected), and "rate-smoothing" mechanisms that prevent abrupt drops in pacing rate when the upper rate limit is exceeded. All of these features tend to be programmable, and can be adjusted or even turned off if necessary.

Pacemaker leads have also undergone important technological advances. Pacing leads have either passive (e.g., tines) or active (e.g., screw-in devices at the tip) fixation mechanisms to prevent dislodgment. There are small pacing electrodes that increase impedance, minimizing current drain and prolonging battery life. Most pacing electrodes contain steroid-eluting reservoirs that decrease inflammation and fibrosis at the electrode-tissue interface, with a resulting reduction in the chronic pacing threshold. Currently under development are single leads that will allow pacing and sensing in both the atrium and ventricle, which would simplify implantation and reduce cost.

AMERICAN COLLEGE OF CARDIOLOGY/ AMERICAN HEART ASSOCIATION GUIDELINES

There are a wide variety of conditions and disorders that can potentially be improved by pacing. In an effort to standardize their recommendations, the American College of Cardiology/American Heart Association (ACC/AHA) Task Force on Practice Guidelines used the following format in their most recent guidelines for pacemaker implantation, published in April 1998 *(1)*:

Class I: there is general agreement that a pacemaker is beneficial, useful, and effective.
Class II: there is divergence of opinion about the usefulness of pacing.
        a: weight of the evidence favors usefulness/efficacy.
        b: usefulness/efficacy is more poorly established.
Class III: it is generally agreed that a pacemaker is not useful and may actually be harmful.

These categories will be referred to in the discussion of each potential indication for pacing.

SINUS-NODE DYSFUNCTION ("SICK SINUS SYNDROME")

Sinus-node dysfunction is a heterogeneous group of disorders of diverse etiologies (*see* Fig. 1). This spectrum of arrhythmias includes sinus and junctional bradycardia, sinus arrest, sinoatrial (SA) block, alternating periods of sinus bradycardia and supraventricular tachyarrhythmias—such as atrial fibrillation (AF) (the "bradycardia-tachycardia syndrome), and AF with a slow ventricular response *(4)*. With chronotropic incompetence, the resting heart rate may be adequate, but the heart rate fails to augment normally with exercise. Thus, the exercise heart rate is inappropriately slow, and the resulting cardiac output is insufficient to meet the metabolic demands of the body. Sinus-node dysfunction is seen with increasing frequency in the elderly, but has also been reported in children and young adults, especially after corrective surgery for congenital heart disease. Because of its abundant blood supply (the sinus node is essentially a specialized adventitia of the large sinus-node artery), the sinus node is relatively resistant to ischemia, and chronic sinus-node dysfunction is not a frequent sequelae of acute MI.

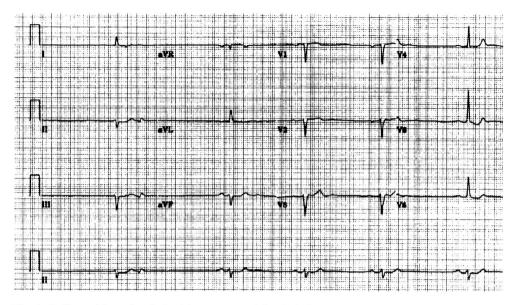

Fig. 1. A 68-yr-old previously healthy man complained of dizzy spells and marked exercise intolerance. His resting heart rate was found to be approx 32 BPM with frequent sinus pauses and junctional escape beats. He was taking no medications. He received a permanent dual-chamber pacemaker.

Sinus-node dysfunction is the most common reason for permanent pacemaker insertion, and accounts for up to 50% of permanent pacemakers implanted in the United States *(3)*. The current ACC/AHA indications for permanent pacing in sinus-node dysfunction are as follows:

Class I: Documented symptomatic bradycardia (or symptomatic chronotropic incompetence), either spontaneous or as a result of necessary drug therapy.

Class IIa: The presence of bradycardia—heart rate <40 beats per minute (BPM)—and symptoms *without* a documented association between the two.

Class IIb: Minimally symptomatic patients with very slow resting heart rates.

Class III: Asymptomatic individuals or those in whom symptoms are documented *not* to be a consequence of a slow heart rate.

Although it is generally accepted that rate-responsive pacing is required in individuals with sinus-node dysfunction because of the high incidence of chronotropic incompetence, there is some controversy about the use of atrial vs ventricular pacemakers. Short-term crossover studies have demonstrated dual-chamber or atrial pacing to be superior to ventricular pacing in improving quality of life, but there is no clear difference in exercise performance when dual-chamber and ventricular rate-responsive units are compared *(5–7)*. Long-term studies, mostly nonrandomized, have consistently demonstrated that dual-chamber pacemakers are associated with a lower incidence of AF, but mortality results have been more equivocal *(8–14)*.

Several large, prospective, and randomized studies have recently been completed. In the Pacemaker Selection in the Elderly (PASE) study, Lamas and colleagues conducted a 30-mo, single-blind, randomized, controlled comparison of ventricular and dual-chamber rate-responsive pacing in 407 patients 65 yr of age or older *(15)*. They also found improved quality of life in patients with sinus-node dysfunction, but could not document any benefit in mortality or cardiovascular events. Recently, Anderson and associates found a significant difference in both morbidity and mortality over a 3.3 (mean)-yr follow-up period in a randomized study of atrial vs ventricular pacing in 225 patients with sick sinus syndrome *(16)*. Preliminary results of the Pac-A-Tach study also show a mortality benefit for physiologic pacing (DDDR) over single-chamber ventricular pacing (VVIR) pacing in 198 patients with bradycardia-tachycardia syndrome *(17)*. In contrast, the Canadian Trial of Physiological Pacing (CTOPP) investigators found that dual-chamber pacing provided no benefit in cardiovascular mortality or incidence of stroke in 2,568 patients followed for a mean period of 3.1 yr *(18)*. This trial did suggest, however, less AF during follow-up in the DDDR group compared to the VVIR group. The preliminary results from the MOST study were similar *(18a)*.

There is also some debate about whether single-chamber atrial pacing (AAI or AAIR) may be superior to dual-chamber pacing in patients with sinus-node dysfunction and intact atrioventricular (AV) conduction *(19)*. Although it would intuitively seem that dual-chamber pacing would be preferable because it would protect patients against the subsequent development of AV block, it has been shown that this complication is unusual in patients with intact AV conduction at the time of implant *(20,21)*, and may not warrant the extra expense and complications associated with inserting an additional pacing lead. In addition, there may be adverse effects resulting from the altered activation pattern associated with ventricular pacing. The answer to this question may be provided by the results of several large ongoing clinical trials (*see* Table 1).

In summary, permanent pacemakers have played a major role in the therapeutic approach to sinus-node dysfunction. The indications for pacing are fairly well delineated, but the *type* of pacemaker that is most appropriate in a given clinical situation remains controversial. Atrial pacing has demonstrated superiority over ventricular pacing in terms of quality of life and the incidence of AF, but the mortality data are less convincing. Current trials focus on the role of AAI or AAIR in individuals with sinus-node dysfunction and intact AV conduction.

ATRIAL FIBRILLATION

AF is the most common sustained arrhythmia encountered in clinical medicine, and it is occurring with increasing frequency in a population that is gradually aging. It is associated with an almost twofold increase in mortality *(23)* and a fivefold increase in the risk of stroke *(24)*. Most studies have suggested that AF is caused by multiple reentrant wavelets within the atrium. The idea that pacing may prevent AF stems from the observation that patients with symptomatic sinus-node dysfunction had a lower incidence of AF with atrial pacing than with ventricular pacing. A number of possible mechanisms may prevent AF by pacing. In patients with vagally mediated AF *(25)*, pacing appears to be beneficial by preventing the initiating bradycardia. Because AF may be initiated by premature atrial beats (by producing atrial distention and dispersion of atrial refractoriness) atrial pacing may be beneficial by suppressing the extra beats or by altering the atrial activation pattern so that premature beats are unable to initiate reentry *(26,27)*. Lastly, there is evidence of anatomic and electrical changes in the fibrillating atrium (e.g., a marked decrease in the effective refractory period) that favor

Table 1
Prospective Randomized Trials of Comparing Pacing Modes in the Prevention of AF

Trial (ref)	# Subjects	Population	Mode	Duration	Results
PASE (15)	407	≥65 & all required PPM	DDDR vs VVIR	≤18 mo	QOL benefits mostly in SSS
Anderson (16)	225	SSS	AAI vs VVI	3.3 yr	AAI superior in morbidity and mortality
CTOPP (18)	2568	PPM for bradycardia	AAIR/DDDR vs VVIR	3.5 yr	QOL/mortality: No difference
STOP-AF (22)	350	SSS	AAIR/DDDR vs VVIR		Unfinished
UKPACE	2000	AV Block	DDD vs VVI		Unfinished
MOST	2000	SSS	DDDR vs VVIR		DDDR reduces AF
DAPPAF			Single vs dual-site pacing		Unfinished
SYNBIAPACE			Single vs dual-site pacing		Unfinished
PAC-A-TACH (17)	198	Brady/tachy syndrome	DDDR vs VVIR	2 years	DDDR reduced mortality but no diff in AF
Saksena (36)	15	Bradycardia requiring pacing	Single vs dual-site RA pacing	> 1 year	Dual-site pacing more effective
DAN-PACE	1900	SSS	AAIR vs DDDR		Unfinished
PA3 (33)	97	Post-AV node ablation	DDI vs DDIR	6 mo	AF incidence the same

PPM = permanent pacemaker; QOL = quality of life; SSS = sick sinus syndrome.

persistence of AF ("atrial fibrillation begets atrial fibrillation") (28). This vicious cycle can potentially be interrupted by an intervention, such as atrial pacing, which helps to maintain sinus rhythm.

The development of automatic mode switching has facilitated the use of permanent pacemakers in patients with recurrent or paroxysmal AF. Mode switching is a feature of dual-chamber pacemakers that allows the pacing mode to change automatically from AV-synchronous to a mode that does not track the atrial rhythm (e.g., VVI, DDI), thus protecting the patient from upper-rate tracking in the event of an atrial tachyarrhythmia. The efficacy of automatic mode switching is highly dependent upon the proper sensing of atrial potentials, and this capability has recently improved (29,30). Although the technique is still evolving, recent studies suggest that automatic mode switching may substantially improve quality of life (31,32).

Randomized studies have clearly demonstrated that atrial pacing may be effective in the long-term prevention of AF, primarily in patients with sinus-node dysfunction (15,17,18). Data from patients with normal sinus-node function are less compelling. In the Peri-Ablation for Paroxysmal Atrial Fibrillation (PA[3]) Trial, 97 patients with symptomatic paroxysmal AF and dual-chamber pacemakers with mode-switching capability were evaluated prior to AV-node ablation using the mode-switch datalogs (33). The investigators found that pacing had no impact upon the total AF burden (time spent in AF), the time to first recurrence of AF, or the frequency of AF episodes. Stabile and colleagues examined the effects of atrial pacing in 47 patients who had dual-chamber pacemakers implanted because of sinus-node dysfunction and/or AV block (34). They found a higher incidence of AF recurrence in those with longer right atrial conduction times and greater dispersion of atrial refractoriness. Therefore, it may be expected that simultaneous pacing from two separate atrial sites might be more effective than single-site pacing in preventing AF because it would create a less favorable milieu for reentry (35). In a preliminary report, Saksena and colleagues found that dual-site atrial pacing (DAP) from the high right atrium and the ostium of the coronary sinus (CS) was associated with a lower incidence of recurrent AF in a group of patients with drug-refractory AF (36). Two recently initiated large prospective trials, the Dual Site Atrial Pacing to Prevent Atrial Fibrillation (DAPPAF) and the SYNBIAPACE study, should help to further elucidate this important issue.

In summary, AF remains one of the most prevalent and treatment-resistant arrhythmias encountered in clinical medicine. Permanent VVIR pacing is clearly indicated in individuals with chronic AF who are symptomatic from a slow ventricular response (or require medications with negative chronotropic properties that cause symptomatic bradycardia). However, despite theoretical advantages and the success of pacing in nonrandomized clinical trials, there is no conclusive evidence that single-site pacing is of benefit in *preventing* AF in patients with no other indication for pacing (e.g., sinus-node dysfunction). Dual-site pacing is a promising technique that is currently under active investigation. A summary of current clinical trials of this important topic is provided in Table 1.

ATRIOVENTRICULAR (AV) BLOCK

The term AV block encompasses a heterogeneous group of disorders of diverse etiologies that all have a delay or block in the transmission of impulses through the

Table 2
Atrioventricular Block

Type	ECG	Level of block	Therapy
First degree	PR prolonged	AVN or HPS	None
Second-degree type I	Gradual PR increase before dropped beat	Usually AVN, but can be in HPS if QRS is wide	None if no sx; PPM if sx; HBE if QRS is wide
Second-degree type II	Dropped beat with no PR increase	HPS	PPM if no reversible cause is found
High-grade—2:1, 3:1, etc.	Every other P not conducted, 2 consec P waves not conducted, etc.	Narrow QRS usually at AVN; Wide QRS usually in HPS	PPM if sx; otherwise PPM if HBE documents HPS block
Third-degree (complete)	No P waves conducted	Narrow QRS usually at AVN; wide QRS usually in HPS	PPM if sx; otherwise PPM if HBE documents HPS block

AVN = atrioventricular node, HPS = His-Purkinje system, PPM = permanent pacemaker, sx = symptoms, HBE = His bundle electrogram.

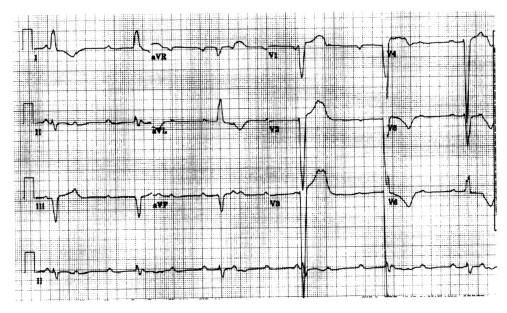

Fig. 2. A 74-yr-old man with a history of right bundle-branch block (RBBB) and left anterior fasicular block was admitted to the hospital after a syncopal episode. Complete heart block with a wide-QRS-complex escape rhythm was noted on his ECG, and a temporary pacemaker and later a permanent pacemaker were inserted. Approximately two-thirds of patients presenting with complete heart block and a wide-complex escape rhythm had antecedent RBBB with left anterior fasicular block.

specialized conduction system. The traditional electrocardiographic categorization of AV block is presented in Table 2. Cells of the conduction system possess a property called automaticity; i.e. the ability to depolarize spontaneously. In general, the rate of depolarization is highest in the SA node and decreases progressively with descent through the conduction system. Thus, from a functional and therapeutic standpoint, the level at which the block is located is more important than the electrocardiographic classification. Block at the level of the AV node is usually associated with a junctional escape rhythm (and a narrow QRS complex). The escape rhythm tends to be reliable, the rate is characteristically adequate (e.g., 50–60 BPM) and responds to autonomic interventions (such as atropine) because the node has extensive sympathetic and parasympathetic innervation. In contrast, block within the His-Purkinje system is associated with an idioventricular escape rhythm characterized by a wide QRS complex (Fig. 2) that is morphologically different from the conducted beats. It tends to be considerably slower and less reliable than a junctional escape rhythm, and is relatively unaffected by autonomic maneuvers.

From a therapeutic standpoint, chronic high-grade block at the level of the AV node is a rare disorder that tends to be relatively benign. The incidence of sudden cardiac death is low in individuals without accompanying severe organic heart disease, and asymptomatic patients can be followed without specific therapy. Individuals who have minimal symptoms can be given conduction-enhancing medications such as theophylline, although these are of questionable efficacy. One possible exception to this approach is the patient with congenital AV block. Although block in this situation characteristically occurs at the level of the AV node, the clinical course may be unpredictable, and sudden cardiac death has been reported (although admittedly, high-grade block has not been documented as the cause), prompting some authorities to routinely recommend permanent pacing for adult patients with congenital second- or third-degree block *(37,38)*. The official ACC/AHA recommendations for permanent pacing in acquired AV block are as follows *(1)*:

Class I: 1. Third-degree AV block at any anatomic level associated with any of the following:
  a. symptomatic bradycardia, either spontaneous or as a result of drug therapy that is required for treatment of other conditions.
  b. Documented periods of asystole ≥3 s or any escape rate <40 BPM.
  c. Following catheter ablation of the AV junction.
  d. Postoperative block that is not expected to resolve.
  e. Neuromuscular diseases with complete AV block such as Kearns-Sayre syndrome.
  2. Second-degree AV block associated with symptomatic tachycardia, regardless of site or type of block.

Class IIa: 1. Asymptomatic complete AV block with an average rate of ≥40 BPM while awake.
  2. Asymptomatic type II second-degree AV block.
  3. Asymptomatic type I second-degree AV block regardless of site.
  4. First-degree AV block with symptoms suggestive of pacemaker syndrome and documented improvement with temporary dual-chamber pacing.

Class IIb: 1. PR interval >0.30 s in symptomatic patients with left ventricular dysfunction in whom it has been demonstrated that shorter AV delays improve hemodynamics.

Class III: 1. Asymptomatic first-degree or type I second-degree AV block.

BUNDLE-BRANCH BLOCK

Patients with bundle-branch block (BBB) are at increased risk of high-grade AV block and sudden cardiac death. Large epidemiologic studies have contributed substantially to our knowledge about the natural history of this disorder. For example, Rotman and Triebwasser reviewed the records of 237,000 presumably healthy personnel at the United States School of Aerospace Medicine *(39)*. They found 394 people with right bundle-branch block (RBBB) and 125 with left bundle-branch block (LBBB), a combined incidence of 0.0002%. Over a 10-yr follow-up period, there were no sudden deaths, and only two people progressed to high-grade AV block. In contrast, in the Framingham study, 5209 people initially free of clinically manifest cardiovascular disease were followed for a period of 18 yr *(40,41)*. The Framingham population was older and had a higher prevalence of cardiac risk factors. BBB developed in 125 people, and in this subgroup, there was a high incidence of sudden cardiac death and four progressions to high-grade block. Thus, it appears that although conduction system disease in these individuals is progressive, the progression is slow and does not warrant prophylactic permanent pacing. The prognosis appears closely related to the presence and severity of underlying cardiovascular disease.

In the 1970s, several large prospective studies were initiated that attempted to identify individuals with BBB who were likely to require permanent pacing *(42–44)*. Since it

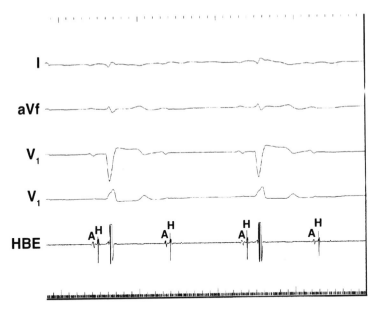

Fig. 3. An intracardiac electrogram recorded with four simultaneous surface leads in a patient with left bundle-branch block (LBBB) and PR prolongation. Type II second-degree atrioventricular (AV) block is shown with every other beat blocked distal to the His bundle depolarization. I, AVF, V1, V6 are standard surface leads, and HBE is the His bundle electrogram. A = atrial depolarization and H = His bundle depolarization.

was recognized that the standard 12-lead electrocardiogram (ECG) provides only limited information about the functional status of the specialized conduction system (it does not differentiate between block at the level of the AV node and block in the His-Purkinje system), intracardiac recordings were utilized (Fig. 3). These studies determined that prolongation of the infranodal conduction time (HV interval) is a significant risk factor for heart block, although the specificity of this finding is relatively low. Based upon this information, it has become common practice to implant permanent pacemakers in individuals with BBB who present with unexplained syncope and are found to have marked (≥100 ms) HV prolongation. However, the validity of this approach remains open to question. Scheinman et al. examined the use of "prophylactic" (defined as the absence of electrocardiographic evidence of high-degree block) permanent pacing in a large, nonrandomized cohort of patients with BBB and HV prolongation, more than one-third of whom had presented with syncope *(44)*. Interestingly, they found no difference in mortality, incidence of sudden cardiac death, or recurrence of syncope in the paced patients compared with a similar group of unpaced patients. A possible explanation of these findings was provided by Morady and colleagues, who performed programmed ventricular stimulation in 25 patients with BBB and unexplained syncope *(45)*. They found inducible ventricular tachycardia (VT) in 14 (56%), suggesting that tachyarrhythmias may be a more common cause of syncope than high-grade AV block in patients with BBB and structural heart disease.

In an effort to improve the diagnostic approach to patients with BBB, especially those with syncope, various techniques have been suggested to "stress" the conduction system. The induction of infranodal block by means of atrial pacing has been reported to be a relatively specific, although insensitive, means of predicting subsequent high-degree block (46,47). Similar findings have been reported for the development of second-degree AV block during exercise stress testing (48). The infusion of various conduction-depressing pharmacologic agents, most notably procainamide, disopyramide, and ajmaline (an investigational drug not commercially available in the United States) has also been suggested as a means of "stressing" the conduction system (49–51). As with the other methods, the induction of high-grade block has been found to be a relatively specific, although insensitive, predictor of future events. The significance of drug-induced HV prolongation is considerably less clear.

The recommended clinical approach to the patient with BBB is summarized in Table 3. It should be noted that to warrant a class I indication for permanent pacing in chronic BBB, even in patients presenting with syncope, high-grade block (Type II second-degree AV block or higher degrees of block) must be documented electrocardiographically (1). AV block, induced by provocative maneuvers in asymptomatic individuals, receives a class IIa indication. Isolated fasicular block, with or without first-degree AV block, is a class III indication for permanent pacing.

NEUROCARDIOGENIC SYNCOPE, CAROTID SINUS HYPERSENSITIVITY, AND RELATED DISORDERS

The term "neurocardiogenic syncope" includes a relatively common group of disorders characterized by abnormalities in autonomic control of the cardiovascular system. Clinically, the spectrum ranges from the person who experiences an occasional vaso-vagal "faint," precipitated by an especially strong stimulus such as fright, severe pain, or emotional upset, to the individual with recurrent disabling syncope without a clear precipitating factor. Although the exact mechanism of neurocardiogenic syncope has not been completely elucidated, the initiating factor appears to involve an exaggerated response of the parasympathetic nervous system to noxious stimuli. The diagnosis of neurocardiogenic syncope usually involves head-up tilt testing, in which an individual is strapped to a specially designed table and tilted up at an angle of 60–80 degrees for a period of time, usually 30–60 min. There are three general types of positive responses: vasodepressor, where there is vasodilatation and symptomatic hypotension without a major change in heart rate; cardioinhibitory, in which the heart rate drops precipitously without accompanying vasodilatation; and mixed response, where there is both bradycardia and vasodilatation. In carotid sinus hypersensitivity and related disorders (such as deglutition syncope, micturition syncope, and post-tussive syncope), symptomatic bradycardia and/or hypotension is elicited by an appropriate stimulus such as pressure on the neck (e.g., wearing a tight collar or using an electric razor), swallowing, bladder emptying, or coughing.

The first line of therapy for neurocardiogenic syncope has traditionally been medication, usually beta-blockers. Other drugs that have been used with variable success included disopyramide, theophylline, steroids that induce salt retention (such as fludrocortisone), serotonin-reuptake inhibitors, alpha agonists (e.g., midodrine), and anticholinergic mediations such as scopolamine.

Initial experience with permanent pacing was relatively discouraging, even with dual-chamber rate-adaptive units. The development of the "rate-drop response" (whereby a

Table 3
Diagnostic and therapeutic approach to BBB

Clinical setting	Syncope	Workup	Therapy
BBB	No	None	None
BBB	Yes	HBE	PPM if HV ≥100 or infranodal block with "stress" of conduction system
		V stim	If SHD, V stim to assess for VT
BBB, second-degree AV block	No	HBE	PPM if infranodal site of block documented or induced
BBB, second-degree AV block	Yes	HBE	PPM if infranodal site of block documented or induced
		V stim	If SHD, V stim to assess for VT
BBB, third-degree AV block	No	HBE	PPM if infranodal site of block documented or induced, no PPM if AV nodal and escape rhythm is adequate
BBB, third-degree AV block	Yes	None	PPM

HBE = His bundle electrogram, PPM = permanent pacemaker, V stim = ventricular stimulation study, SHD = structural heart disease.

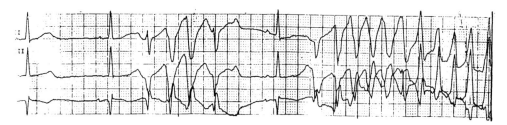

Fig. 4. An individual with recurrent AF was being treated with procainamide. He was noted to have a prolonged QT interval and runs of polymorphic ventricular tachycardia (PVT) (three simultaneous ECG leads are shown here). His ECG normalized when the procainamide was discontinued.

period of rapid pacing is initiated when the rate drops *suddenly* below a certain preset limit) has awakened interest in the use of pacing for these disorders. Recently, the results of the North American Vasovagal Pacemaker Study (VPS) were reported *(52)*. Fifty-four patients with neurocardiogenic syncope and ≥6 syncopal episodes were randomized to dual-chamber pacing with a rate-drop response, or to no pacing. The pacing group experienced an 85.4% reduction in syncopal episodes ($p < 0.00002$). In an accompanying editorial, Benditt agreed that the technique has promise, but cautioned that there was no medical treatment arm for comparison. Moreover, the population was very carefully selected so that the results were not necessarily applicable to the majority of individuals with neurocardiogenic syncope. In addition, treatment groups were not blinded—a potential problem considering the placebo effect of permanent pacing noted in other clinical settings. More recently, the smaller VASIS study yielded similar results *(52A)*. In this trial, the paced patients received a dual-chamber device programmed to the DDI mode with a hysteresis rate of 45 and a pacing rate of 80; the control group received no therapy. Currently, the only class I indication for pacing in these disorders is recurrent syncope caused by carotid sinus hypersensitivity *(1)*. The Vasovagal Pacemaker Study II (VPS II), in which all patients undergo pacemaker implantation, but one-half are randomized to inactive pacing (in a double-blind crossover design), is currently underway. Another multicenter controlled trial, "Syncope and Falls in the Elderly—Pacing and Carotid Sinus Evaluation" (SAFEPACE) is ongoing in the United Kingdom, and should provide additional information.

PROLONGED QT SYNDROME

QT interval prolongation on the standard 12-lead ECG is the hallmark of a heterogeneous group of disorders characterized by malignant ventricular arrhythmias (typically torsades de pointes) and a high incidence of syncope and sudden cardiac death (Fig. 4). Although congenital long QT syndrome (LQTS) was originally reported in children as a genetically transmitted disorder, acquired forms of LQTS have also been described. The pathogenesis of the arrhythmias associated with QT prolongation is incompletely understood, but sympathetic activation and early afterpotentials seem to be involved.

Initial therapy for the congenital LQTS characteristically involves beta-blockers. Other therapeutic modalities include left cervical sympathetic denervation, permanent pacing, and, in cardiac arrest survivors, implantable cardioverter defibrillators (ICDs). Presumably, permanent pacing exerts its beneficial effects by preventing pauses that initiate episodes of torsades, by shortening repolarization and decreasing dispersion of refractoriness, and by eliminating, or diminishing the amplitude of, early afterpotentials. Several studies have found that permanent pacing may be effective in reducing the incidence of syncope in individuals with the LQTS (54–56). However, until mortality benefit has been demonstrated, permanent pacing should be considered to be no more than adjunctive therapy in this syndrome. The 1998 guidelines consider pause-dependent ventricular arrhythmias, with or without LQTS, a class I indication for pacing (1). However, many electrophysiologists presently consider an ICD a more appropriate therapy in high-risk patients with congenital LQTS. Pacing may reduce the risk of torsades in patients treated with QT-prolonging drugs and a tendency to bradycardia. In patients with excessive QT prolongation or torsades, the offending agent should be discontinued.

ORTHOTOPIC CARDIAC TRANSPLANTATION

The vast majority of cardiac transplants today are orthotopic. Bicaval anastamoses are performed and there is retention of a substantial portion of the posterior walls of both atria of the recipient heart, along with their innervation. Bradyarrhythmias have been frequently described following orthotopic cardiac transplant, the majority caused by sinus-node dysfunction (57,58). Sinus-node dysfunction in this setting has been attributed to surgical trauma to the donor sinus node or to interruption of its blood supply (59). As surgical techniques have improved, however, the incidence of sinus-node dysfunction has decreased. There has also been the growing realization that sinus-node dysfunction in this setting is often benign and reversible, and there is currently a tendency to implant pacemakers only in severely symptomatic individuals (60,61). Theophylline may be utilized in the early post-transplant period as a temporary measure until sinus-node function improves (62). Currently, the only class I indication for permanent pacing following cardiac transplant is "symptomatic bradyarrhythmias/ chronotropic incompetence not expected to resolve and other class I indications (e.g., complete atrioventricular block) for permanent pacing" (1).

HYPERTROPHIC CARDIOMYOPATHY

Hypertrophic cardiomyopathy is a disorder of the myocardium characterized by excessive hypertrophy of the left ventricle, especially the interventricular septum. Although in theory there is an obstructive (characterized by a measurable left ventricular outflow gradient) and a nonobstructive form, the distinction between them may be difficult to discern because the gradient is dynamic and is dependent upon preload and the level of sympathetic tone. Both forms of hypertrophic cardiomyopathy are characterized by problems with diastolic relaxation, because the excessively thick ventricular musculature tends to be noncompliant and has difficulty filling. Medical therapy of this disorder is intended to decrease contractility and heart rate (lengthening the diastolic filling period) and to facilitate ventricular relaxation, usually with beta-blockers and/or calcium-channel blockers. The most definitive therapy for the obstructive form of the disease is septal myomectomy with or without mitral-valve replacement, but these procedures have considerable morbidity and mortality. The purpose of pacing in hypertrophic cardiomyopathy, unlike that in dilated cardiomyopathy, is to produce left ventricular dyssynchrony and dilatation, thereby decreasing the outflow gradient and improving ventricular filling.

Much of the interest in pacing therapy for hypertrophic cardiomyopathy stems from the work of Fananapazir, who conducted a nonrandomized study of 44 consecutive patients with hypertrophic obstructive cardiomyopathy (HOCM) and symptoms refractory to medical management (63). With DDDR pacing, there was a dramatic improvement in symptoms, exercise duration, and hemodynamics, including a 50-mmHg reduction in the mean gradient. Surprisingly, the improvement persisted even after discontinuation of pacing, suggesting some type of structural alteration in the myocardium. Their subsequent long-term study, with 84 patients followed for a mean period of more than 2 yr, had similar results (64). Recently, Pak and colleagues studied 11 patients with severe left ventricular hypertrophy (LVH) (65). Five of these individuals had hypertrophic cardiomyopathy, and six had hypertension with left ventricular-cavity obliteration. They found that pacing shifted the end-systolic pressure-volume relation downward and to the right in both groups, improving hemodynamics and reducing the gradient and/or cavity obliteration. In contrast, Nishimura found no significant benefit of DDDR pacing (vs AAI pacing) in a double-blind randomized study of 19 patients with HOCM (66). Similarly, the Multicenter Study of Pacing Therapy for Hypertrophic Cardiomyopathy (M-PATHY) randomized 48 symptomatic patients with drug-refractory hypertrophic cardiomyopathy and resting gradients ≥50 mmHg, to 3 mo of DDDR pacing or "placebo" pacing (AAI pacing at 30 BPM) in a double-blind crossover design (67). They found no significant difference between the two pacing modes in subjective or objective measures of symptoms or exercise capacity, although there was a trend toward improvement in the small subset of patients ≥65 yr of age. Gadler used a randomized double-blind crossover design to study the persistence of clinical improvement in 11 patients who had been paced successfully ≥6 mo (68). All subjects became extremely symptomatic within 20 d, requiring reinitiation of pacing.

How can these apparently conflicting data be reconciled? The Pacing in Cardiomyopathy (PIC) investigators, using a randomized double-blind crossover design, found that pacing was accompanied by a marked placebo effect in 81 patients with severe drug-refractory hypertrophic cardiomyopathy (69). Interestingly, even the outflow-tract gradient was significantly reduced with inactive pacing. Thus, some of the benefits of permanent pacing reported in some of the earlier studies have not been confirmed in rigorously conducted controlled clinical trials. There appears to be considerable variability in the clinical course of hypertrophic cardiomyopathy, even in patients with substantial outflow-tract gradients, so that larger numbers of subjects and longer follow-up periods will be required to adequately assess the response to therapy.

In summary, the role of permanent pacing in hypertrophic cardiomyopathy remains to be elucidated. There are currently no class I or class IIA indications for pacing in these individuals, independent of standard bradycardic indications that are coincident (1). Until definitive information becomes available, permanent pacing should be reserved for severely symptomatic drug-refractory patients who are unwilling or unable to undergo surgical therapy. To date, there are not data suggesting that any of the therapeutic interventions prevent sudden cardiac death or improve survival. Patients with documented malignant ventricular arrhythmias—and probably also those with syncope and inducible VI/VF—should receive ICDs.

LEFT VENTRICULAR SYSTOLIC DYSFUNCTION
(DILATED CARDIOMYOPATHY)

CHF is a problem increasing in frequency, with more than 400,000 new cases diagnosed in the United States every year *(70)*. Although many patients with heart failure require permanent pacemakers because of symptomatic bradyarrhythmias, especially in conjunction with the use of medications with negative chronotropic properties such as beta-blockers or amiodarone, there has been a growing interest in the use of pacing for purely hemodynamic purposes. Initially, this interest was focused on atrioventricular (AV) synchrony, especially in patients with CHF. Atrial contraction has been shown to contribute 15–30% to the total cardiac output in individuals with normal left ventricular function, and it is hypothesized that this percentage may be higher in the setting of CHF, especially if there is concomitant diastolic dysfunction. It is clear that the loss of atrial contraction can adversely affect hemodynamics. The term "pacemaker syndrome" describes a complex of symptoms (such as pulmonary congestion and hypotension) occurring with VVI pacing, probably related to the loss of AV synchrony and contraction of the atrium against closed AV valves *(71)*. This problem was largely remedied by the development of dual-chamber pacing.

It has become apparent that hemodynamics can be adversely affected by a long AV delay, especially when associated with diastolic mitral regurgitation. Accordingly, it was suggested that shortening of the AV delay may be used to improve hemodynamics in heart failure. The early work of Hochleitner and colleagues described dramatic functional improvement using dual-chamber pacing with a very short (100 ms) delay in a group of patients with severe idiopathic dilated cardiomyopathy *(72,73)*. Similar findings were reported by others *(74,75)*. Unfortunately, these findings have not been confirmed by subsequent controlled trials. Gold and colleagues, Innes et al., and Gilligan and colleagues all failed to detect any beneficial effect of short or "optimum" AV delay pacing in patients with severe heart failure using a randomized crossover design *(76–78)*. Thus, the use of short AV-delay pacing cannot presently be recommended as a means of improving hemodynamics in heart failure. It remains to be determined whether there are certain subgroups (e.g., those with severe diastolic mitral regurgitation) who may benefit from this technique.

There has also been considerable interest in the site of ventricular stimulation as a determinant of hemodynamics. When pacing techniques were initially developed, the right ventricular apex was the preferred site of stimulation because it provided an easily accessible and stable position that was usually associated with good pacing and sensing characteristics. It became apparent, however, that apical stimulation altered the pattern of ventricular depolarization, producing paradoxical septal motion and, sometimes, mitral regurgitation. Data from animal models and uncontrolled clinical studies initially suggested that there may be some hemodynamic advantage to pacing from the right ventricular outflow tract (RVOT) or septum *(79–81)*. However, subsequent randomized controlled studies have not confirmed these initial observations *(82,83)*. There are currently few data on the long-term clinical and hemodynamic effects of pacing from the RVOT or septum. The Right Ventricular Outflow Versus Apical Pacing (ROVA) trial, an ongoing study with a randomized double-blind crossover design, should help to provide some of this information.

Despite difficulties in obtaining access, there has been a recent surge of interest in left ventricular or bi-ventricular stimulation as a means of improving hemodynamics in patients with heart failure (i.e., cardiac resynchronization). Many patients with advanced cardiomyopathy have a wide QRS complex, frequently a left bundle-branch block (LBBB), and dyssynchronous left ventricular contraction. Since left ventricular contraction is an important determinant of cardiac output, properly synchronized left ventricular contraction or simultaneous contraction of both ventricles theoretically may enhance cardiac performance. Initial studies with left ventricular epicardial leads (84,85) produced promising results, as did acute studies using endocardial temporary pacing systems (86,87). Subsequently, the feasibility of chronic left ventricular stimulation through the coronary sinus (CS) or a cardiac vein was demonstrated (88–91). In most, hemodynamic and clinical parameters were improved, sometimes dramatically. In the InSync study, the pacing system was successfully implanted in 64 of 81 patients, and these individuals showed improvement in functional class, quality of life, and exercise time (92). Similarly, in the Pacing Therapies for Congestive Heart Failure (PATH-CHF) study, results from the first 27 patients suggested hemodynamic benefit (93). Two randomized trials, MUSTIC (94) and Miracle (95), have shown significant improvement in QOL and heart failure symptoms BiV pacing. The ongoing companion study is powered to determine if BiV pacing offers a survival benefit.

In summary, existing data suggest that manipulation of AV delay and site of stimulation within the right ventricle will not have a major impact upon clinical or hemodynamic parameters. In contrast, left ventricular and bi-ventricular stimulation appear to have considerable potential. Definitive conclusions must await the results of large ongoing randomized clinical trials. Despite the absence of mortality data, the FDA approved the first biventricular pacing system in August 2001.

TEMPORARY PACING

Temporary transvenous pacing is an established technique that can most often be accomplished quickly and easily by appropriately trained individuals. It is often performed under direct fluoroscopic visualization, but positioning flow-directed balloon catheters using electrocardiographic guidance is an acceptable alternative when fluoroscopy is unavailable. There are a number of indications for temporary pacing. In general, temporary pacing is indicated in any person who is markedly symptomatic from a bradyarrhythmia that is not rapidly reversible by the administration of medications or correction of electrolyte abnormalities (Fig. 5). In addition, the use of temporary pacing prophylactically should be considered in certain situations. Patients with underlying conduction system disease who are undergoing general anesthesia for planned surgical procedures have been the topic of several investigations (96–98). In general, the risk of high-degree block is very low and does not warrant prophylactic pacing, even in patients with advanced conduction-system disease, unless there is a history of syncope or second or third-degree AV block has previously been documented. Notably, a recent study by Gauss and associates prospectively studied 106 patients with asymptomatic bifasicular block (99). Progression to high-grade AV block was observed in only one patient. Patients with underlying LBBB who are undergoing right-heart catheterization, especially with endomyocardial biopsy, may also benefit from prophylactic temporary pacing.

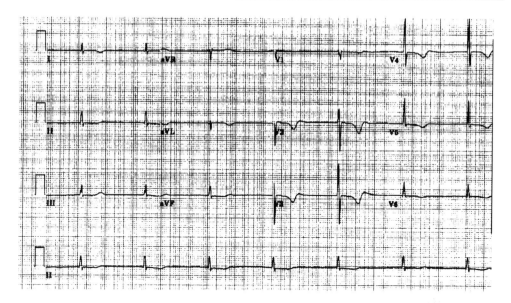

Fig. 5. An elderly woman was inadvertently taking 720 mg of sustained-release verapamil daily. She experienced a syncopal episode, and her ECG revealed a slow junctional rhythm without visible P waves. The verapamil was discontinued, and she received a temporary transvenous pacemaker until the effects of the drug dissipated.

There are other methods of temporary pacing, besides the transvenous route, that are relevant to the present discussion. Transthoracic pacing involves the percutaneous introduction of a pacing catheter directly into the right ventricle. Pacing can be accomplished very rapidly, an advantage for emergency situations, especially when venous access is difficult, but the technique has largely been abandoned because of difficulties in finding a stable pacing position and a high incidence of adverse effects. Transesophageal pacing is a relatively safe and easy technique that is generally well-tolerated. It provides an effective means of atrial pacing, because of the proximity of the esophagus to the left atrium. Ventricular capture is inconsistent, so it should not be used in the setting of AV block. Transcutaneous pacing is an established technique that previously was limited by poor patient tolerance (caused by painful contraction of the chest-wall musculature). It involves connecting several large self-adhesive chest electrodes to an external pulse generator. Recent technical advances have improved patient tolerance, making this a viable alternative to transvenous pacing, especially if used prophylactically when the risk of high-degree block is relatively low. Transcutaneous pacing may be somewhat less effective than transvenous pacing, so consistent ventricular capture should be documented before the device is left on standby.

CONCLUSION

Pacemakers and pacing techniques have undergone enormous changes since their inception in the late 1950s and early 1960s. As the technology has improved, the indications for pacing have widened considerably. However, despite major technological advances, objective data documenting beneficial effect—especially improved survival—has been sometimes lacking, making it somewhat difficult to justify the increasing complexity of newer pacing systems. It is hoped that data documenting survival benefit will be forthcoming with the completion of some of the large clinical trials cited in this chapter.

REFERENCES

1. Gregoratos G, for the Task Force on Practice Guidelines (Committee on Pacemaker Implantation) of the American College of Cardiology/American Heart Association. ACC/AHA guidelines for implantation of cardiac pacemakers and antiarrhythmia devices. J Am Coll Cardiol 1998;31:1175–209.
2. Bernstein AD, Parsonnet V. Survey of cardiac pacing in the United States in 1989. Am J Cardiol 1992;69:331–338.
3. Buckingham TA, Volgman AS, Wimer E. Trends in pacemaker use: results of a multicenter registry. Pacing Clin Electrophysiol 1991;14:1437–1439.
4. Ferrer MI. The sick sinus syndrome. Circulation 1973;47:635–641.
5. Linde C. How to evaluate quality-of-life in pacemaker patients: problems and pitfalls. Pacing Clin Electrophysiol 1996;19:391–397.
6. Adornato E, Bacca F, Polimeni RM. Ventricular single-chamber RR pacing in comparison to dual-chamber RR pacing: preliminary results of an Italian multicenter trial (Abstract). Pacing Clin Electrophysiol 1993;16:1147.
7. Barrington WW, Windle JR, Easley AA, Rundlett R, Eisenger G. Clinical comparison of acute single to dual chamber pacing in chronotropically incompetent patients with left ventricular dysfunction. Pacing Clin Electrophysiol 1995;18:1109–1113.
8. Connolly SJ, Kerr C, Gent M, Yusuf S. Dual-chamber versus ventricular pacing: critical appraisal of current data. Circulation 1996;94:578–583.
9. Brandt J, Schuller H. Pacing for sinus node disease: a therapeutic rationale. Clin Cardiol 1994;17:495–498.
10. Lamas GA, Estes NM, Schneller S, Flaker GC. Does dual chamber pacing prevent atrial fibrillation? The need for a randomized controlled trial. Pacing Clin Electrophysiol 1992;15:1109–1113.
11. Jahangir A, Shen W-K, Neubauer SA, Ballard DJ, Hammill SC, Hodge DO, et al. Relation between mode of pacing and long-term survival in the very elderly. J Am Coll Cardiol 1999;33:1208–1216.
12. Sgarbossa EB, Pinski SL, Maloney JD, Simmons TW, Wilkoff BL, Castle LW, et al. Chronic atrial fibrillation and stroke in paced patients with sick sinus syndrome. Relevance of clinical characteristics and pacing modalities. Circulation 1993;88:1045–1053.
13. Sgarbossa EB, Pinski SL, Maloney JD. The role of pacing modality in determining long-term survival in the sick sinus syndrome. Ann Intern Med 1993;119:359–365.
14. Sgarbossa EB, Pinski SL, Trohman RG, Castle LW, Maloney JD. Single-chamber ventricular pacing is not associated with worsening heart failure in sick sinus syndrome. Am J Cardiol 1994;73:693–697.
15. Lamas GA, Orav J, Stambler BS, Ellenbogen KA, Sgarbossa EB, Huang SKS, et al., for the Pacemaker Selection in the Elderly Investigations. Quality of life and clinical outcomes in elderly patients treated with ventricular pacing as compared with dual-chamber pacing. N Engl J Med 1998;338:1097–1104.
16. Anderson HR, Nielsen JC, Thomsen PE, Thuesen L, Mortensen PT, Vesterlund T, et al. Long-term follow-up of patients with a randomized trial of atrial versus ventricular pacing for sick sinus syndrome. Lancet 1997;350:1210–1216.
17. Wharton JM, Sorentino RA, Campbell P, Gonzalex-Zuelgaray J, Keating E, Curtis A, et al. PAC-A-TACH Investigators. Effect of pacing modality on atrial tachyarrhythmia recurrence in the tachycardia-bradycardia syndrome. Preliminary results of the pacemaker atrial tachycardia trial (Abstract). Circulation 1998;98:I-494.
18. Connolly SJ, Kerr CR, Gent M, Roberts RS, Yusuf S, Gillis AM, Sami Talajic M, Tang AS, Klein GJ, Lau C, Newman DM. Effects of physiologic pacing versus ventricular pacing on the risk of stroke and death due to cardiovascular causes. Canadian Trial of Physiologic Pacing Investigators. N Engl J Med 2000;342(19):1385–1391.
18a. Lamas GA. Presentation at North American Society of Pacing and Electrophysiology, 2001.
19. Anderson HR, Nielsen JC. Pacing in the sick sinus syndrome—need for a prospective randomized trial comparing atrial with dual chamber pacing. Pacing Clin Electrophysiol 1998;21:1175–1179.

20. Anderson HR, Nielsen JC, Thompsen PE, Thuesen L, Vesterlund T, Pedersen AK, et al. Atrioventricular conduction during long-term follow-up of patients with sick sinus syndrome. Circulation 1998; 98:1315–1321.

21. Bohm A, Pinter A, Szekely A, Preda I. Clinical observations with long-term atrial pacing. Pacing Clin Electrophysiol 1998;21:246–249.

22. Charles RG, McComb JM. Systematic trial of pacing to prevent atrial fibrillation (STOP-AF). Heart 1997;78:224–225.

23. Benjamin EJ, Levy D, Vaziri SM, et al. Independent risk factors for atrial fibrillation in a population-base cohort. The Framingham Heart Study. JAMA 1994;271:840–844.

24. Wolfe PA, Abbott RD, Kannel WB. Atrial fibrillation as a risk factor for stroke: the Framingham Heart Study. Stroke 1991;22:983–988.

25. Coumel P, Friocourt P, Mugica J, Attuel P, LeCler JF. Long-term prevention of vagal atrial arrhythmias by atrial pacing at 90/minute: experience with 6 cases. Pacing Clin Electrophysiol 1983;6:552–556.

26. Goel BG, Han J. Atrial ectopic activity associated with sinus bradycardia. Circulation 1970;42:853–858.

27. Mehra R. How might pacing prevent atrial fibrillation? In: Murgatroyd FD, Camm AJ, ed. Nonpharmacologic Management of Atrial Fibrillation. Futura Publishing, Armonk, NY, 1997, pp. 283–307.

28. Wijffels M, Kirchof C, Dorland R, Alessie MA. Atrial fibrillation begets atrial fibrillation: a study in awake chronically instrumented goats. Circulation 1995;92:1954–1958.

29. Palma EC, Kedarnath V, Vankawalla V, Andrews CA, Hanson S, Furman S, et al. Effect of varying atrial sensitivity, AV interval, and detection algorithm on automatic mode switching. PACE 1996; 19:1734–1739.

30. Lam CTF, Lau C-P, Leung S-K, Tse H-F, Ayers G. Improved efficacy of mode switching during atrial fibrillation using automatic atrial sensitivity adjustment. PACE 1999;22:17–25.

31. Kalalvand K, Tan K, Kotsakis A, Bucknall C, Sulke N. Is mode switching beneficial? A randomized study in patients with paroxysmal atrial tachyarrhythmias. J Am Coll Cardiol 1997;30:496–504.

32. Marshall HJ, Harris ZI, Griffith MJ, Holder RL, Gammage MD. Prospective randomized study of ablation and pacing versus medical therapy for paroxysmal atrial fibrillation: effects of pacing mode and mode-switch algorithm. Circulation 1999;99:1587–1592.

33. Gillis AM, Wyse G, Connolly SJ, Dubuc M, Philippon F, Yee R, et al., for the Paroxysmal Atrial Fibrillation Investigators. Atrial pacing periablation for prevention of paroxysmal atrial fibrillation. Circulation 1999;99:2553–2558.

34. Stabile G, Senatore G, De Simone A, Turco P, Coltorti F, Nocerino P, et al. Determinants of efficacy of atrial pacing in preventing atrial fibrillation recurrence. J Cardiovasc Electrophysiol 1999;10:2–9.

35. Guerra PG, Lesh MD. The role of nonpharmacologic therapies for the treatment of atrial fibrillation. J Cardiovasc Electrophysiol 1999;10:450–460.

36. Saksena S, Prakash A, Hill M, Krol RB, Munsif AN, Mathew PP, et al. Prevention of recurrent atrial fibrillation with chronic dual-site right atrial pacing. J Am Coll Cardiol 1996;28:687–694.

37. Michaelson M, Jonzon A, Riesenfeld T. Isolated congenital complete heart block in adult life: a prospective study. Circulation 1995;92:442–449.

38. Friedman RA. Congenital complete AV block: pace me now or pace me later. Circulation 1995;92:283–285.

39. Rotman M, Triebwasser JH. A clinical and follow-up study of right and left bundle branch block. Circulation 1975;51:477–484.

40. Schneider JF, Thomas HE, Kreger BE, McNamara PM, Kannel WB. Newly acquired left bundle branch block: the Framingham study. Ann Intern Med 1979;90:303–310.

41. Schneider JF, Thomas HE, Kreger DE, McNamara PM, Sorlie P, Kannel WB. Newly acquired right bundle branch block: the Framingham study. Ann Intern Med 1980;92:37–44.

42. Dhingra RC, Palileo E, Strasberg, Swiryn S, Bauernfeind RA, Wyndham CRC, et al. Significance of the HV interval in 517 patients with chronic bifasicular block. Circulation 1981;64:1265–1275.

43. McAnulty JH, Rahimtoola SH, Murphy E, DeMots H, Ritzman L, Kanarek PE, et al. Natural history of "high risk" bundle branch block: final report of a prospective study. N Engl J Med 1982;307:137–143.

44. Scheinman MM, Peters RW, Sauve MJ, Desai J, Abbott JA, Cogan J, et al. The value of the HQ interval in patient with bundle branch block and the role of prophylactic pacing. Am J Cardiol 1982; 50:1316–1322.

45. Morady F, Higgins J, Peters RW, Schwartz AB, Shen EN, Bhandari A, et al. Electrophysiologic testing in bundle branch block and unexplained syncope. Am J Cardiol 1984;54:587–591.

46. Dhingra RC, Wyndham C, Bauernfeind, Swiryn C, Amat-y-Leon F, Towne W, et al. Significance of block distal to the His bundle induced by atrial pacing in patients with chronic bifasicular block. Circulation 1979;60:1455–1464.

47. Petrac D, Radic B, Birtic K, Gjurovic J. Prospective evaluation of infrahisal second-degree AV block induced by atrial pacing in the presence of chronic bundle branch block and syncope. PACE 1996;19:784–792.

48. Woelfel AK, Simpson RJ, Gettes LS, Foster J. Exercise-induced distal atrioventricular block. J Am Coll Cardiol 1983;2:578–584.

49. Kaul U, Dev V, Narula J, Malhotra AK, Talwar KK, Bhatia ML. Evaluation of patients with bundle branch block and "unexplained" syncope: a study based on comprehensive electrophysiologic testing and ajmaline stress. PACE 1988;11:289–297.

50. Twidale N, Heddle WF, Tonkin AM. Procainamide administration during electrophysiologic study: utility as a provocative test for intermittent atrioventricular block. PACE 1988;11:1388–1397.

51. Englund A, Bergfeldt L, Rosenqvist. Disopyramide stress test: a sensitive and specific tool for predicting impending high degree atrioventricular block in patients with bifasicular block. Br Heart J 1995;74:650–655.

52. Connolly SJ, Sheldon R, Roberts RS, Gent M, on behalf of the Vasovagal Pacemaker Study Investigators. J Am Coll Cardiol 1999;33:16–20.

52A. Sutton R, Brignole M, Menozzi C, Raviele A, Alboni P, Giani P, Moya A, for the VASIS investigators. Dual chamber pacing in the treatment of neurally mediated tilt positive cardioinhibitory syncope: pacemaker versus no therapy: a multicenter randomized study. Circulation 2000;102:294–299.

53. Benditt DG. Cardiac pacing for prevention of vasovagal syncope. J Am Coll Cardiol 1999;33:21–23.

54. Eldar M, Griffin JC, Abbott JA, Benditt D, Bhandari A, Herre JM, et al. Permanent cardiac pacing in patients with the long QT syndrome. J Am Coll Cardiol 1987;10:600–607.

55. Moss AJ, Liu JE, Gottlieb S, Locati EH, Schwartz PJ, Robinson JL. Efficacy of permanent pacing in the management of high risk patients with long QT syndrome. Circulation 1991;84:1524–1529.

56. Eldar M, Griffin JC, VanHare GF, Witherell C, Bhandarim A, Benditt D, et al. Combined use of beta-adrenergic blocking agents and long-term cardiac pacing for patients with the long QT syndrome. J Am Coll Cardiol 1992;20:830–837.

57. Heinz G, Kratochwill C, Koller-Strametz J, Kreiner G, Grimm M, Grabenwoger M, et al. Sinus node dysfunction after orthotopic cardiac transplantation: postoperative incidence and long-term implications. PACE 1998;21:422–429.

58. Scott, Dark JH, McComb JM. Sinus node function after cardiac transplantation. J Am Coll Cardiol 1994;24:1334–1341.

59. DiBiase, a Tse T-M, Schnittger I, Wexler L, Stinson EB, Valentine HA. Frequency and mechanism of bradycardia in cardiac transplant recipients and need for pacemakers. Am J Cardiol 1991;67:1385–1389.

60. Scott CD, Omar I, McComb JM, Dark JH, Bexton RS. Long-term pacing in heart-transplant recipients is usually unnecessary. PACE 1991;14:1792–1796.

61. Payne ME, Murray KD, Watson KM. Permanent pacing in heart transplant recipients: underlying causes and long-term results. J Heart Lung Transplant 1991;10:738–742.

62. Ellenbogen KA, Szentpetery S, Katz MR. Reversibility of prolonged chronotropic dysfunction with theophylline following orthotopic cardiac transplantation. Am Heart J 1988;202:202–206.

63. Fananapazir L, Cannon RO, Tripodi D, Panza JA. Impact of dual-chamber permanent pacing in patients with obstructive hypertrophic cardiomyopathy with symptoms refractory to verapamil and B-adrenergic blocker therapy. Circulation 1992;85:2149–2161.

64. Fananapazir L, Epstein ND, Curiel RV, Panza JA, Tripodi D, McAreavey D. Long-term results of dual-chamber (DDD) pacing in obstructive hypertrophic cardiomyopathy: evidence for progressive symptomatic and hemodynamic improvement and reduction of left ventricular hypertrophy. Circulation 1994;90:2731–2742.

65. Pak PH, Maughan L, Baughman KL, Kieval RS, Kass DA. Mechanism of acute mechanical benefit from VDD pacing in hypertrophied heart: similarity of responses in hypertrophic cardiomyopathy and hypertensive heart disease. Circulation 1998;98:242–248.

66. Nishimura RA, Trusty JM, Hayes DL, Ilstrup DM, Larson DR, Hayes SN, et al. Dual-chamber

pacing for hypertrophic cardiomyopathy: a randomized, double-blind, crossover trial. J Am Coll Cardiol 1997;29:435–441.

67. Maron BJ, Nishimura RA, McKenna WJ, Rakowski H, Josephson ME, Kieval RS, for the M-PATHY Study investigators. Assessment of permanent dual-chamber pacing as a treatment for drug-refractory symptomatic patients with obstructive hypertrophic cardiomyopathy: a randomized, double-blind, crossover study. Circulation 1999;99:2927–2933.

68. Gadler F, Linde C, Ryden L. Rapid return of left ventricular outflow tract obstruction and symptoms following cessation of long-term atrioventricular synchronous pacing for obstructive hypertrophic cardiomyopathy. Am J Cardiol 1999;83:553–557.

69. Linde C, Gadler F, Kappenberger L, Ryden L. Placebo effect of pacemaker implantation in obstructive hypertrophic cardiomyopathy. Am J Cardiol 1999;83:903–907.

70. Van Orden Wallace CJ. Dual-chamber pacemakers in the management of severe heart failure. Crit Care Nurs Q 1998;18:57–67.

71. Ellenbogen KA, Gilligan DM, Wood MA, Morillo C, Barold SS. The pacemaker syndrome—a matter of definition. Am J Cardiol 1997;79:1226–1229.

72. Hochleitner M, Hortnagl H, Ng C-K, Hortnagl H, Gschnitzer F, Zechmann W. Usefulness of physiologic dual-chamber pacing in drug-resistant idiopathic dilated cardiomyopathy. Am J Cardiol 1990;66:198–202.

73. Hochleitner M, Hortnagl H, Fridrich L, Gschnitzer F. Long-term efficacy of physiologic dual-chamber pacing in the treatment of end-stage idiopathic dilated cardiomyopathy. Am J Cardiol 1992;70:1320–1325.

74. Kataoka H. Hemodynamic effect of physiologic dual chamber pacing in a patient with end-stage dilated cardiomyopathy; a case report. PACE 1991;14:1330–1335.

75. Auricchio Sommariva L, Salo RW, Scafuri A, Chiarello L. Improvement of cardiac function in patients with severe congestive heart failure and coronary artery disease by dual chamber pacing with shortened AV delay. PACE 1993;16:2034–2043.

76. Gold MR, Feliciano Z, Gottlieb SS, Fisher ML. Dual-chamber pacing with a short AV delay in congestive heart failure: a randomized study. J Am Coll Cardiol 1995;26:967–973.

77. Innes D, Leitch JW, Fletcher PJ. VDD pacing at short atrioventricular intervals does not improve cardiac output in patients with dilated heart failure. PACE 1994;17:959–965.

78. Gilligan DM, Sargent DA, Wood MA, Ellenbogen KA. A double-blind, randomized, crossover trial of dual chamber pacing with an "optimized" versus a nominal atrio-ventricular delay in symptomatic left ventricular dysfunction (Abstract). J Am Coll Cardiol 1998;31:389A.

79. Karpawich PP, Vincent JA. Ventricular pacing does make a difference: improved left ventricular function with septal pacing (Abstract). PACE 1994;17:820.

80. Giudici MC, Thornburg GA, Buck DL, Coyne EP, Walton MC, Paul DL, et al. Comparison of right ventricular outflow tract and apical lead permanent pacing on cardiac output. Am J Cardiol 1997; 79:209–212.

81. Cowell R, Morris-Thurgood J, Ilsey C, Paul V. Septal short atrioventricular delay pacing: additional hemodynamic improvements in heart failure. PACE 1994;17:1980–1983.

82. Gold MR, Shorofsky SR, Metcalf MD, Feliciano Z, Fisher ML, Gottlieb SS. The acute hemodynamic effects of right ventricular septal pacing in patients with congestive heart failure secondary to ischemic or idiopathic dilated cardiomyopathy. Am J Cardiol 1997;79:679–681.

83. Brockman RG, Olsovsky MR, Shorofsky SR, Gold MR. The acute hemodynamic effects of pacing site and mode in congestive heart failure (Abstract). J Am Coll Cardiol 1998;31:389A.

84. Foster AH, Gold MR, McLaughlin JS. Acute hemodynamic effects of atrio-biventricular pacing in humans. Ann Thorac Surg 1995;59:294–300.

85. Bakker PF, Meijburg H, de Jonge N, van Mechelen R, Wittkampf F, Mower M, et al. Beneficial effects of biventricular pacing in congestive heart failure (abstract). PACE 1994;17:820.

86. Blanc JJ, Etienne Y, Gilard M, Mansourati J, Munier S, Boschat J, et al. Evaluation of different ventricular pacing sites in patients with severe heart failure: results of an acute hemodynamic study. Circulation 1997;96:3273–3277.

87. Kass DA, Chen C-H, Curry C, Talbot M, Berger R, Fetics B, et al. Improved left ventricular mechanics from acute VDD pacing in patients with dilated cardiomyopathy and ventricular conduction delay. Circulation 1999;99:1567–1573.

88. Cazeau S, Ritter P, Lazarus A, Gras D, Bakdach H, Mundler O, et al. Multisite pacing for end-stage heart failure. PACE 1996;19:1748–1757.
89. Daubert C, Ritter P, Cazeau S, Gras, Lazzarus A, Mabo P. Permanent biventricular pacing in dilated cardiomyopathy: is a totally endocardial approach technically feasible (Abstract) PACE 1996;19:699.
90. Maloney JD, Martin R, Chodinella, Milner L, Emanuele T. Transvenous bi-atrial and biventricular pacing is technically feasible for management of arrhythmias and end-stage heart failure (Abstract). PACE 1996;19:699.
91. Jais P, Douard H, Shah DC, Barold S, Barat J-L, Clement J. Endocardial biventricular pacing. PACE 1998;21:2128–2131.
92. Gras D, Mabo P, Tang T, Luttikuis O, Chatoor R, Pedersen A-K, et al. Multisite pacing as a supplemental treatment of congestive heart failure: preliminary results of the Medtronic Inc. InSync Study. PACE 1998;21:2249–2255.
93. Auricchio A, Stellbrink C, Block M, Sack S, Vogt J, Bakker P, et al., for the Pacing Therapies for Congestive Heart Failure Study Group. Circulation 1999;99:2993–3001.
94. Cazeau S, Leclercq C, Lavergne T, Walker S, Varma C, Linde C, Garrigue S, Kappenberger L, Haywood GA, Santini M, Bailleul C, Daubert J-C. The multisite stimulation in cardiomyopathies (MUSTIC) study investigators. N Engl J Med 2001;344:873–880.
95. Abraham W. MUSTIC Results. Presentation at American College of Cardiology Annual Scientific Session, 2001.
96. Kunstadt D, Punja M, Cagin, Fernandez P, Levitt B, Yuccoglu YZ. Bifasicular block: a clinical and electrophysiologic study. Am Heart J 1973;86:173–181.
97. Santini M, Carrara P, Benhar M. Possible risks of general anesthesia in patients with intraventricular conduction disturbances. PACE 1980;3:130–137.
98. Mikell FL, Weir EK, Chesler E. Perioperative risk of complete heart block in patients with bifasicular block and prolonged PR interval. Thorax 1981;36:14–17.
99. Gauss A, Hubner C, Radermacher P, Georgieff M, Schutz W. Perioperative risk of bradyarrhythmias in patients with asymptomatic chronic bifasicular block or left bundle branch block. Anesthesiology 1998;88:679–687.

12

Approach to the Patient with Ventricular Tachycardia or Ventricular Fibrillation

Reginald T. Ho, MD,
and Francis E. Marchlinski, MD

CONTENTS

INTRODUCTION

Cardiac arrest is the cause of more than 300,000 deaths annually (1). Ventricular tachyarrhythmias are reported in approximately 75% of these cases, with polymorphic ventricular tachycardia (PVT), ventricular fibrillation (VF) and monomorphic ventricular tachycardia (VT) observed with nearly equal frequency (2). VT and VF are therefore the leading causes of death in patients with coronary-artery disease (CAD). The approach to the patient with VT or VF requires a careful evaluation of the clinical history, mode of presentation, underlying cardiac substrate, and ventricular function. For patients who present with VT, electrocardiographic documentation is extremely important. Although most arrhythmic episodes occur in unmonitored settings, the 12-lead electrocardiogram (ECG) provides valuable diagnostic and prognostic information. The fact that a 12-lead ECG could be recorded during the event generally implies that VT is tolerated by the patient. Secondly, the probable diagnosis of right ventricular outflow-tract (RVOT) tachycardia (Fig. 1) and idiopathic left ventricular tachycardia (Fig. 2) is based upon a characteristic morphology recorded on the ECG. Thirdly, the ECG identifies the region of origin for the exit site of VT when ablative therapy is considered. Finally, in some patients, wide-complex tachycardia will be caused by supraventricular tachycardia

From: *Contemporary Cardiology: Management of Cardiac Arrhythmias*
Edited by: L. I. Ganz © Humana Press Inc., Totowa, NJ

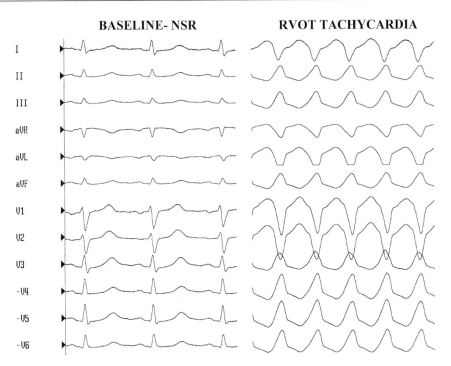

Fig. 1. 12-lead ECG recording of sinus rhythm (left) and VT (right) from a patient with RVOT. Note the left bundle-branch block (LBBB) morphology with right inferior frontal axis during VT. NSR = normal sinus rhythm, RVOT = right ventricular outflow tract.

(SVT) with aberrancy rather than VT; an ECG can be helpful in making this diagnosis. Only after complete assessment of relevant clinical data can a proper therapeutic decision be made regarding the treatment of VT. For patients who are resuscitated from VF, a 12-lead ECG obtained post-resuscitation may offer clues to the cause of the arrest (such as acute myocardial infarction (MI), long QT syndrome (LQTS), or Wolff-Parkinson-White syndrome (WPW)).

The purpose of this chapter is to outline these important clinical variables and to provide an algorithm for the management of patients with VT and VF. The chapter is divided into four sections. The first section discusses the long-term therapeutic options available for patients with VT and VF. The second section discusses the management of patients who have monomorphic VT, with particular emphasis on both primary prevention in the high-risk patient and secondary prevention of the patient who has already suffered a sustained arrhythmic episode. The third section discusses approaches to the patient with documented PVT. The fourth section reviews approaches to patients with VF. The final section discusses the role of electrophysiologic testing in patients with VT and VF.

TREATMENT OPTIONS

Treatment modalities for patients with VT and VF include both substrate modification techniques, which prevent recurrent episodes of tachycardia, and device therapy, which terminates recurrent episodes by either anti-tachycardia pacing (ATP) or internal shocks.

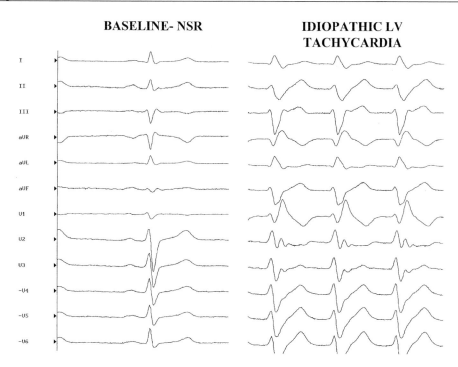

Fig. 2. 12-lead ECG recording of sinus rhythm (left) and VT (right) from a patient with idiopathic left VT arising from the mid-inferior septum. Note the RBBB morphology with left superior frontal axis during VT. NSR = normal sinus rhythm, LV = left ventricular.

Substrate modification techniques include antiarrhythmic drug therapy, catheter and surgical ablative therapy (e.g., encircling ventriculotomy or subendocardial resection). Antiarrhythmic drug therapy functionally modifies the substrate by affecting the electrophysiologic properties of ventricular tissue, prolonging refractoriness and preventing reentry or suppressing automaticity. Catheter and surgical ablation physically disrupt the substrate for VT by either local tissue destruction with radiofrequency energy or excision of critical ventricular sites. Although device therapy does not prevent recurrent episodes of VT or VF, the implantable cardioverter defibrillator (ICD) can effectively terminate ventricular tachyarrhythmias when they occur.

Antiarrhythmic Drug Therapy

Selection of an antiarrhythmic compound for patients with ventricular tachyarrhythmias depends upon several factors: 1) type of arrhythmia; 2) underlying cardiac substrate; 3) left ventricular function; and 4) comorbid diseases, which may be affected by a particular drug or may influence drug metabolism. For VT that occurs without structural heart disease, beta-blockers are standard treatment for RVOT tachycardias (Fig. 1), and verapamil often effectively treats idiopathic left ventricular tachycardias arising from the mid-inferior septum (Fig. 2). Type 1A (e.g., procainamide or quinidine), 1B (e.g., mexiletine), 1C (e.g., propafenone or flecainide) and Type 3 (amiodarone or sotalol) antiarrhythmic drug therapy have been used to successfully prevent recurrent infarct-related VT; and all may be appropriate in patients with an ICD. Because many of these patients have depressed left ventricular function, amiodarone is frequently considered a first-line agent. The results of the AVID study strongly suggest that antiarrhythmic drug therapy alone is inadequate treatment for any patient with structural heart disease who presents with VF or hemodynamically intolerable VT *(3)*. Antiarrhythmic therapy is currently being used as an important adjuvant therapy to the ICD to prevent frequent, symptomatic VT and to control supraventricular arrhythmias. When used primarily as adjuvant therapy coupled with an ICD, any of the Type 1 and 3 antiarrhythmic agents may be appropriate. Selection of antiarrhythmic therapy is frequently based upon the side-effect profile of the particular drug.

Ablative Therapy

Catheter ablative therapy has replaced surgical ablative therapy in the management of frequent, recurrent, drug-refractory VT. The desire to avoid surgical mortality and the success of catheter-based ablation has enabled it to become the standard approach to ablative therapy *(4)*. Catheter ablative therapy typically involves the delivery of radiofrequency energy to ventricular sites crucial for the initiation and/or propagation of VT. Selected areas of ventricular tissue are destroyed by local heating. The ideal VT for catheter ablation has the following features: 1) the tachycardia is easily and reproducibly inducible with programmed stimulation or burst pacing; 2) the tachycardia is associated with a discrete scar (MI) or a structurally normal heart; 3) the VT is monomorphic, with only one tachycardia morphology observed both clinically and in the electrophysiology laboratory; and 4) the tachycardia is well-tolerated hemodynamically. Examples include RVOT tachycardias, idiopathic left ventricular tachycardias, and hemodynamically tolerable infarct-related VT. Bundle-branch reentrant VT is another form of VT that can be successfully treated by ablating the right or left bundle branch, a critical limb of the macroreentrant circuit which involves the His-Purkinje system (Fig. 3). Patients with VT that arises from nonischemic cardiomyopathies are generally more difficult to ablate. Techniques are being developed which target the anatomic substrate for VT. These techniques will undoubtedly extend the clinical applicability of catheter ablation to patients with multiple VT morphologies and VT, which is not mappable using standard mapping techniques. Patients with PVT or VF are not typically candidates for ablative therapy; an important exception is patients with WPW in whom cardiac arrest results from extremely rapid, pre-excited AF or atrial flutter. In these patients, successful ablation of the accessory pathway is curative, and primary therapy for VF is not indicated. Risks of catheter ablation include local complications related to venous and arterial cannulation (bleeding, infection, pseudo-aneurysm formation, thrombosis), cardiac perforation, and stroke.

Implantable Cardioverter-Defibrillator (ICD) Therapy

The first human ICD implantation was performed in 1980 *(5)*. The first ICD systems consisted of both a bulky generator implanted in the abdomen and an epicardial lead system which required an open thoracotomy for implantation. The leads were subcutaneously tunneled to the generator. Implantation required surgical expertise, and was associated with significant morbidity and mortality. ICD implantation has since become simpler and safer. Improvements in capacitor design have allowed for a significant decrease in generator size, and still provides adequate shock energies. Current generators can be implanted subcutaneously in the pectoral region, and improvements in lead design have allowed the development of a non-thoracotomy endocardial system, which

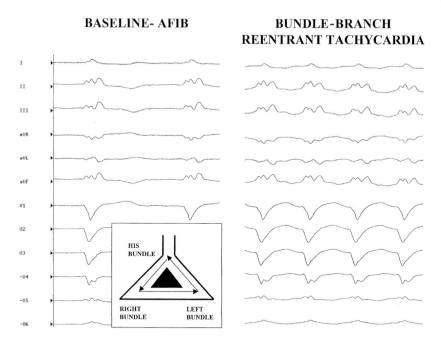

Fig. 3. 12-lead ECG recording during atrial fibrillation (left) and VT (right) from a patient with bundle-branch reentrant tachycardia. Note the similar QRS morphology between baseline and VT complexes. Inset: simplified diagram of the reentrant circuit. AFIB = atrial fibrillation.

is inserted via either the left cephalic (cut-down approach) or subclavian vein (percutaneous approach).

The current ICD system generator houses the sensing and output circuitry in a hermetically sealed titanium shell (can). Electrical signals from the rate-sensing dipole of the defibrillator lead are filtered and amplified for an accurate determination of the ventricular rate. Once the ventricular rate exceeds the programmed detection rate, device therapy is initiated (Fig. 4). The shocking energy is stored within capacitors, which are arranged in series allowing the total output voltage to exceed battery voltage. ICD generators are generally implanted in the left pectoral region because the generator serves as an "active" or "hot" can. The "active" can serve as one of the electrodes in the shocking pathway.

The defibrillator lead system consists of either a single- or double-coil silicone insulated lead with the tip positioned in the trabeculated right ventricular apex. The lead typically contains two smaller electrodes (dipole) for ventricular rate sensing, ATP, and bradycardia pacing. It also contains either one (distal only) or two (proximal and distal) shocking coils. In a single coil defibrillator system, the distal coil and generator serve as the sole shocking vector. In a dual-coil lead system, the shocking pathway is triad or bidirectional: from the distal coil to the generator and proximal coil.

Important ICD options which are critical in selected patients include: 1) an additional atrial lead to provide dual-chamber pacing and improved discrimination of SVT from VT and 2) rate-responsive pacing. Table 1 presents the 1998 American College of Cardiology/American Heart Association (ACC/AHA) Task Force Guidelines for ICD implantation *(6)*.

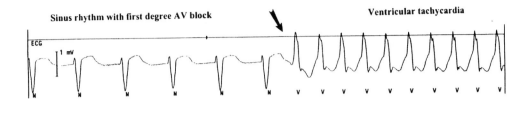

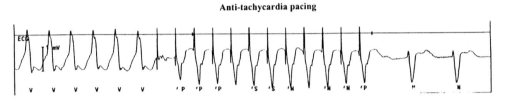

Fig. 4. Rhythm strip recording demonstrating initiation of VT (arrow) followed by a short burst of anti-tachycardia therapy, which terminates the tachycardia.

Hybrid Therapy

This form of therapy refers to combining device therapy with substrate modification techniques to improve survival and decrease the arrhythmic burden. ICD implantation is effective in terminating recurrent VT and VF, and modifying the substrate can be effective in preventing recurrent episodes of VT. Patients with multiple defibrillator shocks caused by ventricular tachyarrhythmias can be treated with various anti-arrhythmic medications. The risk of pro-arrhythmia is lessened because these patients are "protected" by their ICD. When combining antiarrhythmic drug therapy with the ICD, one must anticipate and test for drug effects on tachycardia rate and energy requirement for arrhythmia termination to optimize patient management. Patients with an ICD who have frequent VT can also be safely and successfully treated with catheter mapping and ablative techniques.

MONOMORPHIC VT

Risk-Stratifying Variables

The two most common cardiac disorders associated with sustained monomorphic VT are CAD with prior MI (infarct-related VT) and nonischemic dilated cardiomyopathy. Evidence suggests that the underlying mechanism for sustained VT is reentry involving a fixed substrate consisting of normal myocardium interspersed with islands of poorly conducting fibrotic scar *(7)*. The relatively constant revolution time around the circuit coupled with a fixed exit site results in a uniform tachycardia with a relatively stable rate. Predicting which survivors of MI will develop ventricular tachyarrhythmias is difficult, and risk stratification relies upon the identification of variables associated with increased risk. These variables include:

1) left ventricular dysfunction;
2) nonsustained VT (NSVT);
3) inducibility with nonsuppressibility at electrophysiology study (EPS);
4) abnormal signal-averaged electrocardiograms (SAECG);

Table 1

ACC/AHA Guidelines on Implantation of Implantable Cardioverter-Defibrillators (ICDs)

Class I
1. Cardiac arrest caused by VF or VT not resulting from a transient or reversible cause
2. Spontaneous sustained VT
3. Syncope of undetermined origin with clinically relevant, hemodynamically significant VT or VF induced at EPS when drug therapy is ineffective, not tolerated, or not preferred
4. Nonsustained VT with coronary disease, prior MI, left ventricular dysfunction, and inducible VF or sustained VT at EPS that is not suppressible by a Class I antiarrhythmic drug

Class IIa
None

Class IIb
1. Cardiac arrest presumed to be caused by VF when electrophysiological testing is precluded by other medical conditions
2. Severe symptoms attributable to sustained ventricular tachyarrhythmias while awaiting cardiac transplantation
3. Familial or inherited conditions with a high risk for life-threatening ventricular tachyarrhythmias such as long QT syndrome or hypertrophic cardiomyopathy
4. Non-sustained VT with CAD prior MI, and left ventricular dysfunction, and inducible sustained VT or VF at EPS
5. Recurrent syncope of undetermined etiology in the presence of ventricular dysfunction and inducible ventricular arrhythmia at EPS study when other cause of syncope have been excluded

Class III
1. Syncope of undetermined cause in a patient without inducible ventricular tachy-arrhythmias
2. Incessant VT or VF
3. VF or VT resulting from arrhythmias amenable to surgical or catheter ablation; for example, atrial arrhythmias associated with the WPW, RVOT, VT, idiopathic left ventricular tachycardia, fascicular VT
4. Ventricular tachyarrhythmias caused by a transient or reversible disorder (e.g., AMI, electrolyte balance, drugs, trauma)

Class I:	Conditions for which there is evidence and/or general agreement that a given procedure or treatment is beneficial, useful, and effective
Class II:	Conditions for which there is conflicting evidence and/or divergence of opinion about the usefulness/efficacy of a procedure or treatment
Class IIa:	Weight of evidence/opinion is in favor of usefulness/efficacy
Class IIb:	Usefulness/efficacy is less well established by evidence/opinion
Class III:	Conditions for which there is evidence and/or general agreement that a procedure/treatment is not useful/effective and in some cases may be harmful

From: Gregoratos G, Cheitlin MD, Conill A, et al. ACC/AHA guidelines for implantation of cardiac pacemakers and antiarrhythmia devices. J Am Coll Cardiol 1998;31:1175–1209.

5) reduced heart-rate variability (HRV); and
6) T-wave alternans (TWA) *(8–15)*.

Left ventricular function is the most important determinant of post-infarct survival, and most primary prevention studies have included patients with poor left ventricular function *(8–11)*. Infarct survivors with NSVT are at higher risk than patients without ventricular ectopy. NSVT suggests the presence of a functional reentrant circuit capable of initiation, but without manifest sustained propagation of VT. Similarly, electrophysiology testing exposes a functional reentrant circuit that may or may not be responsible for the clinical arrhythmia. The ability to induce VT or VF (inducibility) despite procainamide therapy (nonsuppressibility) identifies a subset of patients with NSVT after MI who are at high risk *(16)*. The SAECG identifies areas of slow conduction—a criteria for reentry. However, it does not evaluate tissue refractoriness, which is also important for reentry; and therefore does not identify the presence of a viable reentrant circuit. This may partially explain the excellent negative predictive value (absence of slow conduction precludes the presence of a reentrant circuit) but poor positive predictive value (presence of slow conduction is not equivalent to a viable reentrant circuit) in identifying infarct survivors who will develop VT or VF. Inclusion criteria of primary prevention studies have used a combination of these risk-stratifying variables, and left ventricular dysfunction is the most important. Several studies have evaluated the effectiveness of ICD therapy in reducing the mortality of infarct survivors.

Primary Prevention for Patients With Prior MI

THE ROLE OF ANTIARRHYTHMIC DRUG THERAPY IN PRIMARY PREVENTION

The evidence supporting beta-blocker and angiotensin-converting enzyme (ACE)-inhibitor therapy in reducing sudden death after MI is derived from the post-infarct drug trials.

Beta-Blockers. The beneficial effects of beta-blocker therapy in improving survival is partially related to the reduction of sudden cardiac death. The BHAT (Beta-Blocker Heart Attack Trial) Trial was a National Heart, Lung, and Blood Institute-sponsored trial published in 1982, which addressed the efficacy of daily propranolol therapy in reducing all-cause mortality in post-infarct patients *(17)*. Enrolled patients with a documented MI were randomized either to propranolol HCl or placebo. After a mean follow-up of 25 mo in 3,837 patients, total mortality was significantly reduced in the propranolol group compared to placebo (7.2% v. 9.8%, $p < 0.005$). Subset analysis demonstrated that sudden death was significantly lower in the propranolol group (3.3% vs 4.6%, $p < 0.05$).

The Norwegian Multicenter Study Group published a trial hypothesizing that timolol therapy reduces mortality in post-infarct patients *(18)*. Enrolled patients with acute MI were randomized to either timolol therapy or placebo. After a mean follow-up of 17 mo in 1884 patients, total deaths, all cardiac deaths, and sudden cardiac deaths were significantly reduced in the timolol group compared to the placebo group (all $p < 0.001$).

ACE inhibitors. The data on the role of ACE inhibition in the prevention of sudden death in infarct survivors is somewhat disparate. In 1987, the CONSENSUS I (first Cooperative North Scandinavian Enalapril Survival Study) was published, evaluating the effect on mortality of ACE inhibition with enalapril on patients with severe CHF *(19)*. Enrolled patients were randomized to either placebo or enalapril. After a mean follow-up of 188 d in 253 patients, mortality was reduced by 40% ($p = 0.002$) in the enalapril group compared to placebo. The entire reduction in mortality was attributable to a reduction in deaths caused by progressive heart failure and not sudden cardiac death. Similarly, the SOLVD investigators demonstrated that enalapril reduced mortality compared to placebo in patients with CHF and EF ≤35%, with the largest reduction occurring in deaths caused by progressive heart failure *(20)*. Enalapril did not significantly affect deaths caused by arrhythmia without pump failure.

In 1991 the V-HEFT II (second Vasodilator-Heart Failure Trial) was published, comparing the effect on mortality of hydralazine/isosorbide dinitrate combination vs enalapril in patients with congestive heart failure (CHF) *(21)*. Enrolled patients with chronic heart failure were randomized to either hydralazine/isosorbide dinitrate or enalapril therapy. After 2 yr of follow-up in 804 patients, mortality was lower in the enalapril arm ($p = 0.016$), attributable mostly to a reduction in sudden death.

The results of the SAVE (Survival and Ventricular Enlargement) trial suggests that the beneficial effects of ACE inhibitors on infarct survivors may be a reduction in recurrent MI *(22)*. Both the TRACE study *(22a)* and a recent meta-analysis *(22b)* suggested that these agents reduce the incidence of sudden death in infarct survivors.

Type 1 antiarrhythmic agents. Complex ventricular ectopy carries an independent risk for infarct survivors. An important question is whether or not suppression of ventricular ectopy reduces mortality and improves survival in these patients. The original CAST (Cardiac Arrhythmia Suppression Trial) trial, published in 1989, was developed to answer this so-called premature ventricular contraction (PVC) hypothesis *(23)*. Inclusion criteria were ventricular ectopy (>6 PVC/h) with reduced left ventricular function post-MI (EF $\leq$ 40% with remote (>90 d–2 yr) MI or EF $\leq$ 55% with recent (<90 d) MI). Enrolled patients underwent an initial titration phase to establish an effective antiarrhythmic agent (encainide, flecainide, or moricizine) with documented arrhythmia suppression. Patients then underwent the main phase and were randomized to either the effective antiarrhythmic agent or corresponding placebo. After a mean follow-up of 10 mo in 1498 patients, the use of encainide and flecainide was discontinued because of an increased risk of death or cardiac arrest resulting from arrhythmia associated with the active drugs (RR: 2.64, $p = 0.0001$). The CAST trial demonstrated that Type 1C antiarrhythmic agents can be harmful to the post-infarct patient—especially those with reduced left ventricular function—and that arrhythmia suppression does not improve survival. Subsequently, a meta-analysis suggested that all Type 1 agents (Na-channel blockers) are detrimental in the primary prevention of post-infarct patients *(24)*.

Type 3 antiarrhythmic agents. The effectiveness of Type 3 antiarrhythmic agents (K-channel blockers) has been studied, and amiodarone has been the drug best evaluated (*see* Table 2). Besides its direct antiarrhythmic properties, amiodarone also has anti-ischemic and beta-blocking effects. In chronic oral doses, it is not significantly negatively inotropic, and in fact, may improve left ventricular systolic function. Despite its extracardiac side effects, it is generally well-tolerated in patients with CHF.

In 1990, the BASIS (Basel Antiarrhythmic Study of Infarct Survival) study was published *(25)*. This was a three-arm trial, which hypothesized that amiodarone or another antiarrhythmic agent improved survival over placebo in post-infarct patients with high-grade (Lown 3 or 4B) ventricular ectopy. Enrolled patients were randomized to low-dose amiodarone (200mg/d), individualized antiarrhythmic therapy (initial treatment with quinidine or mexiletine), or placebo. During the 1-yr follow-up in 312 patients, amiodarone was associated with a 61% mortality reduction compared to placebo ($p = 0.05$). Patients randomized to the antiarrhythmic arm did not demonstrate improved survival compared to placebo.

In 1995, the CHF STAT (Survival Trial of Antiarrhythmic Treatment-Congestive

Heart Failure) trial was published (26). The CHF-STAT trial hypothesized that amiodarone reduces mortality in patients with CHF, EF ≤40%, and > 10 PVC/h. Enrolled patients were randomized to either amiodarone (300 mg/d) or placebo. Most patients (55%) were New York Heart Association class II. Seventy percent of the patients had ischemic heart disease. After a median follow-up of 45 mo in 674 patients, no difference in mortality was observed between the two treatment groups ($p = 0.6$). Further analysis demonstrated that amiodarone was effective in suppressing ventricular ectopy (arrhythmia suppression), and that there was a trend toward a reduction in overall mortality in patients with nonischemic cardiomyopathy ($p = 0.07$).

In 1997, both the EMIAT (European Myocardial Infarction Amiodarone Trial) and CAMIAT (Canadian Myocardial Infarction Amiodarone Trial) trials were published (27,28). The EMIAT trial tested the ability of amiodarone to improve survival in post-infarct patients with EF ≤40%. Enrolled patients were randomized to either amiodarone (200mg/d) or placebo. After a median follow-up of 21 mo in 1486 patients, no difference in total mortality was observed between the two groups. The CAMIAT trial hypothesized that amiodarone improves survival in post-infarct patients with ventricular ectopy (>10 PVC/h or 1 run of VT). The primary end point was an outcome cluster of arrhythmic death and resuscitated VF. Enrolled patients were randomized to either amiodarone (200 mg/d) or placebo. After a mean follow-up of 1.79 yr in 1202 patients, the amiodarone group was associated with a lower outcome cluster than placebo (0.6% vs 3.3%, ($p = 0.16$). Concomitant beta-blocker therapy with amiodarone further lowered the outcome cluster. In a meta-analysis of this and other trials evaluating amiodarone in patients with prior MI or CHF showed a survival benefit for amiodarone (28a).

In 1998, the SWORD (Survival With Oral D-Sotalol) trial was published (29). The hypothesis of the trial was that prophylactic administration of oral d-sotalol reduced total mortality in survivors of MI (either recent (6–42 d) MI with EF ≤40% or remote (>42 d) MI with symptoms of CHF). Enrolled patients were randomized to either sotalol (up to 200 mg twice daily) or placebo. After enrolling 3,121 patients of the planned 6400, the trial was prematurely terminated because of the increased mortality associated with sotalol (5.0% vs 3.1% p = 0.006).

THE ROLE OF ICD THERAPY IN PRIMARY PREVENTION

The first primary prevention trial demonstrating improved survival with ICD therapy in patients with CAD was MADIT (Multicenter Automatic Defibrillator Implantation Trial) (16) (see Table 3). Published in 1996, the MADIT trial hypothesized that ICD therapy improves survival over conventional medical therapy in high-risk (EF ≤35%, asymptomatic NSVT, and inducible, nonsuppressible ventricular tachyarrhythmias). Enrolled patients were randomized to either ICD implantation or conventional medical therapy. After a mean follow-up of 27 mo in 196 patients, 15 deaths were observed in the ICD group compared to 39 deaths in the conventional group ($p = 0.009$). One criticism of the MADIT trial, however, is that patients randomized to the ICD group were more often on beta-blocker therapy than the conventional group. It has been suggested that the beta-blocker therapy, and not the ICD, conferred the improved survival.

In 1997, the CABG Patch trial was published (30). The CABG Patch trial tested the hypothesis that ICD therapy would improve survival in high-risk (EF≤35%, abnormal SAECG) patients undergoing elective coronary-artery bypass grafts (CABG). Enrolled patients were randomized to either ICD implantation or control. After a mean follow-up of 32 mo in 900 patients, no difference was observed in survival between the two groups ($p = 0.64$). The lack of benefit of ICD therapy may be partly attributable to the poor positive predictive value of the SAECG in identifying patients with CAD who will develop VT or VF, or the improvement in outcome related to coronary revascularization. In fact, in the CABG Patch trial, the ICD did significantly reduce the risk of arrhythmic death, but the proportion of arrhythmic deaths in the trial was too small to cause a difference in overall mortality *(30a)*.

In 1999, the MUSTT (Multicenter UnSustained Tachycardia Trial) trial was published. This trial tested the ability of electrophysiology-guided antiarrhythmic therapy to improve survival in high-risk (EF ≤40%, asymptomatic NSVT) post-infarct patients *(31,32)*. Enrolled patients underwent a baseline EPS and SAECG. Based upon the results of electrophysiology testing alone, patients were divided into a "low-risk" (noninducible) group and "high-risk" (inducible) group. The low-risk group was observed. The high-risk group was further randomized to either electrophysiology-guided antiarrhythmic therapy or standard (no antiarrhythmic) therapy. The group receiving electrophysiology-guided therapy underwent drug evaluation. Drug responders were observed on drug therapy. Drug nonresponders were eligible for ICD implantation. Data from 704 patients demonstrated a significant reduction in overall mortality for the group randomized to electrophysiology-guided antiarrhythmic therapy as compared to the group receiving no antiarrhythmic therapy. Post-hoc analysis revealed that essentially all the benefit was a result of ICD implantation. Overall 5-yr mortality was 24% for patients receiving defibrillators and 55% for those who did not receive an ICD. The results of the MUSTT trial suggest that ICD implantation is warranted in post-infarct patients who have an EF ≤40%, asymptomatic NSVT, and inducible ventricular tachyarrhythmias at EPS. Patients who otherwise qualified for MUSTT but were noninducible at EPS were followed in a registry. Although these patients fared better than the inducible patients who received standard therapy, the risk of sudden death was 12% after 2 yr *(32a)*. Thus, the MUSTT registry suggests that although EPS are useful in risk-stratifying these patients, a single negative EPS does not necessary imply very low risk.

Both MADIT and MUSTT demonstrate that ICD therapy can improve survival in selected post-infarct patients with NSVT. Two studies in progress are investigating the role of the ICD in selected post-infarct patients with no documented ventricular arrhythmias *(33)*. MADIT II (Multicenter Automatic Defibrillator Implantation Trial II) attempts to respond to the criticism that the first MADIT was applicable only to a small subset of patients with CAD. In order to broaden the potential applicability of primary prevention, MADIT II is enrolling infarct survivors with EF ≤30%. Enrolled patients are randomized to either ICD therapy or to a control group. Patients randomized to the ICD group undergo baseline device-based electrophysiology testing at the time of implant to assess the predictive value of the EPS in these patients. All patients also undergo postrandomization noninvasive risk assessment using SAECG, HRV, and TWA. SCD-HeFT (Sudden Cardiac Death-Heart Failure Trial) is a randomized, prospective, three-arm trial comparing ICD therapy, amiodarone, and placebo in patients with either ischemic or nonischemic cardiomyopathy (EF ≤35%, Class II, or III CHF). The results of this trial will hopefully define the role of both ICD and amiodarone therapy in high-risk patients with no "visible" arrhythmic risk and various etiologies of heart failure. Finally, the studies will suggest whether or not the ICD may serve as a bridge to cardiac transplantation in high-risk patients with ischemic cardiomyopathy and advanced CHF who can await heart transplantation from home.

SUMMARY OF PRIMARY PREVENTION FOR PATIENTS WITH PRIOR MYOCARDIAL INFARCTION

ICD therapy has been shown to be beneficial in the primary prevention of selected high-risk post-infarct patients (Table 2) (34–36). All such patients have significantly reduced left ventricular function and documented ventricular ectopy. It remains to be determined whether or not the ICD will be beneficial for patients with left ventricular dysfunction and no documented arrhythmia. Evidence suggests that suppression of PVC's with type 1 antiarrhythmic therapy does not improve survival. Post-infarction beta-blocker therapy reduces sudden death and improves mortality. ACE inhibitors reduce sudden death and improve survival in post-infarct patients with left ventricular dysfunction and CHF. The beneficial effects of prophylactic amiodarone in the post-infarct patient have not been firmly established (Table 3). It may have a more beneficial role in the primary prevention of arrhythmias in patients with nonischemic dilated cardiomyopathy.

Primary Prevention for Patients With Nonischemic Dilated Cardiomyopathy

THE ROLE OF ANTIARRHYTHMIC DRUG THERAPY IN PRIMARY PREVENTION

In 1994, the GESICA (Grupo de Estudio de la Sobrevida en la Insuficiencia Cardiaca en Argentina) trial was published (37). The GESICA trial hypothesized that low-dose amiodarone (300 mg/d) would improve survival in patients with severe CHF (Class II-IV CHF, EF ≤35%). Enrolled patients were randomized to either amiodarone or placebo. Approximately 38% had a prior MI, and 10% had Chagas disease. After a mean follow-up of 2 yr in 516 patients, amiodarone was associated with a 28% mortality reduction compared to placebo (33.5% deaths vs 41.6% deaths ($p = 0.024$). However, mortality in both groups remained high. The results of the GESICA and CHF-STAT trial suggest that amiodarone may be effective in reducing mortality in patients with nonischemic cardiomyopathy (26,37).

THE ROLE OF ICD THERAPY IN PRIMARY PREVENTION

Data evaluating the effectiveness of ICD therapy on the primary prevention of patients with nonischemic dilated cardiomyopathy is scarce. Several trials are currently under investigation to answer this issue. The SCD-HEFT trial has been previously mentioned (33). The ongoing DEFINITE trial hypothesizes the ICD therapy will improve survival in patients with nonischemic cardiomyopathy (EF ≤35%, symptomatic CHF) and NSVT or >10 PVC/h). Enrolled patients are randomized to either ICD therapy with conventional heart-failure treatment or conventional heart-failure treatment alone. The primary end point is overall mortality (37a).

SUMMARY OF PRIMARY PREVENTION FOR PATIENTS WITH NONISCHEMIC DILATED CARDIOMYOPATHY

The role of ICD therapy is unclear, but is under investigation. Amiodarone therapy may be more effective in reducing overall mortality compared to patients with ischemic heart disease.

Table 2
Summary of Primary Prevention Trials of Amiodarone Therapy

Amio trials	No. of patients (Rx arms)	Inclusion criteria	Ejection fraction	% CAD	Amio dose (daily)	Results
BASIS	312 (Individual anti-arrhythmic Rx: 100, low-dose amio: 98, control Rx: 114)	Prior MI, Lown 3 or 4B ectopy	41%/46%/42%	100%	200 mg	1 yr f/u: Control mortality: 13%; amio: 5% (61% reduction in mortality over placebo $p = 0.048$)
CHF STAT	674 (Amio Rx: 336, placebo Rx: 338)	Symptomatic CHF, EF ≤ 40%, > 10 VPD/h	EF < 30%: Amio Rx: 67%; Placebo Rx: 66%	72%/71%	Amio 800 mg × 14 d, then 400 mg × 50 wk, then 300 mg	Median f/u 45 mo: no difference in mortality ($p = 0.6$) with a trend toward mortality reduction in non-ischemic group
GESICA	516 (Amio Rx: 260, standard Rx: 256)	NYHA II advanced, III, iv, EF ≤ 35%	Amio Rx: 19%; Standard Rx: 20%	Prior MI: Amio Rx: 40%, standard Rx; 38% Chagas disease: Amio Rx: 8%, standard Rx: 11%	300 mg	2 yr f/u: Amio Rx deaths: 33.5%; standard Rx deaths: 41.4% (28% risk reduction by amio, $p = 0.024$)
EMIAT	1486 (Amio Rx: 743, placebo Rx: 743)	Prior MI, EF ≤ 40%	EF ≤ 30%: Amio Rx: 48%; Placebo Rx: 45%	100%	Amio 800 mg × 14 d, then 400 mg × 14 wk, then 200 mg	Median f/u 21 mo: No difference of all-cause mortality ($p = 0.96$); 35% risk reduction in arrhythmic death by amio ($p = 0.05$)
CAMIAT	1202 (Amio Rx: 606, placebo Rx: 596)	Prior MI, ≥ 10 VPD/h or ≥ 1 run of VT	—	100%	Amio 10 mg/kg load over 2 wk, then 400 mg	Mean f/u 1.79 yr: resuscitated VF/arrhythmic death: Amio Rx: 3.3%, placebo Rx: 6%, $p = 0.016$

245

Table 3
Summary of Primary Prevention Trials of ICD Therapy

Primary prevention ICD trials	No. of patients (Rx arms)	Inclusion criteria	Ejection fraction	% CAD	Concomitant medications	Results
MADIT I	196 (Conventional Rx: 101 ICD Rx: 95)	Prior MI, EF ≤35%, Asymptomatic NSVT, Inducible nonsuppressible ventricular tachyarrhythmia	Conventional Rx: 25 ± 7%; ICD Rx: 27 ± 7%	100%	Beta-blockers: Conventional Rx: 8.6%; ICD Rx: 28%	Avg. f/u 27 mo: deaths in conventional Rx: 39, ICD Rx: 15 (p = 0.009)
CABG-Patch	900 (Control Rx: 454 ICD Rx: 446)	Elective CABG, EF ≤35%, Abnl SAEKG	Control Rx: 27 ± 6%; ICD Rx: 27 ± 6%	100%	Beta-blockers: Control Rx: 5.4%; ICD RX: 4.2%	Avg. f/u 32 ± 16 mo: deaths in Control RX: 95, ICD Rx: 101 (p = 0.64)
MUSTT	704 (No Rx, EP guided Rx: drug or ICD)	CAD, EF ≤40%, Asymptomatic NSVT	No Rx: 29%; EP-guided Rx: 30%	100%	Beta-blockers: No Rx: 29%; EP-guided Rx: 51%	5-yr mortality: ICD Rx: 24%; Non-ICD Rx: 55% (p < 0.001)
MADIT II	(Conventional Rx, ICD Rx)	Prior MI, EF ≤30%	—	100%	—	—
SCD-Heft	Conventional Rx only, conventional Rx + amio, conventional Rx + ICD	NYHA II, III CHF, EF ≤35%,	—	—	CHF treated with ACE inhibitors	—
DEFINITE	(Conventional RX, ICD Rx)	Symptomatic CHF caused by non-ischemic causes, EF ≤35%, NSVT	—	0%	—	—

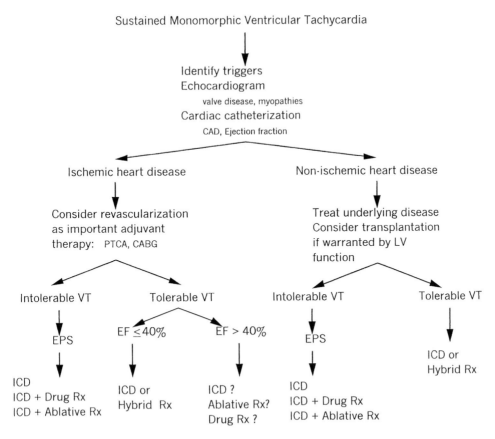

Fig. 5. Management of sustained monomorphic VT in patients with structural heart disease.

Secondary Prevention

IDENTIFICATION OF REVERSIBLE TRIGGERS

Because the management of patients with ischemic and nonischemic heart disease varies considerably, the initial evaluation of patients presenting with sustained monomorphic ventricular tachycardia (SMVT) should include an evaluation for CAD and underlying cardiomyopathic or valvular disorders (Fig. 5). The clinical history should be carefully inspected, and potential triggers should be identified and treated. These triggers include adverse drug effects, electrolyte abnormalities, and ischemia. The proarrhythmic effects of antiarrhythmic drugs are well-known. Drugs can have an adverse effect on the electrophysiologic properties of the reentrant circuit converting NSVT into sustained episodes. Digitalis toxicity manifests in a wide variety of rhythm and conduction disturbances, including VT. VT caused by digitalis toxicity should be recognized because treating the toxicity will effectively terminate VT. This tachycardia typically arises from the fascicles (fascicular tachycardia); and therefore demonstrates a right bundle-branch block (RBBB) morphology with a left superior or right inferior frontal axis when originating from the left posterior or left anterior fascicle, respectively. Rarely, the frontal axis can alternate between left superior and right inferior on a beat-to-beat basis (bi-directional VT) when the VT originates alternately from each fascicle (Fig. 6). Patients can be highly sensitive to potassium levels. A drop in serum potassium

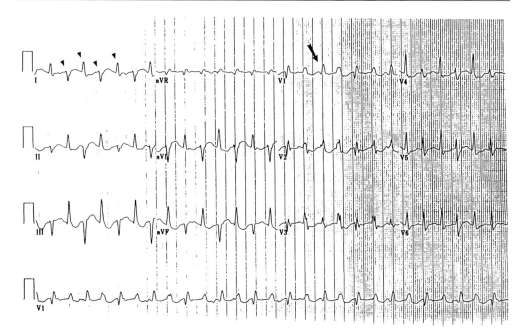

Fig. 6. 12-lead ECG recording of bidirectional VT in a patient with digitalis toxicity. Note the RBBB morphology (arrow) and alternating frontal axis (arrowheads). AV dissociation is evident in the V1 rhythm strip.

may aggravate ventricular arrhythmias by enhancing the binding of digoxin at the level of the Na-K ATPase molecule. Residual ischemia in an area of prior infarction may adversely affect a circuit, resulting in VT. Patients who present with ischemia, VT, and reduced ventricular function should be evaluated for revascularization in an attempt to reduce the ischemic burden, improve ventricular function, and improve survival (38,39). Importantly, the presence of monomorphic VT implies a fixed anatomic substrate for the arrhythmia. Although it may be important to reverse any potential triggers that may result in frequent arrhythmic recurrences, treating the triggers alone does not necessarily eliminate the risk of potentially life-threatening arrhythmia recurrences. Monomorphic VT must be managed with treatment that can effectively alter the anatomic substrate or stop an arrhythmia with appropriate pacing or shock therapy.

HEMODYNAMICALLY INTOLERABLE VT

The mode of presentation and left ventricular function are important determinants of the aggressiveness of therapy. Any patient who presents with hemodynamically intolerable VT (cardiac arrest, syncope) should be considered for device therapy. Substrate modification techniques serve only an adjunctive role to the ICD.

THE ROLE OF ANTIARRHYTHMIC DRUG THERAPY

Drug therapy has a limited role in patients with hemodynamically intolerable VT, serving an adjunctive role to the ICD. Before the AVID trial was published, the CASCADE (Cardiac Arrest in Seattle: Conventional Versus Amiodarone Drug Evaluation) trial was conducted to determine whether empiric amiodarone therapy was more effective than guided (electrophysiologic or electrocardiographic-monitored) anti-arrhythmic therapy in reducing mortality of sudden-cardiac-death survivors *(40)*. A total of 228 enrolled patients were randomized either to empiric amiodarone therapy *(113)* or guided antiarrhythmic therapy *(115)*. Eight-two percent of the patients had CAD. Survival free of cardiac death or sustained ventricular arrhythmias was significantly lower for the amiodarone group (78% vs 52% at 2 yr, 52% vs 36% at 4 yr, 41% vs 29% at 6 yr, $(p = 0.001)$. Although amiodarone was more effective than guided antiarrhythmic therapy, overall mortality remained high.

In 1997, Haverkamp et al. published a trial evaluating the role of d,1-sotalol in patients with inducible VT, VF, or aborted sudden death *(41)*. Enrolled patients were treated with sotalol and underwent programmed ventricular stimulation to document effective suppression of inducibility by sotalol. Only 57% (227) of 396 enrolled patients had effective arrhythmia suppression. Actuarial total survival rates were 94% at 1 yr and 86% at 3 yr. Although oral sotalol can be effective in suppressing ventricular tachyarrhythmias, sudden cardiac death still occurred in a considerable proportion of the study population.

In 1999, Pacifico et al. published a multicenter, double-blinded, placebo-controlled trial demonstrating that sotalol therapy was associated with a lower risk of death and delivery of first shocks from an ICD compared to placebo (risk reduction: 40%, $(p = 0.001)$ *(42)*.

THE ROLE OF CATHETER ABLATIVE THERAPY

At present, only patients with monomorphic VT are candidates for catheter ablation. The standard approach to arrhythmic localization requires induction of the arrhythmia and mapping during the tachycardia to pinpoint the appropriate site for ablation. This standard approach cannot be used in patients with rapid VT that is not tolerated hemodynamically. Voltage-mapping techniques to define the anatomic substrate in conjunction with pace-mapping to regionalize the area of interest have been applied to VT which is not mappable. Linear lesions which cross the densely scarred myocardium through the border zone to normal myocardium appear very effective in treating patients with hemodynamically intolerable VT (Fig. 7).

THE ROLE OF ICD THERAPY

The introduction of the ICD into the armamentarium of available treatment options for VT has raised questions about its effectiveness compared to antiarrhythmic drug therapy in reducing mortality. The CASH (Cardiac Arrest Study Hamburg) trial compared antiarrhythmic therapy (metoprolol, amiodarone, and propafenone) to ICD therapy in mortality reduction of sudden-cardiac-death survivors *(43)*. After baseline clinical testing, enrolled patients were randomized to one of the four regimens. Almost one-half of the patients had CAD. At an interim analysis, propafenone was associated with an increase in mortality, resulting in early termination of the propafenone arm. The final results of the trial were recently published *(43a)*. The total mortality in the ICD group was 23% lower than in the combined amiodarone and metoprolol groups, although this did not reach statistical significance.

In 1997, the larger AVID (Antiarrhythmics Versus Implantable Defibrillator) trial was published comparing antiarrhythmic therapy to ICD in patients with either resusci-

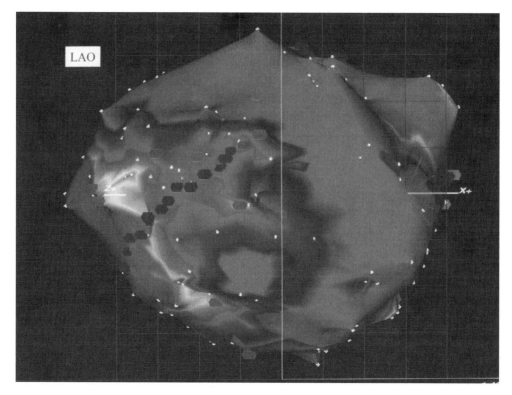

Fig. 7. Electro-anatomic map of the left ventricle in a patient with infarct-related VT, left anterior oblique (LAO) view. Radiofrequency lesions are depicted by dark red dots. Lesions are delivered in a line connecting densely scarred myocardium (red) to normal myocardium (purple). (*See* color plate 4 appearing in the insert following p. 208.)

tated VF or hemodynamically intolerable VT associated with an EF ≤40% *(3)*. Eight-one percent had CAD. Enrolled patients were randomized to either a Type 3 anti-arrhythmic drug (96% amiodarone or 3% sotalol) or ICD implantation. After a follow-up of 3 yr in 1013 patients, ICD therapy was superior to antiarrhythmic therapy in improving survival (75.4% vs 64.1%, p = 0.02).

The CIDS (Canadian Implantable Defibrillator Survival) trial compared amiodarone to ICD therapy in both sudden-cardiac-death survivors and patients suffering from syncopal VT *(44)*. With an enrollment of 659 patients, ICD therapy was associated with a 20% lower total mortality and a 33% lower arrhythmic mortality, although this did not achieve statistical significance.

SUMMARY OF SECONDARY PREVENTION OF HEMODYNAMICALLY INTOLERABLE VT

ICD therapy is the most effective treatment in reducing mortality for patients with hemodynamically intolerable VT or VF (Table 4). Mortality remains high for patients treated with drug therapy alone. Drug therapy should serve an adjunctive role to the ICD to suppress frequent VT recurrences. Catheter ablative therapy guided by a detailed characterization of the anatomic substrate appears to effectively control recurrences that are not responsive to pharmacologic agents alone.

Table 4
Summary of Secondary Prevention Trials of ICD Therapy

Secondary prevention ICD trials	No. of patients	Inclusion criteria	Ejection fraction	% CAD	Medications	Results
CASH	346 (ICD Rx/amio Rx/metoprolol Rx/propafen- one Rx)	SCD survivors	46%	73%	Amio 400-600 mg/d; metoprolol 200 mg/d (max); propafenone 900 mg/d (max)	Propafenone arm terminated because of increased mortality. ICD survival 23% better than combined amiodarone/ metoprolol groups ($p = 0.08$).
AVID	1016 Drug Rx: 509; ICD Rx: 507)	Resuscitated VF/ hemodynamically intolerable VT	Drug Rx: 31 ± 13%, ICD Rx: 32 ± 13%	Drug Rx: 81% ICD Rx: 81%	Drug Rx: amio (95.8%), sotalol (2.8%)	3 yr f/u overall survival drug Rx: 64.1%; ICD Rx: 75.4% ($p = 0.02$)
CIDS	659 ICD Rx vs non- ICD (amio) Rx	SCD survivors/ hemodynamically intolerable VT	34%	82%	Mean amio dose 255 mg/d	All-cause mortality: 20% lower in ICD Rx ($p = 0.14$). 21% amio Rx received ICD within 5 yr

251

Hemodynamically Tolerable VT

The management of patients with CAD or nonischemic dilated cardiomyopathy who present with hemodynamically tolerable VT with no or minimal symptoms is controversial. Studies that evaluate the effectiveness of the ICD in reducing mortality for this group of patients are few. A subset of patients who initially present with hemodynamically tolerable VT treated with drug or ablative therapy may subsequently present with a lethal ventricular event, for which ICD therapy may be useful. We suggest that the treatment strategy for these patients should be based on four guiding principles: 1) the status of left ventricular function; 2) the frequency of arrhythmic recurrences; 3) the inducibility of poorly tolerated arrhythmias; and 4) the outcome of a detailed discussion with the patient in which treatment options and risks are outlined. Left ventricular dysfunction is a poor prognostic variable. Mechanisms of death for patients with cardiomyopathies include both ventricular tachyarrhythmias and progressive CHF. Although the MUSTT trial was a primary prevention study, extrapolating the data to post-infarct patients with sustained tolerable VT suggests that ICD implantation for patients with EF ≤40% is appropriate *(31,32)*. Inducibility of poorly tolerated arrhythmias during electrophysiology testing before and after drug or ablative therapy suggests a higher-risk population.

The management of patients with EF >40% and tolerable VT in the setting of ischemic or nonischemic heart disease is more difficult. Patients with frequent VT episodes need drug or catheter ablative therapy to prevent frequent recurrences. We have been pleased with the outcome of ablation for frequent stable VT; and advocate the approach over chronic drug administration. A final decision should be made on an individual basis after a discussion of options between the patient and physician.

Summary of Secondary Prevention in Patients With Hemodynamically Tolerable VT

The management of patients with ischemic or nonischemic dilated cardiomyopathy with tolerable VT should be approached on an individual basis. Extrapolating from primary prevention studies, it is appropriate to implant defibrillators in post-infarct patients with EF ≤40%. Patients with an EF >40% should be managed based on the frequency of VT occurrences. Those patients with frequent arrhythmias should be considered for catheter ablative therapy. Inducibility of more rapid VT suggests the need for ICD therapy.

VT in the Setting of Other Cardiac Disorders

Monomorphic VT occurs in other cardiac disorders associated with myocardial disease or fibrosis. These include arrhythmogenic RV dysplasia (ARVD), hypertrophic cardiomyopathy, incisional VT related to prior ventriculotomy, infiltrative cardiac disorders (sarcoid, amyloid, or malignancy), and inflammatory disorders (myocarditis). The underlying disease should be treated. Factors that should be considered in the management of these patients include: 1) the overall prognosis; 2) left ventricular function and associated prognostic variables; 3) VT tolerability; and 4) the documented effectiveness of different therapeutic options for the specific disorder.

Arrhythmogenic RV dysplasia. Arrhythmogenic RV dysplasia (ARVD) was first described by Fontaine in 1977 *(45)*. Pathologically, it is associated with fatty infiltration of the right ventricle. The disease has a slight male preponderance. The underlying

BASELINE- NSR   **ARVD TACHYCARDIA**

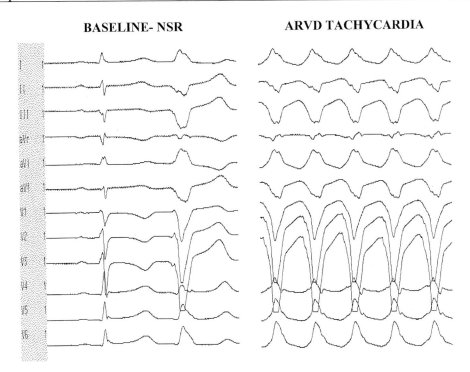

Fig. 8. 12-lead ECG recording of sinus rhythm (left) and VT (right) from a patient with arrhythmogenic right ventricular dysplasia. Note the right precordial T-wave inversion in the sinus rhythm tracing and the spontaneous VPD which matches the VT morphology. NSR = normal sinus rhythm, ARVD = arrhythmogenic right ventricular dysplasia.

mechanism for VT is believed to be reentry. Because the tachycardia typically arises from the RV, it gives rise to a left bundle-branch block (LBBB) morphology with a variable frontal axis, depending upon the site of involvement (Fig. 8). Poor R-wave progression in the precordial leads is expected. The characteristic resting ECG shows right atrial enlargement, right axis deviation, incomplete RBBB, inverted T waves in the right precordial leads and an epsilon wave in lead V_1. The epsilon wave represents slow conduction in the dysplastic RV free wall *(46)*. Treatment options include drugs (beta-blockers, Type 1 and 3 antiarrhythmic agents), catheter ablation *(46a)*, surgery, and ICD implantation.

Hypertrophic cardiomyopathy. Hypertrophic cardiomyopathy is a primary cardiac disease characterized by right or left ventricular hypertrophy (LVH), or both in the absence of another cardiac or systemic cause for hypertrophy. The majority of cases are caused by autosomal dominant inherited mutations in genes encoding cardiac sarcomeric proteins. Rhythm abnormalities include atrial fibrillation (AF), heart block, pre-excitation, VT, and sudden death. VT occasionally originates from left ventricular apical aneurysms in patients with midcavitary obliteration or from the interventricular septum in patients with left ventricular outflow-tract (LVOT) obstruction *(47,48)*. Several risk factors are associated with sudden death, including: 1) severe and diffuse hypertrophy; 2) NSVT; 3) inducible VT/VF; 4) history of syncope; and 5) family history of sudden death. Although prophylactic therapy with amiodarone is associated with a significant reduction in sudden death rate in patients with hypertrophic cardiomy-

BASELINE- AV PACED   SARCOID VT

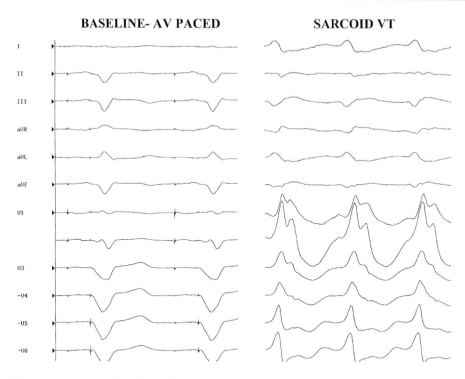

Fig. 9. 12-lead ECG recording of baseline (left) and VT (right) from a patient with cardiac sarcoidosis. Sarcoid VT frequently originates from the basal left ventricle, producing a RBBB VT morphology with positive concordance across the precordial leads.

opathy compared to conventional antiarrhythmic therapy (predominantly disopyramide) *(49)*, patients who are at a substantial risk for sudden death should be considered for ICD therapy *(49a)*.

Sarcoidosis. Sarcoidosis is a chronic, multisystem disorder of unknown etiology characterized by noncaseating granulomas in affected organs. Although 5% of patients with sarcoid have symptomatic cardiac involvement, approx 20% have evidence of cardiac sarcoid at autopsy *(50)*. Cardiac involvement is manifested by myocardial infiltration, CHF, heart block, VT (Fig. 9), and sudden death. Sarcoid granulomas preferentially affect the basal interventricular septum and left ventricular papillary muscles. The right and left ventricular free walls can also be involved. The resting ECG is nonspecific, but frequently abnormal. The mechanism of VT is unclear; but ICD therapy has been advocated because sarcoid-related VT is often difficult to control with antiarrhythmic drug therapy alone *(51)*. As with VT related to chronic CAD, catheter ablation may be important adjunctive therapy in patients with frequent ICD shocks.

Chagas' disease. Chagas' disease (American Trypanosomiasis) is caused by the protozoan parasite, *Trypanosoma cruzi*. Endemic in Central and South America, it is transmitted to humans by the reduviid bug. Cardiac involvement often occurs, and is manifested by biventricular enlargement, apical aneurysms, and mural thrombi that emerge years to decades after the initial infection. Rhythm and conduction disturbances are also prevalent. The most common ECG abnormality is RBBB, but bifascicular block (RBBB/LAFB), AV block, and ventricular tachyarrhythmias are possible. Sudden death has been reported. VT often arises along the epicardial border of the apical aneurysm, and is less effectively treated by endocardial ablative techniques. Epicardial ablative therapy has been advocated *(52)*. A potential danger to epicardial ablation is damage to the coronary arteries. Thus, the procedure is performed with concomitant coronary angiography to avoid damage to large coronary vessels.

VT in the Setting of a Structurally Normal Heart

VTs occurring in patients without structural cardiac abnormalities are generally non-life-threatening arrhythmias, but can be associated with debilitating symptoms such as recurrent palpitations, presyncope, or syncope.

Idiopathic left ventricular tachycardia. Idiopathic left VT, also called Belhassen VT, was described by Zipes in 1979 *(53,54)*. It arises from the left ventricular inferior septum midway between the base and apex, resulting in a tachycardia with RBBB morphology and a left superior axis *(see* Fig. 2). The resting ECG is often normal. The mechanism is controversial, and is believed to be either triggered activity or reentry involving the Purkinje fibers of the left posterior fascicle. Successful ablation sites often reveal a short, sharp, high-frequency potential preceding the QRS during VT, which may represent a Purkinje potential *(55)*. These tachycardias are typically sensitive to verapamil, which provides an alternative therapeutic option to ablation.

RVOT tachycardia. RVOT VT was described by Gallavardin in 1922, who described frequent episodes of NSVT interrupted by short periods of sinus rhythm *(56)*. Patients may also have a pattern of paroxysmal sustained episodes. It typically arises from the outflow tract of the right ventricle, resulting in a LBBB morphology with a right inferior frontal axis *(see* Fig. 1). The tachycardia is often catecholamine-sensitive, precipitated by exercise, and occurring when the heart rate reaches a critical rate (rate-dependent window). RVOT VT can be treated effectively with beta-blockers. Alternative treatment options include calcium-channel-blockers and catheter ablation.

POLYMORPHIC VENTRICULAR TACHYCARDIA

Polymorphic ventricular tachycardia (PVT) can be seen in LQTS (congenital and acquired), acute myocardial ischemia/infarction, and as a primary electrical disturbance in patients with structurally normal hearts *(57–64)*. A particular morphology of PVT associated with QT prolongation has been referred to as torsades de pointes, a term coined by Dessertenne in 1955 *(65)*. The underlying mechanism of PVT is unclear, although the mechanisms for the initiation and propagation of torsades de pointes are believed to differ. Early after-depolarization-induced triggered activity in a milieu of heterogeneous recovery of excitability initiates the tachycardia. This produces a nonstationary excitatory wavefront whose propagation depends upon shifting sites of reentry along the epicardial surface. The dynamic and migratory nature of the reentrant circuit results in the polymorphic morphology of the tachycardia.

Management of patients who present with PVT requires a careful inspection of the patients history, including a search for culprit drugs, electrolyte abnormalities, and ischemia/infarction (Fig. 10). Electrocardiographic documentation of the initiation of the arrhythmia is invaluable. First, temporary pacing may prevent recurrent episodes of pause-dependent PVT (Fig. 11). Secondly, in patients with acute MI, infarction, documentation of the initiation allows differentiation of rapid monomorphic ventricular

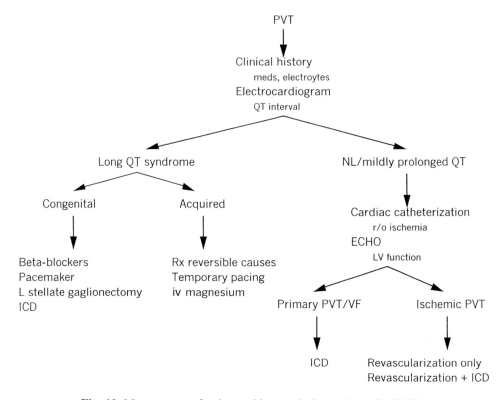

Fig. 10. Management of polymorphic ventricular tachycardia (PVT).

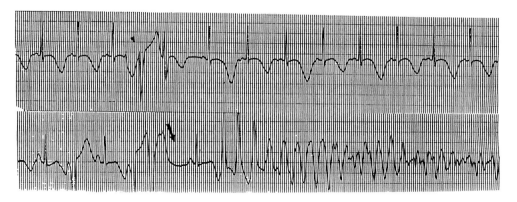

Fig. 11. Pause-dependent initiation (arrow) of PVT. In the upper panel, after a spontaneous VPD (arrowhead), TWA occurs. In the lower panel, torsades de pointes VT is initiated.

tachycardia and subsequent degeneration to PVT from primary PVT. The former suggest the presence of prior MI and a fixed reentrant circuit, in which revascularization alone is insufficient for patient management. ICD therapy should be considered. Patients who develop primary PVT in the setting of acute MI may be treated conservatively with revascularization alone, provided that revascularization is successful and complete (66).

Ischemic PVT

Acute management of patients who present with ischemic PVT is revascularization, reducing the ischemic burden and preventing recurrences with drug therapy. Long-term arrhythmia management depends upon 1) the rhythm at initiation; 2) left ventricular function; and 3) the success of revascularization. Patients with acute ischemia whose PVT results from degeneration of monomorphic VT are unlikely to benefit from revascularization alone, and ICD implantation should be considered. Patients with acute ischemia whose PVT is the initial rhythm may be treated with revascularization alone, if revascularization is complete and LV function preserved. Patients with acute ischemia and PVT whose initial rhythm is not documented should be considered for ICD implantation, especially in the setting of reduced left ventricular function, for which monomorphic VT may have been the precipitating event. After revascularization, electrophysiology testing may be helpful in determining if patients with borderline left ventricular dysfunction are susceptible to SMVT.

Non-Ischemic PVT

Nonischemic PVT is most often seen in the setting of LQTS. Both congenital and acquired causes of QT prolongation have been described *(57)*. PVT in congenital LQTS is often "adrenergically dependent." Treatment of PVT in congenital LQTS should always include beta-blocker therapy. Other adjunctive treatments include pacemaker implantation, left stellate ganglionectomy, and ICD therapy. The major goal for patients with acquired LQTS is to treat any condition causing QT prolongation (e.g., drugs or electrolyte abnormalities). Because PVT in acquired LQTS is often "pause-dependent," acute management to prevent recurrent episodes include temporary pacing or isoproterenol administration to increase heart rate and intravenous (iv) magnesium infusion.

APPROACH TO THE PATIENT WITH VF OR CARDIAC ARREST

Because cardiac arrest may be a presentation of acute MI, once a patient has been resuscitated, it is critical to determine whether or not the patient is having an acute, transmural (i.e., ST elevation or new LBBB) MI. VF that occurs within the first 24–48 h of an acute MI is usually considered to be an epiphenomenon of the MI, and as such does not necessarily require long-term treatment specifically focused on ventricular arrhythmia. Patients with acute MI who are resuscitated from VF and who survive until hospital discharge typically have the same survival as MI survivors who did not have VF *(66,66a)*.

If VF is not caused by acute infarction, specific therapy directed at the arrhythmia will generally be necessary. Patients with unexplained VF should undergo coronary angiography. If there is evidence of significant ischemia, revascularization should generally be carried out. Although in the past revascularization was believed to be adequate therapy for VF presumed ischemic in origin *(66b)*, more recent data has not confirmed this. Natale and colleagues *(66c)* described 58 patients who presented with cardiac arrest caused by VF or PVT. All underwent coronary-artery bypass grafting (CABG) for critical coronary stenoses, and then received ICD implants. In just 2 yr of follow-up, 38% received ICD therapy preceded by symptoms of syncope or presyncope. Several patients who were noninducible at EPS post-CABG had appropriate shocks during follow-up. Thus, revascularization alone is probably not sufficient in this cohort, and EPS does not reliable stratify risk. Thus, even if revascularization is performed, most patients should receive specific therapy for the ventricular arrhythmia.

Several forms of structural heart disease other than CAD should be considered in evaluating patients who present with cardiac arrest. Dilated cardiomyopathy, hypertrophic cardiomyopathy, ARVD, myocarditis, and infiltrative cardiomyopathies (such as sarcoid or amyloid) all may present with ventricular tachyarrhythmias. If myocarditis, sarcoid, or amyloid are in the differential, a myocardial biopsy should be considered, although the yield is uncertain. Even if no structural heart disease is identified, patients should be carefully followed, as some patients may develop manifest structural disease that was absent or subtle at initial evaluation. Coronary spasm may also present with PVT or VF; the role of provocation with ergonovine or other agents to make this diagnosis is unclear.

In addition to associated structural heart disease, patients should be carefully evaluated for primary "electrical disease." Wolff-Parkinson-White syndrome (WPW) and LQTS, both congenital and acquired, can present with cardiac arrest. A short, coupled variant of torsades des pointes has been described. In addition, a catecholamine-mediated PVT has been described in children.

Given the results of AVID, CIDS, and CASH, most patients resuscitated from VF are treated with ICDs. The role of EPS is controversial and is discussed in the following section. In patients not considered candidates for ICD therapy, amiodarone and/or beta-blockers are most commonly used. Such treatment decisions are made on a case-by-case basis.

Idiopathic VF

Idiopathic VF, which is VF in the absence of a precipitating cause, is rare *(66d)*. This diagnosis requires a thorough evaluation to exclude structural heart disease, and primary electrophysiologic abnormalities such as LQTS and WPW *(66c)*. A minority of these patients have the Brugada Syndrome. Although Belhassen and colleagues recently reported their experience using electrophysiology-guided drug therapy in these patients *(66f)*, the usual practice is to recommend ICD implantation *(66g)*.

VF Associated With the Brugada Syndrome

The Brugada Syndrome is characterized by the triad: 1) right precordial (V1–V3) ST-segment elevation (Fig. 12); 2) RBBB (often but not always present); and 3) sudden, unexpected death caused by VF *(67)* (*see* Chapter 18). The incidence is greatest in Asian males, and is a leading cause of sudden death in Japan and Southeast Asia. Although the mechanism of right precordial ST elevation and the genesis of VF is poorly understood, evidence suggests the presence of a prominent, transient outward current (I_{TO}) in the right ventricular epicardium of patients with the Brugada syndrome. Recognition of the characteristic Brugada pattern on the ECG is important for identifying patients at risk for life-threatening ventricular arrhythmias. The ICD has been recommended as the treatment of choice for this syndrome.

ROLE OF ELECTROPHYSIOLOGIC TESTING

Electrophysiologic testing attempts to expose a viable reentrant circuit by the delivery of premature ventricular impulses into the circuit. The goal is induction of SMVT. In

BASELINE- NSR   **PROCAINAMIDE
                           PROVOCATION**

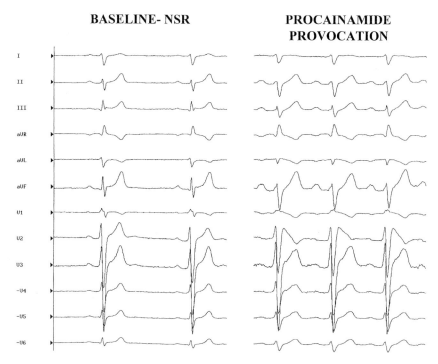

Fig. 12. 12-lead ECG recording during baseline (left) and after procainamide (right) in a patient with the Brugada syndrome. Note the ST-segment elevation in the right precordial leads after procainamide infusion. NSR = normal sinus rhythm.

post-infarct patients without sustained monomorphic VT, it can serve as a risk-stratifying tool. In post-infarct patients with documented SMVT, electrophysiology testing has little role in risk stratification, because these patients are already at high risk by virtue of their clinically manifest arrhythmia. It can, however, provide useful information which is important for optimal management. Electrophysiology testing can 1) exclude the presence of concomitant sustained ventricular tachycardia, which may result in inappropriate ICD therapy; 2) evaluate for conduction disturbances, which may warrant dual-chamber ICD implantation; 3) assist in appropriate ICD programming (tiered therapy); 4) evaluate effectiveness of antiarrhythmic drugs; 4) induce VT for catheter ablation; 5) exclude bundle-branch reentrant tachycardia that can be cured with catheter ablation; and 6) identify induction of more rapid VT, which may be associated with a greater risk of sudden death.

Electrophysiology testing has only a limited role in patients with nonischemic dilated cardiomyopathy and SMVT. Because of patchy areas of fibrosis, electrophysiology testing often results in induction of PVT. It can, however, be helpful in evaluating for bundle-branch reentrant tachycardia.

In patients who present with PVT in which the initiation of the arrhythmia is unknown, electrophysiology testing is useful in identifying patients who are susceptible to monomorphic VT. Induction of monomorphic VT implies the presence of a fixed anatomic substrate; and inducibility in such patients suggests a high risk for sudden cardiac death. If the initiation of the arrhythmia is unknown and myocardial dysfunction is present, a persistent risk of a life-threatening arrhythmia should be assumed; and ICD implantation is the most appropriate treatment option.

Finally, the utility of electrophysiology testing is debatable in patients who present with VF in the absence of acute MI. Most of these patients will be treated with ICDs, whether ventricular arrhythmias are inducible or not in the electrophysiology laboratory. A pre-implant may yield information important to device selection and/or programming. For example, revealing evidence of sinus or A-V conduction disease may lead to dual-chamber ICD implantation. Induction of one or more monomorphic VTs, with evaluation of VT cycle length and response of overdrive pacing, will help to optimize tachycardia detection and therapy parameters post-implant. The need for EPS in cardiac-arrest survivors should therefore be assessed on a case-by-case basis.

FUTURE DIRECTIONS

Although our approach to the patient with VT and VF has rapidly evolved over the last 20 yr, we can anticipate continued advances. Improvements in catheter ablative systems will allow the creation of larger and deeper lesions, and permit mapping of noninducible or hemodynamically intolerable tachycardias to optimize the outcome of catheter ablation. The anatomic substrate of ventricular arrhythmias will be better defined; and successful modification of the anatomic substrate will reduce the number of VT recurrences and subsequent ICD therapies. The results of the multicenter, primary-prevention ICD trials will better define the high-risk patient who will benefit from ICD therapy. Finally, improvements in ICD systems will reduce the number of inappropriate shocks caused by SVT and will allow for a further reduction in generator size while still providing adequate energy for successful internal defibrillation.

REFERENCES

1. Myerburg R, Kessler KM, Castellanos A. Sudden cardiac death: epidemiology, transient risk, and intervention assessment. Ann Intern Med 1993;119:1187–1197.
2. DiMarco JP, Haines DE. Sudden cardiac death. Curr Probl Cardiol 1990:187–232.
3. The Antiarrhythmics Versus Implantable Defibrillators (AVID) Investigators. A comparison of anti-arrhythmic-drug therapy with implantable defibrillators in patients resuscitated from near-fatal ventricular arrhythmias. N Engl J Med 1997;337:1576–1583.
4. Stevenson WG, Friedman PL. Catheter Ablation of Ventricular Tachycardia. In: Zipes DP, Jalife J. Cardiac Electrophysiology: From Cell to Bedside, 3rd ed. WB Saunders Co., Philadelphia, PA, 2000, pp. 1049–1056.
5. Mirowski M. The Automatic implantable cardioverter-defibrillator: an overview. J Am Coll Cardio 1985;6:461–466.
6. Gregoratos G, Cheitlin M, Conill A, et al. ACC/AHA guidelines for implantation of cardiac pacemakers and antiarrhythmia devices. J Am Coll Cardiol 1998;31:1175–1209.
7. Karagueuzian HS, Mandel WJ. Electrophysiologic Mechanisms of Ischemic Ventricular Arrhythmias: Experimental and Clinical Correlations. In: Mandel WJ. Cardiac Arrhythmias: Their Mechanisms, Diagnosis, and Management. J.B. Lippincott Company, Philadelphia, PA, 1995, pp. 563–603.
8. The Multicenter Postinfarction Research Group. Risk Stratification and Survival After Myocardial Infarction. N Engl J Med 1983;309:331–336.
9. Bigger JT, Fleiss JL, Kleiger R, et al. The relationships among ventricular arrhythmias, left ventricular dysfunction, and mortality in the 2 years after myocardial infarction. Circulation 1984;69:250–258.
10. Sanz G, Castaner A, Betriu A, et al. Determinants of prognosis in survivors of myocardial infarction. N Engl J Med 1982;306:1065–1070.
11. Mukharji J, Rude R, Poole W, et al. Risk factors for sudden death after acute myocardial infarction: two-year follow-up. Am J Cardiol 1984;54:31–36.

12. Richards D, Byth K, Ross D, et al. What is the best predictor of spontaneous ventricular tachycardia and sudden death after myocardial infarction. Circulation 1991;83:756–763.

13. Pedretti R, Etro M, Laporta A, et al. Prediction of late arrhythmic events after acute myocardial infarction from combined use of non-invasive prognostic variables and inducibility of sustained monomorphic ventricular tachycardia. Am J Cardiol 1993;71:1131–1141.

14. Denniss AR, Richards DA, Cody DV, et al. Prognostic significance of ventricular tachycardia and fibrillation induced at programmed stimulation and delayed potentials detected on the signal-averaged electrocardiograms of survivors of acute myocardial infarction. Circulation 1986;74:731–745.

15. Kuchar DL, Thorburn CW, Sammel NL. Prediction of serious arrhythmic events after myocardial infarction: signal-averaged electrocardiogram, holter monitoring and radionuclide ventriculography. J Am Coll Cardiol 1987;9:531–538.

16. Moss A, Hall W, Cannom D, et al., for the Multicenter Automatic Defibrillator Implantation Trial (MADIT) Investigators. Improved survival with an implanted defibrillator in patients with coronary disease at high risk for ventricular arrhythmia. N Engl J Med 1996;335:1933–1940.

17. The B-Blocker Heart Attack Trial Research Group. A randomized trial of propranolol in patients with acute myocardial infarction. JAMA 1982;247:1707–1714.

18. The Norwegian Multicenter Study Group. Timolol-induced reduction in mortality and reinfarction in patients surviving acute myocardial infarction. N Engl J Med 1981;304:801–807.

19. The CONSENSUS Trial Study Group. Effects of enalapril on mortality in severe congestive heart failure: results of the Cooperative North Scandinavian Enalapril Survival Study (CONSENSUS). N Engl J Med 1987;316:1429–1435.

20. The SOLVD Investigators. Effect of enalapril on survival in patients with reduced left ventricular ejection fractions and congestive heart failure. N Engl J Med 1991;325:293–302.

21. Cohn J, Johnson G, Ziesche S, et al. A comparison of enalapril with hydralazine-isosorbide dinitrate in the treatment of chronic congestive heart failure. N Engl J Med 1991;325:303–310.

22. Pfeffer M, Braunwald E, Moye L, et al. for the Survival and Ventricular Enlargement Trial (SAVE) Investigators. Effect of captopril on mortality and morbidity in patients with left ventricular dysfunction after myocardial infarction. N Engl J Med 1992;327:669–677.

22a. Kober L, Torp-Pederson C, Carlsen JE, et al. A clinical trial of the angiotensin-converting-enzyme inhibitor trandolapril in patients with left ventricular dysfunction after myocardial infarction. N Engl J Med 1995;333:1670–1676.

22b. Domanski MJ, Exner DV, Borkowf CB, Geller NL, Rosenberg Y, Pfeffer MA. Effect of angiotensin converting enzyme inhibition on sudden cardiac death in patients following acute myocardial infarction: A meta-analysis of randomized clinical trials. J Am Coll Cardiol 1999;33:598–604.

23. Echt D, Liebson P, Mitchell B, et al., for the Cardiac Arrhythmia Suppression Trial (CAST) Investigators. Mortality and morbidity in patients receiving encainide, flecainide, or placebo. N Engl J Med 1991;324:781–788.

24. Teo K, Yusuf S, Furber C. Effects of prophylactic antiarrhythmic drug therapy in acute myocardial infarction: an overview of results from randomized controlled trial. JAMA 1993;270:1589–1595.

25. Burkart F, Pfisterer M, Kiowski W, et al. Effect of antiarrhythmic therapy on mortality in survivors of myocardial infarction with asymptomatic complex ventricular arrhythmias: Basel Antiarrhythmic Study of Infarct Survival (BASIS). J Am Coll Cardiol 1990;16:1711–1718.

26. Singh S, Fletcher R, Fisher S, et al. for the Survival Trail of Antiarrhythmic Therapy in Congestive Heart Failure (CHF-STAT) Investigators. Amiodarone in patients with congestive heart failure and asymptomatic ventricular arrhythmia. N Engl J Med 1995;333:77–82.

27. Julian D, Camm A, Frangin G, et al. for the European Myocardial Infarct Amiodarone Trial (EMIAT) Investigators. Randomized trial of effect of amiodarone on mortality in patients with left ventricular dysfunction after recent myocardial infarction: EMIAT. Lancet 1997;349:667–674.

28. Cairns J, Connolly S, Roberts R, et al. for the Canadian Amiodarone Myocardial Infarction Arrhythmia Trial (CAMIAT) Investigators. Lancet 1997;349:675–682.

28a. Amiodarone Trials Meta-Analysis Investigators. Effect of prophylactic amiodarone on mortality after acute myocardial infarction and in congestive heart failure: meta-analysis of individual data from 6500 patients in randomized trials. Lancet 1997;350:1417–1423.

29. Waldo A, Camm A, deRuyter H, et al. For the Survival With Oral d-Sotalol (SWORD) Investigators. Effect of d-sotalol on mortality in patients with left ventricular dysfunction after recent and remote myocardial infarction. Lancet 1996;348:7–12.

30. Bigger J, for the Coronary Artery Bypass Graft (CABG) Patch Trial Investigators. Prophylactic use

of implanted cardiac defibrillators in patients at high risk for ventricular arrhythmias after coronary artery bypass graft surgery. N Engl J Med 1997;337:1569–1575.

30a. Bigger JT Jr, Whang W, Rottman JN, et al. Mechanisms of death in the CABG Patch trial: a randomized trial of implantable cardiac defibrillator prophylaxis in patients at high risk of death after coronary artery bypass graft surgery. Circulation 1999;99:1416–1421.

31. Buxton A, Fisher J, Josephson M, et al. for the Multicenter Unsustained Tachycardia Trial (MUSTT) Investigators. Prevention of sudden death in patients with coronary artery disease: the Multicenter Unsustained Tachycardia Trial (MUSTT). Prog Cardiovasc Dis 1993;36:215–226.

32. Buxton AE, Lee KL, Fisher JD, et al. for the Multicenter Unsustained Tachycardia Trial Investigators. A randomized study of the prevention of sudden death in patients with coronary artery disease. N Engl J Med 1999;341:1882–1890.

32a. Buxton AE, Lee KL, DiCarlo L, et al. Electrophysiologic testing to identify patients with coronary artery disease who are at risk for sudden death. Multicenter Unsustained Tachycardia Trial Investigators. N Engl J Med 2000 Jun 29;342(26):1937–1945.

33. Klein H, Auricchio A, Reek Sven, et al. New Primary Prevention trial of Sudden Cardiac Death in Patients with Left Ventricular Dysfunction: SCD-HEFT and MADIT-II. Am J Cardiol 1999;83:91D–97D.

34. Gilman J, Jalal S, Naccarelli G. Predicting and preventing sudden death from cardiac causes. Circulation 1994;90:1083–1092.

35. Domanski M, Zipes D, Schron E. Treatment of sudden cardiac death. Circulation 1997;95:2694–2699.

36. Cannom D, Prystowski E. Management of ventricular arrhythmias. JAMA 1999;281:172–179.

37. Doval H, Nul D, Grancelli H, et al., for the Grupo de Estudio de la Sobrevida en la Insuficiencia Cardiaca en Argentina (GESICA) Investigators. Randomized trial of low dose amiodarone in severe congestive heart failure. Lancet 1994;344:493–498.

37a. Kadish A, Quigg R, Schaechter A, Anderson KP, Estes M, Levine J. Defibrillators in nonischemic cardiomyopathy treatment evaluation. PACE 2000;23:338–343.

38. The CASS Investigators. Coronary Artery Surgery Study (CASS): A randomized trial of coronary artery bypass surgery survival data. Circulation 1983;68:939–950.

39. Holmes DR, Davis KB, Mock MB, et al. The effect of medical and surgical treatment on subsequent sudden cardiac death in patients with coronary artery disease: a report from the coronary artery surgery study. Circulation 1986;73:1254–1263.

40. The CASCADE Investigators. Randomized Antiarrhythmic Drug Therapy in Survivors of Cardiac Arrest (the CASCADE Study). Am J Cardiol 1993;72:280–287.

41. Haverkamp W, Martinez-Rubio A, Hief C, et al. Efficacy and safety of d,l-sotalol in patients with ventricular tachycardia and in survivors of cardiac arrest. J Am Coll Cardiol 1997;30:487–495.

42. Pacifico A, Hohnloser SH, Williams JH, et al. Prevention of implantable-defibrillator shocks by treatment with sotalol. d,l-sotalol implantable cardioverter-defibrillator study group. N Engl J Med 1999;340(24):1855–1862.

43. Siebels J, Cappato R, Ruppel R, et al. for the Cardiac Arrest Study Hamburg (CASH) Investigators. Preliminary Results of the Cardiac Arrest Study Hamburg (CASH). Am J Cardiol 1993;72:109F–113F.

43a. Huck K-H, Cappato R, Siebels J, Ruppel R, for the CASH investigators. Randomized comparison of antiarrhythmic drug therapy with implantable defibrillators in patients resuscitated from cardiac arrest: The Cardiac Arrest Study Hamburg (CASH). Circulation 2000;102:748–754.

44. Connolly SJ, Gent M, Roberts RS, et al. Canadian implantable defibrillator study (CIDS): a randomized trial of the implantable cardioverter defibrillator against amiodarone. Circulation 2000 Mar 21; 101(11):1297–1302.

45. Fontaine G, Guiraudon G, Frank R, et al. Stimulation studies and epicardial mapping in ventricular tachycardia: study of mechanisms and selection for surgery. In: Kulbertus HE, ed. Reentrant Arrhythmias. MTP Publishers, Lancaster, 1977, pp. 334–350.

46. Marcus FI, Fontaine G. Arrhythmogenic right ventricular dysplasia. In: Podrid PJ, Kowey PR: Cardiac Arrhythmia: Mechanisms, Diagnosis, and Management. Williams & Wilkins, Baltimore, MD, 1995, pp. 1121–1130.

46a. Ellison KE, Friedman PL, Ganz LI, Stevenson WG. Entrainment mapping and radiofrequency catheter ablation of ventricular tachycardia in right ventricular dysplasia. J Am Coll Cardiol 1998;32:724–728.

47. Alfonso F, Frenneaux MP, McKenna WJ. Clinical sustained uniform ventricular tachycardia in hypertrophic cardiomyopathy: association with left ventricular apical aneurysm. Br Heart J 1989;61:178–181.

48. Borggrefe M, Schwammenthal E, Block M et al. Pre- and Postoperative Electrophysiological Findings in Survivors of Cardiac Arrest and Hypertrophic Obstructive Cardiomyopathy Undergoing Myomectomy (abstract). Circulation 1993;88 (Suppl):1120.

49. McKenna WJ, Oakley CM, Krikler DM, et al. Improved survival with amiodarone in patients with hypertrophic cardiomyopathy and ventricular tachycardia. Br Heart J 1985;53:412–416.

49a. Maron BJ, Shen WK, Link MS, et al. Efficacy of implantable cardioverter-defibrillators for the prevention of sudden death in patients with hypertrophic cardiomyopathy. N Engl J Med 2000 Feb 10;342(6):365–373.

50. Valantine H, McKenna WJ, Nihoyannopoulos P, et al. Sarcoidosis, a pattern of clinical and morphological presentation. Br Heart J 1987;57:256–263.

51. Winters SL, Cohen M, Greenberg S, et al. Sustained ventricular tachycardia associated with sarcoidosis: assessment of the underlying cardiac anatomy and the prospective utility of programmed ventricular stimulation, drug therapy, and an implantable antitachycardia device. J Am Coll Cardiol 1991;18: 937.

52. Sosa E, Scanavacca M, D'Avila A, et al. Endocardial and epicardial ablation guided by non-surgical transthoracic epicardial mapping to treat recurrent ventricular tachycardia. J Cardiovasc Electrophysiol 1998;9(3):229–239.

53. Belhassen B, Rotmensch HH, Laniago S. Response of recurrent sustained ventricular tachycardia to verapamil. Br Heart J 1981;46:679–682.

54. Zipes DP, Foster PR, Troup PJ. Atrial induction of ventricular tachycardia: reentry versus triggered automaticity. Am J Cardiol 1978;44:1–8.

55. Nakagawa H, Beckman KJ, McClelland JH, et al. Radiofrequency catheter ablation of idiopathic left ventricular tachycardia guided by a purkinje potential. Circulation 1993;88:2607–2617.

56. Gallarvardin Ll. Extrasystolie Ventriculaire a Paroxysmes Tachycardiques Prolonges. Arch Mal Coeur 1922;15:298.

57. Jackman W, Friday K, Anderson J, Aliot E, Clark M, Lazzara R. The Long QT Syndromes: A critical review, new clinical observations and a unifying hypothesis. Prog Cardiovasc Dis 1988;31:115–172.

58. Napolitano C, Priori S, Schwartz P. Torsade de pointes: mechanisms and management. Drugs 1994;47:51–65.

59. Kay G, Plumb V, Arciniegas J, Henthorn R, Waldo A. Torsade de pointes: the long-short initiation sequence and other clinical features: observations in 32 patients. J Am Coll Cardiol 1983;2:806–817.

60. Keren A, Tzivoni D, Gavish D, Levi J, Gottlieb S, Benhorin J, et al. Etiology, warning signs and therapy of torsade de pointes. Circulation 1981;64:1167–1174.

61. Saxon L, Wiener I, Natterson P, Laks H, Drinkwater D, Stevenson W. Monomorphic versus polymorphic ventricular tachycardia after coronary artery bypass grafting. Am J Cardiol 1995;75:403–405.

62. Wolfe C, Nibley C, Bhandari A, Chatterjee K, Scheinman M. Polymorphous ventricular tachycardia associated with acute myocardial infarction. Circulation 1991;84:1543–1551.

63. Carter J, Childers R. Torsade de pointes complicating acute myocardial infarction. the importance of autonomic dysfunction as assessed by heart rate variability. Clin Cardiol 1992;15:769–772.

64. Eisenberg SJ, Scheinman MM, Dullet NK, et al. Sudden cardiac death and polymorphous ventricular tachycardia in patients with normal QT intervals and normal systolic cardiac function. Am J Cardiol 1995;75:687–692.

65. Dessertenne F. La Tachycardie Ventriculaire a Deux Foyers Opposes Variable. Arch Mal Coeur 1966;59:263–272.

66. Dhurandhar RW, Macmillan RL, Brown KW. Primary ventricular fibrillation complicating acute myocardial infarction. Am J Cardiol 1990;66:1208–1211.

66a. Volpi A, Cavalli A, Santoro L, et al. Incidence and prognosis of early primary ventricular fibrillation in acute myocardial infarction—results of the gruppo italiano per lo studio della sopravvivenza nell'infarcto miocardico (GISSI-2) database. Am J Cardiol 1998;82:265–271.

66b. Kelly P, Ruskin J, Vlahakes GJ, Buckley MJ, Freeman CS, Garan H. Surgical coronary revascularization in survivors of prehospital cardiac arrest: its effect on inducible ventricular arrhythmias and long-term survival. J Am Coll Cardiol 1990;15:267–272.

66c. Natale A, Sra J, Axtell K, et al. Ventricular fibrillation and polymorphic ventricular tachycardia with critical coronary artery stenosis: does bypass surgery suffice? J Cardiovasc Electrophysiol 1994;5:988–994.

66d. Marcus FI. Idiopathic ventricular fibrillation. J Cardiovasc Electrophysiol 1997;8:1075–1083.

66e. Consensus statement. Survivors of out-of-hospital cardiac arrest with apparently normal heart. Circulation 1997;95:265–272.

66f. Belhassen B, Viskin S, Fish R, Glick A, Setbon I, Eldar M. Effects of electrophysiologic-guided therapy with Class IA antiarrhythmic drugs on the long-term outcome of patients with idiopathic ventricular fibrillation with or without the Brugada syndrome. J Cardiovasc Electrophysiol 1999; 10:1301–1312.

66g. Ruskin JN. Idiopathic ventricular fibrillation: is there a role for electrophysiologic-guided antiarrhythmic drug therapy? J Cardiovasc Electrophysiol 1999;10:1313–1315.

67. Antzelevitch C. The Brugada Syndrome. J Cardiovasc Electrophysiol 1998;9:513–516.

13 Nonsustained Ventricular Tachycardia

Evaluation and Treatment

Brian Olshansky, MD

INTRODUCTION

Nonsustained ventricular tachycardia (NSVT) refers to three or more consecutive ventricular beats with a rate greater than 100 beats per minute (BPM) that does not: cause hemodynamic collapse, require cardioversion, or last more than 30 s. Although it is not life-threatening, NSVT can cause symptoms requiring suppressive, or curative treatment. NSVT can also carry a high risk of sudden death.

Strategies have been proposed to risk-stratify patients with NSVT, and offer high-risk patients therapy that reduces the risk of sudden cardiac death. However, prophylactic therapy is not well-defined in all patient subgroups. Even "definitive" studies provide incomplete guidance. Cogent data from clinical trials now indicate that substantial risk reduction can be achieved in some patients with proper prophylactic treatment. Although earlier clinical trials have focused on pharmacologic prophylaxis, more recent trials have evaluated the implantable cardioverter defibrillator (ICD). Despite the results of these trials, NSVT remains a common clinical problem that can be difficult to evaluate and treat *(1,2)*.

From: *Contemporary Cardiology: Management of Cardiac Arrhythmias*
Edited by: L. I. Ganz © Humana Press Inc., Totowa, NJ

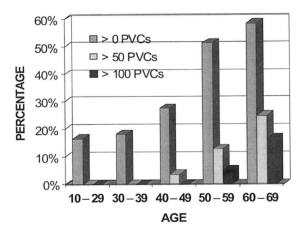

Fig. 1. Density of ventricular ectopy in unselected patients undergoing 24-h Holter monitoring as a function of age. (From: Kostis JB. Circulation 1981;63:1353.)

Incidence of NSVT

The actual incidence of NSVT in the general population is unknown (*see* Fig. 1). In asymptomatic individuals with no apparent heart disease, NSVT is rare (1–4%) *(3,4–10)*. NSVT may occur in the general population at a frequency too small to be detectable during an average 24-h observational period. Treadmill testing can detect NSVT in about 1% of an unselected population *(7,8)*.

A relationship does exist between the extent of structural heart disease and the prevalence of NSVT *(11–13)*. In the CHF STAT trial, 80% of patients with congestive heart failure (CHF) had NSVT on routine 24-h Holter monitoring *(14)*. Other studies of patients with heart failure confirm a high frequency of NSVT with routine monitoring *(15,16)*. In the GESICA trial, the incidence of NSVT was 50.3%. Prolonged monitoring of most patients with cardiomyopathy and CHF will reveal NSVT. NSVT is commonly associated with many forms of heart disease, including ischemic heart disease, cardiomyopathy (dilated, infiltrative, and hypertrophic), congenital heart disease, valvular heart disease, myocarditis, long QT syndrome (LQTS), and right ventricular dysplasia. Approximately 35–50% of patients with acute myocardial infarction (MI) have NSVT during the acute phase of the MI, and 5–10% of those with history of MI will have NSVT in the chronic phase *(17–19,20–23)*.

CLASSIFICATION OF NSVT

NSVT can be categorized by morphology, clinical presentation, underlying substrate, and symptoms.

Morphology

Nonsustained tachycardias may present many appearances. The possibility that a nonsustained wide-complex tachycardia may be caused by supraventricular tachycardia with aberrancy should also be considered (*see* Fig. 2B). Multiple algorithms have been proposed to aid in diagnosis; from a practical perspective, wide-complex tachycardia is more likely VT than SVT with aberrancy, particularly in patients with structural heart disease. In addition, motion or tremor artifact can occasionally "masquerade" as

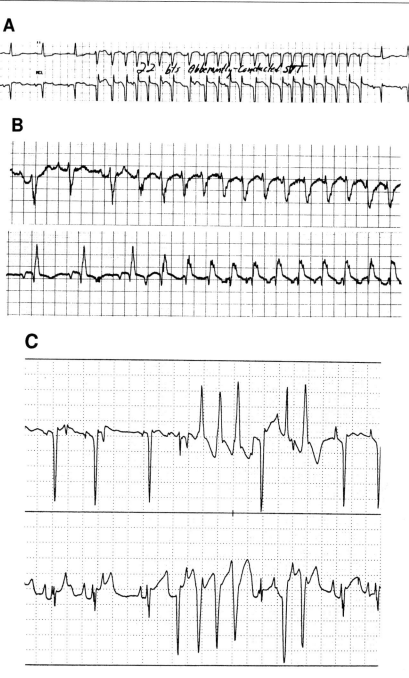

Fig. 2. Diagnosis of nonsustained wide-complex tachycardia:

(**A**) Nonsustained wide-complex tachycardia in a patient with remote MI. Although the tachycardia is relatively narrow and somewhat irregular, dissociated P waves are evident in the lower rhythm strip, making the diagnosis nonsustained VT. Note that this was misdiagnosed as SVT with aberrancy.

(**B**) Two separate rhythm steps of nonsustained wide-complex tachycardia in a patient 48 hours into MI, with RBBB at baseline. During tachycardia, the QRS complex is slightly wider than at baseline. The tachycardia was initiated by a PAC, and is supraventricular in nature.

(**C**) On this Holter monitor, the baseline rhythm is sinus with frequent PAC's. Note that during the wide-complex tachycardia there is a narrow complex capture beat, making the tachycardia diagnosis NSVT.

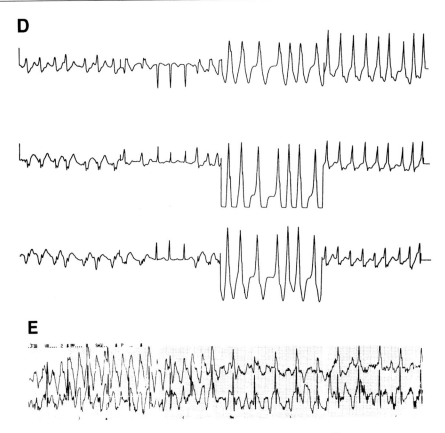

Fig. 2. (*Continued*) Diagnosis of nonsustained wide-complex tachycardia:
(D) An irregular, mostly wide-complex tachycardia. Note the variable QRS width, as well as several narrow beats. This is pre-excited atrial fibrillation (AF) in a young patient with Wolff-Parkinson-White Syndrome (WPW).
(E) Tremor artifact on inpatient telemetry misdiagnosed as NSVT. Note that the narrow QRS complexes march through the "wide-complex tachycardia" at a rate of about 100 BPM.

wide-complex tachycardia (*see* Fig. 2E). The electrocardiographic tracing must be inspected carefully to ascertain the diagnosis. The rate and the regularity of the rhythm does not necessarily help in the diagnosis, since NSVT may be irregular and mono-morphic, irregular and polymorphic, apparently polymorphic (beat-to-beat changes resulting from capture and fusion beats), fast, or relatively slow (*see* Figs. 3A–3K).

Monomorphic NSVT

Monomorphic NSVT originates from a single focal source or single reentrant circuit (*see* Figs. 2A,3A,3B,3H,3I,3K). A focal source can be caused by enhanced automaticity, or triggered activity caused by delayed after-depolarizations (DADs) or early after-depolarizations (EADs). Chung and Pogwizd, using a 3-dimensional mapping technique, evaluated the mechanisms of NSVT and compared the initiation of nonsustained tachy-cardia with sustained VT in the same patients *(24,25)*. The mechanisms of NSVT and sustained VT were different. NSVT was initiated from discordant sites caused by either a macro-reentrant or a focal mechanism. Monomorphic VT can present as a single morphology or as multiple morphologies. Multiple monomorphic morphologies may

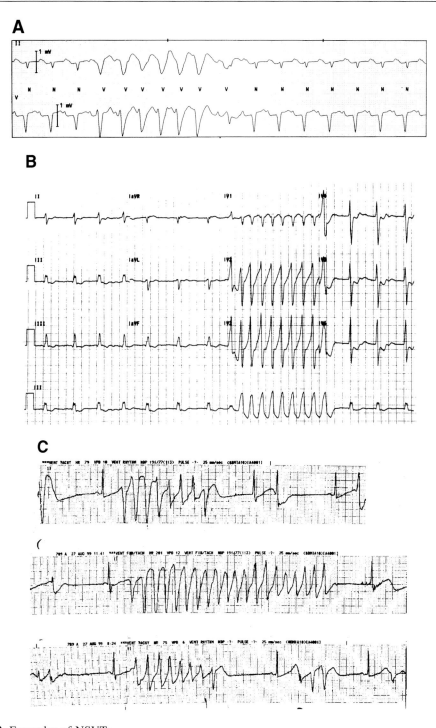

Fig. 3. Examples of NSVT:

(A) Monomorphic NSVT in a patient with ischemic cardiomyopathy. The patient fit the MADIT/MUSTT profile. During EPS, rapid VT was induced, and the patient received an ICD.

(B) Monomorphic NSVT in a patient with underlying nonischemic cardiomyopathy and AF. Note that the PVC that initiates NSVT has a different morphology than the subsequent salvo of NSVT.

(C) Torsades de pointes PVT in a patient with acquired LQTS caused by quinidine therapy. Note the recurrent paroxysms of NSVT following "long-short" sequences.

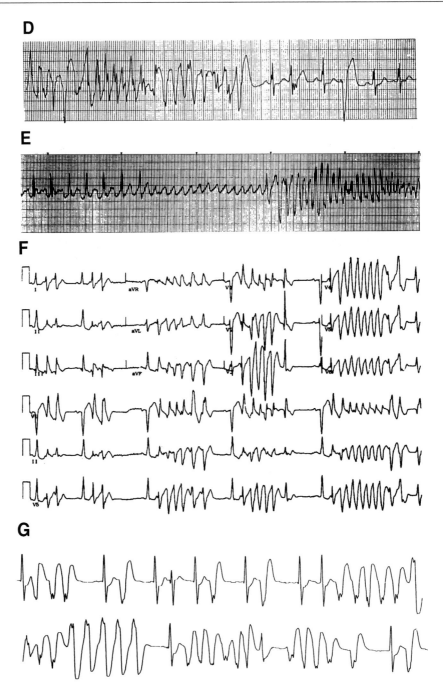

Fig. 3. (*Continued*) Examples of NSVT:

(**D**) Polymorphic NSVT in a patient with acute MI. Although the morphology is suggestive of torsades, marked QT prolongation is absent. The etiology was believed to be acute ischemia.

(**E**) Pause-dependent torsades de pointes, in a patient with atrial flutter treated with iv procainamide and verapamil.

(**F**) Incessant nonsustained torsades de pointes VT, in a patient early after mitral-valve surgery. Atrial overdrive pacing suppressed further episodes.

(**G**) Incessant nonsustained polymorphic VT in a patient with nonischemic cardiomyopathy. Acutely, the VT was suppressed by IV amiodarone, and the patient received an ICD.

H

I

J

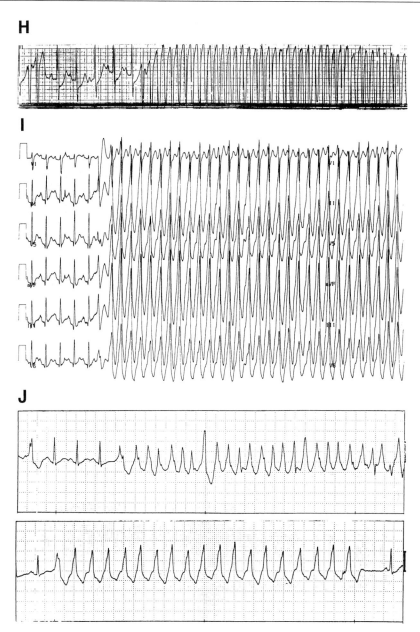

Fig. 3. (*Continued*) Examples of NSVT:

(**H**) Spontaneous recording in an 11-yr-old female with syncope and "probable" hypertrophic cardio-myopathy. She received an ICD, and has had no recurrent syncope or ICD discharges during 10 yr of follow-up.

(**I**) Young athlete with palpitations during exercise. Work-up was negative for structural heart disease. During a treadmill exercise test, this rhythm was recorded. VT seemed to be triggered by sinus rates above 160 BPM. The patient was treated with a beta-blocker, and was unable to achieve this sinus rate. He has done well, without symptomatic VT recurrences.

(**J**) Young athlete with palpitations and syncope, which occurred while playing hockey. No structrual heart disease was detected during a thorough evaluation. Two rates of tachycardia were recorded (top and bottom panels). Diagnostic EPS was unrevealing. Though this appears monomorphic, simultaneous recording in multiple leads revealed polymorphic VT. The patient was treated with a beta-blocker, and no recurrences were observed during follow-up.

K

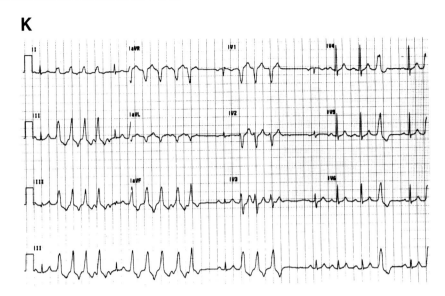

Fig. 3. (*Continued*) Examples of NSVT:
(K) 12-Lead ECG in a patient with repetitive, nonsustained idiopathic VT of right ventricular outflow tract (RVOT) origin. Note the characteristic LBBB, normal-axis morphology.

indicate either multiple discrete circuits or multiple breakthrough sites from the same circuit. Alternatively, this may indicate the presence of various arrhythmia mechanisms.

POLYMORPHIC NSVT

Polymorphic NSVT does not originate from a single focal source. Electrical activation is not uniform (*see* Figs. 3C–3G,3J). Polymorphic ventricular tachycardia (PVT) can occur with a normal or prolonged QT interval, and generally carries a poor prognosis. If PVT occurs in a young individual with no obvious structural heart disease, it is frequently exercise- or stress-induced, and potentially life-threatening (*see* Fig. 3J). A beta-blocker may be life-saving *(26–29)*. Polymorphic NSVT can occur with arrhythmogenic right ventricular dysplasia/cardiomyopathy (ARVD), Brugada's syndrome, acute myocardial ischemia (or infarction), sarcoidosis, myocarditis, and hypertrophic and dilated cardiomyopathies *(30)*.

PVT associated with a long QT interval at the onset of the arrhythmia and occurring in repetitive paroxysms is known as torsades de pointes (*see* Figs. 3C,3E,3F). Torsades de pointes is likely caused by dispersion between local refractory periods, and can be initiated by EADs *(27,31–34)*. If torsades de pointes occurs in relation to the congenital long QT interval syndrome (LQTS), then the baseline QT interval is generally long. When torsades de pointes is initiated by a drug pro-arrhythmia or an electrolyte abnormality, QT prolongation may be dynamic and rate-related; slow rates or a long pause can precipitate marked QT-interval prolongation. Correction of the responsible electrolyte abnormality or discontinuation of the inciting drug will improve the arrhythmia and the prognosis. Conversely, in PVT not indicative of torsades de pointes and not caused by QT prolongation (*see* Figs. 3D,3G), amiodarone, a drug which lengthens the QT interval, may be beneficial. Ironically, a prolonged episode of a rapid polymorphic NSVT, in the setting of a long QT interval, may be life-threatening, but if an underlying

Table 1
Clinical Presentations of NSVT

1. Asymptomatic monomorphic short duration (<10–20 beats) NSVT associated with chronic heart disease (the most common form).
2. Repetitive monomorphic "idiopathic" (often catecholamine sensitive) NSVT originating primarily from the right ventricular outflow tract (RVOT), and, less commonly, from other anatomic locations.
3. NSVT caused by an acute precipitant (MI, CHF, or cardiac surgery) that resolves spontaneously.
4. Symptomatic NSVT.
5. NSVT associated with congenital LQTS.
6. Polymorphic, exercise-induced, NSVT in children without heart disease (potentially life-threatening).
7. PVT associated with heart disease (long or short QT interval) and/or antiarrhythmic drugs.
8. Prolonged, frequent, or incessant NSVT interspersed with infrequent sinus or supraventricular rhythm that is difficult to distinguish from sustained VT.

cause (e.g., a proarrhythmic drug) is identified and eliminated, the prognosis is good. In contrast, a single 3-beat run of relatively slow, asymptomatic, monomorphic NSVT in a patient with coronary-artery disease (CAD) and left ventricular dysfunction may portend a poor prognosis.

Clinical Presentation

The clinical presentation can dictate the need for and urgency of therapy. Many scenarios exist; these are described in Table 1.

Underlying Condition

The underlying substrate is important in assessing the prognosis and management options for a particular patient with NSVT. Various underlying and associated conditions are listed in Table 2.

Table 2
Underlying Conditions Associated With NSVT

1. No apparent structural or electrical heart disease (i.e., idiopathic VT).
2. CAD (chronic).
3. Cardiomyopathy: hypertrophic, dilated, or infiltrative (i.e., sarcoidosis, hemochromatosis).
4. Drug proarrhythmia.
5. Toxic/metabolic causes.
6. Exercise.
7. Repaired congenital conditions (e.g., tetrology of Fallot).
8. Primary "electrical disorders" (congenital LQTS Brugada's syndrome).
9. Arrhythmogenic right ventricular dysplasia.
10. Myocardial ischemia/infarction (acute).
11. Myocarditis.
12. Noncardiac disease.

Symptoms

Many patients who have NSVT are asymptomatic. Since NSVT can cause loss of AV synchrony, rate irregularity, abrupt change in rate, and a rapid heart rate, it can alter hemodynamics and cause symptoms. The symptom severity depends on the duration and rate of NSVT, associated heart disease, and patient-specific issues that are poorly characterized. Common symptoms associated with NSVT include: palpitations (frequently perceived as "skipped beats" or missed beats rather than extra beats), irregular heart action, chest and neck discomfort, dyspnea, dizziness, weakness, lightheadedness, near syncope, anxiety, and hypertension. Symptoms may be more severe, and rarely include syncope. NSVT can influence sympathetic and parasympathetic tone, cause hormonal fluctuations, elevate central venous pressure, and lower cardiac output to cause an even longer list of symptomatic presentations. In addition, symptoms may be unrelated to NSVT.

It is important to recognize a hierarchy of symptom severity; this will dictate the urgency for evaluation and treatment. No specific clinical classification schema exists to categorize the type and severity of symptoms of patients with NSVT. Careful clinical assessment is crucial to determine the need for treatment based on symptoms and to determine that the symptoms are indeed caused by NSVT. Symptoms should be shown to be a result of the arrhythmia before treating the patient for this reason alone.

Treatment for symptoms should be prescribed if symptoms are recurrent and if symptoms impact on the patient's "quality-of-life," as long as treatment is safe and effective. Such therapy includes suppression of NSVT by a drug or elimination by catheter ablation. Both approaches have risks, and neither should be assumed to improve survival. An implantable cardioverter defibrillator (ICD) will not supress symptomatic NSVT. If hemodynamic collapse is caused by NSVT, suppressive therapy is required.

PROGNOSIS

NSVT is one of several risk factors for sudden death and death resulting from heart disease, but by itself, NSVT has little predictive value (35–37). In combination with specific conditions (acute MI, hypertrophic cardiomyopathy, impaired left ventricular function caused by CAD or LQTS), NSVT can be a major concern (38–42). In a "normal" population, NSVT recorded on a Holter monitor is associated with a significantly higher risk of early death, although causality has not clearly been established. Some studies show as much as a doubling in mortality and an association with CAD ultimately diagnosed (36). However, other studies have yielded contradictory results (43). In patients with CHF, some studies have linked NSVT with a higher risk of death (3,44–46). The GESICA trial showed that NSVT imparted an excess mortality risk of 69% (15,16). In the CHF STAT trial, NSVT was associated with an insignificant trend toward worsened survival (14,47). In another trial, NSVT was associated with higher pulmonary-artery pressures, higher pulmonary wedge pressures, and more pronounced sympathetic activation (47A). These data suggest that the NSVT may be a marker for a more diseased heart, which results in a poorer outcome.

In contrast to patients with heart failure, NSVT has consistently been shown to be a marker of risk for death for patients with CAD and reduced left ventricular ejection fraction (LVEF) (48) (see Fig. 4). These patients have a doubling or tripling in risk

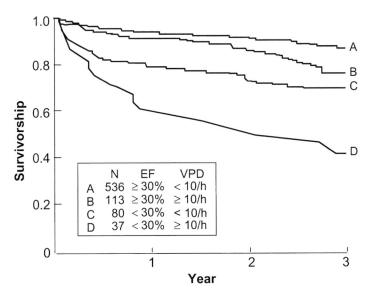

Fig. 4. Survival after acute MI, stratified by left ventricular fraction and density of ventricular ectopy. (From: Bigger et al. Am J. Cardiol 1986;57:12B.)

of sudden cardiac death *(49)*. Even a single 3-beat recording of NSVT on a 24-h Holter monitor has prognostic significance. When the LVEF is <0.35, mortality can exceed 20% in 2-yr follow-up, clearly greater than if no NSVT is present. In this population, the length and frequency of the episodes have not reproducibly been linked to prognosis, although recent data from the MUSTT trial indicates that NSVT runs >8 beats are associated with a poorer prognosis *(50,51)*. The presence of NSVT in patients with CAD and impaired left ventricular function (LVEF <0.40 or 0.35) remains a nonspecific marker for sudden and total cardiac death. To this end, other prognostic markers have been considered to further define risk.

The prognostic significance of NSVT during the acute phase of a myocardial infarction is controversial even if impaired left ventricular function is present *(39,52)*. In patients with hypertrophic cardiomyopathy, NSVT has been associated with higher risk for cardiac death in some, but not all studies *(53)*. Some series suggest that NSVT imparts a several-fold increase in mortality in hypertrophic cardiomyopathy. Exercise-induced NSVT can have prognostic importance *(8,54–61)*. While it may be caused by a benign condition ("idiopathic VT") *(62)*, it can be associated with arrhythmogenic right ventricular dysplasia, LQTS, an aberrant coronary artery, hypertrophic cardiomyopathy or dilated cardiomyopathy. An athlete with NSVT requires restriction from athletics until the problem is evaluated fully and treated based on the Bethesda guidelines *(62a)*.

Refining risk in patients with cardiac disease may extend beyond the diagnosis of NSVT, symptoms of CHF, and presence of ventricular dysfunction. Other risk-stratifiers currently being investigated include heart-rate variability (HRV), signal-averaged electrocardiography (SAECG), baroreflex responses, spectral turbulence, QT dispersion, and T-wave alternans (TWA). Even if better predictors become available, the magnitude of absolute-risk "high" enough to warrant ICD implantation must be defined.

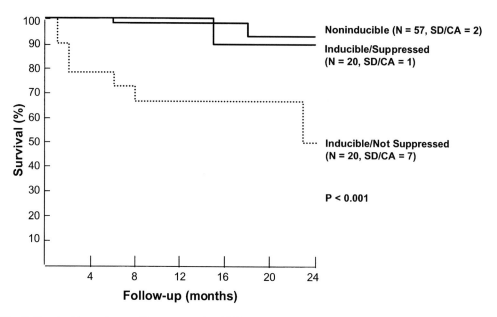

Fig. 5. Survival in patients with nonsustasined VT, coronary disease, and left ventricular dysfunction, stratified by results of electrophysiologic testing. (From: Wilber DJ. Circulation 1990;82:350–358.)

Risk Stratification—Electrophysiologic Testing

Electrophysiology study (EPS) has been used to assess risk of life-threatening arrhythmias in patients with NSVT. The use of such testing is based on the premise that if a sustained, potentially life-threatening, ventricular arrhythmia is induced in the electrophysiology laboratory, it may occur spontaneously. After extensive study, it appears that this approach has no important predictive value in patients without CAD *(63,64)*. In the absence of CAD, even if there is a high risk for sudden arrhythmic death, the likelihood of inducing such an arrhythmia in the electrophysiology laboratory is small. Thus, EPS is not generally recommended to assess risk in patients with NSVT who do not have CAD.

Electrophysiologic testing for NSVT has prognostic value when CAD and left ventricular dysfunction are present. In the MUSTT trial, about one-third of the patients with impaired ventricular function, coronary disease, and NSVT had inducible sustained ventricular tachyarrhythmias. No clinical parameters predicted inducibility *(50)*. Several studies have assessed the efficacy of electrophysiology testing to predict the risk of sustained VT or ventricular fibrillation (VF) in post-MI patients with mixed results *(65–73)*. Prior to the era in which ICD implantation was commonplace, we evaluated 100 patients with NSVT, CAD, and a LVEF less than 0.40 *(74)*. Forty-three had inducible sustained VT at electrophysiology testing. Of these, 20 became noninducible with serial antiarrhythmic drug testing, and 20 patients remained inducible, but with a slower ventricular tachycardia (VT) rate. The 1- and 2-yr mortality in the inducible group, despite drug treatment, was 38% and 50%, respectively (*see* Fig. 5). Patients who did not have inducible VT fared better.

More recent data call into question the value of EPS to define risk in this population *(75)*. In MUSTT (Multicenter Unsustained Tachycardia Trial), patients with prior myo-

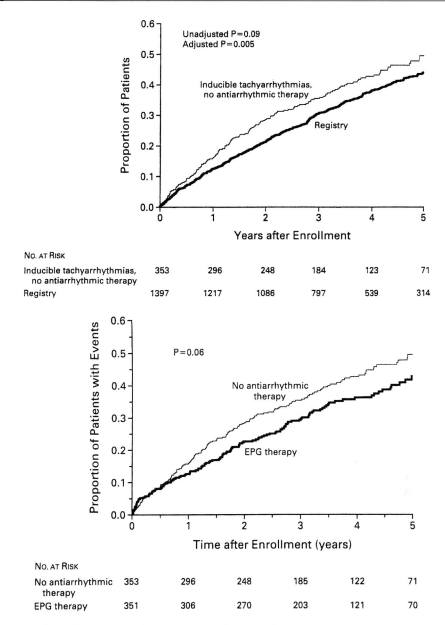

Fig. 6. Data from the MUSTT trial—Kaplan-Meier mortality curves:
(A) Total mortality in patients who met trial inclusion criteria, but were noninducible at EPS (registry) compared with patients who were inducible but randomized to no arrhythmic therapy. (From: Buxton A. N Engl J Med 2000;342:1942.)
(B) Total mortality in patients randomized to EP-guided therapy vs no antiarrhythmic therapy. (From: Buxton A. N. Engl J Med 1999;341:1855.)

cardial infarction, EF ≤ 0.40, and NSVT underwent EPS. The 1-yr mortality in such patients who had a negative electrophysiology test and received no specific anti-arrhythmic treatment was 12% *(76)* (*see* Fig. 6A). Although this was better than the 18% risk if the EPS were positive and no antiarrhythmic therapy was administered, *all* such patients with NSVT, CAD, and left ventricular dysfunction are at risk. A

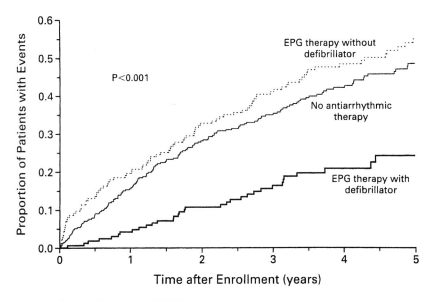

Fig. 6. (*Continued*) Data from the MUSTT trial—Kaplan-Meier mortality curves:
(**C**) Total mortality in patients randomized to EP-guided therapy vs no antiarrhythmic therapy, stratified by whether the patient eventually received an ICD or not. (From: Buxton A. N Engl J Med 1999;341:1886.)

generous interpretation was that EPS differentiated high-risk from moderate-risk patients in this study. Some have advanced the position that EPS is of little benefit in this population *(77)*.

PHARMACOLOGIC TREATMENT OF PATIENTS WITH NSVT

For patients at high risk, the concept of primary prevention of death is valid as long as an effective, proven, prophylactic approach exists. Several methods have been attempted: antiarrhythmic drug suppression and ICD therapy.

ACE inhibitors, spironolactone, and beta-blockers improve survival in "high-risk" patients with NSVT who have CAD, heart failure and/or impaired ventricular function. Even so, death rates in these high-risk groups remain high. Beta-blockers are effective in reducing overall *and* sudden death mortality among survivors of MI. Whether or not beta-blocker therapy suppresses NSVT or has particular benefit in the NSVT population remains unclear. Nevertheless, beta-blockers improve survival, and should therefore be part of the treatment regimen in post-infarct patients unless contraindications exist.

Antiarrhythmic drugs can suppress NSVT, but they can also increase ectopy and cause sustained VT, torsades de pointes, bradycardia, VF, and death. The empiric use of an antiarrhythmic drug to suppress asymptomatic NSVT is not recommended, and probably never will be. Suppressive antiarrhythmic drug use tested in post-infarct patients has shown no benefit thus far, and in several instances has demonstrated harm *(78–82)*. Antiarrhythmic drug risk is lowest when there is no structural heart disease, and in this setting can be used with more impunity when there is need to suppress symptomatic NSVT ("idiopathic" NSVT).

The Cardiac Arrhythmia Suppression Trial (CAST I) tested the hypothesis that suppression of ventricular arrhythmias after MI with a class I antiarrhythmic drug would improve survival *(80,83,84)*. The trial was terminated early because arrhythmic death and total mortality were substantially higher among those receiving encainide and flecainide compared to those receiving placebo, despite effective suppression of ventricular ectopy. Similarly, CAST II was stopped because of early excess mortality in those receiving moricizine compared with placebo despite arrhythmia suppression. These data support the concept that antiarrhythmic drug suppression of ventricular arrhythmias, including NSVT, can be harmful. As a low mortality rate was present in the placebo group, CAST may have targeted a population at a risk too low to benefit from antiarrhythmic prophylaxis. The sickest patients (e.g., those with NYHA class IV CHF or sustained VT) were excluded from CAST. Despite these limitations, the increased mortality rate in the empirically drug-treated patients focused on the dangers of arrhythmia suppression by an antiarrhythmic drug.

Drug suppression with other antiarrhythmic drugs, and in different patient populations, highlight the global dangers of antiarrhythmic drugs used "empirically" in patients with NSVT. A pure class III drug, D-sotalol, tested in a post-MI population, showed similar results to CAST. The Survival with ORal D-Sotalol (SWORD) trial was designed to test the hypothesis that d-sotalol would reduce all-cause mortality in patients with previous MI and left ventricular dysfunction *(79)*. Many patients in SWORD had NSVT. The trial was terminated prematurely because of a higher mortality among those randomized to d-sotalol. Excess mortality occurred in the "less sick" patients with more preserved left ventricular function, suggesting that the risk of pro-arrhythmia because of D-sotalol was higher than the baseline risks in these patients.

Post-MI studies of empiric amiodarone (BASIS, EMIAT, CAMIAT) and dofetilide (DIAMOND), however, showed a neutral effect on mortality DIAMOND-MI *(81,85–87)*. There was no difference in all-cause or cardiac mortality between the amiodarone and placebo. As many of patients in these trials had NSVT, it is likely that amiodarone use is safe for patients with CAD and NSVT (although not necessarily beneficial). The Canadian Amiodarone Myocardial Infarction Arrhythmia Trial (CAMIAT) enrolled 1,202 post-MI patients with frequent or repetitive ventricular premature depolarizations, and randomly assigned them to amiodarone or placebo. The primary end point was the combination of resuscitated VF and arrhythmic death, which occurred in 6% of the group receiving placebo and 3.3% of the group receiving amiodarone (RR reduction 48.5%, $p = 0.016$) over a mean follow-up of 1.8 yr. The study lacked power to detect a reduction in all-cause mortality. The European Myocardial Infarct Amiodarone Trial (EMIAT) enrolled 1,486 patients 5–21 d after MI with a LVEF ≥ 0.40. The results were nearly identical to those of CAMIAT; there was a decrease in resuscitated cardiac arrest and arrhythmic death, but not total morbidity in patients randomized to amiodarone. In a meta-analysis of these two studies, and several smaller studies evaluating amiodarone in post-infarct and heart-failure patients, total mortality was decreased slightly in patients randomized to amiodarone *(87a)*.

To assess whether beta-blockers used with amiodarone in post-MI patients could improve survival, a post-hoc, intention-to-treat analysis was performed from pooled CAMIAT and EMIAT data. Unadjusted and adjusted relative risks for total mortality, cardiac death, arrhythmic death, non-arrhythmic cardiac death, and resuscitated cardiac arrest or arrhythmic death were lower for patients taking beta-blockers at entry and randomized to amiodarone than for those receiving amiodarone alone. Although these findings require further confirmation, they support the idea that a beta-blocker works synergistically with amiodarone *(87b)*.

The Congestive Heart Failure Survival Trial of Antiarrhythmic Therapy (CHF-STAT) randomized 674 patients with heart failure, cardiac enlargement, ≥ 10 premature ventricular contractions (PVCs)/h, and a LVEF of ≤ 0.40 to either amiodarone or placebo *(47)*. Overall mortality was the primary end point. Although amiodarone effectively suppressed ventricular ectopy and improved the LVEF, the 2-yr actuarial survival rate was the same in both groups (69.4% amiodarone vs 70.8% placebo, $p = 0.6$).

An antiarrhythmic drug for NSVT can be a double-edged sword—although the symptoms may be improved, survival may be worsened. No study has shown that empiric suppression of NSVT with an antiarrhythmic drug improves survival. If there is a need to suppress NSVT for symptoms in a high-risk patient or to treat other arrhythmias, amiodarone is the drug of choice.

IMPLANTABLE CARDIOVERTER DEFIBRILLATORS (ICDs) IN NSVT PATIENTS

The ICD is highly effective in terminating life-threatening "malignant" ventricular arrhythmias, and, as such, can lower mortality rates in select populations. As NSVT can be an indicator of risk of arrhythmic death, it has been postulated that ICD implantation may improve survival. The ICD is not meant to treat spontaneously terminating (i.e., nonsustained) VT. An ICD could have a proarrhythmic effect, transforming a benign episode of NSVT into life-threatening VF. Also, ICD shocks may be triggered for a benign arrhythmia (such as AF or sinus tachycardia) or for NSVT that would stop, or does stop, spontaneously, with a negative impact on quality of life. Finally, lead malfunction can cause spurious shocks which detract from quality of life, and may pose risk.

ICD Clinical Trials

To evaluate the survival benefits from ICD implantation, the only end points of importance are all-cause or total mortality. Any other end point ("appropriate shock," treated VT, arrhythmic death, or sudden death) is inadequate and of less importance. As Milton Packer has said: *"All deaths are sudden: one minute you are alive. The next you are dead."*

Two multicenter primary prevention ("prophylactic") trials have been completed in high-risk patients with NSVT, impaired ventricular function, and ischemic heart disease: the MADIT (Multicenter Automatic Defibrillator Implant Trial) *(88)* and the MUSTT (Multicenter UnSustained Tachycardia Trial) trials *(89)*. Several important ICD trials are in progress: SCD-HeFT, DEFINITE, COMPANION, MADIT II, and others.

The MADIT trial assessed patients who had CAD and a prior MI. To be enrolled, patients were required to have a LVEF ≤ 0.35, asymptomatic NSVT on a Holter recording, and inducible, nonsuppressible (by procainamide) VT or VF induced during electrophysiology testing. Patients with an acute infarction or recent surgery or angioplasty were excluded. Patients were assigned randomly to ICD implant or "conventional" medical therapy. "Conventional" therapy was not specified, but consisted initially of

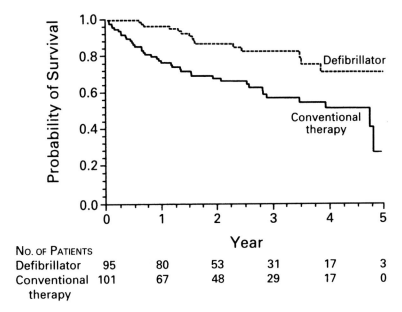

No. of Patients

Defibrillator	95	80	53	31	17	3
Conventional therapy	101	67	48	29	17	0

Fig. 7. Data from the MADIT trial—Kaplan-Meier survival curve, depicting total survival in patients randomized to ICD therapy vs conventional therapy. (From: Moss AJ. N Engl J Med 1996;335:1938.)

amiodarone in 74% of the patients (45% of whom were taken off amiodarone within 6 mo). One hundred ninety-six patients (16 women, mean age 63 yr) were enrolled from 32 centers over a 5-yr period (on average, slightly more than one patient enrolled per center per yr) with most patient enrollment concentrated at 2 sites (63 patients, 32% of the study population). The mean ejection fraction was 0.26. Seventy-five percent were randomized ≥6 mo after an acute MI.

The trial was terminated because of a dramatic decrease in total mortality in the ICD arm (*see* Fig. 7). The mortality reduction was 54% at 27 mo ($p = 0.009$). A powerful triangular statistic used to analyze the data in MADIT. Although rarely used in cardiac research, this methodology yielded a statistically significant result with the smallest number of patients enrolled. Most of the benefit of the ICD occurred early after implantation.

The 24-mo mortality in the "conventional arm" was high: 32%. This high mortality may reflect a selection bias, as this mortality was greater than expected based on studies of patients who had survived sustained VT or cardiac arrest (*88a*). The MADIT population, as a highly selective referral population, was difficult to quantify. These enrolled patients may therefore not represent all patients who could satisfy the enrollment criteria.

Therapy in the non-ICD ("conventional") group was left to the individual investigator to decide. Thus, there was no true control group. Many standard therapies, including beta-blockers, ACE inhibitors, diuretics, and digoxin were relatively underused in the "conventional" group. Drug therapy, dosing, or monitoring were not controlled or even assessed. In the ICD arm, there was more frequent use of beta-blockers (26% vs 8%).

Despite these limitations, electrophysiologists were quick to embrace the results of MADIT, citing its randomized nature and the magnitude of the benefit. The provocative implications of this trial, however, are tempered by several important considerations:

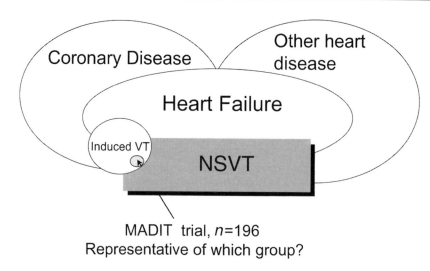

Fig. 8. Venn diagram "identifying" the MADIT patient population.

1) NSVT can be a nonspecific marker; 2) Electrophysiology testing was not shown to enhance patient selection for ICD implantation; and 3) The applicability of these results remains questionable, even in patients with CAD. Nevertheless, the American College of Cardiology/American Heart Association (ACC/AHA) guidelines indicate that a class I indication for an ICD is inducible, nonsuppressible, VT in a patient with NSVT and ischemic cardiomyopathy (90).

The common problem of NSVT in patients with structural heart disease can be a highly visible reminder of risk of death. Although MADIT focused attention on this issue, controversy persists. The high mortality in MADIT may simply reflect the patient selection and enrollment specific to this trial and not represent the larger population of patients who appear to satisfy the enrollment criteria (see Fig. 8). Giorgberidze et al. showed that "MADIT-type" patients have a low mortality if they are simply treated with a beta-blocker and no antiarrhythmic therapy (91).

The Multicenter Unsustained Tachycardia Trial (MUSTT), the second important multicenter NSVT trial, tested the hypothesis that electrophysiology-guided anti-arrhythmic therapy would reduce the risk of sudden cardiac death or cardiac arrest (89). A total of 2,202 patients were enrolled from 85 centers. All had CAD, a LVEF ≤ 0.40, and asymptomatic NSVT. Of the patients enrolled, thirty-two percent (704) had inducible sustained ventricular tachyarrhythmias, and were randomized to anti-arrhythmic therapy (drugs or an ICD) or to no antiarrhythmic therapy. A total of 1,435 patients did not have an inducible sustained tachyarrhythmia and were followed without antiarrhythmic therapy in a registry, as were 63 patients with inducible tachyarrhythmias who refused randomization. Therapy with ACE inhibitors and beta-blockers was recommended for all patients.

Patients designated for no antiarrhythmic therapy had 2-yr and 5-yr rates of cardiac arrest or arrhythmic death of 18% and 32%, respectively. Corresponding rates for patients assigned to electrophysiology test-guided therapy were 12% and 25% ($p = 0.04$). Overall mortality rates for patients assigned to no antiarrhythmic therapy were 28% at 2 yr and 48% at 5 yr, compared with 22% and 42%, respectively, for those assigned to electrophysiology test-guided therapy ($p = 0.06$, *see* Fig. 6B). At 5 yr, the death rate from cardiac causes was significantly higher in the group randomized to no antiarrhythmic therapy, compared with those assigned to electrophysiology test-guided treatment (40% vs 34%, $p = 0.05$). There was no significant difference in the prevalence of spontaneous, sustained VT between the two groups. Inducibility was not associated with the length of the qualifying run of NSVT *(49)*.

The lower incidence of arrhythmic death and cardiac arrest among patients randomized to electrophysiology-guided therapy was attributable entirely to the ICD. There was no specific randomization to ICD, but among patients assigned to electrophysiology-guided therapy who received an ICD because of drug inefficacy, the 5-yr sudden death or cardiac arrest rate was 9%, compared with 37% among those in the group who were treated with antiarrhythmic drugs ($p < 0.001$). The total mortality at 5 yr was 24% among the group receiving an ICD vs 55% among those who did not ($p < 0.001$, *see* Fig. 6C). Thus, all of the benefit in the EP-guided group was attributable to ICD therapy; patients in the EP-guided group who did not receive ICDs fared worse than patients randomized to conventional therapy.

The results of MUSTT confirmed the results of MADIT: patients with CAD, left ventricular dysfunction, asymptomatic NSVT, and inducible sustained VT have a high arrhythmic and total mortality. MUSTT provided evidence that therapy with an ICD, but not with an antiarrhythmic drug, reduces the risk of death. Lingering questions after these studies center on how best to identify patients that will benefit from prophylactic ICD implantation (*see* Fig. 8). Questions include: should screening Holter monitors be performed? If so, how often? Can these results be extrapolated to slightly different populations (e.g., patients who have undergone recent revascularization or those with LVEF of 0.45%)? How should patients with NSVT and non-ischemic cardiomyopathy be managed?

Several ongoing trials are attempting to define other high-risk populations. The Sudden Cardiac Death Heart Failure Trial (SCD-HeFT) is evaluating 2,500 patients with class II or III heart failure and a LVEF of ≤0.35 *(91a)*. This primary prevention placebo-controlled trial is designed to test the hypothesis that an ICD or amiodarone can improve survival in patients already treated with the optimal pharmacologic therapy, including an ACE inhibitor an a beta-blocker. The SCD-HeFT trial has the potential to target a large, less selective high-risk population and with less bias than previous primary prevention trials. While NSVT is not required for enrollment, the actual incidence of NSVT in the study population is likely to be high.

The MADIT II trial is evaluating patients with ischemic cardiomyopathy, New York Heart Association (NYHA) functional class I–III, and LVEF ≤0.30, to test the hypothesis that these patients will have a lower total mortality with an ICD implant *(91b)*. MADIT II is comparing ICD therapy to no specific additional therapy in this high-risk population. No specific Holter or electrophysiology test criteria are required for enrollment, although device-based EPS is performed at the time of ICD implantation in patients randomized to device therapy. Patients who meet MADIT I ICD implant criteria are excluded from MADIT II.

Another trial which may provide clues to the treatment of high-risk patients with NSVT is the DEFINITE (DEFibrillators In Non-Ischemic Cardiomyopathy Treatment Evaluation) trial *(91c)*. This trial tests the hypothesis that an ICD will improve survival in patients with a history of symptomatic CHF non-ischemic dilated cardiomyopathy

(LVEF ≤0.35), and spontaneous ventricular arrhythmias >10 PVCs/h or NSVT documented on telemetry or Holter monitoring). Exclusion criteria include: CAD, symptomatic ventricular arrhythmias, unexplained syncope within the past 6 mo, prior cardiac arrest, NSVT ≥15 beats at a rate ≥120/min, and NYHA functional class IV CHF. All patients will receive standard therapy for CHF, including beta-blockers. One group will receive an ICD. The primary end point is total mortality. Secondary end points include cost-effectiveness, quality-of-life, and cause-specific mortality. There is a 2-yr enrollment with an 18-mo follow-up. The investigators hope to enroll more than 400 patients.

Data from recent clinical trials provide strong evidence that the ICD is useful in patients with NSVT, CAD, impaired ventricular function, and a positive electrophysiology test. This is the only group of patients that should be considered for a prophylactic ICD based on the present data. There is no other group with asymptomatic NSVT for whom prophylaxis with an antiarrhythmic drug or an ICD has been proven to be beneficial. Ongoing trials will define which other patient groups will benefit from prophylactic ICD implantation.

Guidelines for Prophylactic ICD Implantation

In 1998, the joint ACC/AHA task force deemed the MADIT profile a class I indication (evidence and/or general agreement that the ICD is beneficial, useful, and effective) for ICD implantation: *Non-sustained ventricular tachycardia with coronary disease, prior myocardial infarction, left ventricular dysfunction, and inducible ventricular fibrillation or sustsained ventricular tachycardia at electrophysiologic study that is not suppressible by a class I antiarrhythmic drug (90)*. A class IIb indication (conflicting evidence and/or a divergence of opinion with usefulness of the ICD less well-established) includes nonsustained ventricular tachycardia with CAD, prior MI, and left ventricular dysfunction, and inducible sustained VT or VF at EPS *(90)*. The subgroup, like the MADIT population, differs because an antiarrhythmic drug has not been tested. Many electrophysiologists are now performing EPS in patients who fit the MADIT profile, but are implanting ICDs without testing procainamide. The value of drug testing is questionable. Even if a patient responds beneficially to procainamide during electrophysiology testing, there are no data indicating that chronic treatment with procainamide will provide a benefit, or that the patient is at a lower risk than patients who do not respond to procainamide.

A number of situations involving NSVT have been deemed class III indications, such as when an ICD is not indicated *(90)*. These include NSVT amenable to surgical or catheter ablation (e.g., idiopathic right ventricular outflow tract (RVOT) or left ventricular septal tachycardias), NSVT caused by a transient or reversible disorder, patients with a terminal illnesses (projected life expectancy <6 mo) and drug-refractory NYHA functional class IV heart failure in patients who are not candidates for cardiac transplantation. Ironically, patients with profound heart failure, cardiomyopathy, and prolonged QRS duration are the focus of studies with biventricular pacing ICDs, to determine whether this device improves survival rates in these high-risk patients.

Caveats Regarding Prophylactic ICD Therapy

A therapy must be evaluated based on its ability to improve longevity and symptoms, but other variables must also be considered: risk, quality of life, and cost. Many patients

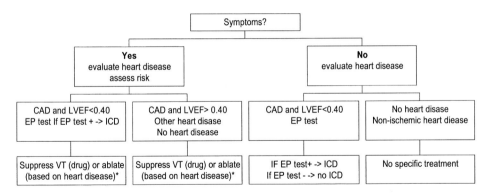

Fig. 9. Algorithm for the management of patients with NSVT.

do not fit clearly into trial inclusion criteria, and extrapolation of study results can be difficult. For example, is it appropriate to evaluate a 90-yr-old with NSVT for prophylactic ICD implantation? Enthusiasm for ICD use has led to attempts to treat patients with more complex medical problems. In such settings, the ICD may or may not prolong overall survival. In some patients, ICD therapy may impair the quality of remaining life without increasing longevity. In addition, patients with multisystem diseases may have problems that complicate the use of the ICD and increase the risk of device implantation.

Quality-of-Life Issues

Although the ICD clearly has the potential to reduce sudden cardiac death and total morbidity in high-risk patients with NSVT, the impact of the ICD on quality of life is not fully understood. Based on a recent review of published studies that address the psychosocial effects of ICDs, Sears et al. concluded that patients who experience high discharge rates, as well as young ICD recipients, appear to be at highest risk for impaired quality of life (92–94). The incidence of psychological disorders, including depression, appears high. Issues include fear of a shock and/or device malfunction, fear of death, and fear of embarrassment. Between 13% and 38% of ICD recipients experience high levels of anxiety, but these studies are not conclusive, and results vary. Additional investigations concerning the effects of ICD therapy on quality of life are needed.

A PRACTICAL APPROACH TO NSVT

Practical clinical issues include patient identification and screening, diagnostic evaluation, and treatment selection (*see* Fig. 9).

Patient Identification

The population which requires aggressive diagnostic and therapeutic interventions includes patients with CAD and impaired left ventricular function. In this patient population, NSVT can reflect a significantly increased mortality risk. At present, the majority of these potentially high-risk patients with NSVT are not being referred for ICD implantation or electrophysiology testing. There are several potential explanations. It is possible that the MADIT and MUSTT trials are perceived as not representing the average patient with CAD impaired left ventricular function, and NSVT, even if ventricular tachycardia was induced in the electrophysiology laboratory. In addition, it is likely that patients who fit the MADIT/MUSTT profile are not being routinely screened for the presence of NSVT.

Screening is not necessarily a straightforward issue. Patients were not routinely screened for inclusion in the MUSTT and MADIT trials, so it is not clear which patients these trials actually represent. The AHA/ACC guidelines for ambulatory monitoring consider a "high-risk" profile to be a class IIb indication for a Holter monitor *(95,96)*. Thus, routine Holter monitoring of high-risk patients has not yet been formally endorsed, although many electrophysiologists recommend this practice.

More frequently, NSVT is identified on an inpatient monitor when a patient is admitted for an acute issue such as exacerbation of CHF, MI, myocardial ischemia, revascularization syncope, surgery, or another issue. NSVT is also identified in outpatients with cardiovascular disease who are undergoing outpatient ambulatory monitoring or treadmill testing. The frequency with which NSVT is documented depends on the aggressiveness of inpatient and outpatient monitoring.

Evaluation of Patients with NSVT

The assessment begins with a history and physical examination to determine the symptoms and detect the potential presence of heart disease. Several questions help to focus the approach:

1) Is the NSVT benign?
2) Are there symptoms attributable to NSVT?
3) Is NSVT caused by a treatable cause?
4) Is there immediate danger to the patient?

It must be determined whether the problem is potentially life-threatening and requires urgent evaluation, or if the NSVT can be managed out of the hospital. The presence of structural heart disease is a key issue that often dictates the urgency of intervention, evaluation, therapy, and the prognostic importance of the arrhythmia.

NSVT Documentation

If available, an ECG recording NSVT provides more information than a rhythm strip. An ECG may help to identify the site of origin of NSVT. Many patients present with palpitations. If patients describe symptoms linked to exertion, an exercise tolerance test is appropriate. If the symptoms are sporadic, but occur daily, a Holter monitor is the approach of choice. An event monitor can help make the diagnosis in a patient with less frequent palpitations. This device comes in two forms: an endless loop recorder worn continuously, which stores information only when activated, or a recorder which is applied intermittently when symptoms occur. An implantable loop recorder (ILR) is now available for less frequent symptoms, although utility in screening for NSVT has not been established. Some ILRs, and even cardiac pacemakers, have automatic recording modes for tachyarrhythmias in addition to patient-activated event storage. A Holter monitor can be used to screen asymptomatic patients.

Further Testing

It is important to evaluate underlying heart disease and to assess the frequency, severity, length and triggers of the episodes. A baseline 12-lead ECG should be analyzed for signs of MI or ischemia, conduction system defects, QT prolongation, ventricular pre-excitation, Brugada's syndrome, or right ventricular dysplasia. A 12-lead ECG of the NSVT, if available, may provide clues about the site of origin of the tachycardia and the prognosis. Idiopathic VT has a characteristic electrocardiographic appearance. A noninvasive assessment of the left and right ventricular function is the next step. An echocardiogram or gated radionuclide ventriculogram are generally appropriate. If right ventricular dysplasia is suspected, however, an angiogram of the right ventricle, MRI, and/or SAECG may be needed.

Assessment for CAD is frequently needed. In patients with normal left ventricular function and presumed idiopathic VT, a nuclear perfusion study is generally adequate. If there is evidence of left ventricular dysfunction, however, coronary angiography is frequently recommended. Revascularization, if indicated, should generally be performed prior to further evaluation of the NSVT.

At present, electrophysiology testing has only been shown to be of benefit in the risk stratification of patients with CAD, reduced left ventricular function, and NSVT. Few data exist supporting the use of electrophysiology testing for risk stratification in patients with other forms of heart disease, or patients with CAD and preserved left ventricular function.

INPATIENT VS OUTPATIENT MANAGEMENT

The role of hospital admission for evaluation of NSVT must be carefully considered. If the patient has significant concurrent problems such as heart failure or angina, hospital admission is required. If an arrhythmia is uncontrollable or uncontrolled, highly symptomatic, frequent, prolonged, rapid, or potentially life-threatening, hospital admission is required. In other patients, electrophysiology testing for risk stratification can generally be performed on an outpatient basis. If radiofrequency ablation is performed for idopathic VT, an observational (23-h) admission is usually adequate.

REFERRAL TO AN ELECTROPHYSIOLOGIST

Any patient with NSVT will need a carefully directed evaluation of both general cardiac issues and the specific arrhythmia. The basic cardiac evaluation can be performed by a general cardiologist, but the management of NSVT should generally be referred to an electrophysiologist. Certainly, if there is impaired (right or left) ventricular function, heart failure, or severe symptoms, if the patient is an athlete, or if the diagnosis is in question (i.e., is it supraventricular or VT), the patient should be referred to an electrophysiologist. Invasive electrophysiology testing and ICD implantation, as well as ICD follow-up, are performed by electrophysiologists. In addition, the use of antiarrhythmic drugs is becoming more complex. Some drugs are now mandated by the FDA to be initiated in the hospital, and there is a movement (by the FDA) to certify doctors in the use of specific antiarrhythmic drugs because of their potential risk. Drug interactions and metabolism must be considered. The risks of torsades de pointes can outweigh any benefit of the drugs in some instances. For these and other reasons, it makes sense to refer to an electrophysiologist any patient in whom antiarrhythmic drug therapy for NSVT is considered.

SPECIFIC CONDITIONS ASSOCIATED WITH NSVT

Acute precipitants of NSVT include MI, cardiac surgery, electrolyte and metabolic abnormalities, antiarrhythmic drugs, QT prolongation, and pulmonary edema. NSVT caused by an acute precipitant often resolves promptly with resolution of the precipitating condition. Chronic treatment depends on the continued presence of the arrhythmia, patient age, heart disease, and symptoms. After patient stabilization and after correction of potential precipitants, evaluation and long-term therapy should be considered if NSVT persists.

Acute Myocardial Infarction

The prognostic significance of NSVT that occurs early after an acute MI remains uncertain (see Fig. 3D). Monomorphic NSVT after acute MI has been reported to occur in as few as 1% and as many as 75% of the patients. In a recent report, 10 ± 6 d after an acute MI, (52) 9% of 325 consecutive patients had NSVT. The predictive value of NSVT increases the further out from MI it occurs. Initially, conservative management is generally indicated: beta-blocker therapy (but not titrated to suppress NSVT), assessment of ischemia, and determination of left ventricular function. Revascularization should be undertaken if indicated. If NSVT persists and impaired left ventricular function (LVEF ≤0.4) is present, electrophysiology testing for risk stratification should be considered. Potential causes of polymorphic NSVT include ischemia, electrolyte disturbance, drug pro-arrhythmia, and coronary reperfusion (see Fig. 3D). Supplementation with magnesium sulfate may reduce ventricular ectopy, but data on improved survival are questionable. Lidocaine, or any antiarrhythmic drug, does not appear to improve survival when given acutely or chronically.

Limited data address the prognostic significance of NSVT in acute infarction. In one study of 112 patients with NSVT within 72 h of an acute MI, in-hospital VF occurred more frequently in the NSVT group (9% vs 0% in the control group; $p < 0.001$), but total mortality during hospitalization and after discharge did not differ significantly (39). Multivariate analysis identified time from presentation to occurrence of NSVT as an important predictor of mortality ($p < 0.0001$). The increased relative risk of NSVT first became significant at 13 h from presentation; this risk increased as the interval from presentation to occurrence of NSVT increased. The risk plateaued at 24 h with a relative risk of 7.5. Contrary to prevailing clinical opinion, NSVT that occurs in the setting of acute MI may have important prognostic significance. Notably, in this group, beta-blocker usage at hospital discharge was also significant predictor of survival ($p < 0.0001$).

Peri-Operative NSVT

In a report of 185 patients with ventricular arrhythmias after coronary-bypass graft (CABG) surgery, 108 had NSVT (97). NSVT did not predict early mortality, and usually disappeared late after the operation. If NSVT is present preoperatively, and the LVEF is ≤0.40, postoperative monitoring for NSVT is recommended. If NSVT persists, a postoperative electrophysiology test should be considered, although recent CABG excluded patients from enrolling in MADIT and MUSTT (98). If noncardiac surgery is planned and NSVT is present, the patient's symptoms, chronicity of the problem, medical regimen, and underlying heart disease should be considered. Ischemia and a progression of cardiac disease should be excluded prior to surgery. If the LVEF is ≤0.40 in the setting of CAD, EP testing should be considered preoperatively. If there is an inducible sustained ventricular tachyarrhythmia, ICD implantation should be considered prior to elective surgery. If there is new-onset NSVT after cardiac surgery, without an acute change in cardiac condition, the prognostic significance is unclear. Beta-blocker therapy may be useful in this setting. In many patients, NSVT resolves spontaneously within 7–14 d. If NSVT persists in the setting of left ventricular dysfunction, an electrophysiology test is indicated, with ICD implantation if positive.

Idiopathic VT

The prognosis is generally excellent in patients with idiopathic VT (IVT). Idiopathic NSVT usually arises from the RVOT (repetitive monomorphic, or exercise-induced) (*see* Fig. 3K) or the left ventricular apical septum ("Bellehassen's" tachycardia) *(98a)*. The 12-lead ECG characterization of the morphology of the NSVT is useful to determine the location of the NSVT if ablative therapy is considered. If NSVT is an incidental finding in a patient with no known heart disease, an appropriate evaluation includes an echocardiogram and a treadmill test. Given the excellent prognosis in the absence of structural heart disease, therapy is usually directed at symptoms. If tachycardia is frequent or incessant, however, patients may be at risk of tachycardia-induced cardiomyopathy, and therapy should be recommended. Idiopathic RVOT tachycardia frequently responds to a beta-blocker, and idiopathic left ventricular VT may be more responsive to verapamil. If ineffective and/or intolerable symptoms occur, other drugs to consider include propafenone or flecainide (second-line), sotalol (third-line), and amiodarone. Ablation is a highly effective therapy for these patients, and should also be considered a first-line therapy. Referral to an electrophysiologist is recommended for these patients. Optimal management of patients with atypical forms of IVT is not clear (*see* Fig. 3I).

Polymorphic VT

Bidirectional or polymorphic NSVT in a young individual, even if there is no apparent heart disease, may be life-threatening (*see* Fig. 3J). Treatment with a beta-blocker may be effective. Similarly, the presence of nonsustained PVT in a patient with congenital LQTS requires initial treatment with a beta-blocker and referral to an electrophysiologist. These patients are now being treated with ICDs more frequently when a significant risk of sudden cardiac death is suspected *(98b)*. Discontinuation of the offending agent, and avoidance of QT-prolonging drugs in the future, are frequently sufficient in patients with acquired LQTS.

Cardiomyopathy

An exacerbation of heart failure can trigger NSVT. Treatment with intravenous (iv) inotropic agents, diuretics, digoxin, and antiarrhythmic drugs may trigger or exacerbate ventricular arrhythmias. Toxid and metabolic disturbances (e.g., hypoxia, hypokalemia, or acidosis) may be contributory. Pharmacologic therapy should be optimized in all of these patients.

CHRONIC ISCHEMIC CARDIOMYOPATHY

NSVT is not rare in patients with ischemic cardiomyopathy (*see* Figs. 2A, 3A). If there are no symptoms, a SAECG or other noninvasive marker (such as TWA or HRV) may give further prognostic information when the ejection fraction is greater than 0.40, but there is no evidence thus far that any therapy—pharmacologic or ICD—will improve the prognosis in this patient group. In general, the noninvasive tests are relatively nonspecific and insensitive. Beta-blockers are recommended unless contraindications exist. If there are severe symptoms associated with NSVT, beta-adrenergic blockers sotalol or amiodarone (started in the hospital) may be needed to suppress frequent recurrences. If the LVEF is <0.40, patients should be referred for electrophysiology testing, with ICD implantation if positive. Screening for NSVT in this cohort is reasonable. It is still premature to suggest that all patients with NSVT, CAD and impaired left ventricular function require ICD implantation.

NON-ISCHEMIC CARDIOMYOPATHY

The best long-term therapy for NSVT in patients with dilated (i.e., nonischemic) cardiomyopathy (*see* Figs. 3B, 3G) is a matter of debate, because of conflicting data. Based on available data, asymptomatic NSVT does not require antiarrhythmic therapy for suppression or protection. Ongoing ICD trials such as DEFINITE may help to define the efficacy of ICD implantation *(91c)* in this setting. Preliminary results of the AMIOVERT trial suggest no benefit to ICD implantation compared with amiodarone *(91d)*. If there are symptomatic episodes of NSVT, empiric treatment with amiodarone is reasonable. This may improve symptoms; the effect on prognosis is unclear. Few data guide the management of patients with infiltrative cardiomyopathies and NSVT.

HYPERTROPHIC CARDIOMYOPATHY

NSVT can potentially forecast a malignant, life-threatening ventricular arrhythmia, and occurs in 10–20% of patients with hypertrophic cardiomyopathy (*see* Fig. 3H). It is premature to suggest that ICD implantation is needed in all asymptomatic patients with hypertrophic cardiomyopathy and NSVT. No specific antiarrhythmic therapy is recommended, but restriction from athletics is mandatory and a beta-adrenergic blocker is the recommended first-line option. Amiodarone has been used in some patients with NSVT. ICD implantation is controversial in this patient population for NSVT, although the trend is to implant "high-risk" patients *(98c)*. Electrophysiology testing is of no proven benefit in this setting. NSVT may indicate higher mortality than patients without VT, but no drug therapy has been proven to improve survival.

RIGHT VENTRICULAR DYSPLASIA

If there are severe symptoms or family history of sudden death, an ICD should be considered. If there are episodes of frequent NSVT, a beta-blocker is an appropriate initial therapy. If symptoms persist, sotalol or amiodarone may be beneficial. The implantation of an ICD may be appropriate, but little data exists.

ACUTE MYOCARDITIS

Few data guide the management of patients with NSVT in the setting of acute myocarditis *(98d)*. The fact that many patients will have significant or even complete recovery of ventricular function tempers enthusiasm for very early ICD implantation.

CONCLUSION

NSVT must be evaluated and treated in order to improve symptoms and to reduce the risk of sudden death. For those patients with severe symptoms, treatment is necessary to reduce or eliminate symptoms; however, most episodes of NSVT are asymptomatic. An asymptomatic patient with ischemic cardiomyopathy and NSVT should be referred to an electrophysiologist for EPS and possible ICD implantation. In all patient groups, antiarrhythmic drug therapy is indicated only to treat symptoms; it should not be expected to prolong survival. Results of ongoing and planned randomized clinical trials will provide useful information on the management of a number of patient groups with NSVT, particularly those with nonischemic cardiomyopathy.

REFERENCES

1. Olshansky B, Gunnar RM. Asymptomatic nonsustained ventricular arrhythmias. Hosp Pract (Off Ed), 1993;28(5):129–132,135–136,139–141.
2. Marinchak RA, Rials SW, Filart RH, et al. The top ten fallacies of nonsustained ventricular tachycardia. Pacing Clin Electrophysiol 1997;20(11):2825–2847.
3. McHenry PL, Fisch C, Jordan JW, et al. Cardiac arrhythmias observed during maximal treadmill exercise testing in clinically normal men. Am J Cardiol 1972;29(3):331–336.
4. Sobotka PA, Mayer JH, Bauernfeind RA, et al. Arrhythmias documented by 24-hour continuous ambulatory electrocardiographic monitoring in young women without apparent heart disease. Am Heart J 1981;101(6):753–759.
5. Brodsky M, Wu D, Denes P, et al. Arrhythmias documented by 24 hour continuous electrocardiographic monitoring in 50 male medical students without apparent heart disease. Am J Cardiol 1997;39(3):390–395.
6. Montague TJ, McPherson DD, MacKenzie BR, et al. Frequent ventricular ectopic activity without underlying cardiac disease: analysis of 45 subjects. Am J Cardiol 1983;52(8):980–984.
7. Fleg JL, Kennedy HL. Cardiac arrhythmias in a healthy elderly population: detection by 24-hour ambulatory electrocardiography. Chest 1982;81(3):302–307.
8. Fleg JL, Lakatta EG. Prevalence and prognosis of exercise-induced nonsustained ventricular tachycardia in apparently healthy volunteers. Am J Cardiol 1984;54(7):762–764.
9. Fleg JL. Ventricular arrhythmias in the elderly: prevalence, mechanisms, and therapeutic implications. Geriatrics 1988;43(12):23–29.
10. Romhilt DW, Chaffin C, Choi SC, et al. Arrhythmias on ambulatory electrocardiographic monitoring in women without apparent heart disease. Am J Cardiol 1984;54(6):582–586.
11. Maskin CS, Siskind SJ, LeJemtel TH. High prevalence of nonsustained ventricular tachycardia in severe congestive heart failure. Am Heart J 1984;107(5 Pt 1):896–901.
12. Meinertz T, Hofmann T, Kasper W, et al. Significance of ventricular arrhythmias in idiopathic dilated cardiomyopathy. Am J Cardiol 1984;53(7):902–907.
13. Meinertz L, Treese N, Kasper W, et al. Determinants of prognosis in idiopathic dilated cardiomyopathy as determined by programmed electrical stimulation. Am J Cardiol 1985;56(4):337–341.
14. Singh SN, Fisher SG, Carson PE, et al. Prevalence and significance of nonsustained ventricular tachycardia in patients with premature ventricular contractions and heart failure treated with vasodilator therapy. Department of Veterans Affairs CHF STAT Investigators. J Am Coll Cardiol 1998;32(4):942–947.
15. Doval HC, Nul DR, Grancelli HO, et al. Randomised trial of low-dose amiodarone in severe congestive heart failure. Grupo de Estudio de la Sobrevida en la Insuficiencia Cardiaca en Argentina (GESICA). Lancet 1994;344(8921):493–498.
16. Doval HC, Nul DR, Grancelli HO, et al. Nonsustained ventricular tachycardia in severe heart failure. Independent marker of increased mortality due to sudden death. GESICA-GEMA Investigators. Circulation 1996;94(12):3198–3203.
17. Campbell RW. Ventricular ectopic beats and non-sustained ventricular tachycardia. Lancet 1993; 341(8858):1454–1458.
18. Bigger JT, Jr. Relation between left ventricular dysfunctioni and ventricular arrhythmias after myocardial infarction. Am J Cardiol 1986;57(3):8B–14B.
19. Maggioni AP, Zuanetti G, Franzosi MG, et al. Prevalence and prognostic significance of ventricular arrhythmias after acute myocardial infarction in the fibrinolytic era. GISSI-2 results. Circulation 1993;87(2):312–322.
20. Brugada P, Andries EW. Early postmyocardial infarction ventricular arrhythmias. Cardiovasc Clin 1992;22(1):165–180.
21. Ruberman W, Weinblatt E, Frank CW, et al. Ventricular premature beats and mortality of men with coronary heart disease. Circulation 1975;52(6 Suppl):III199–III203.

22. Ruberman W, Weinblatt E, Goldberg JD, et al. Ventricular premature beats and mortality after myocardial infarction. N Engl J Med 1977;297(14):750–757.

23. Ruberman W, Weinblatt E, Goldberg JD, et al. Ventricular premature complexes and sudden death after myocardial infarction. Circulation 1981;64(2):297–305.

24. Pogwizd SM, McKenzie JP, Cain ME. Mechanisms underlying spontaneous and induced ventricular arrhythmias in patients with idiopathic dilated cardiomyopathy. Circulation 1998;98(22):2404–2414.

25. Chung MK, Pogwizd SM, Miller DP, et al. Three-dimensional mapping of the initiation of non-sustained ventricular tachycardia in the human heart. Circulation 1997;95(11):2517–2527.

26. Coume P. Polymorphous ventricular tachyarrhythmias in the absence of structural heart disease (editorial). Pacing Clin Electrophysiol 1995;18(4 Pt 1):633–636.

27. Coumel P. Polymorphous ventricular tachyarrhythmias in the absence of structural heart disease. Pacing Clin Electrophysiol 1997;20(8 Pt 2):2065–2067.

28. Coumel P, Jazra C. Ventricular tachyarrhythmias in the absence of structural heart disease. J Med Liban 1999;47(3):178–180.

29. Coumel P, Leclercq JF, Zimmerman M. The clinical use of beta-blockers in the prevention of sudden death. Eur Heart J 1986;7 Suppl A:187–201.

30. Brugada J, Brugada R, Brugada P. Right bundle-branch block and ST-segment elevation in leads V1 through V3: a marker for sudden death in patients without demonstrable structural heart disease. Circulation 1998;97(5):457–460.

31. Roden DM. Torsade de pointes. Clin Cardiol 1993;16(9):683–686.

32. Sanguinetti MC. Long QT syndrome: ionic basis and arrhythmia mechanism in long QT syndrome type 1 (In Process Citation). J Cardiovasc Electrophysiol 2000;11(6):710–712.

33. Roden DM. Ionic mechanisms for prolongation of refractoriness and their proarrhythmic and antiarrhythmic correlates. Am J Cardiol 1996;78(4A):12–16.

34. Antzelevitch C, Sicouri S. Clinical relevance of cardiac arrhythmias generated by afterdepolarizations. Role of M cells in the generation of U waves, triggered activity and torsade de pointes. J Am Coll Cardiol 1994;23(1):259–277.

35. Fleg JL, Kennedy HL. Long-term prognostic significance of ambulatory electrocardiographic findings in apparently healthy subjects greater than or equal to 60 years of age. Am J Cardiol 1992;70(7):748–751.

36. Bikkina M, Larson MG, Levy D. Prognostic implications of asymptomatic ventricular arrhythmias: the Framingham Heart Study (see comments). Ann Intern Med 1992;117(12):990–996.

37. Cullen K, Stenhouse NS, Wearne KL, et al. Electrocardiograms and 13 year cardiovascular mortality in Busselton study. Br Heart J 1982;47(3):209–212.

38. Castelli G, Cinccheri M, Cecchi F, et al. Nonsustained ventricular tachycardia as a predictor for sudden death in patients with idiopathic dilated cardiomyopathy. The role of amiodarone treatment. G Ital Cardiol 1999;29(5):514–523.

39. Cheema AN, Shev K, Parker M, et al. Nonsustained ventricular tachycardia in the setting of acute myocardial infarction: tachycardia characteristics and their prognostic implications. Circulation 1998;98(19):2030–2036.

40. Bjerregaard P, Sorensen KE, Molgaard H. Predictive value of ventricular premature beats for subsequent ischaemic heart disease in apparently healthy subjects. Eur Heart J 1991;12(5):597–601.

41. Abdalla IS, Prineas RJ, Neaton JD, et al. Relation between ventricular premature complexes and sudden cardiac death in apparently healthy men. Am J Cardiol 1987;60(13):1036–1042.

42. Wilber DJ, Kopp D, Olshansky B, et al. Nonsustained ventricular tachycardia and other high-risk predictors following myocardial infarction: implications for prophylactic automatic implantable cardioverter-defibrillator use. Prog Cardiovasc Dis 1993;36(3):179–194.

43. Gardner RA, Kruyer WB, Pickard JS, et al. Nonsustained ventricular tachycardia in 193 U.S. military aviators: long-term follow-up (In Process Citation). Aviat Space Environ Med 2000;71(8):783–790.

44. Kostis JB, Byington R, Friedman LM, et al. Prognostic significance of ventricular ectopic activity in survivors of acute myocardial infarction. J Am Coll Cardiol 1987;10(2):231–242.

45. Packer M. Lack of relation between ventricular arrhythmias and sudden death in patients with chronic heart failure. Circulation 1992;85(1 Suppl):150–156.

46. Chakko S, de Marchena E, Kessler KM, et al. Ventricular arrhythmias in congestive heart failure. Clin Cardiol 1989;12(9):525–530.

47. Singh SN, Carson PE, Fisher SG. Nonsustsained ventricular tachycardia in severe heart failure. Circulation 1997;96(10):3794–3795.

47a. Mortara A, LaRovere MT, Pinna GD, et al. Depressed arterial baroreflex sensitivity and not reduced heart rate variability identifies patients with chronic heart failure and nonsustained ventricular tachycardia: the effect of high ventricular filling pressure. Am Heart J 1997;134:879–888.

48. Vismara LA, Amsterdam EA, Mason DT. Relation of ventricular arrhythmias in the late hospital phase of acute myocardial infarction to sudden death after hospital discharge. Am J Med 1975;59(1):6–12.

49. Buxton AE, et al. Nonsustained ventricular tachycardia in coronary artery disease: relation to inducible sustained ventricular tachycardia. MUSTT Investigators. Ann Intern Med 1996;125(1):35–39.

50. Buxton AE, Duc J, Berger EE, Torres V. Nonsustained ventricular tachycardia. Cardiol Clin 2000; 18(2):327–336,

51. Buxton AE, Hafley GE, Lehmann MH, et al. Prediction of sustained ventricular tachycardia inducible by programmed stimulation in patients with coronary artery disease. Utility of clinical variables. Circulation 1999;99(14):1843–1850.

52. Hohnloser SH, Klingenheben T, Zabel M, et al. Prevalence, characteristics and prognostic value during long-term follow-up of nonsustained ventricular tachycardia after myocardial infarction in the thrombolytic era. J Am Coll Cardiol 1999;33(7):1895–1902.

53. Spirito P, Rayezzi C, Autore C, et al. Prognosis of asymptomatic patients with hypertrophic cardiomyopathy and nonsustained ventricular tachycardia. Circulation 1994;90(6):2743–2747.

54. Henry RL, Kennedy GT, Crawford MH. Prognostic value of exercise-induced ventricular ectopic activity for mortality after acute myocardial infarction. Am J Cardiol 1987;59(15):1251–1255.

55. Faris JV, McHenry PW, Jordan JW, et al. Prevalence and reproducibility of exercise-induced ventricular arrhythmias during maximal exercise testing in normal men. Am J Cardiol 1976;37(4):618–622.

56. Hoch DH, Rosenfeld LE. Tachycardias of right ventricular origin. Cardiol Clin 1992;10(1):151–164.

57. Yli-Mayry S, Huikury HV, Korhonen VR, et al. Prevalence and prognostic significance of exercise-induced ventricular arrhythmias after coronary artery bypass grafting. Am J Cardiol 1990;66(20):1451–1454.

58. McHenry PL, Morris SN, Kavalier M. Exercise-induced arrhythmias—recognition, classification, and clinical significance. Cardiovasc Clin 1974;6(1):245–254.

59. McHenry PL, Morris SN, Kavalier M, et al. Comparative study of exercise-induced ventricular arrhythmias in normal subjects and patients with documented coronary artery disease. Am J Cardiol 1976;37(4):609–616.

60. Lerman BB, Stein K, Engelstein ED, et al. Mechanism of repetitive monomorphic ventricular tachycardia. Circulation 1995;92(3):421–429.

61. Proclemer A, Ciani R, Feruglio GA. Right ventricular tachycardia with left bundle branch block and inferior axis morphology: clinical and arrhythmological characteristics in 15 patients. Pacing Clin Electrophysiol 1989;12(6):977–989.

62. Ritchie AH, Kerr CR, Qi A, et al. Nonsustained ventricular tachycardia arising from the right ventricular outflow tract. Am J Cardiol 1989;64(10):594–598.

62a. Zipes DP, Garson A Jr. 26th Bethesda conference: recommendations for determining eligibility for competition in athletes with cardiovascular abnormalities. Task Force 6: arrhythmias. J Am Coll Cardiol 1994;24:892–899.

63. Grimm W, Hoffmann J, Menz V, et al. Programmed ventricular stimulation for arrhythmia risk prediction in patients with idiopathic dilated cardiomyopathy and nonsustained ventricular tachycardia. J Am Coll Cardiol 1998;32(3):739–745.

64. Stamato NJ, O'Connell JB, Murdock DK, et al. The response of patients with complex ventricular arrhythmias secondary to dilated cardiomyopathy to programmed electrical stimulation. Am Heart J 1986;112(3):505–508.

65. Spielman SR, Greenspan AM, Kay HR, et al. Electrophysiologic testing in patients at high risk for sudden cardiac death. I. Nonsustained ventricular tachycardia and abnormal ventricular function. J Am Coll Cardiol 1985;6(1):31–40.

66. Hammill SC, Trusty JM, Wood DL, et al. Influence of ventricular function and presence or absence of coronary artery disease on results of electrophysiologic testing for asymptomatic nonsustained ventricular tachycardia. Am J Cardiol 1990;65(11):722–728.

67. Turitto G, Fontaine JM, Ursell S, et al. Risk stratification and management of patients with organic heart disease and nonsustained ventricular tachycardia: role of programmed stimulation, left ventricular ejection fraction, and the signal-averaged electrocardiogram. Am J Med 1990;88(IN):35N–41N.

68. Manolis AS, Estes NAD. Value of programmed ventricular stimulation in the evaluation and management of patients with nonsustained ventricular tachycardia associated with coronary artery disease. Am J Cardiol 1990;65(3):201–205.

69. Furukawa T, Rozanski JJ, Moroe K, et al. Predictors of sustained ventricular tachycardia inducibility in patients with nonsustained ventricular tachycardia and chronic artery disease. Am Heart J 1989;117(5):1050–1059.

70. Kim SG, Mercando AD, Fisher JD. Comparison of the characteristics of nonsustained ventricular tachycardia on Holter monitoring and sustained ventricular tachycardia observed spontaneously or induced by programmed stimulation. Am J Cardiol 1987;60(4):288–292.

71. Buxton AE, Marchlinski FE, Flores BT, et al. Nonsustained ventricular tachycardia in patients with coronary artery disease: role of electrophysiologic study. Circulation 1987;75(6):1178–1185.

72. Sulpizi AM, Friehling TD, Kowey PR. Value of electrophysiologic testing in patients with non-sustained ventricular tachycardia. Am J Cardiol 1987;59(8):841–845.

73. Veltri EP, Platin EV, Griffith LS, et al. Programmed electrical stimulation and long-term follow-up in asymptomatic, nonsustained ventricular tachycardia. Am J Cardiol 1985;56(4):309–314.

74. Wilber DJ, Olshansky B, Moran JF, et al. Electrophysiological testing and nonsustained ventricular tachycardia. Use and limitations in patients with coronary artery disease and impaired ventricular function. Circulation 1990;82(2):350–358.

75. Hernandez M, Taylor J, Marinchak R, et al. Outcome of patients with nonsustained ventricular tachycardia and severely impaired ventricular function who have negative electrophysiologic studies. Am Heart J 1995;129(3):492–496.

76. Buxton AE, Lee KL, DiCarlo L, et al. Electrophysiologic testing to identify patients with coronary artery disease who are at risk for sudden death. Multicenter Unsustained Tachycardia Trial Investigators. N Engl J Med 2000;342(26):1937–1945.

77. Kowey PR, Taylor JE, Marinchak RA, et al. Does programmed stimulation really help in the evaluation of patients with nonsustained ventricular tachycardia? Results of a meta-analysis. Am Heart J 1992;123(2):481–485.

78. Yap YG, Camm AJ. Lessons from antiarrhythmic trials involving class III antiarrhythmic drugs. Am J Cardiol 1999;84(9A):83R–89R.

79. Waldo AL, Lamm AJ, de Ruyter H, et al. Effect of d-sotalol on mortality in patients with left ventricular dysfunction after recent and remote myocardial infarction. The SWORD Investigators. Survival With Oral d-Sotalol (published erratum appears in Lancet 1996 Aug 10;348(9024):416). Lancet 1996;348(9019):7–12.

80. Echt DS, Liebson PR, Mitchell LB, et al. Mortality and morbidity in patients receiving encainide, flecainide, or placebo. The Cardiac Arrhythmia Suppression Trial. N Engl J Med 1991;324(12):781–788.

81. Naccarelli GV, Wolbrette DL, Dell'Orfano JT, et al. Amiodarone: what have we learned from clinical trials? Clin Cardiol 2000;23(2):73–82.

82. Farre J, Romero J, Rubio JM, et al. Amiodarone and prevention of sudden death: critical review of a decade of clinical trials. Am J Cardiol 1999;83(5B):55D–63D.

83. Preliminary report: effect of encainide and flecainide on mortality in a randomized trial of arrhythmia suppression after myocardial infarction. The Cardiac Arrhythmia Suppression Trial (CAST) Investigators. N Engl J Med 1989;321(6):406–412.

84. Effect of the antiarrhythmic agent moricizine on survival after myocardial infarction. The Cardiac Arrhythmia Suppression Trial II Investigators. N Engl J Med 1992;327(4):227–233.

85. Cairns JA, Connolly SJ, Roberts R, Gent M. Randomised trial of outcome after myocardial infarction in patients with frequent or repetitive ventricular premature depolarisations. CAMIAT. Lancet 1997;349:675–682.

86. Julian DG, Camm AJ, Frangin G, et al. Randomised trial of effect of amiodarone on mortality in patients with left-ventricular dysfunction after recent myocardial infarction: EMIAT. Lancet 1997;349:667–674.

87. Burkart E, Pfisterer M, Kiowski W, et al. Effect of antiarrhythmic therapy on mortality in survivors of myocardial infarction with asymptomatic complex ventricular arrhythmias: Basel Antiarrhythmic Study of Infarct Survival (BASIS). J Am Coll Cardiol 1990;16(7):1711–1718.

87a. Amiodarone Trials Meta-Analysis Investigators. Effect of prophylactic amiodarone on mortality after acute myocardial infarction and in congestive heart failure: Meta-analysis of individual data from 6500 patients in randomised trials. Lancet 1997;350:1417–1424.

87b. Boutitie F, Boissel JP, Connolly SJ, et al. Amiodarone interaction with beta-blockers: analysis of the merged EMIAT (European Myocardial Infarct Amiodarone Trial) and CAMIAT (Canadian Amiodarone Myocardial Infarction Trial) databases. The EMIAT and CAMIAT Investigators. Circulation 1999;99:2268–2275.

88. Moss AJ, Hall WJ, Cannorm DS, et al. Improved survival with an implanted defibrillator in patients with coronary disease at high risk for ventricular arrhythmia. Multicenter Automatic Defibrillator Implantation Trial Investigators (see comments). N Engl J Med 1996;335(26):1933–1940.

88a. AVID Investigators. A comparison of antiarrhythmic-drug therapy with implantable defibrillators in patients resuscitated from near-fatal ventricular arrhythmias. The Antiarrhythmics versus Implantable Defibrillators (AVID) Investigators. N Engl J Med 1997;337:1576–1583.

89. Buxton AE, Lee KL, Fisher JD, et al. A randomized study of the prevention of sudden death in patients with coronary artery disease. Multicenter Unsustained Tachycardia Trial Investigators (published erratum appears in N Engl J Med 2000 Apr 27;342(17):1300). N Engl J Med 1999;341(25):1882–1890.

90. Gregoratos G, Cheitlin MD, Conill A, et al. ACC/AHA Guidelines for Implantation of Cardiac Pacemakers and Antiarrhythmia Devices: Executive Summary—a report of the American College of Cardiology/American Heart Association Task Force on Practice Guidelines (Committee on Pacemaker Implantation). Circulation 1998;97(13):1325–1335.

91. Giorgberidze I, Saksena S, Krol RB, et al. Risk stratification and clinical outcome of minimally symptomatic and asymptomatic patients with nonsustained ventricular tachycardia and coronary disease: a prospective single-center study. Am J Cardiol 1997;80(5B):3F–9F.

91a. Klein H, Auricchio A, Reek S, Geller C. New primary prevention trials of sudden cardiac death in patients with left ventricular dysfunction. SCD-HeFT and MADIT-II. Am J Cardiol 1999;83:91D–97D.

91b. Moss AJ, Cannom DS, Daubert JP, et al. Multicentre automatic defibrillator implantation trial II (MADIT II). Ann Noninvas Electrocardiol 1999;4:83–91.

91c. Kadish A, Quigg R, Schaechter A, Anderson KP, Estes M, Levine J. Defibrillators in nonischemic cardiomyopathy treatment evaluation. PACE 2000;23:338–343.

91d. Strickberger SA. Presentation at American Heart Association Scientific Sessions 2000, New Orleans, LA.

92. Sears SF, Jr, Conti JB, Curtis AB, et al. Affective distress and implantable cardioverter defibrillators: cases for psychological and behavioral interventions. Pacing Clin Electrophysiol 1999;22(12):1831–1834.

93. Sears SF, Jr, Todaro JF, Lewis TF, et al. Examining the psychosocial impact of implantable cardioverter defibrillators: a literature review. Clin Cardiol 1999;22(7):481–489.

94. Sears SF, Todaro JF, Vrizar G, et al. Assessing the psychosocial impact of the ICD: a national survey of implantable cardioverter defibrillator health care providers. Pacing Clin Electrophysiol 2000;23(6):939–945.

95. Crawford MH, Bernstein SJ, Veedwania PC, et al. ACC/AHA guidelines for ambulatory electrocardiography: executive summary and recommendations. A report of the American College of Cardiology/American Heart Association task force on practice guidelines (committee to revise the guidelines for ambulatory electrocardiography). Circulation 1999;100(8):886–893.

96. Crawford MH, Bernstein SJ, Deedwania PC, et al. ACC/AHA Guidelines for Ambulatory Electrocardiography. A report of the American College of Cardiology/American Heart Association Task Force on Practice Guidelines (Committee to Revise the Guidelines for Ambulatory Electrocardiography). Developed in collaboration with the North American Society for Pacing and Electrophysiology. J Am Coll Cardiol 1999;34(3):912–918.

97. Pinto RP, Romerill DB, Nasser WK, et al. Prognosis of patients with frequent premature ventricular complexes and nonsustained ventricular tachycardia after coronary artery bypass graft surgery. Clin Cardiol 1996;19(4):321–324.

98. Olshansky B. Ventricular arrhythmias and the use of antiarrhythmic drugs after cardiovascular surgery. Am J Manag Care 1998;4(11):1603–1610; quiz 1611–1612.

98a. Iwai S, Lerman BB. Management of ventricular tachycardia in patients with clinically normal hearts. Curr Cardiol Rep 2000;2:515–521.

98b. Moss AJ, Zareba W, Hall WJ, et al. Effectiveness and limitations of beta-blocker therapy in congenital long-QT syndrome. Circulation 2000;101:616–23.

98c. Maron BJ, Shen WK, Link MS, et al. Efficacy of implantable cardioverter-defibrillators for the prevention of sudden death in parents with hypertrophic cardiomyopathy. N Engl J Med 2000;342:365–373.

98d. Feldman AM, McNamara D. Myocarditis. N Engl J Med 2000;343:1388–1393.

14 Indications for Implantable Cardioverter Defibrillators

Current and Emerging

Richard N. Fogoros, MD

CONTENTS

INTRODUCTION
WHY INDICATIONS FOR THE ICD HAVE BEEN CONTROVERSIAL
RANDOMIZED TRIALS WITH THE ICD
ACCEPTED INDICATIONS FOR THE ICD
REFERENCES

INTRODUCTION

Although the implantable cardioverter defibrillator (ICD) has been in clinical use for nearly 20 years, the appropriate indications for this device—and how we arrive at those indications—remain controversial. The controversy has nothing to do with how well the device works, since the ICD has long been known to be extremely effective in its goal: to automatically terminate life-threatening ventricular arrhythmias.

Instead, the controversy stems from three general factors: the relative expense and inconvenience of using the ICD as opposed to other available therapies; confusion as to the most appropriate definition of "efficacy" for this device; and until relatively recently, the widespread notion that insufficient data existed to document the efficacy of the ICD.

This chapter reviews the present and emerging indications for the ICD. Before discussing the indications, however, we must first address the three general factors that render these indications controversial.

WHY INDICATIONS FOR THE ICD HAVE BEEN CONTROVERSIAL

The Expense and Inconvenience of ICDs

There would be little controversy over its clinical indications if the ICD were relatively cheap and easy to use. The ICD, however, is very expensive. The hardware itself costs between $15,000 and $30,000 (US), and the total cost of implanting the defibrillator system often exceeds $40,000.

From: *Contemporary Cardiology: Management of Cardiac Arrhythmias*
Edited by: L. I. Ganz © Humana Press Inc., Totowa, NJ

Furthermore, despite improvements in implantation techniques over the past 15 years, neither the implantation of the device nor the long-term management of its recipients are simple endeavors. Device selection, lead placement, intra-operative and postoperative testing, optimal programming of the device, follow-up, and troubleshooting all remain very complex (much more than for permanent pacemakers, for instance), and yet critically important tasks. Physicians who have not dedicated themselves to the treatment of complex arrhythmias and the use of antitachycardia devices are unlikely to have favorable results in managing patients with ICDs.

Both the expense and the continued complexity of the ICD create a persistent inclination among policymakers and physicians alike to seek alternative therapies, even when a suitable alternative may not exist. Thus, it has been relatively difficult to establish and expand the formal indications for use of this device.

Confusion as to the Most Appropriate Definition of "Efficacy"

Progress in establishing firm indications for the ICD has been hindered by a disagreement among electrophysiologists as to what constitutes "efficacy" for this device.

When the ICD first came into clinical use in the early 1980s, its efficacy seemed entirely obvious to most physicians. Both in laboratory testing and in the clinical arena, the defibrillator quickly proved itself to be extremely efficient at automatically recognizing and terminating ventricular tachyarrhythmias. Most clinicians who implanted defibrillators in more than a handful of patients rapidly saw firsthand examples of the life-saving capabilities of these devices. The ability of the ICD to prevent sudden death became immediately and dramatically obvious.

For early proponents of the ICD, it came as something of a surprise when, at the end of the 1980s, the efficacy of this device was challenged by serious and well-respected electrophysiologists (1–2).

The challenge went something like this: Although the ICD indeed prevents sudden death by terminating ventricular arrhythmias, that does not necessarily mean it also prolongs overall survival. Until well-designed studies show that the ICD significantly improves overall survival and prevents sudden death, its efficacy remains an open question.

The confusion created by this new definition of efficacy assured that, for much of the next decade, the indications for the ICD remained controversial.

There is no doubt that prolongation of overall survival is the outcome that must concern us the most. After all, it does little good to prevent sudden death if doing so fails to yield an overall survival benefit. Yet, although this is true, prolongation of overall survival nonetheless does *not* define the efficacy of the ICD.

The confusion in defining efficacy arises from mixing the concept of efficacy with that of outcome. The *outcome* one achieves with any treatment in medicine is different from the *efficacy* of that treatment. Penicillin is effective in treating infections with many gram-positive cocci. Yet, giving penicillin to a patient who has pseudomonas sepsis—despite the efficacy of the drug when it is used appropriately—will yield a poor outcome. This poor outcome does not mean the drug itself is inherently "ineffective"—it merely means that we have used it badly. We have achieved a poor outcome through our inappropriate use of this effective drug. The question when using penicillin is not whether the drug is effective in people with infections, but in which people with infections will this effective drug give us the outcome we desire?

Similarly, the ICD is designed to terminate ventricular arrhythmias and thus to prevent sudden death. It is demonstrably effective in doing this. The fact that we also want to prolong overall survival (i.e., the fact that we desire a particular outcome) simply means that we must pay attention to how we use it.

The relationship of the defibrillator's ability to prevent sudden death to its ability to prolong overall survival (i.e., the relationship between efficacy and outcome) can be stated as an axiom, the Axiom of Overall Survival *(3)*: *In a given population of patients followed over time* t, *the implantable cardioverter defibrillator will measurably prolong overall survival as long as the risk of sudden death from ventricular tachyarrhythmias is sufficiently greater than the risk of death from all other causes combined.*

In other words, the ability of the ICD to prolong overall survival depends, completely and solely, on the population of patients in which it is used. Despite the proven efficacy of the device, the outcome will be unfavorable if either of two conditions is not met: that is, if the risk of sudden death is not high, or the risk of death from other causes is not low.

Fig. 1 illustrates how the outcome with the ICD depends entirely on the risk of sudden death (dark circles) and the risk of death from all other causes (white circles) in the population receiving the device.

Population 1 is analogous to the population at large. In this population, over time *t,* the risk of both sudden death and death from all other causes is low. Implanting defibrillators in such a population will not have a measurable effect on overall survival—survival will be good with or without the defibrillator.

Patients in Population 2 carry a high risk of sudden death (over time *t*) but a relatively low risk of death from other causes. This sort of risk profile may be seen, for instance, in patients who present with ventricular fibrillation (VF) in the face of normal or near-normal cardiac function. In such patients, eliminating the risk of sudden death with the ICD would significantly reduce overall mortality and improve overall survival over time *t.*

In Population 3, the risk of sudden death is also quite substantial. However, the risk of death from other causes is even higher—and furthermore, the risks overlap, so that death is likely over time *t* even if sudden death can be prevented. Although an ICD may prevent numerous episodes of sudden death, overall survival may not be measurably improved. Patients with severe end-stage cardiac disease may fit into such a risk profile.

Population 4 represents the group of patients frequently referred to electrophysiologists, either for evaluation of arrhythmia risk or management of documented arrhythmia. This population has varying degrees of risk and varying securities of underlying structural heart disease and comorbid conditions. The effect of the defibrillator on overall survival depends specifically on which patients are selected for implantation in this heterogeneous population.

These examples graphically illustrate how the ability of the ICD to prolong overall survival (the outcome one obtains with the device) is intrinsically dependent on the population in which the device is used, and not on the device itself.

Therefore, if a clinical trial fails to show a benefit in overall survival with the ICD this result simply indicates a failure to apply the defibrillator to a population of patients who meet the two criteria given by the Axiom of Overall Survival. Conversely, a clinical trial that does show an overall survival benefit does not "prove" the efficacy of the ICD itself. Instead, it merely indicates that a population of patients who meet

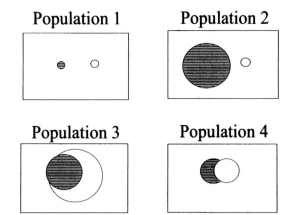

Fig. 1. The dark circles represent the risk of sudden death, and the white circles represent the risk of death from all other causes, over time t. Time t is represented by the area of the rectangle.

In Population 1, the risks of both sudden death and death from all other causes over time t are relatively small. In Population 1, the ICD would not measurably improve overall survival. The risk profile of Population 1 is representative of the population at large.

In Population 2, the risk of sudden death over time t is relatively large, and is substantially larger than the risk of death from all other causes. The ICD would significantly improve overall survival in this population over time t. Population 2 represents survivors of cardiac arrest whose electrical disease predominates over their structural heart disease.

In Population 3, the risk of sudden death is also high (similar to Population 2). But here, the risk of non-sudden death is even higher, and the two risks largely overlap. The area in which the circles overlap represents patients at high risk for both sudden death and non-sudden death. While implantation of a defibrillator would undoubtedly prevent many instances of sudden death in Population 3, overall survival for the group would not be measurably improved. Population 3 represents many patients with end-stage cardiac disease.

Although Populations 1–3 represent idealized subsets of patients, Population 4 is representative of the heterogeneous group of patients commonly referred to electrophysiologists for documented or suspected ventricular tachyarrhythmias. These patients have varying degrees of arrhythmias (and thus a spectrum of risks for sudden death), and also varying degrees of underlying cardiac and other organic disease (and thus a spectrum of risks for non-sudden death). The effect of the ICD on overall survival in Population 4 would depend on which patients in this group were "selected" to receive the device.

the criteria given by the Axiom has been successfully identified. In other words, clinical trials with the ICD are not actually measuring the efficacy of the device at all (since that efficacy was established long ago). Instead, they are simply measuring the efficiency of patient selection—the clinical outcome achieved when the ICD is used in selected populations of patients.

Unfortunately, because of the confusion over the definition of efficacy, electrophysiologists spent much of the 1990s trying to "prove" the efficacy of the defibrillator, instead of working to identify subsets of patients who would benefit from this remarkably effective device. Progress in firmly establishing indications for the ICD has thus been delayed.

Perceived Inadequacy of Data Documenting the Efficacy of the ICD

To those who entered the 1990s assuming the efficacy of the ICD had been firmly established by its unquestioned ability to prevent sudden death, the indications for using this device seemed relatively clear. Namely, (and in accordance with the Axiom), these individuals sought to offer the defibrillator to patients whose risk for arrhythmic sudden death was substantially increased, and whose risk for early death from other causes appeared low. For these clinicians, deciding whether an ICD was likely to be beneficial was simply a matter of estimating the relative risks for sudden death and death from other causes.

These clinicians were quite taken aback when several very prominent electrophysiologists—well-known experts in the field—demurred on this point of view, publicly stating that there was no useful data demonstrating the efficacy of the ICD and furthermore, the only way to get such data would be to conduct randomized clinical trials. Only when randomized trials demonstrated that the defibrillator prolonged the overall survival of its recipients could the device be said to be effective (1–2).

We have already addressed the point that defining "efficacy" of the defibrillator in this way is incorrect. Now added to this mistaken premise was the assertion that to demonstrate such efficacy, only data from randomized clinical trials could be considered.

This assertion, since it claimed the scientific high ground, carried the day. Accordingly, randomized trials with the ICD were organized, and during the 1990s considerable efforts were devoted to conducting these trials with the full support of the government, industry, and professional organizations.

Some of these trials have added materially to our ability to use the ICD effectively. Others (in the author's opinion) served only to confuse clinicians, for much of the 1990s, in regard to acceptable indications for the ICD.

It is important to consider how randomized trials with the ICD may not always be useful. Consider a clinical trial in which all patients who have survived a cardiac arrest are randomized to receive either the ICD or drug therapy. Such an indiscriminately selected group of subjects is likely to include individuals from each of Populations 1, 2, and 3 (Fig. 1). Taken as a group, the risk profile of this composite population will probably resemble Population 4 (Fig. 1). These patients will have varying degrees of arrhythmic risk, and varying degrees of underlying cardiac disease (and thus varying risks of death from nonarrhythmic causes). Taken as a group, there will be a relatively high risk of sudden death, a relatively high risk of death from all other causes, and a relatively high overlap between the risks.

Will the ICD significantly prolong survival in such a clinical trial? The answer depends on the precise mixture of patients from the heterogeneous population eligible for this trial that is finally selected for enrollment. If enrolled patients include a fairly high proportion of individuals from Population 2, overall survival will be prolonged for the group. But if enrolled patients include a fairly high proportion of individuals from Population 3, overall survival may not be prolonged. A positive outcome will depend solely on whether a sufficient proportion of patients from Population 2 are enrolled by design, by chance, or by covert preselection.

Depending on the variables of study design and of patient selection, the results easily come out either way, and either way, the study will tell us nothing about the efficacy of the ICD. Worse, since what this trial would tell us is merely the effect of using the ICD indiscriminately, its outcome would be of little practical use.

Since randomized trials with the ICD only give us outcome data—they merely tell us how well we are using this highly effective tool—to be useful such trials should be designed to measure the efficacy of the defibrillator on reasonably well-defined and

Table 1
Secondary Prevention Trials With the ICD

	Patient population	Test-group therapy	Control-group therapy	Survival benefit with ICD
Utrecht	Survivors of cardiac arrest	ICD	"Conventional therapy"	Yes, improvement in overall survival
AVID	Life-threatening sustained ventricular tachyarrhythmias	ICD	Amiodarone or sotalol	Yes, improvement in overall survival
CASH	Survivors of cardiac arrest	ICD	1 of 3 drug treatment arms	Yes, improvement in overall survival
CIDS	Sustained ventricular tachyarrhythmias	ICD	Amiodarone	Yes, trend toward improvement in overall survival

Utrecht = Utrecht study; AVID = Antiarrhythmics vs Implantable Defibrillator trial; CASH = Cardiac Arrest Study—Hamburg; CIDS = Canadian Implantable Defibrillator Study.

circumscribed populations of patients. The randomized trials that have done this have proven very helpful in defining the indications for this device.

RANDOMIZED TRIALS WITH THE ICD

Secondary Prevention Trials

Secondary prevention trials enroll patients who have already presented with a life-threatening ventricular arrhythmia. These patients, since they have already "declared" themselves to be prone to such arrhythmias, tend to have a very high risk of recurrent tachyarrhythmias, and therefore a high risk of sudden death.

These, of course, are the very patients whom the ICD is most likely to help. They usually fall into Population 2, unless the extent of their underlying heart disease pushes them into Population 3. According to the Axiom, deciding whether to implant a defibrillator should be based not on the results of a randomized trial, but on the clinician's assessment of whether a particular patient is likely to survive for a substantial period of time if sudden death can be prevented.

Nonetheless, four large, randomized secondary prevention trials are now in progress. These trials are summarized in Table 1.

THE UTRECHT STUDY

The first such trial was published in 1995 by Wever et al. *(4)*. These investigators randomized 60 consecutive patients who had survived cardiac arrest to either therapy with the ICD or to "conventional therapy" in accordance with a relatively complex treatment algorithm (typical for the times) that incorporated drugs, catheter ablation, and map-guided surgical ablation. Subjects randomized to conventional therapy could also receive the ICD but only as a last resort. Eventually, almost half of the control patients in this trial received defibrillators.

After a mean follow-up of 27 mo, only 14% of the patients randomized to receive the ICD died, compared to 35% of patients treated with the conventional strategy ($p = 0.02$). These results, although impressive, did not have much impact on clinical practice.

The Antiarrhythmics vs Implantable Defibrillator (AVID) Trial

For many, the question of whether the ICD prolongs survival when used as secondary prophylaxis was finally answered by the AVID trial (5). AVID was a large, multicenter (NIH)-sponsored study that enrolled 1016 patients who had experienced sustained ventricular tachyarrhythmias. Patients were randomized to receive either the ICD or antiarrhythmic drug therapy (with either amiodarone or sotalol). The primary end point of the study was overall mortality.

The results of AVID showed the overall survival among patients randomized to the ICD to be 89.3% at 1 yr, compared to 82.3% in the drug-treated patients. At 2 yr, survival was 81.6% for the defibrillator vs 74.7% for drug therapy; and at 3 yr those values were 75.4% vs 64.1% respectively. The corresponding reductions in mortality with the ICD (with 95% confidence limits) at 1,2, and 5 yr was $39 \pm 20\%$, $27 \pm 21\%$, and $31 \pm 21\%$. It is notable, however, that the average duration of benefit (extension of survival) conferred by the defibrillator in this trial was less than 3 mo. Fig. 2 shows the actuarial survival of the defibrillator group and the control group in the AVID trial.

Although AVID generated significant controversy within the electrophysiology community (6–7), this trial has clearly had a significant impact on clinical practice. With the publication of results from the AVID trial, the ICD became rapidly accepted as the treatment of first choice for survivors of cardiac arrest.

Cardiac Arrest Study—Hamburg (CASH)

CASH, a study conducted in Hamburg, Germany, examined the early use of the ICD in survivors of tachyarrhythmic cardiac arrest (8). In this trial, 346 survivors of cardiac arrest were randomly assigned to one of four treatment arms—amiodarone, metoprolol, propafenone, or the ICD. The propafenone arm of the study, however, was dropped in 1993 because of excess mortality in patients randomized to this drug. The results from the three remaining arms of the study were finally reported at the 1998 Scientific Sessions of the American College of Cardiology (ACC) and then recently published (9). The results were favorable to the ICD.

At a mean follow-up of 57 ± 34 mo, the overall mortality reported for patients randomized to the ICD was 36.4%, compared to 44.4% for patients who were medically managed with either amiodarone or metoprolol ($p = 0.081$). There was also a significant reduction in sudden death with the ICD (13.0% vs 33.0%, $p <0.005$).

The Canadian Implantable Defibrillator Study (CIDS)

CIDS was another randomized, multicenter clinical trial designed to test whether the ICD prolongs overall survival when used as secondary prophylaxis (10). More than 600 patients presenting with sustained ventricular tachyarrhythmias were randomized to receive either the ICD or amiodarone. The results of this trial were presented at the 1998 Scientific Sessions of the ACC, and recently published (11).

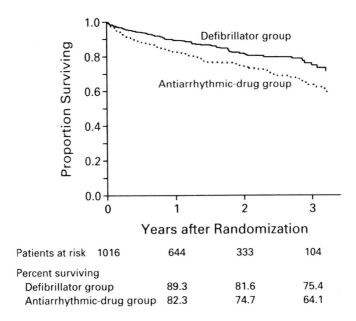

Fig. 2. AVID trial results: Actuarial survival curves for patients treated with the ICD and for patients treated with antiarrhythmic drugs in the AVID trial. There is a small but statistically significant increase in survival in the defibrillator group. (From: The Antiarrhythmics Versus Implantable Defibrillator (AVID) Investigators. A comparison of antiarrhythmic-drug therapy with ICDs in patients resuscitated from near-fatal ventricular arrhythmias. N Engl J Med 1997;337:1576–1583. Copyright © 1997 Massachusetts Medical Society.)

The results of CIDS failed to reach statistical significance, but were still consistent with the other secondary prophylaxis trials. After 3 yr of follow-up, patients who were randomized to receive the ICD had a 25% overall mortality, compared to a 30% overall mortality in patients randomized to amiodarone ($p = 0.072$). The patients in the defibrillator group had a 19.6% reduction in their relative risk of overall mortality.

SECONDARY PREVENTION TRIALS—SUMMARY

These secondary prevention trials, once again, were meant to test the ability of the ICD, as compared to more conventional therapy, to prolong the overall survival of a population of patients presenting with life-threatening ventricular tachyarrhythmias. As we have seen in our prior discussion, however, the ability of the ICD to prolong survival is a given—whether it actually does so or not depends on how we use it.

According to the Axiom, the issue in conducting an indiscriminate clinical trial with the defibrillator (i.e., one that allows enrollment of essentially all comers) is whether enough patients from Population 2 will be enrolled to counterbalance the effect of patients enrolled from Population 3. Indeed, there is anecdotal evidence suggesting that patients who could easily be identified as belonging to Population 2 often were systematically withheld from these studies, because their doctors strongly believed they should receive a defibrillator. If so, these studies would have enrolled a disproportionate share of Population 3 patients. This is a particularly intriguing possibility, given the finding in the AVID trial that the average prolongation of survival conferred by the ICD although statistically significant, was of short duration. (Fig. 2 demonstrates the significant but relatively small difference in survival curves between the two treatment groups in AVID.) This is exactly what the Axiom predicts will happen with Population 3 patients.

In each of these trials except CIDS, a statistical benefit was observed with the defibrillator. The medical community has chosen to interpret these results at face value. "For the first time," wrote National Heart, Lung, and Blood Institute Director Lenfant, the ICD has been proven to "improve overall survival in patients with serious ventricular arrhythmias" *(12)*.

Others are less sanguine, thanking our lucky stars that we dodged a bullet. In any case, evidence from randomized clinical trials now firmly supports the use of the ICD as therapy of first choice in survivors of symptomatic, sustained ventricular tachyarrhythmias. Although perhaps for the wrong reasons, at least this area of controversy over indications for the ICD seems to have been resolved. Ironically, several years after the AVID study was published, two articles in the *New England Journal of Medicine* supported the importance and veracity of carefully conducted observational studies as an alternative to randomized controlled clinical trials *(12a)*.

Primary Prevention Trials

Patients who already have had sustained ventricular tachyarrhythmias have a high risk of recurrence, and it is to be expected that in this high-risk population, the ICD should measurably prolong overall survival.

The issue is much less obvious, however, when one is dealing with patients whose risk of sudden arrhythmic death, although substantially higher than normal, is still only *relatively* high. Such patients would include those whose underlying cardiac disease places them at risk for ventricular arrhythmias, but in whom those arrhythmias have never actually manifested. The risk of sudden death in such patients has been relatively difficult to quantify, and as a result, the potential benefit of an ICD has been much more difficult to predict.

Thus, at least conceptually, randomized trials using the ICD in such patients— primary prophylaxis trials—are usually much less controversial than the trials we have just considered. Three such primary prevention trials have now been reported, and two additional trials are ongoing (see Table 2).

MULTICENTER AUTOMATIC DEFIBRILLATION IMPLANTATION TRIAL (MADIT)

In MADIT *(13–14)*, patients who had a prior MI, a left ventricular ejection fraction (LVEF) of less than 0.35, and a documented episode of nonsustained ventricular tachycardia (NSVT) were eligible for screening by means of electrophysiologic testing. Those who had inducible ventricular tachycardia (VT) during baseline testing, and in whom the inducible tachycardia was not suppressed with iv procainamide in subsequent testing, were then eligible for randomization. Overall, 196 patients were randomized to receive either the ICD vs whatever drug therapy the physician considered appropriate. Approximately 80% of the patients randomized to drug therapy received amiodarone.

MADIT was ended in early 1996 (a little more than 5 yr after its inception) by the trial's Safety Monitoring Committee, when a highly significant survival benefit became apparent in patients randomized to the ICD. Patients randomized to drug therapy had 2.6-fold more deaths overall than patients randomized to the defibrillator. The Kaplan-Meier cumulative mortality curves for the two groups (Fig. 3) showed an early and

Table 2
Primary Prevention Trials With the ICD

| | Selection criteria | | | | Treatment and outcome | | |
	Heart Disease	Election fraction (LV)	NSVT?	Other	Study group therapy	Control group therapy	Survival benefit with ICD?
MADIT	Prior MI	<0.35	Yes	+EPS failed drug trial	ICD	Anti-arrhythmic drugs	Yes, improved overall survival
CABG Patch	Ischemic heaert disease	<0.36	No	+SAECG	ICD	Conventional therapy	No
MUSTT	CAD	<0.4	Yes	+EPS failed drug trial	ICD	Conservative therapy	Yes, arrhythmic survival
SCD-HeFT	CMP	<0.35	No		ICD	Amiodarone or conventional therapy	Ongoing trial
MADIT II	CAD	<0.3	No		ICD	Conventional therapy	Ongoing trial
DEFINITE	Non-ischemic CMP	<0.35	Yes	>10 PVC/hr or NSVT to qualify	ICD	Conventional therapy	Ongoing trial

MADIT = Multicenter Automatic Defibrillator Implantation Trial; CABG Patch = Coronary Artery Bypass Graft Patch trial; MUSTT = Multicenter Unsustained Tachycardia Trial; SCD HeFT = Sudden Cardiac Death in Heart Failure Trial; MADIT II = Multicenter Automatic Defibrillator Implantation Trial-II; MI = myocardial infarction; CMP = cardiomyopathy; ICD = implantable cardioverter defibrillator; EPS = electrophysiology study; SAECG = signal-averaged electrocardiogram; LV = left ventricle.

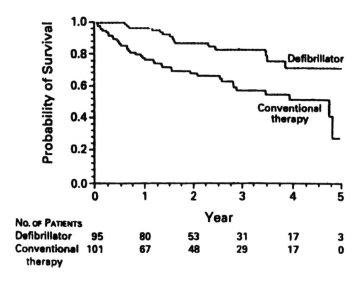

No. of Patients

Defibrillator	95	80	53	31	17	3
Conventional therapy	101	67	48	29	17	0

Fig. 3. MADIT trial results: Actuarial survival curves for patients treated wtih the defibrillator and with conventional therapy. (From: Moss AJ, Hall J, Cannom DS, Daubert JP, et al. Improved survival with an implanted defibrillator in patients with coronary artery disease at high risk for ventricular arrhythmia. N Engl J Med 1996;335:1933–1940. Copyright © 1996 Massachusetts Medical Society.)

substantial separation in favor of the defibrillator, which was maintained throughout the follow-up period, and was highly significant ($p = 0.009$).

The results of MADIT were sufficiently striking that in a highly unusual move, the Food and Drug Administration (FDA) was compelled to rapidly expand the indications for the ICD to include patients who met the MADIT entrance criteria.

The Coronary-Artery Bypass Graft (CABG) Patch Trial

CABG Patch *(15)* enrolled patients who were scheduled to have coronary-artery bypass grafting for ischemic heart disease, who had LVEFs of less than 0.36, and who had positive signal-averaged electrocardiograms (SAECGs). Randomization itself took place in the operating room, once the revascularization was completed and the patient was deemed stable. Patients deemed eligible at that point were randomized to either receive or not receive the ICD.

A total of 1055 patients were enrolled during the 4 years of the study, and were followed for a mean of 32 mo postoperatively. In April 1997, the study's Data Safety Monitoring Board terminated the trial when it was determined that no survival benefit was provided by the ICD in this population. In fact, the survival curves from both the defibrillator and control groups were virtually identical (Fig. 4). Subsequent analyses showed that the ICD reduced the risk of sudden cardiac death significantly, but the risk of arrhythmic death in this population was lower than expected, leaving the trial inadequate to detect a difference in total mortality *(15a)*.

Multicenter Unsustained Tachycardia Trial (MUSTT)

MUSTT was not specifically designed to test whether the ICD can prolong overall survival when used as primary prophylaxis *(16)*. Instead, it was designed to test the hypothesis that antiarrhythmic therapy guided by electrophysiologic testing can benefit patients with NSVT, left ventricular dysfunction, coronary-artery disease (CAD) and

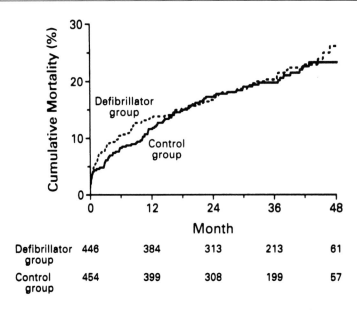

Fig. 4. CABG Patch results: Actuarial survival curves for patients treated with the defibrillator and with conventional therapy. See text. (From: Bigger TJ, for the Coronary Artery Bypass Graft (CABG) Patch Trial Investigators. Prophylactic use of implanted cardiac defibrillators in patients at high risk for ventricular arrhythmias after CABG surgery. N Engl J Med 1997;337:1569–1575. Copyright © 1997 Massachusetts Medical Society.)

inducible ventricular arrhythmia during electrophysiologic studies. The ICD in this trial was simply one of the forms of antiarrhythmic therapy to which patients might be guided when relying on electrophysiologic testing.

In MUSTT, patients with CAD, NSVT, and a LVEF less than 0.4 underwent electro-physiologic testing to see if sustsained VT could be induced. If VT was inducible, patients were then randomized to "conservative treatment" with beta-blockers and angiotensin-converting enzyme (ACE) inhibitors, or to therapy guided by electrophysio-logic testing (including serial drug testing with up to three antiarrhythmic drugs, or an ICD after at least one failed antiarrhythmic drug test).

The results of MUSTT were recently published (17). Of 2202 patients enrolled in the study, 704 who had inducible VT were randomized. Patients randomized to the antiarrhythmic therapy group had a significantly reduced arrhythmic mortality compared to the conservative therapy group at both 24 and 60 mo of follow-up (12% vs 18% at 24 mo, and 25% vs 32% at 60 mo; $p = 0.043$). There was also a trend toward a reduction in all-cause mortality in the antiarrhythmic therapy group, although a statistical significance was not reached.

Most remarkably, 46% of patients in the antiarrhythmic therapy group who received the ICD had a 92% 60-mo survival. Furthermore, when patients with the defibrillator were removed from the analysis, there was no significant difference in outcome between the antiarrhythmic therapy group and the conservative group. Thus, virtually all of the survival benefit in the antiarrhythmic therapy group appears to have been imparted by the ICD. In fact, patients treated with antiarrhythmic drugs appeared to do worse than the conventionally treated patients. Fig. 5 illustrates the results of MUSTT.

The results of MUSTT are therefore entirely consistent with those of MADIT.

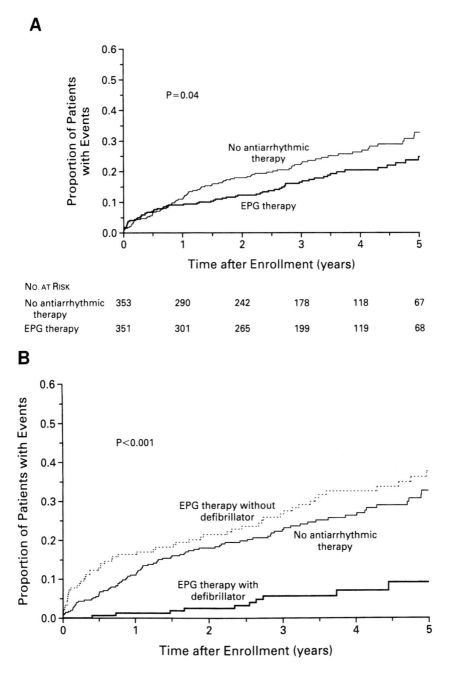

Fig. 5. MUSTT results: Actuarial estimates of event rates (cardiac arrest or death from arrhythmia). **(A)** EPG (electrophysiologically guided therapy) vs conventional therapy. See text. **(B)** The EPG group is divided into patients with and without ICDs. Note that all of the benefit is in the ICD group, and that the EPG patients without ICDs did worse than the conventional group. See text. (From: Buxton A, Lee KL, Fisher JD, et al. A randomized study of the prevention of sudden death in patients with coronary artery disease. N Engl J Med 1999;341:1882–1890. Copyright © 1999 Massachusetts Medical Society.)

MUSTT confirms that, in patients with NSVT, CAD, and depressed LVEFs, the EPS may identify a subset with a substantial risk of sudden arrhythmic death; and the ICD is effective in significantly reducing that risk and prolonging overall survival.

Reconciling MADIT, MUSTT, and CABG Patch

Both MADIT and MUSTT showed a strong benefit in using the ICD as primary prophylactic therapy, whereas CABG Patch showed no benefit at all. How can studies that randomize seemingly similar groups of patients (i.e., patients with ischemic heart disease, the presence of left ventricular dysfunction, and a marker for arrhythmic risk) yield such different results? The answer is that the patients studied in these trials, although superficially similar, were actually quite different, and that given those differences, the Axiom of Overall Survival predicts these results.

Simply put, the patients finally enrolled in the CABG Patch trial had a low arrhythmic event rate, and so were not eligible to have their lives significantly prolonged by the ICD. In contrast, patients in MADIT and MUSTT had a relatively high arrhythmic event rate, so that removing the risk of arrhythmic death with the ICD significantly prolonged overall survival.

Why was the prognosis of patients eligible for CABG Patch so much better than for patients eligible for the other two trials? First, the screening for eligibility to MADIT and MUSTT was far more rigorous than for CABG Patch. Specifically, it appears likely that the EPS has a much higher predictive value at an indicator of arrhythmic risk than does a positive SAECG. And secondly, all patients randomized in the CABG Patch trial had successful revascularization surgery. Indeed, successful revascularization was a criterion for randomization. This systematic elimination of ischemia is very likely to have had at least some antiarrhythmic value.

In any case, the MADIT and MUSTT screening criteria were much more effective in identifying a high-risk subgroup of enrollees than those used in CABG Patch. The first criterion of the Axiom (the risk of sudden death must be sufficiently high) was met in these two trials; it was not in CABG Patch. Thus, the reduction in sudden death provided by the ICD had a measurable effect on overall survival in MADIT and MUSTT, whereas it did not in CABG Patch.

Summary of Primary Prevention Trials

Two well-designed multicenter trials have now shown that the ICD can significantly increase overall survival in carefully selected patients who have not yet experienced a sustained ventricular tachyarrhythmia. Based on the results of both MADIT and MUSTT, electrophysiologic testing should be strongly considered in patients with coronary CAD, depressed left ventricular function, and NSVT. If sustained VT is induced, those patients should receive an ICD.

How important is electrophysiologic testing in selecting patients for primary prophylaxis with the ICD? This question remains open. In the MUSTT trial, the EPS identified patients at high risk of arrhythmic death. Patients who met the clinical criteria for inclusion but were not inducible at EPS also had a significant risk of arrhythmic death (and total mortality) during follow-up (17a). A similar registry had not been published for the MADIT study. Although it is likely that the EPS (or lack thereof) accounts for at least some of the difference in outcomes between MADIT and MUSTT on one hand, and CABG Patch on the other, we cannot yet prove this theory.

Three ongoing trials will give us more insight as to whether electrophysiologic testing is necessary in identifying patients who will benefit from primary prophylaxis with the implantable ICD. The Sudden Cardiac Death in Heart Failure Trial (SCD HeFT) *(17b)* is enrolling 2400 patients with either CAD or dilated cardiomyopathy and a LVEF of less than 0.35. Patients will simply be randomized to therapy with conventional drugs, amiodarone, or the ICD. The MADIT II trial *(17b)* is enrolling patients with CAD and a LVEF of less than 0.3. These patients will be randomized to either conventional therapy or the ICD. DEFINITE *(17c)* randomizes patients with nonischemic cardiomyopathy and NSVT to either an ICD or conventional therapy. If inducibility during electrophysiologic testing really is an important prognostic indicator, then MADIT II may have difficulty demonstrating a significant survival benefit with the ICD. Since electrophysiologic testing is less sensitive and less specific in nonischemic compared with ischemic myopathies, the effect of omitting this "qualifying" test is less clear in DEFINITE and SCH HeFT.

It is interesting to speculate what the Axiom of Overall Survival may predict about the outcome of SCD HeFT, DEFINITE, and MADIT II. Since these trials enroll very broad populations of patients, it seems likely that (unlike MADIT and MUSTT) they will tend to dilute Population 2 patients with patients from Population 3—and even Population 1. Thus, the Axiom seems to suggest that these trials will either be negative, or like AVID, will show a significant but short-lived benefit from the ICD.

ACCEPTED INDICATIONS FOR THE ICD

We are finally ready to consider the indications for the ICD, as currently accepted by the ACC and by the American Heart Association (AHA) *(18)*.

Class I indications. Class I indications are those for which a broad consensus exists. These include:

1. Patients who have had cardiac arrest caused by VT or VF that is not the result of a transient or reversible cause
2. Patients with spontaneous sustained VT
3. Patients with syncope of undetermined origin who have clinically relevant inducible sustained VT or VF induced during electrophysiologic testing
4. Patients with NSVT who have CAD, prior myocardial infarction (MI), left ventricular dysfunction, and inducible VT or VF during electrophysiologic testing that is not suppressed by Class I antiarrhythmic drug

Class II indications. Class II indications are those for which a consensus does not exist. These include:

1. Patients with cardiac arrest presumed to be the result of VF when electrophysiologic testing is precluded by other medical conditions
2. Patients with severe, symptomatic sustained ventricular tachyarrhythmias that occur while awaiting cardiac transplantation
3. Patients with familial or inherited conditions with a high risk of life-threatening ventricular tachyarrhythmias, such as long QT syndrome (LQTS) or hypertrophic cardiomyopathy
4. Patients with NSVT who have CAD, prior MI, left ventricular dysfunction, and inducible sustained VT during electrophysiologic testing
5. Patients with recurrent syncope of unknown etiology who have ventricular dysfunction

and inducible ventricular arrhythmias during electrophysiologic testing when other causes of syncope have been excluded

Discussion

The accepted indications for the ICD are much more grounded on the results of controlled, randomized trials than at any time in the past. Yet these indications remain imperfect and incomplete.

PATIENTS WHO MEET THE ACCEPTED INDICATIONS BUT ARE UNLIKELY TO BE HELPED

The most striking drawback to these generally accepted indications for the defibrillator is that they tend to address only the characteristics of patients' arrhythmias, and not the characteristics of the patients themselves. In terms of the Axiom of Overall Survival, they address only one of the two criteria necessary for prolongation of survival, namely, that recipients of the defibrillator should have a high risk of sudden death from ventricular arrhythmias.

The accepted indications generally fail to address the second criterion: the likelihood of early death from other causes. Conceivably, one could implant the defibrillator in a large population of patients who all meet the acceptable indications, and still fail to achieve a favorable overall result.

It is the obligation of the clinician to always ask that second question when faced with a decision as to whether to implant a defibrillator: "Yes, the patient has a life-threatening arrhythmia that meets acceptable implantation criteria for the device. But is he or she likely to have significant overall benefit if prevention of sudden death can be achieved?" Unless the answer to this question is also yes, the ICD should not be used in most cases.

PATIENTS WHO DO NOT MEET ACCEPTED INDICATIONS BUT MAY BE HELPED BY THE ICD—EXPANDING THE INDICATIONS

Presently, only a few tens of thousands of patients worldwide receive the ICD each year, in contrast to the more than 300,000 individuals who die suddenly each year in the United States alone, and in contrast to the vastly larger number who (by virtue of their underlying cardiac disease) are at high risk for sudden death. Can we expand the use of the ICD to impact on these grim statistics?

Except for the relatively small subset of high-risk patients who meet the MADIT/MUSTT profiles, in order for an ICD to be indicated, candidates must have already experienced (and survived) sustained ventricular tachyarrhythmias. Notably, the huge majority of individuals who die suddenly never experience prior sustained arrhythmias, and therefore are never candidates for an ICD until it is too late.

Most victims of sudden death come from the large pool of patients who have significant underlying cardiac disease, such as prior MI, a history of congestive heart failure (CHF), or reduced LVEF. It is very likely that some subsets of these patients (i.e., patients with risk factors but no manifest sustained arrhythmias) would benefit from an ICD. MADIT was the first trial to successfully identify such a subset, a result that was apparently confirmed (and possibly enlarged) by MUSTT. Ongoing trials are attempting to expand the population that can be helped by insertion of one of these devices, and in a few years we may know more. But insisting on randomized trials as the only means to expand the indications for the ICD will continue to be an excruciatingly

Table 3
Projected Cost of ICD Per Life-Year Saved, Group A

Yearly mortality risk, Group A	Probability				
Sudden death	0.1				
Non-sudden death	0.05				

	Year 1	Year 2	Year 3	Year 4	Year 5
Pts alive at beginning of year	100	95	90.3	85.7	81.4
Non-sudden death, projected	5	4.75	4.51	4.29	4.07
Sudden death, projected	9.5	9.03	8.57	8.15	7.74
Total death without ICD, projected	14.5	13.8	13.1	12.4	11.8
Total death with ICD, projected	5	4.75	4.51	4.29	4.07
Pts saved this year	9.5	9.03	8.57	8.15	7.74
Saved pts from last year still alive	0	9.03	17.1	24.4	31.0
Total saves pts still alive	9.5	18.1	25.7	32.6	38.6
Total life-years saved this year*	4.75	13.5	21.4	28.5	34.8
Cumulative life-years saved	4.75	18.2	39.7	68.2	103
Pts alive at end of year, projected	95	90.3	85.7	81.4	77.4

5-year projection					
Total life-years saved	103				
Life-years saved per patient	1.03				
Cost of implantable defibrillator	$30,000				
Cost per life-year saved	$29,000				

*Calculation assumes 0.5 additional life-year saved for year in which life was saved.
ICD = implantable cardioverter defibrillator.

slow and expensive method. For some disease processes, randomized trials are not feasible, because of the small numbers of patients affected. Observational studies of high-risk patients with hypertrophic cardiomyopathy (18a) and congenital LQTS (18b) are cited when high-risk patients are implanted with defibrillators, although defining "high risk" for primary prevention in these patients admittedly remains difficult.

However, there is an alternative method. We could use the Axiom of Overall Survival to determine indications. To do so, we would need to develop sufficient epidemiological data to predict the survival of various subsets of patients who have a relatively high risk of life-threatening ventricular arrhythmias. Much work has already been done in quantifying the risk of sudden arrhythmic death in various populations using combinations of noninvasive measures such as ejection fraction, degree of ectopy, SAECGS, heart rate variability (HRV), and T-wave changes. Work has also been done in quantifying the risk of death from heart failure in certain subsets of patients with cardiac dysfunction. If these two measures of risk (i.e., the yearly risk of sudden death and the yearly risk of death from other causes) could be firmed up sufficiently for various subsets of patients, then we would have all the information we needed to apply the Axiom to calculate whether to implant a defibrillator.

Examples of such a calculation are shown in Tables 3 and 4. These tables compute a projected cost-effectiveness for a 5-yr ICD, as applied to two different populations of patients. Patients in Group A (Table 3) are predicted to have an annual 10% risk

Table 4
Projected Cost of ICD Per Life-Year Saved, Group B

Yearly mortality risk Group A	Probability				
Sudden death	0.1				
Non-sudden death	0.33				

	Year 1	Year 2	Year 3	Year 4	Year 5
Pts alive at beginning of year	100	67	44.9	30.1	20.2
Non-sudden death, projected	33	22.1	14.8	9.93	6.65
Sudden death, projected	6.7	4.5	3.0	2.0	1.4
Total death without ICD, projected	39.7	26.6	17.8	11.9	8.0
Total death with ICD, projected	33	22.1	14.5	9.93	6.65
Pts saved this year	6.7	4.5	3.0	2.0	1.4
Saved pts from last year still alive	0	4.5	6.0	6.0	5.4
Total saves pts still alive	6.7	9.0	9.0	8.1	6.8
Total life-years saved this year*	3.4	6.7	7.5	7.0	6.1
Cumulative life-years saved	3.4	10.1	17.6	24.7	30.7
Pts alive at end of year, projected	67	44.9	30.1	20.2	13.5

5-year projection					
Total life-years saved	30.7				
Life-years saved per patient	0.31				
Cost of ICD	$30,000				
Cost per life-year saved	$97,621				

* Calculation assumes 0.5 additional life-year saved for year in which life was saved.
ID = implantable cardioverter defibrillator.

of sudden death, and an annual 5% risk of death from other causes (i.e., patients are similar to those in Population 2). Patients in Group B (Table 4) also have a 10% yearly risk of sudden death, but their risk of death from other causes is much higher: 33% yearly (similar to Population 3). During the 5 yr after implantation, the defibrillator would add a net of 1.03 life-years per patient in Group A, but only 0.31 life-years per patient in Group B. At a cost of $30,000 per implantation, the cost per life-year saved would be approx $29,000 for Group A and $98,000 for Group B.

Note that the data used to calculate these values are epidemiological data, similar to that available from the Framingham study. With such data in hand, we only need to decide how much we are willing to spend to prolong a patient's life by 1 yr (the going rate, unofficially, is $50,000 per life-year saved), and plug the numbers into a spreadsheet. If a patient's statistical risk of sudden death is high enough, and the risk of death from other causes low enough, the cost will fall under the threshold value and we would implant a defibrillator. If not, patients would receive alternative therapy.

Such a methodology admittedly may sound radical. It does, however, bring a fundamental fact about how we use the defibrillator into the light of day. Namely, our use of the ICD meets the "but for" test for rationing: Since ICDs are unsurpassed at preventing sudden arrhythmic death, then *but for the expense,* we would implant these devices in *everybody* who has a substantially increased risk for sudden death.

This suggested methodology does not introduce rationing to our use of the defibrillator—it simply makes the rationing we are doing more open, and arguably more fair. It also would be relatively quick and simple to implement, and would save us the time and expense of conducting a score of randomized trials, one for each identifiable subset of potentially eligible patients, to determine who gets the defibrillator.

Given the continued high cost and complexity of the ICD however, no matter how we ultimately decide to expand its indications, making an appreciable impact in the worldwide incidence of sudden death will probably never be possible with this device. Such an impact will almost certainly require a breakthrough outside the realm of implantable antitachycardia devices.

REFERENCES

1. Epstein AE. AVID Necessity. PACE 1993;16:1773–1775.
2. The Antiarrhythmic versus Implantable Defibrillator (AVID) Trial Executive Committee. Are implantable cardioverter-defibrillators or drugs more effective in prolonging life? Am J Cardiol 1997;79:661–663.
3. Fogoros RN. The impact of the implantable defibrillator on mortality: the axiom of overall implantable cardioverter-defibrillator survival. Am J Cardiol 1996;78:57–61.
4. Wever EFD, Hauer RNW, van Capelle FJL, et al. Randomized study of implantable defibrillator as first-choice therapy versus conventional strategy in postinfarct sudden death survivors. Circulation 1995;91;2195–2203.
5. The Antiarrhythmics Versus Implantable Defibrillator (AVID) Investigators. A comparison of antiarrhythmic-drug therapy with implantable defibrillators in patients resuscitated from near-fatal ventricular arrhythmias. N Engl J Med 1997;337:1576–1583.
6. Josephson ME, Nisam S. The AVID Trial: evidence-based or randomized control trials—is the AVID study too late? Am J Cardiol 1997;80:194–197.
7. Fogoros RN. Why the antiarrhythmics versus implantable defibrillator (AVID) trial sets the wrong precedent. Am J Cardiol 1997;80:762–765.
8. Siebels J, Kuck KH, and the CASH Investigators. Implantable cardioverter defibrillator compared with antiarrhythmic drug treatment in cardiac arrest survivors (the Cardiac Arrest Study Hamburg). Am Heart J 1994;127:1139–1144.
9. Huck K-H, Cappato R, Siebels J, Ruppel R, for the CASH investigators. Randomized comparison of antiarrhythmic drug therapy with implantable defibrillators in patients resuscitated from cardiac arrest: The Cardiac Arrest Study Hamburg (CASH). Circulation 2000;102:748–754.
10. Cannom DS. A review of the implantable defibrillator trials. Curr Opin Cardiol 1998;13:3–8.
11. Connolly SJ, Gent M, Roberts RS, Dorian P, et al. Canadian implantable defibrillator study (CIDS): A randomized trial of the implantable defibrillator against amiodarone. Circulation 2000;101:1297–1302.
12. National Institutes of Health (NIH) News Release: NHLBI stops arrhythmias study—implantable cardiac defibrillator reduces death. NHLBI communications. April 4, 1997.
12a. Benson K, Hartz AJ. A comparison of observational studies and randomized, controlled trials. N Engl J Med 2000;342:1878–1886.
12b. Concato J, Shah N, Horowitz RI. Randomized, controlled trials, observational studies, and the hierarchy of research designs. N Engl J Med 2000;342:1887–1892.
13. Moss AJ, Hall J, Cannom DS, Daubert JP, et al. Improved survival with an implanted defibrillator in patients with coronary artery disease at high risk for ventricular arrhythmia. N Engl J Med 1996;335:1933–1940.
14. Moss AJ. Background, outcome, and clinical implications of the Multicenter Automatic Defibrillator Implantation Trial (MADIT). Am J Cardiol 1997;80:28F–32F.
15. Bigger TJ, for the Coronary Artery Bypass Graft (CABG) Patch Trial Investigators. Prophylactic use of implanted cardiac defibrillators in patients at high risk for ventricular arrhythmias after coronary artery bypass graft surgery. N Engl J Med 1997;337:1569–1575.
15a. Bigger JT, Whang W, Rottman JN, et al. Mechanisms of death in the CABG Patch trial: a randomized trial of implantable cardiac defibrillator prophylaxis in patients at high risk of death after coronary artery bypass grafting. Circulation 1999;99:1416–1421.

16. Buxton AE. Ongoing risk stratification trials: the primary prevention of sudden death. Control Clin Trials 1996;17:47S–51S.

17. Buxton A, Lee KL, Fisher JD, et al. A randomized study of the prevention of sudden death in patients with coronary artery disease. N Engl J Med 1999;341:1882–1890.

17a. Buxton AE, Lee KL, DiCarlo L, et al. Electrophysiologic testing to identify patients with coronary artery disease who are at risk for sudden death. N Engl J Med 2000;342:1937–1945.

17b. Klein H, Auricchio A, Reek S, Geller C. New primary prevention trials of sudden cardiac death in patients with left ventricular dysfunction: SCD-HeFT and MADIT-II. Am J Cardiol 1999;83:91D–97D.

17c. Kadish A, Quigg R, Schaechter A, et al. Defibrillators in nonischemic cardiomyopathy treatment evaluation. PACE 2000;23:338–343.

18. American College of Cardiology/American Heart Association Task Force on Practice Guidelines. ACC/AHA Guidelines for implantation of cardiac pacemakers and antiarrhythmia devices. J Am Coll Cardiol 1998;31:1175–1209.

18a. Maron BJ, Shen W-K, Link MS, et al. Efficacy of the implantable cardioverter-defibrillators for the prevention of sudden death in patients with hypertrophic cardiomyopathy. N Engl J Med 2000;342:365–373.

18b. Moss AJ, Zareba W, Hall WJ, et al. Effectiveness and limitations of beta-blocker therapy in congenital long-QT syndrome. Circulation 2000;101:616–623.

15 Implantable Cardioverter Defibrillator Therapy

Technical and Implant Issues

Ralph S. Augostini, MD,
Robert A. Schweikert, MD,
and Bruce L. Wilkoff, MD

CONTENTS

INTRODUCTION
INDICATIONS
CONTRAINDICATIONS
DEVICE SELECTION
IMPLANTATION
DEVICE REPLACEMENT
TACHYCARDIA DETECTION AND THERAPY
BRADYCARDIA DETECTION AND THERAPY
MAGNET FUNCTION
MANAGING AND FOLLOWING PATIENTS
FREQUENT THERAPIES
ELECTROMAGNETIC INTERFERENCE (EMI)
INSTRUCTIONS TO PATIENTS
FUTURE OF THE ICD
REFERENCES

INTRODUCTION

The implantable cardioverter defibrillator (ICD) was initially designed to automatically detect and treat tachyarrhythmias *(1,2)*. The modern ICD has evolved into a multifunctional, multiprogrammable electronic device designed to treat episodes of ventricular tachycardia (VT) and ventricular fibrillation (VF), and to support bradycardia. The ICD consists of a pulse generator and a lead system with electrodes for pacing and coils for defibrillation. Current ICDs have the programming potential to deliver multi-level therapies, which may include a combination of anti-tachycardia pacing, cardioversion, or defibrillation. Contemporary ICDs also have extensive bradycardia

From: *Contemporary Cardiology: Management of Cardiac Arrhythmias*
Edited by: L. I. Ganz © Humana Press Inc., Totowa, NJ

functionality, which may include single-chamber pacing, dual-chamber pacing, automatic mode-switching, and sensor-driven rate-responsive pacing. ICDs incorporate sophisticated algorithms to detect and differentiate supraventricular tachycardia (SVT) from ventricular arrhythmias. Additionally, some models deliver pacing or defibrillation therapy for atrial arrhythmias. Multiple clinical trials have demonstrated the efficacy of ICDs to accurately detect and treat VT and to reduce the risk of sudden cardiac death.

In 1972, the concept of an ICD was first introduced following the development of external defibrillation to terminate life-threatening ventricular arrhythmias in the intensive-care-unit setting. First-generation ICDs were non-programmable, provided only the basic function of defibrillation, and required a thoracotomy approach for placement of an epicardial lead system. The size of the pulse generator limited placement to an abdominal site. Subsequent advancements in electronic technology over the past 20 yr have drastically reduced the size of the pulse generator yet improved the programmability, diagnostic data storage, and longevity of the device. A heightened understanding of cardiac pacing, VF, and defibrillation has resulted in the development of multiphasic shock waveforms and transvenous pace/defibrillation lead systems which preclude the need for a thoracotomy. As a result, the typical ICD is a much smaller device with expansive programming capability that can be implanted in a pectoral location with low surgical morbidity.

Like a cardiac pacemaker, the ICD incorporates a microprocessor, capacitors, an energy source, and memory in a pulse generator that attaches to a lead system which interfaces with the heart. New implants are almost exclusively implanted transvenously, with the pulse generator placed in a left pectoral position. Some systems incorporate a single right ventricular coil with an active pulse generator. Other configurations use a right ventricular coil combined with a superior vena cava (SVC) coil and an active pulse-generator can. Ventricular sensing and pacing are achieved either through two "dedicated bipolar" electrodes at the tip of the right ventricular lead or via "integrated bipolar" electrodes that incorporate a single right ventricular tip electrode with the right ventricular coil. As with a pacemaker, communication with the ICD system is established with a bedside programmer incorporating a radiofrequency wand to encode and transmit data. Finally, the development of event memory storage of ICDs has greatly enhanced our understanding of ongoing device and lead function. A review of the episode data helps to distinguish between appropriate and inappropriate device therapy.

INDICATIONS

An ICD system is indicated for patients who are at high risk of sudden cardiac death caused by ventricular arrhythmias. The combined American College of Cardiology/American Heart Association (ACC/AHA) Task Force has published guidelines for the implantation of cardiac pacemakers and anti-arrhythmia devices. The 1998 updated report reflects several recent prospective randomized clinical trials for primary and secondary prevention of sudden cardiac death (3–5). Current indications for ICD implantation are summarized in Table 1.

Dual-chamber pacemaker ICDs have not yet been introduced and tested in randomized clinical trials, but have been used to treat bradycardia and to improve the specificity of ventricular tachyarrhythmia detection and to exclude false detections of SVTs as ventricular events. Prophylactic ICD implantation for patients with coronary-artery

Table 1
Indications for ICD Implantation *(3)*

Indication Class	*Indication Description*
I.	Cardiac arrest resulting from VF or VT, not caused by a transient or reversible cause.
	Spontaneous sustained VT.
	Syncope of undetermined origin with clinically relevant, hemodynamically significant sustained VT or VF induced at electrophysiology study (EPS) when drug therapy is ineffective, not tolerated, or not preferred.
	NSVT with CAD, prior MI, left ventricular dysfunction, and inducible VF or sustained VT at EPS that is not suppressible by a Class I antiarrhythmic drug.
II.	Cardiac arrest presumed to be caused by VF when EP testing is precluded by other medical conditions.
	Severe symptoms attributable to sustained ventricular tachyarrhythmias while awaiting cardiac transplantation.
	Familial or inherited conditions with a high risk for life-threatening ventricular tachyarrhythmias such as long QT syndrome (LQTS) or hypertrophic cardiomyopathy.
III.	Syncope of undetermined cause in a patient without inducible ventricular tachyarrhythmias.
	Incessant VT or VF.
	VF or VT resulting from arrhythmias amenable to surgical or catheter abalation; for example, atrial arrhythmias associated with the Wolff-Parkinson-White syndrome (WPW), right ventricular outflow tract VT (ROVT), idiopathic left VT, or fascicular VT.
	Ventricular tachyarrhythmias caused by a transient or reversible disorder (e.g., acute MI, electrolyte imbalance, drugs, trauma).
	Significant psychiatric illnesses that may be aggravated by device implantation or may preclude systematic follow-up.
	Terminal illnesses with projected life expectancy ≤ 6 mo.
	Patients with CAD with left ventricular dysfunction and prolonged QRS duration in the absence of spontaneous or inducible sustained or nonsustained VT who are undergoing coronary bypass surgery.
	NYHA Class IV drug-refractory CHF in patients who are not candidates for cardiac transplantation.

Class I: Evidence and general agreement regarding the benefit, usefulness, and effectiveness of ICD therapy.

Class II: Conflicting evidence and divergence of opinion regarding usefulness or effectiveness of ICD therapy.

Class III: Evidence and general agreement regarding the lack of usefulness or effectiveness of ICD therapy.

VF = ventricular fibrillation, VT = ventricular tachycardia, EP = electrophysiology, NYHA = New York Heart Association.

With permission from the American College of Cardiology (Gregoratos G, et al. ACC/AHA guidelines for implantation of cardiac pacemakers and antiarrhythmia devices. J Am Coll Cardiol 1998;31:1199.)

disease (CAD), ventricular systolic dysfunction, nonsustained VT (NSVT), and induc-ible sustained VT/VF at electrophysiologic testing has been shown to improve survival in the MADIT and MUSTT studies (6,7). Further clinical trials are underway to test the use of prophylactic ICDs for patients with dilated cardiomyopathy regardless of the cause. The CABG Patch trial made clear that prophylactic ICD implantation is not useful as an adjunct to bypass surgery (8).

Candidates for ICD implantation should be carefully screened to determine whether the prescribed therapy is appropriate. Patient education regarding the implantation, maintenance, and follow-up of an implantable device should be initiated pre-operatively. A thorough discussion of potential therapies is helpful in alleviating fear for some patients. The candidate should be allowed to make an informed choice prior to implanta-tion of a device.

CONTRAINDICATIONS

Currently, ICD implantation is contraindicated for remedial causes of ventricular arrhythmia such as acute myocardial infarction (MI), myocardial ischemia, electrolyte imbalance, drug toxicity, hypoxia, or sepsis. Transient ventricular tachyarrhythmia secondary to electrocution or drowning is a contraindication for ICD placement. Patients with incessant ventricular arrhythmias are not candidates for an ICD.

DEVICE SELECTION

Once a decision is made to proceed with ICD implantation, several considerations must guide device selection. The patient's body habitus must be considered, as available devices vary in size, shape, and thickness. Because device longevity also varies, the patient's age and comorbid conditions should also be considered. Output also varies among devices. Unfortunately, predicting which patients are likely to have a high defibrillation threshold at implant is extremely difficult (9).

Firm guidelines for choosing between single- and dual-chamber devices have not yet been developed. Dual-chamber devices offer more sophisticated pacing support, discrimination algorithms to withhold therapy for supraventricular tachyarrhythmias, and stored electrograms to assess the appropriateness of therapy. Dual-chamber devices are preferred in patients who have or are at risk for sick sinus syndrome and/or heart block, as well as patients with paroxysmal supraventricular tachyarrhythmias. Conversely, single-chamber devices are appropriate for patients with chronic atrial fibrillation (AF), patients not likely to require back-up pacing, and many patients who receive prophylactic ICDs.

IMPLANTATION

ICD implantation using the transvenous approach has evolved into a well-tolerated procedure with low surgical morbidity. Operative risks involved with implantation of an ICD are similar to the risks of pacemaker insertion, and are primarily related to lead placement. Pneumothorax, air embolism, bleeding, deep-vein thrombosis, hemothorax, infection, myocardial damage, vascular/cardiac perforation, tamponade, thromboemboli, and acceleration of arrhythmias are reported with an overall mortality rate of less than 1%. Late complications include infection, chronic nerve damage, erosion, extrusion, fluid accumulation, formation of hematomas/cysts, keloids, lead migration, lead dislodgment, and venous occlusion. Many physicians have switched to conscious sedation rather than general anesthesia during implantation and testing procedures to reduce operative risk. Because of the nature of the procedure, a separate standby external pacemaker/defibrillator should always be immediately available for rescue therapy, in case the implanted device fails to appropriately treat an arrhythmia during the testing procedure *(10)*.

Currently available devices are small enough to allow subcutaneous (SC) pectoral placement in most patients. As contemporary devices utilize "active can" technology, a left pectoral location is preferred for defibrillation therapy. A right pectoral or epicardial system may be needed in a patient who has an existing left-sided pacemaker or in a patient who has undergone prior pectoral surgery (e.g., mastectomy). Rarely, a SC patch or array of coils is necessary to achieve an acceptable defibrillation threshold. Epicardial patch placement is generally reserved for patients who have failed to meet implant criteria with a transvenous lead system or if there has been prior bilateral pectoral surgery. Occasionally, subpectoral placement of the generator is appropriate for cosmetic or size considerations, but that is rare because of the dramatic reduction in generator size. This was important when the majority of ICD implantations occurred with the ICD leads tunneled to an abdominal pocket. The reduction in size and the implementation of the ICD can as a shock electrode, or "active can," has made the SC pectoral implant approach almost universal.

A single 2–3 inch incision is made transversely below the clavicle or over the deltopectoral groove with access for transvenous lead placement achieved through either subclavian puncture or cephalic-vein cutdowns. Because of the occasional lack of venous access, some physicians prefer to achieve subclavian access prior to creation of the pectoral incision. Either a pre-pectoral (SC) or sub-pectoral pocket is created with blunt dissection. The lead is advanced to the right ventricular apex under fluoroscopic guidance, where the tip is secured via an active fixation screw or embedded in trabeculi with passive fixation tines. If there is already a pacemaker lead in the right ventricular apex, then septal placement of the lead tip is chosen. Ideally, the lead tips are placed at maximal distance from each other to avoid device-device interaction. The advanced pacing capabilities of fourth-generation ICDs has promoted the elective removal of a chronically implanted pacemaker and lead prior to ICD system implantation.

The lead is tested for pace/sense thresholds utilizing a pacing-system analyzer (PSA) or high-voltage system analyzer. An acute pacing threshold < 2 V, R-wave amplitude > 5 mV and lead impedance within the accepted range of the manufacturer (300–1200 ohms) are typical implant criteria. The lead is then secured to the posterior wall of the pocket with a suture sleeve tie-down. If the device requires an atrial lead, then it is deployed at this time. The lead is attached to the pulse generator, and the system is placed in the pocket. The pulse generator should be placed with the logo "up" toward the skin and excess lead coiled posterior to the can to maximize the ability to communicate with an external programming wand and to avoid trauma to the lead. The device is then interrogated to assure appropriate communication. Pace/sense thresholds are tested again. Capture of a real-time electrogram may identify signal noise in the shock sensing leads.

Defibrillation testing may be achieved either through a high-voltage system analyzer or through device-based testing; the latter approach is the most common today. Many manufacturers recommend a synchronized sinus test shock to assess the integrity of the device/lead system prior to induction of VF. This is achieved by delivery of a low-energy (<1 J) synchronized shock delivered on the QRS complex. This low-energy test allows assessment of appropriate sensing as well as shock impedance (typically 30–90 ohms). Many devices are now capable of delivering a "painless" low-energy discharge without requiring patient sedation to test shock impedance. VF is usually induced with ultrafast burst pacing (30-ms intervals), shock on T-wave, or application of AC (or DC) current. Appropriate ICD detection and effective therapy is verified. Typically, a step-down protocol is incorporated to determine the defibrillation threshold. Two successful therapies that are at least 10 J less than the maximal output of the device are required to meet implant criteria. Defibrillation therapy is then programmed at a level at least 10 J above the defibrillation threshold. Rarely, a patient may require the addition of a shocking coil in the SVC/SC patch, or an array to achieve an adequate safety margin. Among patients receiving current biphasic ICDs, clinical characteristics do not seem to predict which patients will have high defibrillation thresholds requiring additional shocking electrodes (9).

ICD therapy includes low-energy shocks and antitachycardia pacing. It is usually not necessary to test these functions during the implantation procedure. Empiric programming of an antitachycardia burst therapy seems to be as effective as testing the termination of induced VT. Whether antitachycardia pacing or cardioversion shock therapy is tested or not, effective defibrillation must be programmed to be delivered in an expeditious manner.

DEVICE REPLACEMENT

Pulse-generator replacement represents a vulnerable period for the ICD/lead system. A fourfold increased risk of infection has been reported with ICD pulse-generator replacement. Additionally, manufacturers have had multiple-lead models of variable pin lengths and diameters before adopting the 3.2-mm international pace/sense standard (IS-1) and 3.2-mm defibrillation standard (DF-1) in 1991. Prior to an attempted device replacement, assessment of the chronic lead models should be performed to verify that the appropriate replacement header or adapters are available at the time of surgery (11).

Leads may be inadvertently damaged during exploration of the pocket or during the exchange of pulse generators. Intra-operative assessment of lead function is imperative prior to introducing the replacement generator to the operative field. Replacement of a pace/sense or defibrillation lead may be necessary, and may require the use of a different header. Replacement of an abdominal device should be coordinated with a physician capable of tunneling a new transvenous lead to the abdominal pocket. If the operative plan includes adding a new lead(s) to an existing transvenous system (such as atrial lead or new ventricular pace-sense lead), a pre-operative venogram is useful to document patency of the subclavian vein. Increasingly, epicardial systems are abandoned and capped with placement of a new transvenous lead system.

TACHYCARDIA DETECTION AND THERAPY

The ICD senses the intracardiac electrogram signal via the implanted ventricular sensing electrodes. The determination of a ventricular arrhythmia is recognition of a specified number of V-V intervals that fall within the programmed detection rate and duration criteria. Each V-V interval that falls inside a therapy zone increments the ICD event counter. When the device reaches a specified number of intervals for detection, the ICD will deliver the prescribed therapy. After delivery of therapy, the device either confirms termination of the episode or meets criteria for redetection, and the next programmed therapy is delivered. Some devices are committed to deliver secondary therapy if redetection is met. This is an important aspect of multiple therapies and is designed to assure tachycardia termination. However, it may lead to multiple ICD therapies for NSVT following initial ICD therapy. The ICD automatically adjusts its sensitivity thresholds following sensed and paced events through an auto-gain mechanism. This allows the device to automatically adjust its sensitivity during the tachycardia episode in response to the amplitude of the ventricular signal. For example, the auto-gain may rapidly increase sensitivity to detect small amplitude V-signals during VF rather than interpreting no signal and begin pacing. This auto-gain feature also allows the device to reduce the incidence of T-wave oversensing as well as cross-chamber sensing, particularly with paced events.

Atrioventricular-sequential devices incorporate supraventricular criteria that consider the atrial rhythm and exclude supraventricular tachyarrhythmias when detection of a high ventricular rate is observed. Some single-chamber ventricular devices have morphology discrimination algorithms, which assess the morphology of the ventricular sensed electrogram in order to withhold therapy for supraventricular tachyarrhythmias. Rate stability, sudden-onset, V>A event counters are all helpful in discrimination of SVT from VT.

Most devices allow programming of multiple VT zones. The VT zone is programmed with a lower detection cutoff, which would include any clinical VT events. Ideally, the cutoff rate for detection of tachycardia should be above the patient's maximal heart rate to avoid therapy for sinus tachycardia. Anti-tachycardia pacing schemes with burst pacing, ramp pacing, and inter-burst decrement are all currently available features. Burst pacing sequences consist of a set of ventricular pulses delivered at equal intervals to treat VT. Ramp pacing consists of a set of ventricular pulses delivered at decreasing intervals to treat VT. Following a failed anti-tachycardia pacing (ATP) attempt, inter-burst decrement allows a more aggresssive shortening of the intervals during either a burst or ramp attempt. The first pulse of a burst or ramp sequence (S1) is delivered at a calculated percentage of the tachycardia cycle length. The S1 percentage cycle lengths, number of pulses, interburst decrement, and number of ATP attempts are all programmable features. Additionally, cardioversion therapy (1–38 J) can be programmed in a VT zone. All VT zones have a programmable time limit on episode duration, when the device defaults to the next zone. Also, if a tachycardia is accelerated to a faster arrhythmia, then the ICD will deliver the therapy appropriate for the rate of the accelerated tachycardia.

Successful ICD treatment of VF occurs with defibrillation therapy. All devices are programmed with a VF zone because of the risk of acceleration with anti-tachycardia pacing or cardioversion. Because of the hemodynamic instability observed with fast VT or VF, the device is typically programmed to treat any sustained episode with intervals <300 ms (heart rate >200 beats per minute (BPM)) with defibrillation therapy. The device should be programmed with at a least 10-J safety margin over the defibrillation threshold observed either at implant or during follow-up testing. Up to six additional shocks may be programmed with maximal outputs programmed at the second or third

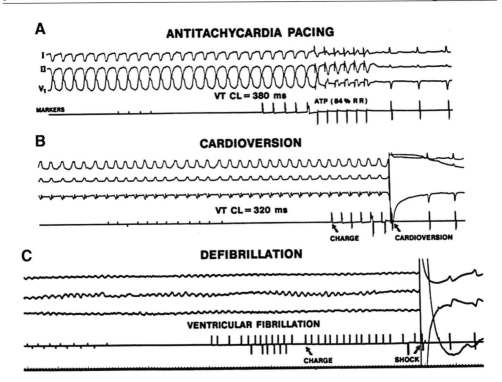

Fig. 1. Various ICD therapies for VT and VF demonstrated during device-based ICD testing. All panels show, from top to bottom, surface electrocardiographic leads I, II, and V_1 and ICD marker channel. CL = cycle length. **(A)** ICD delivery of antitachycardia pacing (ATP) for termination of VT. **(B)** ICD delivery of cardioversion for termination of VT. **(C)** ICD delivery of defibrillation shock for termination of VF.

shock and onward. Once a device exhausts its programmed therapies for a single episode, it quits *(12)*.

Fig. 1, 2, and 3 illustrate the various ICD therapies available for VT and VF.

BRADYCARDIA DETECTION AND THERAPY

All currently available ICDs provide basic single-chamber ventricular (VVI) pacing with separate programmable post-shock lower rate limit and output. Recently, dual-chamber devices have been introduced with use of an atrial lead for diagnostic use only or for atrioventricular (AV) synchronized pacing. These devices allow multiple programmable pacing modes including DDDR, DDD, DDIR, DDI, AAIR, AAI, VVIR, and VVI. These expanded pacing modes have obviated the need for a separate dual-chamber pacemaker that is sometimes necessary in the chronically ill patients who typically receive ICDs. Additionally, they will likely be shown to reduce the incidence of inappropriate shocks attributed to SVT.

In AV-synchronized devices, the ICD continues to sense in both chambers for tachyarrhythmias regardless of the programmed bradycardia pacing mode. To maintain proper sensing, both atrial and ventricular sensing thresholds are adjusted with auto-gain. The ICD has multiple blanking periods to avoid post-pacing depolarization, T-wave oversensing, and cross-communication between chambers. To avoid undersensing

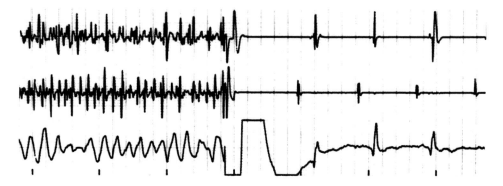

Fig. 2. ICD delivery of defibrillation shock for termination of VF. From top to bottom, intracardiac ventricular electrogram, intracardiac atrial electrogram, and ventricular shock electrocardiogram. Note that in addition to VF there is atrial fibrillation (AF) that was also terminated with the defibrillation shock.

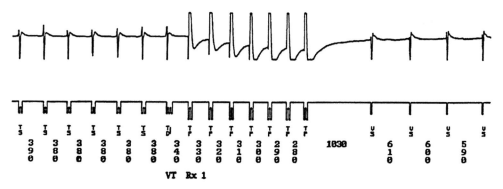

Fig. 3. ICD electrogram showing ATP terminating VT. From top to bottom, intracardiac ventricular electrogram and ICD marker channel with annotations and intervals in ms. VT Rx = VT therapy, TS = VT sense, TD = VT detection, TP = VT pace (ATP), VS = ventricular sense.

of tachyarrhythmias, short cross-chamber blanking periods after paced-events and no cross-chamber blanking after sensed events are necessary. AV synchronous devices have programmable refractory periods available for bradycardia functions, but these refractory periods do not affect tachyarrhythmia detection.

MAGNET FUNCTION

Confusion abounds concerning the function of a magnet with ICDs. The pulse generator contains a reed switch that is closed when a magnet is placed over the device. Closure of the reed switch prevents delivery of tachyarrhythmia therapy. Unlike pacemakers, bradycardia pacing is not affected by the use of a magnet in ICDs. Normal device therapy resumes when the magnet is removed and the reed switch opens.

One manufacturer, Cardiac Pacemakers, Inc./Guidant, has developed two expanded functions during magnet application. In addition to the inhibition of tachyarrhythmia therapy, magnet application can be used to determine the tachycardia mode of the ICD. If a continuous tone is heard, then the tachycardia mode is programmed "off" (off, storage-only, or monitor-only modes). Alternatively, if a series of intermittent tones (synchronized to the R-wave) are heard, then the tachycardia mode is programmed "on" and the device will deliver therapy once the magnet is removed and detection is met. The second additional magnet feature is the change of tachycardia mode with a magnet. If this feature is programmed "on," the application of a magnet for more than 30 S will change the tachycardia mode. If the device is programmed to "off" or "monitor only" (continuous tone), then the device will be programmed "on" (intermittent tone). If the ICD is programmed "on" (intermittent tone), subsequent application of a magnet for > 30 s will program the device "off" (continuous tone). If the device is programmed to storage mode, application of a magnet has no effect on tachycardia mode, and a continuous tone will be heard.

MANAGING AND FOLLOWING PATIENTS

In the United States, patient registration and tracking is mandated United States government. Once registered, a patient receives a permanent identification card to carry with them at all times. A Medic Alert is strongly encouraged and provided by some manufacturers. Patients should be followed initially every 3 mo for at least 6 mo and then at 6-mo intervals. They should be advised they are likely to receive therapies. At the follow-up visitation, a history of symptoms that might suggest tachyarrhythmias should be obtained. The diagnostic and episode data should be reviewed. Current data also include stored episode electrograms to allow review of NSVT as well as delivered therapies for sustained arrhythmias. Device sensing, pacing thresholds, and lead imped-ances should be obtained.

In general, ICD pulse generators have 3–6-yr longevity depending on usage. The programmer allows evaluation of battery status. As the device approaches the elective replacement interval (ERI), follow-up visits should be intensified. In general, once the device reaches ERI, it will operate normally for at least 3 mo, depending upon frequency of therapy. Capacitor deformation occurs during periods when no shocks are delivered, and will result in longer charge times as well as decreased battery longevity. Current ICDs perform an automatic capacitor re-formation that charges the capacitors and delivers the energy to an internal test load. This function improves subsequent charge times and battery longevity. Capacitor re-formations should be conducted manually every 3–6 mo if they are not automatically conducted.

Typically, 40% of patients receive a therapy within the first year after implant, and 10% per yr thereafter. Fig. 4 shows the percentage of patients without ICD shock therapy over time. After a patient experiences a first therapy, they should seek medical attention for assessment of the appropriateness of the therapy. If multiple ICD discharges are experienced, medical attention should be immediately sought. Failure to discriminate between ventricular and supraventricular arrhythmias is the most common reason for inappropriate shocks. Indeed, up to 40% of shocks are delivered inappropriately for supraventricular rhythms. Irregular V-V intervals with a variability greater than 30 ms suggest a SVT such as AF. Rate stability is a commonly used enhancement to improve the appropriateness of device therapy observed in AF with a rapid ventricular response.

Therapy that is conducted during physical exertion and is noted to have gradually increasing V-V intervals, failure of device therapy, and gradual decreasing V-V intervals

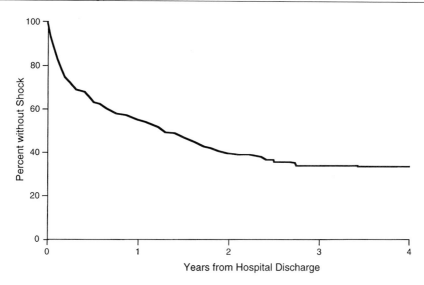

Fig. 4. Time to first shock after hospital discharge in 449 patients after ICD implantation.

suggests sinus tachycardia. Ideally, the cut-off rate for detection of tachyarrhythmias should be greater than the patient's maximal heart rate. In many cases, the VT rate falls within the patient's achievable sinus rate. Enhancements such as sudden-onset and sustained high-rate can allow sinus tachycardia overlap into the VT zone without delivery of an inappropriate shock. Additional enhancements such as morphology discrimination of the ventricular electrogram, as well as the introduction of dual-chamber devices with timing intervals, marker channels, and mode-switching capabilities, are likely to improve the specificity of device therapy. Beta-blocker therapy may help prevent sinus tachycardia from rising into the programmed VT zones.

In the event of multiple ICD discharges, a magnet can be used to inhibit ICD therapy so that the underlying rhythm can be appropriately assessed and treated. The device should be interrogated as soon as possible to assess ICD function and facilitate diagnosis. If a SVT is present, it should be managed as medically appropriate. For patient comfort, the magnet should be left in place to inhibit ICD therapy until the device can be reprogrammed or the SVT is terminated. If VF is present, the device is deemed inoperable and cardiopulmonary resuscitation (CPR) with external defibrillation should be performed.

FREQUENT THERAPIES

Episodes of ventricular tachyarrhythmias sometimes come in storms or bunches. Antitachycardia pacing can reduce the frequency of shocks, but usually antiarrhythmic medications such as amiodarone are required to reduce the frequency of therapy *(13)*. Sotalol has also been shown to be effective in reducing the frequency of shocks in ICD patients *(14)*. In addition, VT ablation, particularly the ablation of bundle-branch reentry VT, can be a useful adjunct. It is important to understand that amiodarone and VT ablation do not prolong life, and that their use is only adjunctive to ICD therapy.

ELECTROMAGNETIC INTERFERENCE (EMI)

Patients should be counseled to avoid sources of EMI, because it may cause the pulse generator to become inhibited, fail to deliver appropriate therapy, or deliver inappropriate therapy. Potential sources of EMI include industrial transformers, radiofrequency transmitters such as RADAR, therapeutic diathermy equipment, arc welding equipment, toy radiotransmitters, anti-theft devices such as electronic article surveillance systems, and magnetic wands. The safe use of medical technologies such as electrosurgery, lithotripsy, external defibrillation, and ionizing radiation can be accomplished by deactivating the device prior to the event. Shielding the device is also appropriate when possible. The device should be evaluated for appropriate operation following exposure. Magnetic resonance imaging (MRI) is contraindicated. Recent reports of interference created by cellular phones may be related to either a magnetic field from within the phone or the radiofrequency signal generated by the phone. It is suggested that if an ICD patient wishes to use a cellular phone, it should be held to the ear opposite the device and carried at least 6–12 inches away from the pulse generator (15).

INSTRUCTIONS TO PATIENTS

The implantation of an ICD is a dramatic intervention for patients and their families. It is important to counsel the patient about their heart disease as well as the consequences of ventricular arrhythmias with and without the ICD. The patient needs to know what to expect when there is a therapy from the ICD. The average time to the first shock is 7 mo, with a clustering of shocks early after implantation and trailing off during the ensuing months. This has been the basis for the recommendation that patients not drive for the first 6 mo after implantation of an ICD (16). This suggestion is appropriate for patients who have had syncopal VT or cardiac arrest. After ICD implantation, it is much less likely, but still possible, that the patient may lose consciousness with an event. Patients with prophylactic ICDs should be told what to expect with a shock, but should be allowed to drive. The patient should also be told to contact their physician each time they feel a shock from their device. If the patient feels well after ICD therapy, it is not an emergency and the patient does not need to go to the emergency room. However, if the patient is in any distress or multiple shocks are delivered, the patient should not waste time contacting their physician, but instead call for an ambulance to be taken directly to an emergency department (17).

FUTURE OF THE ICD

It is likely that the indication and role of ICD implantation will continue to evolve. Several studies are currently being conducted to assess the expanded use of prophylactic ICDs for primary prevention of sudden cardiac death in selected patient populations. Improvements in electronic technology will continue to expand the programming capabilities of these devices, while reducing their size. An atrial defibrillator for therapy of AF is currently in clinical trials. Also, auto-capture algorithms and multi-sensor units are anticipated. Continuous hemodynamic monitoring with the addition of sensors as well as multi-site pacing, resulting in automatic changes in dual-chamber pacing to improve cardiac function, are likely to be instituted in the near future. The storage of hemodynamic data may prove useful in the ongoing management of patients with congestive heart failure (CHF). Suggested future directives incorporate alternative pacing algorithms to suppress foci of automaticity, as well as overdrive suppression of reentrant circuits involved in the generation of tachycardia. Automatic pharmacological infusion therapy commanded by the device has been suggested.

REFERENCES

1. Lown B, Axelrod P. Implanted standby defibrillators. Circulation 1972;46:637–639.
2. Mirowski M, Reid PR, Mower MM, et al. Termination of ventricular arrhythmias with an implanted automatic defibrillator in human beings. N Engl J Med 1980;303:322–324.
3. Gregoratos G, Cheitlin MD, Conill A, Epstein AE, Fellows C, Ferguson TB Jr, et al. ACC/AHA guidelines for implantation of cardiac pacemakers and antiarrhythmia devices: a report of the American College of Cardiology/American Heart Association Task Force on Practice Guidelines (Committee on Pacemaker Implantation). J Am Coll Cardiol 1998 Apr;31(5):1175–1209.
4. Antiarrhythmics versus Implantable Defibrillators (AVID) Investigators. A comparison of antiarrhythmic drug therapy with implantable defibrillators in patients resuscitated from near-fatal ventricular arrhythmias. N Engl J Med 1997;337:1576–1583.
5. Connolly SJ, Gent M, Roberts RS, Dorian P, Roy D, Sheldon RS, et al. Canadian Implantable Defibrillator Study (CIDS): A randomized trial of the implantable cardioverter defibrillator against amiodarone. Circulation 2000 Mar 21;101(11):1297–1302.
6. Moss AJ, Hall WJ, Cannom DS, et al. Improved survival with an implanted defibrillator in patients with coronary disease at high risk for ventricular arrhythmias. N Engl J Med 1996;335:1933–1940.
7. Buxton AE, Fisher JD, Lee KL, et al. for the MUSTT Investigators. A randomized study of the prevention of sudden death in patients with coronary artery disease. N Engl J Med 1999;341:1882–1890.
8. Bigger JT Jr. Prophylactic use of implanted cardiac defibrillators in patients at high risk for ventricular arrhythmias after coronary-artery bypass graft surgery. N Engl J Med 1997;337:1569–1575.
9. Trusty JM, Hayes DL, Stanton MS, Friedman PA. Factors affecting the frequency of subcutaneous lead usage in implantable defibrillators. PACE 2000;23:842–846.
10. Belott PH, Reynolds DW. Permanent Pacemaker and Implantable Cardiovertor-Defibrillator Implantation. In: Clinical Cardiac Pacing and Defibrillation, 2nd ed. W.B. Saunders Publications, Philadelphia, PA, p. 573.
11. Kutalek SP, Kantharia BK, Maquilan JM. Approach to Generator Change. In: Clinical Cardiac Pacing and Defibrillation, 2nd ed. W.B. Saunders Publications, p. 645.
12. Kroll MW, Tchou PJ. Testing of implantable defibrillator functions at implantation. In: Clinical Cardiac Pacing and Defibrillation, 2nd ed. W.B. Saunders Publications, p. 540.
13. Pinski SL, Simmons TW, Maloney JD. Troubleshooting antitachycardia pacing in patients with defibrillators. In: Estes NAM, Wang P, Manolis A, eds. Implantable Cardioverter-defibrillators: A Comprehensive Textbook. Marcel Dekker, New York, NY, 1994, pp. 445–477.
14. Pacifico A, Hohnloser SH, Williams JH, Tao B, Saksena S, Henry PD, et al. Prevention of implantable-defibrillator shocks by treatment with sotalol. N Engl J Med 1999;340:1855–1862.
15. Hayes DL, Strathmore NF. Electromagnetic interference with implantable devices. In: Clinical Cardiac Pacing and Defibrillation, 2nd ed., W.B. Saunders Publications, p. 939.
16. Epstein AE, Miles WM, Benditt DG, Darling EJ, Friedman PL, Garson A, Jr., et al. Personal and public safety issues relates to arrhythmias that may affect consciousness: implications for regulations and physician recommendations. A medical/scientific statement from the American Heart Association and the North American Society of Pacing and Electrophysiology. Circulation 1996;94:1147–1166.
17. Pinski SL, Trohman RG. Implantable cardioverter-defibrillators: implications for the non-electrophysiologist. Ann Intern Med 1995;122:770–777.

16

Pharmacologic Therapy of Ventricular Tachyarrhythmias

Kelley P. Anderson, MD, Susan Brode, MD,
Venkateshwar Gottipaty, MD, PhD,
Alaa Shalaby, MD,
Vladimir Shusterman, MD, PhD,
and Raul Weiss, MD

CONTENTS

Half of what we know in medicine today is wrong.
The trouble is we don't know which half.

INTRODUCTION

Quinidine in the form of cinchona bark has been used to treat palpitations since at least 1749 *(1)*. Its first use for ventricular tachyarrhythmias (VTA) is uncertain because the clinical distinction between supraventricular tachycardia (SVT) and ventricular tachycardia (VT) was probably not appreciated before it was hypothesized by Mackenzie on the basis of venous pulsation in 1908 *(2)*. VT was first demonstrated electrocardiographically by Lewis in 1909 in the first issue of *Lancet (3)*. The first case of control of VT by quinidine was reported in 1921 *(4)*. Fifty years ago, in the first issue of *Circulation,* a series of cases of "paroxysmal ventricular tachycardia" collected between 1915 and 1948 at the Peter Bent Brigham Hospital in Boston, was reported by Armbrust and Levine *(5)*. They examined the efficacy of various medications, including quinidine,

From: *Contemporary Cardiology: Management of Cardiac Arrhythmias*
Edited by: L. I. Ganz © Humana Press Inc., Totowa, NJ

procainamide, magnesium sulfate, potassium salts, atropine, and morphine. Quinidine was the most effective, demonstrating benefit in 46 of 57 treated episodes with oral administration. Additional cases were controlled using rectal and intravenous (iv) administration. However, of 31 patients treated with iv quinidine, six died, two in incessant VT and four of "quinidine toxicity." Single oral doses of quinidine ranged between 200 and 2,500 mg and single iv doses ranged between 200 and 1,500 mg. In retrospect, the ability to make diagnostic and treatment conclusions based on such a varied collection of VT origins and mechanisms demonstrates not only insight and clinical acumen, but some naïveté as well. The administration of such high doses of quinidine seems cavalier in view of the caution we now believe is essential to the safe use of antiarrhythmic drugs. Before the availability of electrical defibrillators, however, the risk of iv quinidine seemed appropriate, given the high likelihood of death associated with "paroxysmal ventricular tachycardia." We now recognize the existence of benign forms of VT that would be refractory to the medications available 50 years ago, and could be rapidly converted into a malignant form if high doses of antiarrhythmic drugs were administered. On the other hand, our early colleagues would likely be both amazed and dubious about the value and ethics of an implanted device that delivers powerful and painful shocks automatically to unanesthetized patients. It is sobering to consider that before the first publication of the Cardiac Arrhythmia Suppression Trial (CAST) *(6)* in 1989, it was standard practice to prescribe the most potent antiarrhythmic drugs to suppress ventricular ectopic activity regardless of the presentation. The spirits of our predecessors and the specters of their errors should remind us that much of what we think accurate today may be proven wrong tomorrow. We must be skeptical of our knowledge, and be ready to change when we are satisfied that the evidence from well-conducted studies provides a better guide than the untrustworthy anecdotes of our own experience and intuition.

GENERAL PRINCIPLES OF ANTI-ARRHYTHMIC THERAPY

Steps in the Selection of Antiarrhythmic Therapy

Thorough evaluation of the individual patient and the clinical context is the essential first step in the selection of the optimal treatment strategy. This includes a determination of the underlying cardiac disorder and its severity, comorbid conditions, response to previous therapy, and other factors that affect prognosis and the response to various treatment alternatives. The second step includes risk assessment for each mode of death: arrhythmic, nonarrhythmic cardiovascular, and noncardiac. The third step is to determine possible treatment strategies. The fourth step is a risk-to-benefit analysis of each of the possible treatment alternatives. This is based on an estimate of impact of therapy on the risk of death and on quality of life. It must be acknowledged that it is rarely possible to comprehensively address any one of the "essential steps," much less all four. Nevertheless, a methodological approach is needed to select the therapy that will achieve the ultimate goal: prolongation of life and enhancement of quality of life. In the midst of the drama of a cardiac arrest and the urgency associated with VT, it is sometimes forgotten that the arrhythmia itself may be a secondary issue and may or may not be the only important target of therapy. The risk of another episode of VTA may be lower than other modes of death. The priorities of care should always be set after the physician defines 1) the ultimate goal (i.e., prolongation of life vs improving quality of life, 2) the specific therapeutic target (e.g., reduction of palpitations, elimination of syncope, reduction of shocks from an implantable cardioverter defibrillator (ICD), prevention of sudden death), 3) the target arrhythmia (e.g., sustained monomorphic VT (SMVT), recurrent ventricular fibrillation (VF), 4) the method to be used to evaluate the drug (e.g., symptoms (PVC) frequency on Holter monitoring, frequency of ICD interventions), and 5) the criteria to be used to define drug success (e.g., 80% reduction in PVC frequency, inability to induce SMVT with programmed electrical stimulation, ICD shock frequency $\leq$ 1 per yr). Even after considerable experience, many of the elements defined before therapy is initiated will change during the course of treatment. However, this initial step provides a framework for subsequent changes, and a basis for educating and informing the patient, health care workers, and payers about the process that is necessary for optimal outcome.

Pharmacological Principles

In an effort to advance antiarrhythmic drug therapy past the traditional empiric approach, the "Sicilian Gambit" was proposed in 1980 *(7)*. This paradigm professed to allow antiarrhythmic drug choice based on arrhythmia mechanisms, vulnerable sites, and pharmacokinetic and pharmacodynamic considerations. Unfortunately, despite substantial progress in the understanding of arrhythmias, it is rarely possible to accurately determine an effective therapy on the basis of known actions on known mechanisms of specific arrhythmias. Moreover, the expanding array of approaches is indicative of the limited effectiveness, safety, and tolerance of current choices. Therefore, antiarrhythmic therapy selection remains largely empiric. The therapeutic range of most antiarrhythmic drugs is severely limited by low efficacy at small doses and the potential for toxicity at high doses. The most important adverse reactions are proarrhythmic effects. It is often difficult to distinguish between failure of therapy resulting from inadequate drug effect and drug-induced proarrhythmias. Too often, several trials must be conducted, which results in a time-consuming and costly process that tests the will and confidence of patients and referring physicians. Antiarrhythmic drugs are highly sensitive to factors that alter concentrations, are highly interactive, and have substantial interindividual variation. Because treatment options are often very limited, it is as important to avoid rejection of a potentially effective drug as it is to reject a toxic drug. Incorrect administration is often responsible for inadequate or excessive effects. For these reasons, an understanding of pharmacological principles and the specific pharmacological properties of each drug is critical to safe, predictable use of antiarrhythmic medications *(8)*.

Interactions

Interactions of antiarrhythmic drugs are an important source of treatment failures and dangerous reactions. Three general categories can be observed: *Pharmacokinetic interactions* may occur with other drugs, foods, and other substances. These interactions can increase or decrease the concentration of the drug at the effector site by altering bioavailability, volume of distribution, protein binding, formation of metabolic products, or clearance. *Pharmacodynamic interactions* refer either to inhibition or augmentation of the physiological response to the drug as a consequence of the pharmacological properties of another drug or endogenous substance, or as a consequence of a change in physiological phenomena such as heart rate. *Drug-device interactions* are a type of pharmacodynamic effect in which a function of a device (ICD or pacemaker) is altered *(9,9a)*. Drugs may alter the characteristics of spontaneous defibrillation energy requirements, capture threshold, or intracardiac signal amplitude or duration. Devices are usually set with wide margins of safety. Therefore, small changes caused by antiarrhythmic drugs are usually of no clinical consequence. However, if the thresholds for an individual patient are near the maximum capacity of the device, there is a risk of failure to properly detect and terminate the arrhythmia. The effects may be of greater significance in the future, when devices will be programmed with narrower tolerances to reduce energy consumption. Of greater clinical significance are the effects of antiarrhythmic drugs on the spontaneous VTA. Drugs can slow the rate of VTA, increase the beat-to-beat variability, and render the presumed reentrant circuit refractory to penetration by paced impulses. These changes can alter the detection and termination of VTA.

Hemodynamic Effects

All antiarrhythmic drugs can reduce cardiac output as a consequence of alterations of contractility, vascular resistance, or the neurohormonal milieu. The mechanisms are complex and interdependent. Contractility may be diminished as a consequence of reduced intracellular calcium ion activity caused by sodium- or calcium-channel blockade. Action-potential prolongation can increase intracellular calcium and partially restore contractility. However, contractility is rate-dependent. In normal hearts, contractility rises at rates as high as 180/min. In heart failure, however, contractility is reduced, and the heart rate at which it peaks may also be reduced to less than 100 beats per minute (BPM). Contractility would be expected to decline during faster rates. Sodium-channel blockade is also increased at faster rates while the influence of action-potential prolongation diminishes. It is probably for a combination of these reasons that hemodynamic collapse may occur with drugs that are widely believed to be hemodynamically neutral, such as lidocaine. If VTA recur despite the presence of an antiarrhythmic drug, the hemodynamic consequences may be more severe. In some cases, hemodynamic properties can be used to select therapy. For example, vasodilation maybe the mechanism by which quinidine is better tolerated than disopyramide (which causes vasoconstriction) in patients with heart failure.

Proarrhythmic Effects

Exacerbation or facilitation of existing arrhythmias or provocation of new arrhythmias are frequent and life-threatening complications of antiarrhythmic drugs *(10)*. Most antiarrhythmic drugs depress normal automatically and may cause bradyarrhythmias. This complication is relatively rare in patients with normal sinus-node function. Indeed, drugs with atropine-like effects (muscarinic-receptor blockade) such as disopyramide and quinidine may cause an increase in heart rate. The calcium-channel blockers diltiazem and verapamil cause variable responses in heart rate. Although calcium-channel blockade reduces automaticity, increased sympathetic tone caused by vasodilation may result in an increase in heart rate. Beta-blockers usually decrease heart rate, but this is rarely clinically significant in patients with normal sinus-node function. Although drug-induced bradyarrhythmias are relatively rare, even in patients with sinus-node dysfunction, such patients are at risk for severe bradyarrhythmias. Evidence suggests that drug-induced bradycardia is a rare cause of death. In contrast, bradyarrhythmia-

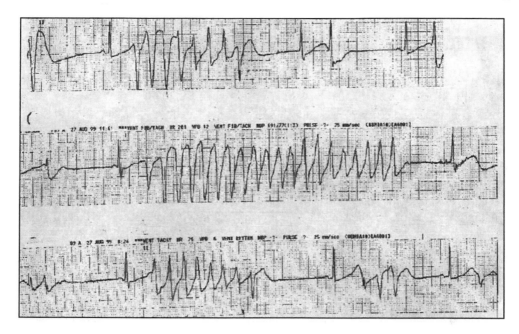

Fig. 1. Episodes of nonsustained torsades de pointes in a patient with acquired LQTS caused by quinidine. Note the excessive QT prolongation following the longer R-R intervals, with the first beat of VT falling on the T wave. Quinidine was discontinued, and the patient was treated acutely with iv magnesium and temporary transvenous pacing. Once the quinidine washed out, the patient's QT interval returned to normal and no further torsades de pointes occurred.

induced VTA may not be a rare mechanism of drug-associated sudden death, and is usually related to treatment with class IA and III drugs. This drug-associated arrhythmia is polymorphic, often resembling torsades de pointes (*see* Fig. 1). This arrhythmia may account for some reports of drug-induced long QT syndrome (LQTS) associated with drugs that would not be expected to cause this complication, such as mexiletine and flecainide. Bradycardia-induced VTA also occur in patients who develop severe brady-arrhythmias in the absence of antiarrhythmic drugs. It is possible that this complication results from a genetic predisposition for LQTS. If so, advance prediction may be possible in the future. Although there has been concern that sodium-channel blockers will cause complete heart block in patients with conduction-system disease, this compli-cation has rarely been observed. Unfortunately, the extent to which bradyarrhythmias are responsible for out-of-hospital drug-associated sudden death is unknown. Nevertheless, based on current knowledge, the presence of sinus-node dysfunction or severe atrioven-tricular (AV) conduction-system disease should not be considered contraindications to antiarrhythmic drug therapy. Such patients should be observed closely during initiation of antiarrhythmic drugs. Periodic monitoring during long-term treatment would seem prudent—e.g., 24-hour Holter monitoring at least every 6 mo. Unfortunately, no infor-mation exists to guide selection of the ideal method of repeat monitoring, the frequency, or the yield. Patients with ICDs should have their devices programmed for backup pacing at an appropriate lower rate limit to protect against significant bradycardia.

VTA associated with drug-induced LQTS, i.e., torsades de pointes (*see* Fig. 1), is relatively frequent with drugs that prolong action-potential duration (class IA and III drugs) and may occur with an expanding group of noncardiac drugs and conditions *(11,12)*. Precautions should be taken to minimize the incidence. The risk of this complication is related to the specific drug, the severity of myocardial dysfunction, the presenting arrhythmia, the sex of the patient, the genetic background ("reduced repolarization reserve"), heart rate, concomitant medications, and electrolyte disturbances (hypokalemia and hypomagnesemia). The long-term risk is related to the chance that risk factors will coincide in the future. For instance, alterations in diuretic dose and adequacy of supplementation with potassium and magnesium increase the likelihood of electrolyte disturbances. Drugs that delay repolarization should be used cautiously or not at all in patients with multiple risk factors for this form of the acquired LQTS. The type and intensity of monitoring should be proportional to the risk of torsades de pointes. The 12-lead ECG should be used to monitor QT duration. Rhythm monitoring is needed to assess danger signs including self-terminating runs of polymorphic VT (PVT), postpause U-wave accentuation, QT prolongation, T-wave alternans (TWA), and bradycardia. Patients at high risk should be continuously monitored in-hospital, and monitor staff should be trained to recognize the characteristic electrocardiogram (ECG) warning signs. The initiation of antiarrhythmic drugs to out-patients is debated, but this may be acceptable in patients at low risk of drug-induced LQTS. Nevertheless, it would seem prudent to obtain 12-lead ECGs and use other rhythm-monitoring methods at critical times—e.g., upon initiation of medications, achievement of steady-state concentrations, and during dose changes. Risk-factor minimization is essential during long-term therapy. Care must be taken to avoid electrolyte disturbances and exposure to drugs that augment the effects on repolarization by increasing concentration (usually by inhibition of metabolism) or by additive pharmacodynamic activity.

Excessive sodium-channel blockade is believed to be the mechanism of the most important arrhythmias caused by class IC drugs, flecainide, propafenone, and moricizine *(13)*, but all of the sodium-channel blockers are capable of this reaction. Although presentation may consist of asymptomatic nonsustained ventricular arrhythmias, this complication requires immediate attention in order to prevent the highly malignant intractable VTA that characterizes this disorder. The appearance of these VTA may vary in a single episode from incessant SMVT to repeated runs of polymorphic VT (PVT) that degenerates into VF only to recur shortly after countershock. For this reason, the presence of an ICD may not provide adequate protection for this form of pro-arrhythmia. It is critical to distinguish this form of drug-induced proarrhythmia from torsades de pointes. Pacing therapy is indicated in the latter, but contraindicated in the former. Instead, efforts are directed toward maneuvers that reduce sodium-channel binding (e.g., heart-rate reduction, competition with fast-on, fast-off sodium-channel-binding drugs) and that restore the inward sodium current (infusion of hypertonic sodium solutions). Risk factors include the presence of structural heart disease, especially coronary artery disease (CAD), and a history of VTA. The presence of these risk factors are considered strong contraindications to therapy with class IC agents. Precipitating factors include tachycardia, myocardial ischemia, high concentrations of the drug, and addition of another sodium-channel blocker. Tachycardia and ischemia are especially provocative, because both cause increased binding of the drug to sodium channels, and they can establish a positive feedback process whereby tachycardia increases ischemia, and ischemia increases tachycardia (by augmenting sympathetic activity). Increasing sodium-channel blockade makes the arrhythmias more difficult to terminate and reduces contractility and systemic pressure, which further reduces myocardial perfusion. Careful avoidance of the precipitating factors is required in all patients receiving class IC agents. Steps must be taken to avoid tachycardia that may occur in several circumstances. A stress test may be useful for estimating the likelihood for high heart rates during daily activities. Implanted devices should be tested and adjusted to avoid excessive pacing rates during antitachycardia pacing, tracking of atrial arrhythmias, high sensor-mediated rates, and pacemaker-mediated-tachycardia. Concomitant administration of beta-blockers is highly recommended, and may be considered mandatory. Exercise-testing or 24-h monitoring should be considered to verify adequate beta-blockade.

Another form of proarrhythmia that may occur with any sodium-channel blocker—but is most often observed in patients receiving flecainide and propafenone—is a sudden increase in the ventricular-rate response to atrial tachyarrhythmias, especially atrial fibrillation (AF) or atrial flutter. The proposed mechanism is that the antiarrhythmic drug converts AF or rapid atrial flutter to a slow atrial flutter, which results in one-to-one activation of the ventricles. Often a wide QRS tachycardia is observed, which is difficult to distinguish from a SMVT.

There is uncertainty about the spectrum, frequency, and impact of proarrhythmic effects in patients with ICDs (9). Patients with ICDs may be protected from drug-related bradycardia-induced VTA because of backup pacing or by detection and termination of the sustained VTA. However, some drug-induced arrhythmias may be refractory to antitachycardia pacing and defibrillation, or be exacerbated by the programmed algorithms. AF or atrial flutter may result in heart rates that meet detection criteria and cause inappropriate and ineffective ICD pacing or defibrillation that could precipitate proarrhythmic effects. As noted earlier, antiarrhythmic drugs may alter myocardial properties and native VTA characteristics resulting in failure to detect and terminate spontaneous arrhythmias. Devices are not routinely programmed specifically for drug-induced arrhythmias. These concerns emphasize the need for careful monitoring of patients with ICDs who require antiarrhythmic drug therapy. Strong consideration should be given to reassessment of pacing, sensing, and defibrillation energy parameters. Retesting of detection and termination algorithms in the presence of antiarrhythmic drugs should be considered, but is often not possible in patients who do not have inducible arrhythmias. The distinction between arrhythmia recurrence resulting from ineffectiveness of the drug and proarrhythmia is critical, but may be difficult. Changes in the pattern of arrhythmias detected and treated based on symptoms, stored data, and electrograms, supplemented by Holter or event-monitor recordings, should be helpful.

There are major gaps in our understanding of proarrhythmic effects, particularly with regard to risks during long-term treatment. The strongest evidence for this are the inconsistencies between our current understanding, which is based on observations obtained at the time of initiation of drugs and on in-hospital observations, and the pattern of excess mortality associated with antiarrhythmic drugs in the CAST (6) and Survival with Oral d-Sotalol (SWORD) trial in patients with left ventricular dysfunction after myocardial infarction (MI) (14). There may be forms and mechanisms of fatal proarrhythmic effects that have not been discovered.

Implantable Cardioverter Defibrillators

For many clinicians, no other therapy provides as much assurance for an individual patient as an implantable cardioverter defibrillator (ICD). The results of recent clinical trials substantiate superiority over standard antiarrhythmic therapy in selected patients. There is a temptation to use the ICD in any patient with a significant risk of arrhythmic death. However, the Coronary Artery Bypass Graft—Implantable Defibrillator (CABG Patch) trial demonstrated that certain groups of patients do not benefit from ICD implantation *(15)*. Subgroup analysis of the Antiarrhythmics Versus Implantable Defibrillator (AVID) trial indicated no benefit of ICD over amiodarone therapy in patients with ejection fractions greater than 0.35 *(16);* a similar conclusion has emerged from the CIDS study *(17)*. Clinical trials that have demonstrated its successful application excluded categories of patients who were unlikely to benefit from protection against arrhythmic death. Appropriate application and informed consent required a thorough appreciation of the disadvantages and risks of current-generation ICDs. A partial list includes: 1) life-long complications of device-lead systems that require periodic replacement; 2) continued need for antiarrhythmic drugs for adequate arrhythmia control with exposure to risks of long-term drug use; 3) painful shocks caused by recurrent ventricular tachyarrhythmia (VT), atrial arrhythmias, or spurious signals and artifacts; 4) risk of interference from other devices and electromagnetic fields; 5) exclusion from tests and treatments that cannot be performed in patients with implanted devices; 6) psychological effects from anxiety related to unpredictable shocks, embarrassment, loss of control, dependency, humiliation, and other feelings that can lead to depression and psychosis; 7) driving, travel, and restrictions on other activities; 8) occupational effects such as job restrictions, time lost from work, reduced occupational status, and advancement; and 9) social exclusion.

Necessity should take precedence over cost. However, in many countries the patient bears the cost of the ICD. Also significant is the fact that health costs are controlled in most countries so that a high expense in one area forces a reduction in other areas. Rough calculations indicate the enormity of the problem: The United States has the highest ICD implantation rate in the world: about 40,000 devices in 1999. This rate would have to increase sevenfold if ICDs were provided to all patients who are expected to die suddenly in the coming year—i.e., 300,000 persons in the United States alone. Many clinicians consider a patient to be a candidate for an ICD if the risk of sudden death is between 1% and 10% per yr. This would increase the rate of implantation by 10–100 times over that limited to 100% risk. In addition, most patients in whom ICDs are implanted receive no benefit but are at risk for all of the complications—e.g., 90 out of every 100 patients in the 10% risk category. These facts are presented here to emphasize the importance of careful patient selection. Fortunately, it is likely that many of the problems with current-generation ICDs, including the cost, will be substantially reduced with a few years by the remarkable pace of technical advances.

Pharmacological agents play a major role in patients with ICDs. Amiodarone and sotalol are frequently used in ICD patients *(18)*. Indications for antiarrhythmic therapy in patients with ICDs include: 1) to reduce the frequency of VTA events requiring ICD therapy, especially painful and battery-depleting shocks; 2) to slow the rate of VTA in order to increase the efficacy of antitachycardia pacing and reduce the need for shock; 3) to reduce the recurrence of supraventricular tachyarrhythmias that may cause inappropriate ICD therapies; 4) to reduce the ventricular-rate response to atrial tachyarrhythmias that may cause inappropriate ICD therapies; 5) to reduce the maximum sinus rate to avoid inappropriate ICD therapy; 6) to reduce the frequency and duration of nonsustained VT (NSVT) events to avoid unnecessary ICD therapy; and 7) to decrease defibrillation thresholds. The potential for proarrhythmic effects and drug-device interactions discussed here should be used to guide drug selection, administration of selected drugs, ICD programming, and the frequency and extent of periodic follow-up and monitoring.

Catheter Ablation and Operative Intervention

Operative and catheter-based ablation, excision, and interruption of tachycardia foci and circuits provide an opportunity for permanent cure. Catheter ablation appears to be highly effective for idiopathic SMVT and is considered first-choice therapy by many clinicians. In patients with ischemic heart disease, however, catheter ablation is often used adjunctively to control incessant VTA or to reduce the recurrence rate in patients with ICDs. Often, pharmacologic therapy does not result in adequate control, but is maintained at the time of ablation and often continued after the procedure *(19)*. Antiarrhythmic drugs are often helpful in reducing the rate of VTA and improving hemodynamic stability. This allows electrical activation-sequence mapping and better control of ablation. There are reports of improved responsiveness of antiarrhythmic drugs after catheter-based and operative interventions, but the extent to which the beneficial effects of antiarrhythmic drugs are improved or adverse effects increased has not been established.

IMMEDIATE MANAGEMENT OF VENTRICULAR TACHYARRHYTHMIAS

Initial management of the patient who presents with a sustained VTA is guided by advanced cardiac life support (ACLS) recommendations. National guidelines vary, and specific aspects—particularly adjunctive pharmacological therapy—are controversial. This is largely because of the lack of controlled trials, which are difficult to perform in victims of VTA *(20)*. The International Liaison Committee on Resuscitation (ILCOR) was formed to create a consensus guideline from the diverse guidelines established in different countries *(21)*. The American Heart Association (AHA) has recently published recommendations entitled "Guidelines 2000 for Cardiopulmonary Resuscitation and Emergency Cardiovascular Care." These recommendations represent an international consensus, and include a comprehensive discussion of the rationale of treatments, as well as alternative treatments and their indications classified according to the confidence of scientific data supporting the recommendation *(22)*.

Defibrillation is performed as soon as possible in patients who present with pulseless VTA or VF. If the initial three attempts at defibrillation fail, they are repeated after intravenous (iv) administration of epinephrine 1 mg every 3–5 min, or a single dose of vasopressin (40 units iv). Reversible causes of the VTA should be found and corrected. Sodium bicarbonate administration should be considered in refractory VTA, or in situations such as tricyclic overdose, hyperkalemia, and prolonged resuscitative efforts. Special situations may require alterations in management that deviate from the basic algorithm *(23)*. Some authorities have recommended higher doses of epinephrine (up to 0.1 mg/kg), although clinical trials have not shown a significant improvement in survival until hospital discharge.

Although arbitrary, an arrhythmia may be considered intractable if there is failure to convert the rhythm after several attempts of defibrillation, epinephrine, or vasopressin,

Table 1
Dosages of Antiarrhythmic Drugs for VF/Pulseless VT

Drug	Bolus	Rebolus	Infusion	Comments
Amiodarone	300 mg iv push	150 mg iv push if needed	1 mg/min for 6 h	Maximum cumulative dose 2.2 mg/kg/24 h
Lidocaine	1.0–1.5 mg/kg iv push	Consider 1.0–1.5 mg/kg in 5 min	1–4 mg/min	Maximum cumulative dose 3.0 mg/kg
Magnesium sulfate	1.0–2.0 g			For torsades and refractory VF
Procainamide	30 mg/min (total 10–17 mg/kg)		1–4 mg/min	Maximum rate 50 mg/min; Maximum dose 17 mg/kg
Bretylium*	5 mg/kg	10 mg/kg after 5 min	1–2 mg/min	See below*

*Removed from Guidelines 2000 for Cardiopulmonary Resuscitation and Emergency Cardiovascular Care (22); currently unavailable in United States.

and attempts at correction of potential causes—or if there is initial conversion but repeated reinitiation of the VTA. For persistent pulseless VTA, the recent recommendations classify antiarrhythmic drugs as either class IIB (unproven, but acceptable, possibly helpful) or indeterminate agents (22). The recommended drugs are amiodarone, lidocaine, magnesium (for torsades de pointes or refractory VF), and procainamide (see Table 1). Notably, bretylium has been removed from these most recent guidelines because of its high rate of adverse effects, the availability of other agents with a more favorable intended/adverse effect profile, and lack of availability of bretylium from the manufacturer. For persistent VTA, defibrillation shocks are given after administration of each dose of the antiarrhythmic drug. After return of spontaneous circulation, patients are generally maintained initially on a continuous infusion of an antiarrhythmic drug; dosages are given in Table 1.

For treatment of the patient who presents with a VTA that is hemodynamically stable, AHA/ACLS recommendations are that the basic "ABC" (Airway, Breathing, Circulation: i.e., secure airway, administer oxygen, start iv, attach monitor) be followed by assessment of vital signs, review of history, physical examination, a 12-lead ECG, and a portable chest X-ray. Although lidocaine had traditionally been used first in previous ACLS algorithms in the United States, it appears less effective in VT not caused by acute ischemia or infarction. In a randomized study, Goergels et al. found iv procainamide more likely than lidocaine to terminate monomorphic VT in the non-AMI setting (24). The most recent guidelines do not recommend lidocaine initially in all VT patients. Rather, antiarrhythmic drug recommendations in these guidelines are based on cardiac function (22). For patients with normal cardiac function, procainamide and sotalol are recommended as initial agents, with amiodarone and lidocaine also listed as acceptable options. Intravenous sotalol is not approved for use in the United

Table 2
Antiarrhythmic Drug Dosing for Hemodynamically Tolerated VT

Drug	Bolus	Rebolus	Infusion	Comments
Procainamide	20–50 mg/min (total 17 mg/kg)		1–4 mg/kg	Monitor BP and QRS width; contraindicated in torsades des pointes
Sotalol†	10 mg/min (total 1.0–1.5 mg/kg)			iv form not available in US; contraindicated in torsades des pointes
Amiodarone	150 mg over 10 min	As 150 mg over 10 min every 10–15 min as needed	10 mg/min for 6 h, then 0.5 mg/min	Maximum cumulative dose 2.2 mg/kg/24 h
Lidocaine	0.5–0.75 mg/kg	0.5–0.75 mg/kg every 5–10 min	1–4 mg/kg	Maximum bolus total 3.0 mg/kg over 1 h
Bretylium*	5–10 mg/kg over 8–10 min	5–10 mg/kg	1–2 mg/kg	Maximum bolus 30 mg/kg/24 h

*Removed from Guidelines 2000 for Cardiopulmonary Resuscitation and Emergency Cardiovascular Care (22); currently unavailable in United States.
†iv sotalol not available in United States.

States; oral sotalol will not acutely terminate VT. Procainamide and sotalol are contraindicated in torsades de pointes VT. For patients with impaired cardiac function, amiodarone and lidocaine are recommended. Guidelines for the specific drugs and doses are presented in Table 2. Antiarrhythmic drugs often decrease the rate of SMVT without terminating it (see Fig. 2). If sinus rhythm is not restored with antiarrhythmic therapy, patients should be cardioverted.

Approved for use in the United States in 1995, iv amiodarone's pivotal role in the immediate management of sustained VTA has not been fully established. The recent guidelines, however, support the use of iv amiodarone early in the acute management of sustained VTA. Evidence from controlled studies supports the use of iv amiodarone. In a randomized controlled trial, amiodarone (300 mg iv) or placebo was administered to patients when VF or pulseless VT persisted after ≥3 unsuccessful DC shocks and epinephrine 1 mg iv (25). Amiodarone administration led to a significantly increased survival to reach hospital (44% vs 34%, p = 0.02). Survival to hospital discharge rate was similar (13.4% vs 13.2%), but the study was not powered to detect a difference. There was also an increased rate of hypotension and bradycardia in patients treated with amiodarone. Preliminary data from the ALIVE trial suggests the iv amiodarone is superior to lidocaine in cardiac arrest refractory to initial shocks. In this trial, iv amiodarone (5 mg/kg bolus) increased survival to hospital admission by 52% (25a). Two multicenter prospective trials evaluated iv amiodarone in patients refractory to (or intolerant of) lidocaine, procainamide, or bretylium (26,27). The majority of these

A

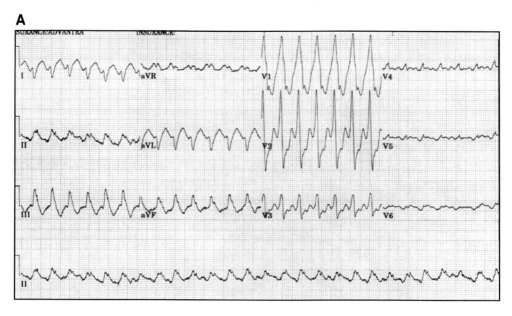

B

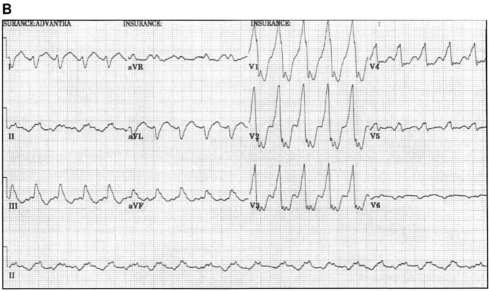

Fig. 2. Monomorphic VT in a patient with prior MI. **(A)** The initial rate of VT was 163 BPM. **(B)** Following a procainamide load, the VT has slowed to 118 BPM, and the QRS has widened.

patients had previous MI, and many had incessant VT or were receiving cardiopulmonary resuscitation (CPR). Both studies demonstrated a dose-dependent beneficial effect on mean time to first recurrence of VTA. Neither study demonstrated a statistically significant dose-related trend in mortality. Another trial compared iv amiodarone to standard-dose iv bretylium in patients refractory to lidocaine and procainamide *(28)*. At a dose of 1 g/24 h iv amiodarone was equivalent to standard-dose bretylium (2500 mg/24 h) with respect to arrhythmia event rate, the time to first arrhythmia recurrence, and

48-h survival. However, significantly more patients receiving bretylium developed hypotension or heart failure.

Although generally supportive, these trials failed to demonstrate the superiority of iv amiodarone to standard therapy based on "hard" survival end points. On the other hand, given the heterogeneous nature of the patients and disorders for whom the interventions were applied, the results seem impressive. In any case, iv amiodarone has achieved widespread acceptance and usage. Part of the enthusiasm for iv amiodarone may result from the positive reputation of the oral form. Many authorities believe that oral amiodarone is the drug with the best risk-to-benefit performance in control of sustained VTA. However, many of its electrophysiological effects develop weeks after initiation. It is not known which of the many effects of amiodarone are essential to its success, and it is probable that the critical elements vary according to the type and degree of cardiac dysfunction and arrhythmia characteristics. Therefore, the electrophysiological profile of iv amiodarone differs from that of the oral form, and it can be expected to change over time. The rationale for early administration is not limited to the immediate effects of iv amiodarone; rather the more quickly amiodarone is administered, the sooner the effects on repolarization and other slowly developing properties will exert their benefits. The initial dose recommended by the Intravenous Amiodarone Multicenter Investigators Group is a bolus of 150 mg over 10 min followed by a 6-h infusion period at 1 mg/min, followed by a maintenance rate of 0.5 mg/min. This provides 1 g in the first 24 h. Supplemental doses of 150 mg iv are recommended to achieve suppression of breakthrough arrhythmias. The "Guidelines 2000" recommend an initial 300 mg bolus of iv amiodarone for VF/VT cardiac arrest with additional boluses of 150 mg as necessary/maximum cumulative dose 2.2g over 24 h (22).

Standard ACLS guidelines were developed to address the majority of cardiac-arrest cases, which are usually out-of-hospital events and often unwitnessed. In contrast, clinicians are more likely to encounter sustained VTA in the hospitalized patient. In such cases, more information and more therapeutic options may be available, such as circulatory assist devices, rapid-rate pacemakers, and access to catheter-based therapies (including revascularization and radiofrequency ablation). Because the distribution of response varies widely between situations, optimal treatment guidelines may differ from those proposed by national organizations.

Gillis has proposed an approach to intractable VTA (IVTA) directed toward the hospitalized patient (29). Patients who present with VTA are treated according to standard guidelines, and receive at least one trial of either lidocaine or procainamide and correction of immediately reversible causes. If beta-blockers are not contraindicated, atrial pacing is performed at 80–100 beats per minute (BPM), and 3 to 5 doses of the β_1-selective beta-blocker metoprolol 5 mg iv are administered every 5 min. Alternatively, a nonselective agent such as esmolol (0.5 mg/kg over 1 min, then 0.05–0.3 mg/kg/min continuous infusion) or propranolol (1 mg iv every min to total initial dose of 0.1 mg/kg) may be used. Beta-blockers can be administered to most patients with heart failure. Small doses of beta-blockers are often tolerated, and are beneficial in patients with cardiogenic shock.

Nadamanee and colleagues (30) recently published their findings in 49 patients with electrical storm, defined as recurrent, multiple VF episodes. Patients treated with sympathetic blockade fared better than those treated according to ACLS algorithms with lidocaine, procainamide, and bretylium. Sympathetic blockade consisted of iv esmolol or propranolol, as well as left stellate ganglionic blockade in some patients; these patients also received oral amiodarone.

If beta-blockers are contraindicated or a trial is unsuccessful, Gillis recommends amiodarone iv at twice the dose recommended by the Intravenous Amiodarone Multicenter Investigators Group. The prospective multicenter study reported that patients initiated on higher doses had longer times to first ventricular tachyarrhythmia (VTA) recurrences and required fewer supplemental infusions, and that hypotension, which occurred in approx 25% of patients, was not significantly more frequent in the high-dose group. The suggested dosing schedule, based on a pharmacokinetic study, provides an iv dose of 2100 mg in the first 24 h, 300 mg iv over 10–20 min followed by an initial infusion rate of 2 mg/min for 6 h (720 mg), then a maintenance rate of 1 mg/min. The iv infusion at 1 mg/kg is then continued for 3 d (1440 mg/d) (29). The Gillis algorithm does not include the use of bretylium. The Intravenous Amiodarone Multicenter Investigators Group observed that amiodarone was as effective as bretylium, but was associated with fewer adverse effects. Other considerations could also guide the early use of amiodarone. If oral amiodarone therapy is a long-term option, then early use of iv amiodarone should accelerate the slowly developing antiarrhythmic effects of oral amiodarone. On the other hand, amiodarone has a very long elimination half-life. This can result in prolonged adverse effects, which may be particularly serious in the rare case of proarrhythmic properties and interactions that occur between amiodarone and many forms of therapy. The extended effects may also affect electrophysiological evaluation and complicate the use of other antiarrhythmic drugs.

Other pharmacological therapies may also play an important role in IVTA. Heavy sedation or general anesthesia (combined with assisted ventilation) could reduce sympathetic activity, energy utilization, myocardial oxygen demand, and congestive heart failure (CHF). Inotropic drugs and pressors are often necessary, although they may have proarrhythmic actions. Pharmacological therapy is only one element of the total approach to IVTA. Other strategies include internal defibrillation, cardiac pacing to inhibit or to terminate VTA, ablation of culprit myocardial tissue by catheter-based radiofrequency ablation, or surgical ablation and excision. Circulatory assist devices are of particular importance in reducing sympathetic drive, myocardial stretch, and oxygen demand, and allowing the use of medications that cause hypotension (31).

LONG-TERM MANAGEMENT OF VTA

Initial Evaluation

Errors in the long-term management of patients who present with VTA often result from the failure to delineate the goals and targets of therapy. Most patients who present with VTA have severe underlying structural heart disease and comorbid conditions that may constitute risks for multiple mechanisms of death. A therapeutic strategy focused solely on the presenting arrhythmias may not fully address the ultimate goal: prolongation of survival. In some circumstances, effective prevention of the VTA increases the risk of other mechanisms of death. In other circumstances, risk modification reduces the risk of recurrent VTA so that additional specific treatment is unnecessary. The optimal treatment strategy provides the greatest reduction of all causes of mortality, with modifications for quality of life and other patient preferences. Risk assessment is the key step that ascertains the potential benefit of a therapeutic strategy. Unfortunately, adequate information regarding risk is almost always lacking. This results in estimates of arrhythmic death with large confidence intervals resulting from the inaccuracies of current data. The clinical response to this uncertainty is to offer ICD therapy, which is believed to be the most secure treatment available.

Overview

The last 10 yr have witnessed a tremendous change in approaches to the long-term management of VTA. Guided therapy of antiarrhythmic drugs, usually by serial invasive electrophysiologic studies (EPS), but sometimes by Holter monitoring, was the paradigm until the early 1990s. The CASCADE trial, however, showed that empiric amiodarone therapy was superior to electrophysiology-guided therapy with class I agents in cardiac-arrest survivors *(32)*. The ESVEM trial showed that guided therapy with sotalol was superior to guided therapy with class I agents, either using electrophysiology or Holter guidance *(33,34)*. These trials led to a marked decrease in class I drug use and guided therapy in general. Randomized trials such as AVID *(16)*, CIDS *(34a)*, and CASH *(35)*, which documented the superiority of ICD therapy to amiodarone in patients with VTA, have led to a marked decrease in the use of pharmacologic therapy as a primary measure in patients with a history of VT or VF. Amiodarone continues to be used in patients for whom ICDs are not a good option or are undesirable.

Ischemic Heart Disease

Ischemic heart disease is the most common etiology of VTA. It is an extraordinarily complex syndrome with many potential influences that contribute to arrhythmogenesis. Four general processes can be considered: ischemia-reperfusion, acute MI, healed MI, and remodeling of noninfarcted myocardium. Ischemia followed by reperfusion is an extremely potent cause of arrhythmias. The resulting ventricular arrhythmia is usually a polymorphic VTA (i.e., polymorphic VT or VF). SMVT is rarely observed in the absence of a pre-existing scar. Ischemia-reperfusion VTA can occur in the absence of ischemic heart disease (IHD) because of vasospasm, thromboembolism followed by lysis, and other mechanisms. Because it may be transient, asymptomatic and completely reversible, ischemia-reperfusion can rarely be completely excluded as a possible contributor to arrhythmogenesis. The potential for ischemia should be evaluated in most cases. Although proper precautions must be taken, provocation of ischemia for diagnostic purposes is rarely contraindicated in patients who present with VTA. VTA are rarely induced during physical or pharmacological stress tests for ischemia. Failure to reproduce a VTA during provoked ischemia does not exclude a contribution of ischemia for the previous event or a future event. Therefore, prevention of ischemia is appropriate in most patients with IHD who present with VTA.

Cardiac arrest or VTA in the context of an acute MI is generally attributed to the electrophysiological and neurohormonal changes related to ischemia-reperfusion, followed by those caused by the acute necrotic process. About 65% of deaths from MI occur within the first few hours of symptoms, and most are a result of VF *(36)*. Patients who develop sustained VT are older, have larger infarctions, and have high mortality rates. In one study, mortality was 27%, 39% and 45% at 7 d, 30 d, and 1 yr, respectively. This was higher than in patients who develop in-hospital VF or NSVT *(37)*. This is clearly a group in which aggressive evaluation and therapy is warranted.

Ventricular tachyarrhythmia that occurs during an acute MI can be classified as early (<24 h) or late (>24 h after admission), and as primary (i.e. Killip class I), or secondary (i.e., Killip class II–IV). Patients with primary VF tend to have a more extensive infarction. In one report, in-hospital mortality was high if the arrhythmias occurred within 4 h of acute MI, but even higher if VF occurred between 4 and 48 h. On the other hand, after discharge, patients with primary VF have a similar 6-mo, 1-yr, and 5-yr mortality compared to controls. The in-hospital and 1-yr mortality of patients with secondary VF is very high: 58% at 1 yr in one study *(37)*. Lidocaine is recommended for prevention of further episodes in patients who with VTA early after acute MI. The need for lidocaine should be reevaluated after about 12–24 h when the risk of recurrence of VTA declines markedly *(36)*. Presentation with early primary VTA does not appear to select patients who will benefit from long-term antiarrhythmic drug treatment beyond standard therapy after MI.

Patients who develop late VF (>24 h after admission) have a worse in-hospital and subsequent prognosis than those with early VF. It is not known what time cut-off point after acute MI provides the most reliable segregation of low- and high-risk patients. Patients were excluded from the Canadian Implantation Defibrillator Study (CIDS) *(38)*, and the AVID trial *(16)* if the presenting VTA occurred less than 3 d and 5 d after MI, respectively. The purpose was to exclude patients who would be unlikely to benefit from ICD therapy because of low risk for subsequent arrhythmic events.

The transition between acute, healing, and chronic MI is a continuum during which risk for VTA varies. Moreover, there are large interindividual differences in the pattern of variation. Risk is high during the first 6 mo after an acute MI, and usually declines. However, in some patients, remodeling results in continuous changes in the MI scar, which may form into a substrate for reentry at any time from days to decades after the acute MI. This process results in regions of unexcitable tissue that can form anatomic barriers, and areas of viable tissue with altered cell-to-cell coupling and other nonuniform properties that form the basis for slow conduction, unidirectional block and other factors that promote reentry. This underlies SMVT in many patients with ischemic heart disease. Remodeling also occurs in noninfarcted myocardium caused by an extensive acute MI, progressive ischemia, or concomitant cardiovascular disease such as hypertensive cardiovascular disease or superimposed dilated cardiomyopathy. This type of remodeling is a process associated with anatomic, electrophysiological, and neurohormal changes—all of which may facilitate arrhythmogenesis. The electrophysiological changes include reduction of potassium currents and action-potential prolongation. One theory is that this process results in an acquired form of LQTS because of reduced repolarization reserve. The observed arrhythmias are usually polymorphic VT (PVT) or VF with mechanisms similar or identical to those observed in some forms of LQTS.

Although separation of the various arrhythmogenic influences is helpful in understanding the pathogenesis of VTA in IHD, it oversimplifies the interactions between the electrophysiological, neurohormonal, and anatomical changes. In practice, it is rarely possible to distinguish between the four major influences or to completely exclude any single influence in the genesis of a clinical event. Most patients with ischemic heart disease (IHD) have multiple mechanisms or potential paths to arrhythmic death. This necessitates a comprehensive search for risk factors. All patients with IHD who present with VTA should undergo a careful evaluation to determine current symptoms, the degree of functional impairment, the presence of risk factors, evidence of other cardiovascular disease, and the presence of comorbid conditions. Most patients should undergo tests for risk stratification, including quantification of left ventricular function and a provocative test for myocardial ischemia. In some patients, assessment of neuro-hormonal function by heart-rate variability (HRV) and baroreflex sensitivity (BRS) analysis may be useful, although these techniques remain largely investigational. Invasive tests including cardiac catherization, coronary angiography, and EPS should be strongly considered. Treatment alternatives should address all modifiable risk factors. Most patients are candidates for optimal adjunctive therapy (lifestyle modifications, exercise programs, lipid-lowering therapy, platelet inhibitors or other anticoagulants, angiotensin-converting enzyme (ACE) inhibitors or related compounds, and beta-blockers). Complete revascularization is indicated in patients with evidence of stress-induced ischemia and significant coronary-artery stenoses. Although the role of EPS is debated, there is evidence that inducible SMVT predicts arrhythmic death in patients with NSVT and after acute MI. It is also probable that the induction of SMVT in patients who present with VTA indicates a heightened risk for arrhythmic death. This may affect the choice of long-term therapy and motivate more aggressive risk modification. Randomized clinical trials have established the benefit of ICD therapy over treatment with amiodarone in patients who present with cardiac arrest or hemodynamically significant VTA in the absence of reversible causes (16). However, the benefit of ICD therapy was marginal, patients with severe functional limitations were excluded, and subgroup analyses indicate that some categories of patients do not benefit from ICD implantation over treatment with amiodarone. Therefore, the decision for ICD therapy should be placed in the context of the overall treatment strategy. A risk-to-benefit analysis is used to develop the optimal treatment strategy for the individual patient.

An illustrative example is the patient who presents with symptomatic SMVT, or VF with a history of previous MI and class II heart failure. The patient often has a number of risk factors for progression of CAD, such as hypertension or smoking, but no major comorbid conditions such as terminal cancer. Risk assessment may demonstrate no provocable ischemia, moderately reduced left ventricular function (e.g., left ventricular ejection fraction (LVEF) 0.25–0.35), depressed HRV (SDNN <70 ms) and low BRS (≤3 ms/mmHg). SMVT is induced at EPS. This patient has a substantial risk of total mortality (nonarrhythmic cardiovascular causes and arrhythmic death), but little contribution from noncardiovascular causes. The treatment strategy should include an aggressive program to reduce cardiovascular events caused by recurrent VTA, ischemia, thrombosis, and progressive myocardial remodeling. Optimal adjunctive therapy, as described here, is an essential component of long-term treatment. Many clinicians would recommend an ICD to reduce the risk of arrhythmic death from any cause (ischemia, acute MI, chronic MI, or remodeled ventricular myocardium).

The major treatment alternative to ICD therapy is amiodarone. Amiodarone therapy should be considered for patients who are not likely to benefit from ICD therapy because of a high risk of nonarrhythmic death or a low risk of arrhythmic death. Patients with severe functional limitations (e.g., NYHA class 4) or another condition with a poor 1-yr survival would fit into the former category. Patients with preserved left ventricular function (e.g., LVEF ≥0.40) and patients with possible transient factors that could have caused the presenting VTA may fit into the low arrhythmic death risk category. Patients at high risk for complications because of ICD therapy and patients who prefer pharmacologic therapy should also be considered for amiodarone therapy.

Racemic sotalol has been shown to reduce the recurrence rate of VTA and death compared to type I antiarrhythmic drugs. Although small studies suggest that it may be less effective than ICD therapy, a rigorous comparison has not been performed. The risk of proarrhythmia is increased in patients with significant left ventricular dysfunction and VTA, but it does not have many of the side effects associated with long-term use of amiodarone. If other therapeutic options are contraindicated, or if the contribution of risk of arrhythmic death to the overall mortality is small, then consideration could be given to treatment with beta-blockers plus optimal adjunctive therapy without additional specific antiarrhythmic drugs. The addition of beta-blockers to the other elements of optimal adjunctive therapy has demonstrated a marked reduction in sudden death in patients after MI and in patients with heart failure. Treatment with amiodarone was not superior to metoprolol therapy in the Cardiac Arrest Study of Hamburg (CASH) *(35)*. Treatment with sodium-channel-blocking agents is not recommended in patients with IHD with VTA because of the high risk of proarrhythmic effects and relatively poor efficacy. Catheter-based ablation therapy may be useful for reducing the frequency of recurrent VTA, but in isolation probably does not protect against the multiple sources of risk for arrhythmic death in patients with IHD. Many patients with VTA associated with IHD who are treated with ICDs also require antiarrhythmic drug therapy for a number of indications discussed earlier. Amiodarone is often used with generally satisfactory results, but potential adverse effects on ICD function include an increase in defibrillation energy requirement *(9,9a)*. Racemic sotalol has several characteristics that make it well-suited for this form of combination therapy: it inhibits ventricular and supraventricular arrhythmias and reduces the ventricular rate response to AF. As a beta-blocker, sotalol has antisympathetic activity which reduces the sinus rate and myocardial oxygen demand. Sotalol reduces the defibrillation energy requirement. Compared to other antiarrhythmic drugs, sotalol is less likely to interfere with capture thresholds, to cause QRS prolongation, to cause excessive reduction of the VTA rate, and to cause variability in the VTA cycle length *(39)*. These characteristics could result in more uniform, predictable ICD function *(18)*. Class Ib antiarrhythmic drugs should also be considered, particularly in combination *(40)*. Class Ia antiarrhythmic drugs are used primarily when other therapies have failed. The risk of intractable or incessant ventricular arrhythmias would make class Ic drugs less than ideal for patients with IHD whether or not they had an ICD.

Coronary Artery Anomalies, Spasm, and Myocardial Bridges

Abnormal origin and course of coronary arteries and vasospasm are rare but important causes of sustained VTA. Myocardial bridging has been reported to cause acute myocardial ischemia, but this concept has been challenged. Therefore, although a contribution of myocardial bridging to VTA resulting from ischemia cannot be excluded, other mechanisms should be sought. Therapy of coronary spasm has included nitrates and calcium-channel blockers. Refractory cases have been reported, and some patients have been treated with ICDs. Amiodarone has vasodilatory and antifibrillatory properties that may be beneficial. However, class I and III antiarrhythmic drugs would not be expected to have a favorable risk-to-benefit ratio. The use of beta-blockers has been questioned because they could inhibit catecholamine-induced vasodilation, and lead to unopposed alpha-receptor mediated vasoconstriction.

Nonischemic Dilated Cardiomyopathies

Dilated cardiomyopathies arise in a number of clinical contexts, including valvular heart disease, the dilated phase of hypertrophic cardiomyopathies, and various neuromuscular disorders. The etiologies of the most common varieties—i.e., the idiopathic dilated cardiomyopathies—are unknown. Mortality is high in these conditions, and arrhythmic death constitutes a large percentage of total mortality. In patients with significant left ventricular dysfunction, the risk of arrhythmic death remains high even if reversible triggers of the presenting VTA are identified. Although a number of noninvasive methods for determining risk appear promising, none has been widely accepted. The imprecision of risk assessment has resulted in the recommendation for ICD therapy in most patients with dilated cardiomyopathy who present with VTA. It is important to recognize that most patients will not require an ICD. All patients should receive optimal medical therapy with beta-blockers, ACE inhibitors and, possibly spironolactone and angiotensin II-receptor blockers. Alternative pharmacological approaches would include amiodarone therapy. Nonpharmacological therapies include cardiac transplantation and permanent circulatory-assist devices. Bundle-branch reentry can be induced in some patients with dilated cardiomyopathies, and may be efficiently prevented (with low risk) by radiofrequency ablation. However, this form of therapy does not address other potential mechanisms of arrhythmic death. Therefore, if the risk of arrhythmic death is estimated to be high despite treatment—e.g., in the presence of moderate or severe ventricular dysfunction—then additional therapy with ICD or amiodarone should be considered. In the CHF-STAT trial, amiodarone appeared more effective in patients with nonischemic compared with ischemic cardiomyopathies *(41)*.

Congenital Heart Diseases

Success in the management of congenital heart disease (CHD) has increased longevity and more physicians are encountering GUCH (Grown-Up Congenital Heart) patients, many of whom have undergone operative correction or palliation of the CHD. VTA and sudden death are relatively uncommon in congenital heart disease. Possible mechanisms are surgical scar and patch-related reentrant VTA, and VTA related to remodeling of ventricular myocardium that can occur after years of abnormal hemodynamic forces. Patients with VTA may present with syncope, but atrial arrhythmias may also be responsible and must be excluded. Excessive ventricular rates caused by atrial arrhythmias may also cause malignant VTA. The appearance of atrial and ventricular arrhythmias often reflects severe deterioration in hemodynamic function. Appropriate therapy requires a comprehensive evaluation of hemodynamic function and underlying anatomic abnormalities (congenital and iatrogenic) by experienced GUCH clinicians. The accumulated experience in management of VTA and outcome in patients with congenital heart disease is limited. Practice is often guided by experience in other more common disorders, such as ischemic heart disease. However, the youthful ages of many of the patients require special considerations for long-term medical therapy. Thus, antiarrhythmic therapy with amiodarone, sotalol, and other beta-blockers would be considered. Catheter ablation of surgical-scar-related VTA has been performed. ICD therapy probably provides the most reliable protection, but implantation may be complicated by the abnormal course of vessels and inaccessibility of specific cardiac chambers. In addition, anecdotal evidence suggests a high rate of psychiatric complications in ICD-treated young patients, particularly adolescents. Finally, heterodynamic abnormalities may require operative correction that could offer opportunities for ablation or better access to sites for pacing and defibrillation leads.

Hypertrophic Cardiomyopathies

Hypertrophic cardiomyopathies may exist in asymmetric forms with or without left ventricular outflow tract (LVOT) obstruction and concentric forms. These disorders are associated with multiple abnormalities that could contribute to arrhythmogenesis, including myocardial hypertrophy, myofiber disarray, fibrosis, myocardial ischemia, autonomic dysfunction, and abnormalities of cellular and subcellular functions (42). Some patients have genetic mutations associated with a high risk of sudden death but relatively few anatomic changes. Several reports indicate that supraventricular arrhythmias are important triggers of VTA. An unusual presentation of SMVT is observed in patients with midventricular obstruction who develop apical aneurysms. Risk assessment requires evaluation of the individual factors, family history, and results of noninvasive and invasive examinations. Methods of risk stratification have included long-term Holter monitoring to detect NSVT, TWA, exercise testing to identify abnormal hemodynamic-autonomic reflexes, and stress imaging to detect myocardial ischemia. EPS has been used to assess the ventricular response rate to induced supraventricular arrhythmias, evidence of AV conduction disturbances, fractionation of ventricular electrograms, and inducible VTA. For most patients who present with VTA, the indication for ICD therapy is so strong that further risk assessment would seem superfluous (43). However, some elements of evaluation may affect the type of ICD or additional therapy. Additional therapy could include catheter-based or operative reduction of septal hypertrophy and interruption of AV conduction. ICD selection could include dual-chamber pacing and capacity for AF. Many patients with malignant forms of hypertrophic cardiomyopathy are very young, and may have anatomical and psychological contraindications for ICD therapy. Amiodarone has been reported to be successful in preventing arrhythmic death, but a major problem exists in the inability to test its effectiveness in individual patients (44). Beta-blockers, calcium antagonists, and operative methods do not prevent arrhythmic death, but may be indicated to prevent ischemia, outflow-tract obstruction, and excessive sympathetic activity. Myocardial hypertrophy results in action-potential prolongation. Drugs that prolong action-potential duration (class IA and III) are relatively contraindicated caused by increased risk of pro-arrhythmia. Class Ic antiarrhythmic drugs are also contraindicated in the presence of ventricular hypertrophy. Adjunctive medical therapy is important in patients with hypertensive cardiomyopathy. Blood pressure control may reduce progression of ventricular hypertrophy, and experimental evidence suggests that ACE-inhibitors reduce vulnerability to VF (45).

Myocarditis and Inflammatory Cardiomyopathies

Myocarditis should be considered in patients who present with VTA or sudden death in the absence of other causes (45a). This suspicion should be confirmed with endomyocardial biopsy. Because there is often spontaneous resolution, antiarrhythmic control may be required only temporarily. There are several progressive disorders associated with varying degrees of active inflammation and fibrosis. Chaga's disease is an important cause of VTA in some South American countries, but it is a relatively rare cause of VTA elsewhere. Amiodarone is reported to be more effective than other antiarrhythmic drugs, but reliable comparisons with ICD therapy and catheter ablation have not been published *(46)*. The optimal strategies for VTA associated with sarcoid heart disease and giant-cell myocarditis are unclear. Some inflammatory disorders respond to immunosuppression. Selection of therapy should be based on an estimate of reversible and permanent damage. Unfortunately, there are few guides to risk assessment or to pharmacological therapy. ICD therapy is likely to dominate the selection process in patients who present with VTA. Amiodarone is the major pharmacological alternative.

Arrhythmogenic Right Ventricular Cardiomyopathy (Dysplasia)

Arrhythmogenic right ventricular cardiomyopathy is a disorder—often familial—of unknown mechanism, which is characterized by fatty tissue replacement of myocardium in the free wall of the right ventricle *(47)*. Several configurations of ventricular arrhythmias occur in this syndrome, and SMVT—usually with a left bundle-branch block (LBBB) morphology—is not an uncommon presentation. Unfortunately, cardiac arrest and sudden death, sometimes in association with physical activity, may be the initial presentation. Arrhythmogenic right ventricular cardiomyopathy is an important cause of sudden death in athletes. The substrate for VTA may be reentrant circuits created by separation of muscle bundles by fatty tissue. Optimal therapy has not been determined. Patients should be advised to avoid competitive athletic activity. Amiodarone—alone and in combination with beta-blockers and d,l-sotalol—has been successfully used to control VTA in this disorder. However, these drugs do not provide complete protection against sudden death. Suggested indicators of high risk include previous cardiac arrest, syncope, and left ventricular involvement. EPS has been suggested as a method for risk stratification and for guiding antiarrhythmic drug selection. However, based on the limited experience available and on poor results of EPS in other nonischemic disorders, these suggestions should be considered preliminary. Operative excision and catheter ablation have been reported to be effective for preventing recurrent SMVT. However, one problem with local ablation is arrhythmia recurrence caused by the development of sources and circuits at new locations. Complete operative disarticulation of the right ventricular free wall has also been used to control VTA. Reliable methods of identifying patients at particularly high risk or at very low risk have not been developed. The uncertain level of control with other methods promotes recommendation for ICD therapy in patients who present with VTA. The distinction between arrhythmogenic right ventricular dysplasia and right ventricular outflow-tract tachycardia (RVOT) is critical because the latter disorder is treated differently; RVOT VT has an excellent prognosis, is not associated with structural heart disease, and is not heritable.

Idiopathic VF and RBBB ST Elevation (Brugada) Syndrome

Idiopathic VF (IVF) is used to describe disorders in which unexplained VF occurs in patients without detectable structural heart disease *(48)*. No pharmacological therapy is widely accepted. There are reports of favorable responses to quinidine, but data from the European registry suggests that antiarrhythmic drugs and beta-blockers do not provide reliable protection. The reported recurrence rate of VF is 30%. ICD therapy is currently recommended for this syndrome. Brugada syndrome is a variety of IVF with a distinctive ECG pattern appearance of complete or partial right bundle-branch block (RBBB) and ST-segment elevation *(49)*. Several genetic abnormalities produce the disorder, and the expression varies considerably. The characteristic ECG pattern is often intermittent, but can be elicited with variable reliability with certain class I antiarrhythmic drugs, including ajmaline, flecainide, pilsicainide, and procainamide. Quinidine has been reported to be effective in a small number of patients, and a theory exists to explain its therapeutic effect *(50)*. Amiodarone and beta-blockers have not been found to be protective. No pharmacological approach has received widespread acceptance. ICDs are recommended for patients with a history of VTA *(51)*.

Congenital and Acquired Long QT Syndromes

LQTS has been divided into congenital and acquired forms. The latter consists mostly of drug-induced LQTS. Drug-related LQTS is a common cause of polymorphic VTA and VF in hospitalized patients, and probably accounts for a significant number of sudden deaths because a large number of drugs cause this syndrome. Nevertheless, multiple contributing factors may be involved, including female gender, electrolyte disturbances (hypokalemia or hypomagnesemia), bradycardia, heart failure, and myocardial hypertrophy. An important cause is the administration of a drug or other substance (e.g., grapefruit juice) that interferes with elimination of a drug that delays repolarization. The interaction of several factors may explain why some patients develop LQTS weeks or years after initiation of the offending drug. It may be a challenge to determine each of the factors, avoid their repetition in the future and select safe alternatives to the culprit drugs. There is speculation that a genetic predisposition or "reduced repolarization capacity" accounts for the sensitivity of some persons to this complication. If true, it may become possible to identify susceptible patients.

Although remarkable progress has been made in the understanding of congenital LQTS, better information about the natural history and response to treatment has exposed deep uncertainties about identifying and treating individuals at risk for VTA *(52)*. Only about 70% of carriers have unequivocal QT prolongation, and approx 12% have a normal QT interval. In addition, sudden death is the first manifestation of the syndrome in at least 10% of affected persons. There are probably several undiscovered genetic defects and sporadic mutations that cause this disorder. Moreover, the types of provocative factors, the long-term risk of sustained VTA, and the response to therapy varies with the specific genetic defect. Finally, severe myocardial dysfunction is often associated with action-potential prolongation, and could exacerbate arrhythmias associated with excessive delay of repolarization. Therefore, the possibility of LQTS should be considered in any patient who presents with VTA, if not as the primary disorder, then perhaps as a contributor. Therapy for LQTS depends on the estimated risk of sudden death based on the individual history of signs or symptoms of VTA, the family history, genetic subtype, and other considerations such as the patients' age and preference for type of therapy. Beta-blockers are the mainstay of treatment, and are usually prescribed to all affected patients *(52a)*. Education about risk-factor avoidance is essential. Patients who present with VTA or syncope, those who experience symptoms despite beta-blockers, and other individuals at high risk are candidates for ICD therapy. Left cervicothoracic ganglionectomy and permanent pacing cannot be relied upon to prevent sudden death, but may be useful alternatives to patients who are intolerant of beta-blockers or who do not comply with drug therapy. Experimental therapies include administration of supplemental potassium chloride for HERG mutations and mexiletine for LQT subtypes 3, 2, and possibly 1. The presence of provocative factors should be sought in patients who present with VTA, as this may affect selection of long-term therapy. Many of the patients at risk are infants, young children, adolescents, and young adults. Poor compliance may be more prevalent in certain age groups of patients. Concern about effects of medications during pregnancy may result in inappropriate termination of therapy. Device therapy can improve compliance, and advanced ICDs can provide the sophisticated pacing programs to prevent VTA. However, the size of current-generation ICDs and lack of lead systems that meet the demand for the small physical size and rapid growth of young patients must be considered. The special psychological problems of ICDs in young persons are relevant, as noted earlier.

Short-Coupled Variant of Torsades de Pointes

This rare malignant arrhythmia usually occurs in the absence of detectable structural heart disease. Transient global hypokinesis has been noted in at least one case *(53)*. Some authorities reserve the term "torsades de pointes" for the characteristic pattern that occurs in the presence of a prolonged QT. However, the name given by the authors of the first systematic characterization of the disorder highlights the essential feature needed to distinguish it from LQTS *(54)*. There is little experience with this disorder. Given this uncertainty, ICD therapy may be recommended to patients who request maximum protection against sudden death. However, control of arrhythmias may still be required to reduce symptoms and ICD discharges. Anecdotal reports suggest that verapamil and amiodarone inhibit VTA in this syndrome.

Catecholaminergic PVT

Another disorder that occurs in children without detectable structural heart disease and a normal QT interval is called catecholaminergic PVT because of its strong relationship to exercise and provocation with isoproterenol. Although beta-blockers are recommended, experience with this disorder is very limited.

Idiopathic Ventricular Tachycardias and RVOT

Idiopathic VT refers to disorders in which VT, sustained or unsustained but generally monomorphic, occurs in association with no or minimal detectable structural changes. Patients with idiopathic VT account for approx 10% of VTA that present for evaluation. RVOT VT accounts for about 80% of idiopathic VT. The underlying etiology of RVOT VT is unknown, but the evidence indicates that the mechanism is cyclic adenosine monophosphate (cAMP)-mediated delayed after-depolarizations, a form of triggered activity *(55)*. VTA with identical electrophysiological characteristics have been found to originate from the LVOT, epicardial locations, and other sites. Termination in response to adenosine is characteristic, and strongly supports the diagnosis of RVOT VT. Sudden cardiac death caused by RVOT VT is a rare event, but accumulated experience is insufficient for accurate determination of the risk. Treatment is indicated for patients with syncope, intolerable palpitations, and other disabling symptoms. The initial choice of pharmacological therapy is usually a beta-blocker or calcium-channel blocker. Flecainide and d,l-sotalol may also be effective. In a series of pediatric patients, the most effective control was observed with amiodarone followed by verapamil, class IC drugs, and sotalol. Other beta-blockers were associated with a low rate of effectiveness *(56)*. Preliminary results suggest that nicorandil, an ATP-sensitive potassium-channel opener, may be effective in this disorder. Catheter ablation is often the therapy selected first because of the high rate of permanent correction with few adverse sequellae. However, experience is required to avoid injury to coronary arteries and other complications. The distinction between RVOT VT and VT caused by ARVD is often difficult but essential because of the differences in treatment and prognosis.

Less commonly, idiopathic VT originates from the left ventricular septum. The mechanism is believed to be re-entry involving Purkinje fibers near the left posterior fascicle, which generates a RBBB/left axis morphology of VT. Pharmacologic therapy with verapamil and catheter ablation are first-line therapies.

THE FUTURE OF PHARMACOLOGICAL THERAPY

The antiarrhythmic drugs that are currently available do not provide satisfactory protection against malignant VTA. There are three general explanations for this: 1) The drugs are the problem: They lack the necessary therapeutic actions to prevent arrhythmic death and/or they are too toxic, thus negating any beneficial effects. 2) Patient selection is the problem: The drugs are effective for specific arrhythmia mechanisms, but available methods cannot distinguish between those who will and those who will not benefit. Patients likely to have a proarrhythmic response also cannot be reliably identified in advance of treatment. 3) The paradigm is the problem: The concept that reversible binding to membrane channels, receptors, and pumps can prevent arrhythmic death is incorrect. There may be too many arrhythmogenic mechanisms, too many promoters, too many interactions, and too many changes over time for a simple pharmacological approach to result in a satisfactory solution.

If explanation #1 is true, then new antiarrhythmic drugs will be developed that provide satisfactory protection. If explanation #2 is correct, then new methods of assessing physiologic changes may provide a more accurate selection of patients. However, if explanation #3 is correct, then many current efforts may be misdirected and new approaches are needed. The effectiveness of amiodarone and beta-blockers could be cited as support for explanation #1, 2, or 3. Explanation #1 is supported because both amiodarone and beta-blockers have been shown to reduce arrhythmic death in some clinical settings. Explanation #2 is supported because amiodarone and beta-blockers do not protect all patients from arrhythmic death. Amiodarone has been shown to provide only weak protection against arrhythmic death in some populations such as patients with ventricular arrhythmias and ischemic cardiomyopathy. However, some of the beneficial effects of amiodarone and beta-blockers appear over weeks and months. Prolongation of repolarization, for instance, associated with amiodarone occurs over several weeks. Although numerous explanations exist, a slowly developing structural change with functional consequences may be responsible. Studies in animal models indicate that a process called electrophysiological remodeling may account for reduced vulnerability to atrial and ventricular arrhythmias. Studies in patients with CHF have shown that beta-blockers result in partial restoration of anatomic and neurohormonal abnormalities, a process called reverse remodeling. It is plausible that reverse remodeling of anatomic and neurohormonal abnormalities in CHF could be accompanied by electrophysiological changes that lessen vulnerability to VTA. If true, this may be an important mechanism by which beta-blockers exert their protective effects. It is our hypothesis that reverse remodeling provides the optimal long-term solution to antiarrhythmic therapy. It is not likely to be proarrhythmic, and it may reduce the propensity for ventricular tachyarrythmia (VTA) resulting from multiple mechanisms. Moreover, it is accompanied by improvements in myocardial function. If this can be demonstrated, then current antiarrhythmic methods—i.e., drugs and ICDs—would be considered bridges or adjuncts to the long-term strategy of inhibiting remodeling and promoting reverse remodeling.

REFERENCES

1. Lüderitz B. History of the Disorders of Cardiac Rhythm. Futura Publishing, Armonk, NY, 1998.
2. Mackenzie J. Diseases of the Heart. Oxford University Press, London, 1908.
3. Lewis T. Single and successive extrasystoles. Lancet 1909;1:382.
4. Scott RW. Observations on a case of ventricular tachycardia with retrograde conduction. Heart 1921; 9:297.
5. Armbrust CA, Levine SA. Paroxysmal ventricular tachycardia: a study of one hundred and seven cases. Circulation 1950;1:28–40.
6. The Cardiac Arrhythmia Suppression Trial (CAST) Investigators: Preliminary report: effect of encainide and flecainide on mortality in a randomized trial of arrhythmic suppression after myocardial infarction: Effect of the antiarrhythmic agent moricizine on survival after myocardial infarction. N Engl J Med 1989;321:406–412.
7. Task force of the working group of arrhythmias of the European Society of Cardiology. The Sicilian gambit: a new approach to the classification of antiarrhythmic drugs based on their actions on arrhythmogenic mechanisms. Circulation 1991;84:1831–1851.
8. Anderson KP, Freedman RA, Mason JW. Use of antiarrhythmic drugs: general Principles. In Parmley WW, Chatterjee K, eds. Cardiology, JB Lippincott Company, Philadelphia, PA, 1988, pp. 837–849.
9. Dorian P. Interactions between implantable devices and pharmacological agents. Cardiac Electrophysiol Rev 1998;2:151–153.
9a. Pelosi F, Jr, Oral H, Kim MH, et al. Effect of chronic amiodarone therapy on defibrillation energy requirements in humans. J Cardiovasc Electrophysiol 2000;2:736–740.
10. Grant AO. Proarrhythmia: classification, incidence, risk factors, monitoring, prevention and management. Cardiac Electrophysiol Rev 1998;2:127–131.
11. Makielski JC, January CT. Proarrhythmia related to prolongation of repolarization: mechanisms, monitoring, prevention and management. Cardiac Electrophysiol Rev 1998;1:132–134.
12. Chen SA, Chen Y. Proarrhythmic activity and interactions of non-cardiac drugs and other substances. Cardiac Electrophysiol Rev 1998;2:147–150.
13. Wilde AAM. Proarrhythmia related to sodium channel blockade: mechanisms, monitoring, prevention and management. Cardiac Electrophysiol Rev 1998;2:136–141.
14. Waldo AL, Camm AJ, DeRuyter H, Friedman PL, MacNeil DJ, Pauls JF, et al. Effect of d-sotalol on morality in patients with left ventricular dysfunction after recent and remote myocardial infarction. Lancet 1996;348:7–12.
15. Bigger JT Jr, for the Coronary Artery Bypass Graft Patch Trial Investigators: Prophylactic use of implanted cardiac defibrillators in patients at high risk for ventricular arrhythmias after coronary-artery bypass graft surgery. N Engl J Med 1997;337:1569–1575.
16. AVID Investigators. A comparison of antiarrhythmic-drug therapy with implantable defibrillators in patients resuscitated from near-fatal ventricular arrhythmias. N Engl J Med 1997;337:1576–1583.
17. Sheldon R, Connolly S, Krahn A, Roberts R, Gent M, Gardner M. Identification of patients most likely to benefit from implantable cardioverter-defibrillator therapy: the Canadian Implantable Defibrillator Study. Circulation 2000;10:1660–1664.
18. Pacifico A, Hohnloser SH, Williams JH, Tao B, Saksena S, Henry PD, et al. Prevention of implantable-defibrillator shocks by treatment with sotalol. N Engl J Med 1999;340:1855–1863.
19. Langberg JL. Modification of response to antiarrhythmic drugs after catheter ablation. Cardiac Electrophysiol Rev 1998;2:154–156.
20. Johnston PW, O'Kane D, Adgey AJJ. Immediate evaluation and management of sudden death: cardiopulmonary resuscitation. Cardiac Electrophysiol Rev 1997;1:155–158.
21. Kloeck W, Cummins RO, Chamberlain D, Bossaert L, Callanan V, Carli P, et al. The universal

advanced life support algorithm: an advisory statement from the advanced life support working group of the international liaison committee on resuscitation. Circulation 1997;95:2180–2182.

22. Guidelines 2000 for cardiopulmonary resuscitation and emergency cardiovascular care. Circulation 2000;102 (suppl I):I1–I394.

23. Kloeck W, Cummins RO, Chamberlain D, Bossaert L, Callanan V, Carli P, et al. Special resuscitation situations: an advisory statement from the advanced life support working group of the international liaison committee on resuscitation. Circulation 1997;95:2196–2210.

24. Goergels AP, van den Hofs A, Mulleneers R, Smeets JL, Vos MA, Wellens HJ. Comparison of procainamide and lidocaine in terminating sustained monomorphic ventricular tachycardia. Am J Cardiol 1996;78:43–46.

25. Kudenchuk PJ, Cobb LA, Copass MK, Cummins RO, Doherty AM, Fahrenbruch CE, et al. Amiodarone for resuscitation after out-of-hospital cardiac arrest due to ventricular fibrillation. N Engl J Med 1999; 341:871–878.

25a. Dorian P. ALIVE trial results. North American Society of Pacing and Electrophysiology Annual Scientific Sessions, 2001.

26. Levine JH, Massumi A, Scheinman MM, Winkle RA, Platia EV, Chilson DA, et al. Intravenous amiodarone for recurrent sustained hypotensive ventricular tachyarrhythmias. J Am Coll Cardiol 1996 Jan;27:67–75.

27. Scheinman MM, Levine JH, Cannom DS, Friehling T, Kopelman HA, Chilson DA, et al. Dose-ranging study of intravenous amiodarone in patients with life-threatening ventricular tachyarrhythmias. Circulation 1995;92:3264–3272.

28. Kowey PR, Levine JH, Herze JM, Pacifico A, Lindsay BD, Plumb VJ, et al. Randomized, double-blind comparison of intravenous amiodarone and bretylium in the treatment of patients with recurrent, hemodyamically destabilizing ventricular tachycardia or fibrillation. Circulation 1995;1901;92:3255–3263.

29. Gillis AM. Intractable ventricular tachyarrhythmias: immediate evaluation and management: role of pharmacological therapy. Cardiac Electrophysiol Rev 1997;1:136–139.

30. Nadamanee K, Taylor R, Bailey WE, Rieders DE, Kosar EM. Treating electrical storm: sympathetic blockade versus advanced cardiac life support-guided therapy. Circulation 2000;102:742–747.

31. Bolooki H. Circulatory assist devices for the management of intractable ventricular tachyarrhythmias. Cardiac Electrophysiol Rev 1997;1:140–141.

32. The CASCADE investigators. Randomized antiarrhythmic drug therapy in survivors of cardiac arrest A (the CASCADE study). Am J Cardiol 1993;72:280–287.

33. Mason JW, et al. A comparison of electrophysiologic testing with Holter monitoring to predict antiarrhythmic-drug efficacy for ventricular tachyarrhythmias. N Engl J Med 1993;329:445–451.

34. Mason JW, et al. A comparison of seven antiarrhythmic drugs in patients with ventricular tachyarrhythmias. N Engl J Med 1993;329:452–458.

34a. Connolly SJ, Gent M, Roberts RS, et al. Canadian implantable defibrillator study (CIDS): a randomized trial of the implantable cardioverter defibrillator against amiodarone. Circulation 2000;101(11):1297–1302.

35. Hack K-H, Cappato R, Siebels J, Ruppel R, for the CASH investigators. Randomized comparison of antiarrhythmic drug therapy with implantable defibrillators in patients resuscitated from cardiac arrest: the Cardiac Arrest Area Study Hamburg (CASH). Circulation 2000;102:748–754.

36. Gottlieb S, Eldar M, Stern S, Behar S. Ventricular tachyarrhythmias complicating acute myocardial infarction. Cardiac Electrophysiol Rev 1997;1:182–192.

37. Eldar M, Gottlieb S, Harpaz D, Avidov A, Behar S. Arrhythmias associated with acute myocardial infarction. Cardiac Electrophysiol Rev 1999;3:174–176.

38. Connolly SJ, Gent M, Roberts RS, Dorian P, Green MS, Klein GJ. Canadian Implantation Defibrillator Study (CIDS): study design and organization. Am J Cardiol 1993;72:103F–108F.

39. Brode S, Singh B, Anderson KP. Sotalol. Cardiac Electrophysiol Rev 1998;2:211–214.

40. Duff HJ. Antiarrhythmic drug combination therapy. Cardiac Electrophysiol Rev 1998;2:142–146.

41. Singh S, Fletcher R, Fisher S, et al., for the Survival Trial of Antiarrhythmic Therapy in Congestive Heart Failure (CHF-STAT) Investigators. Amiodarone in Patients With Congestive Heart Failure and Asymptomatic Ventricular Arrhythmia. N Engl J Med 1995;333:77–82.

42. Anderson KP. Mechanisms of sudden death in patients with hypertrophic cardiomyopathy. In: Akhtar M, Myerburg RJ, Ruskin JN, eds. Sudden Cardiac Death. Williams & Wilkins, Philadelphia, PA, 1994, pp. 163–189.

43. Maron BJ, Shen W-K, Link MS, et al. Efficacy of the implantable cardioverter-defibrillators for the prevention of sudden death in patients with hypertrophic cardiomyopathy. N Engl J Med 2000;342:365–373.

44. McKenna WJ, Oakley CM, Krikler DM, et al. Improved survival with amiodarone in patients with hypertrophic cardiomyopathy and ventricular tachycardia. Br Heart J 1985;53:412–416.

45. Srikanthan VS, Dunn FG. Arrhythmias, sudden death and syncope in hypertensive cardiovascular disease. Cardiac Electrophysiol Rev 1997;1:233–236.

45a. Feldman AM, McNamara D. Myocarditis. N Engl J Med 2000;343:1388–1398.

46. Doval H, Nul D, Grancelli H, et al., for the Grupo de Estudio de la Sobrevida en la Insuficiencia Cardica en Argentina (GESICA) Investigators. Randomized Trial of Low Dose Amiodarone in Severe Congestive Heart Failure. Lancet 1994;344:493–498.

47. Marcus FI. Arrhythmogenic right ventricular dysplasia. Cardiac Electrophysiol Rev 1997;1:255–257.

48. Priori SG, Paganini V. Idiopathic ventricular fibrillation: epidemiology, pathophysiology, primary prevention, immediate evaluation and management, long-term evaluation and management, experimental and theoretical developments. Cardiac Electrophysiol Rev 1997;1:244–247.

49. Brugada P, Brugada J, Brugada R. The Brugada syndrome. Cardiac Electrophysiol Rev 1999;3:202–204.

50. Belhassen B, Viskin S, Fish R, Glick A, Setbon I, Eldar M. Effects of electrophysiologic-guided therapy with class IA antiarrhythmic drugs on the long-term outcome of patients with idiopathic ventricular fibrillation with or without the Brugada syndrome. J Cardiovasc Electrophysiol 1999; 10:1301–1312.

51. Ruskin JN. Idiopathic ventricular fibrillation: is there a role for electrophysiologic-guided antiarrhythmic drug therapy? J Cardiovasc Electrophysiol 1999;10:1313–1315.

52. Vincent GM, Timothy K, Zhang L. Congenital long QT syndrome. Cardiac Electrophysiol Rev 1999; 1:207–209.

52a. Moss AJ, Zareba W, Hall WJ, et al. Effectiveness and limitations of β-blocker therapy in long QT syndrome. Circulation 2000;101(6):616–623.

53. Anderson KP, Friedman A. Unpublished observations.

54. Leenhardt A, Glaser E, Burguera M, Nuernberg M, Maison-Blanche P, Coumel P. Short-coupled variant of torsade de pointes: a new electrocardiographic entity in the spectrum of idiopathic ventricular tachyarrhythmias. Circulation 1994;89:206–215.

55. Lerman BB, Stein KM, Markowitz SM. Right ventricular outflow tract tachycardia. Cardiac Electrophysiol Rev 1997;1:251–254.

56. Lerman BB, Stein KM, Markowitz SM, Mittal S, Slotwiner DJ. Recent advances in right ventricular outflow tract tachycardia. Cardiac Electrophysiol Rev 1999;3:210–214.

17 Catheter Ablation of Ventricular Tachycardia

William G. Stevenson, MD

CONTENTS

INTRODUCTION

Catheter ablation plays a role in the management of selected patients with monomorphic ventricular tachycardia. The efficacy and safety depend on the type and location of origin of the ventricular arrhythmia, which can be predicted from the nature of the underlying heart disease and tachycardia characteristics (Table 1).

The QRS morphology identifies a ventricular tachycardia (VT) as either polymorphic or monomorphic. Polymorphic ventricular tachycardias (PVTs) are those in which the QRS morphology is continuously changing because of a changing sequence of ventricular activation. With PVT, a consistent site of origin that can be targeted for ablation is unlikely.

Monomorphic ventricular tachycardias are those in which the morphology of each QRS complex resembles that of the preceding and following QRS. The ventricles are repetitively activated in the same sequence. An arrhythmia focus or structural substrate is present, which can potentially be targeted for catheter ablation. The QRS morphology provides an indication of the probable location of the arrhythmogenic region *(1)* (Fig. 1). Tachycardias that have a left bundle-branch block (LBBB)-like configuration in V_1 have an origin in the right ventricle or the interventricular septum (either the right or left side of the septum). Conversely, a right bundle-branck block (RBBB)-like morphology in V_1 suggests a left ventricular origin. A frontal plane axis directed inferiorly (dominant R-waves in leads II, III, AVF) indicates an origin in the cranial aspect of the heart, such as the anterior wall of the left ventricle or the right ventricular outflow tract

From: *Contemporary Cardiology: Management of Cardiac Arrhythmias*
Edited by: L. I. Ganz © Humana Press Inc., Totowa, NJ

Table 1
Catheter Ablation of Ventricular Tachycardia: Approximate Effectiveness and Risks of
Major Complications

	Efficacy	*Risk*
Incessant VT	High	2–10%
Idiopathic VT		
RV Outflow Tract	80–90%	Low, but rare fatalities
Left ventricular verapamil-sensitive	90%	Low
Post-MI slow VT		
Reduction of VT episodes	70–80%	5–10%
Prevention of all VT	50–67%	5–10%
Post-MI fast VT	?	?
Other scar-related VTs		
RV dysplasia + RV dilation	Palliative	?
Nonischemic cardiomyopathy	~50%	?Low
Bundle-Branch reentry VT	100%	Low-pacemaker

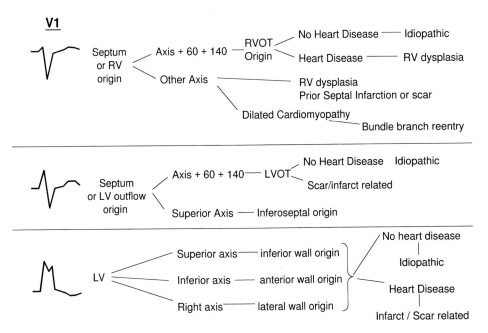

Fig. 1. The QRS morphology suggests the probable origin and often the type of VT. The morphology of V_1 is illustrated at left. *See* text for discussion LV = left ventricle, RV = right ventricle, OT = outflow tract.

(RVOT). A frontal-plane axis directed superiorly (dominant S-waves in leads II, III, and AVF), indicates initial depolarization of the inferior wall of the left or right ventricle. Dominant R-waves in leads V3–V4 favor a location of the focus nearer the base of the heart than the apex. Dominant S-waves in these leads favor a more apically placed focus. The QRS morphology is an excellent marker of the arrhythmia site of origin when the ventricles are structurally normal, but much less reliable when tachycardia is associated with regions of infarction or scar.

Precise localization of the arrhythmia origin requires catheter mapping. The specific approach to mapping is determined by the nature of the arrhythmia. Ideally, mapping requires that the tachycardia be stable and sustained, allowing a catheter to be moved from point to point during the tachycardia. This is facilitated by hemodynamic stability during tachycardia. Tachycardias that produce hemodynamic collapse requiring immediate termination are not amenable to point-by-point mapping of the activation sequence, but can sometimes be targeted by other approaches.

Once the region giving rise to the tachycardia has been located, ablation of the tissue in the region is accomplished by radiofrequency current application that heats the tissue. A temperature in excess of 48°C irreversibly damages the tissue (2). A fibrous scar forms at the ablation site (3–5). The ablation lesion is initially accompanied by some edema and hemorrhage into the tissue. With time, healing occurs accompanied by resolution of the edema. Occasionally, healing of the lesion is followed by recovery of the tissue in the border of the lesion, and the arrhythmia returns. Alternatively, microvascular damage produced by the lesion can cause it to expand during the healing phase, increasing lesion size. Individual radiofrequency ablation lesions are typically less than 1 cm in diameter. Small focal lesions are ideal for ablation of supraventricular tachycardias (SVT) and small foci. However, VTs that are related to areas of scar often require larger lesions. When a large number of radiofrequency lesions is required to ablate a large region, late changes are not uncommon. Occasionally, an arrhythmia recurs early and then disappears. Ablation failure is often caused by inadequate lesion size or penetration.

Whether VT can be ablated depends on the location and size of the region that causes the arrhythmia. Most VTs originate from sites on the endocardial surface of the heart, which can be reached with an electrode catheter. For the purposes of ablation, VTs can be divided into three types: focal origin, bundle-branch reentry, and scar-related (Table 2). Focal-origin tachycardias arise from a small region; the excitation wavefront spreads out across the ventricles from a focal point that is often amenable to ablation. Most VTs in patients who do not have structural heart disease (idiopathic ventricular tachycardias (IVTs)) are of this type. The mechanism may be automaticity or reentry. Bundle-branch reentry is caused by circulation of the excitation wavefronts through the bundle branches; a bundle branch can be targeted for ablation. Scar-related reentry circuits occur in various configurations and locations, and are the most challenging to ablate.

Patients with VT also fall into three major groups according to underlying heart disease: patients without structural heart disease, in whom tachycardias are referred to as idiopathic; those with a clear region of scar, such as that prior myocardial infarction (MI); and patients with nonischemic cardiomyopathies, including valvular heart disease.

IDIOPATHIC VENTRICULAR TACHYCARDIAS

These tachycardias usually occur in patients who do not have other structural heart disease, and have a focal origin (6–8). The prognosis is good—sudden death is very rare, but symptoms can be severe. Occasionally tachycardia is incessant, and causes

Table 2
Catheter Ablation of VT Definition of Terms

Types of VT	Mapping
Focal Origin Tachycardia originates from a small focus, usually not associated with scar. The QRS morphology is a good indicator of the location of the focus and type of tachycardia. **Bundle-branch reentry** Tachycardia caused by circulation of the excitation wavefront down one bundle branch, through the interventricular septum, and up the contralateral bundle branch to complete the circuit. **Scar-Related reentry** Tachycardia caused by circulation of the excitation wavefront through and around regions bordered by scar, often from prior MI.	**Mapping** The process of localizing the source of the tachycardia, usually by moving an electrode catheter around the ventricles. **Activation Sequence Mapping** Recording activation during tachycardia at multiple sites to determine the pattern of ventricular activation. Focal-origin tachycardias can be located by identifying the earliest site of activation. **Pace-Mapping** Pacing from the mapping catheter during sinus rhythm and comparing the resulting QRS morphology to that of the VT. For focal-origin tachycardias pacing at or near the tachycardia focus produces a QRS morphology identical to that of the tachycardia. **Entrainment Mapping** Pacing from the mapping catheter during tachycardia. The effect of pacing can be analyzed to determine the proximity of the pacing site to the tachycardia circuit.

dilated cardiomyopathy. This tachycardia-induced cardiomyopathy may resolve if the tachycardia is suppressed before irreversible left ventricular dilation has occurred *(9,10)*.

Idiopathic RVOT Tachycardia

The most common IVT originates from a focus in the outflow tract of the right ventricle *(7,11–13)* (Fig. 2). This tachycardia has LBBB configuration in ECG lead V1. The frontal plane axis is directed inferiorly or inferiorly and to the right. Tall monophasic R-waves are present in leads II, III, and AVF. Tachycardia may occur in repetitive bursts (referred to as repetitive monomorphic ventricular tachycardia) *(14)*. Sustained episodes are often precipitated by exercise or emotion. Unifocal premature ventricular contractions (PVCs) with a morphology identical to that of the tachycardia are often present during sinus rhythm. In some patients, the premature beats are severely symptomatic and warrant therapy *(15)*. This tachycardia is most likely caused by a form of automaticity linked to intracellular calcium increases that provoke spontaneous depolarizations known as after-depolarizations *(13,14)*. Initiation often requires bursts of rapid pacing and/or administration of isoproterenol, and usually terminates in response to administration of adenosine *(13)*. Although evidence of heart disease by echocardiogram, electrocardiogram (ECG), and angiography is generally absent, the possibility of a focal structural abnormality is suggested by one study in which cardiac magnetic resonance imaging (MRI) identified focal areas of thinning, hypokinesis, or fatty infiltration *(16)*. The major differential diagnosis is arrhythmogenic right ventricular dysplasia.

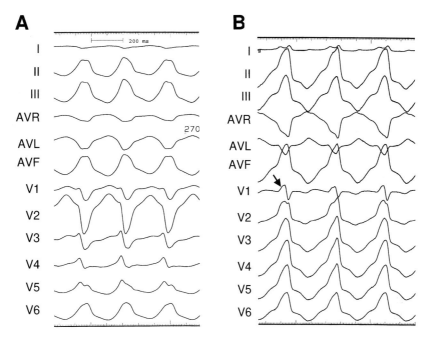

Fig. 2. Two different IVTs. Both have a LBBB configuration and frontal plane axis directed inferiorly, consistent with an origin in the RVOT. The tachycardia in (**A**) was successfully ablated from the RVOT. Ablation in the RVOT failed to interrupt the tachycardia in (**B**). This tachycardia has an initial prominent R-wave in V_1 (arrow), suggesting a more leftward origin (*see* text).

Right ventricular dysplasia is suggested by multiple morphologies of VT, usually with a LBBB-type configuration, because of reentry (as assessed in the electrophysiology laboratory). Idiopathic tachycardia is often controlled by chronic therapy with verapamil, diltiazem, or beta-blockers. Catheter ablation is a reasonable consideration when pharmacologic therapy is not effective.

Catheter ablation targets the focus. Isoproterenol combined with ventricular pacing is often required for initiation. If VT or frequent premature ventricular contractions (PVCs) are present, activation-sequence mapping can be used to locate the focus. During sinus rhythm, pace-mapping can be used to attempt to locate the arrhythmia focus. Sites which pacing exactly reproduces the tachycardia QRS morphology are at or near the arrhythmia focus. Ablation is successful in approx 85% of patients (7,11,17–20). Failures occur because of two major problems. The first is an inability to reproducibly provoke the tachycardia in the electrophysiology laboratory, preventing adequate localization. The second problem is the occasional location of the focus deep within the septum, or possibly epicardial over the septum, where ablation from the endocardial surface is difficult. Occasionally, ablation from the left side of the interventricular septum is effective (21). Electrocardiographic findings suggestive of an atypical location and lower likelihood of success include a slurred downstroke of the S-wave in lead V1 and a large initial r-wave in lead V_1 or V_2 (7,11) (Fig. 2, panel B). Complications are rare, but fatal cardiac perforation has been reported (18). Rare cases of coronary-artery occlusion during radiofrequency ablation in the left ventricular outflow tract (LVOT) have also been reported (22).

Idiopathic Left Ventricular, Verapamil-Sensitive Tachycardia

The most common form of idiopathic left ventricular tachycardia has a RBBB configuration with a frontal plane axis that is directed superiorly *(8,23)* (Fig. 1, middle). This tachycardia can be terminated by administration of intravenous (iv) verapamil, suggesting that slow calcium-channel-dependent tissue is involved. The mechanism is reentry, probably involving the distal fascicles of the posterior division of the LBB. Rarely, tachycardia arises from the anterior division of the LBB and has a RBBB configuration with the frontal plane axis directed to the right *(7,24,25)*. If specifically sought with echocardiography, more than 90% of patients have a left ventricular false tendon identifiable *(26)*. These false tendons can contain Purkinje tissue, raising the possibility that the tendon is involved in causing the tachycardia *(27)*. False tendons are not specific for this arrhythmia; they are also seen in patients without this tachycardia. Similar to idiopathic right ventricular tachycardia, this idiopathic left ventricular tachycardia rarely, if ever, leads to sudden death. Chronic therapy with beta-adrenergic blockers and/or the calcium-channel blockers verapamil or diltiazem often prevents episodes. Catheter ablation is a reasonable therapy for patients who do not respond to or do not wish to take antiarrhythmic medications.

Ablation targets a discrete Purkinje potential that precedes the onset of the QRS complex during tachycardia *(23)*. The target is usually identified along the inferior aspect of the left ventricular septum. When the tachycardia originates from the anterior division of the LBB, the target can be on the anterior wall *(24,25,28)*. Ablation is successful in more than 90% of patients *(8,23,24,26,29,30)*. Occasional failures are usually caused by catheter-induced trauma or "bumping" the arrhythmia focus, preventing its initiation to allow mapping *(27)*. Complications are rare, but damage to the aortic or mitral valve from catheter manipulation can occur *(18)*.

Idiopathic focal tachycardias can occur in other locations, such as along the ventricular aspect of the mitral annulus, and in the epicardial portion of the LVOT *(21,31)*. Successful ablation depends on whether the focus is sufficiently close to the endocardium to allow damage with present catheter techniques. Success is often unpredictable without performing catheter mapping.

BUNDLE-BRANCH REENTRANT VT

The most common form of bundle-branch reentrant tachycardia is caused by circulation of the excitation wavefront up the LBB, down the RBB, and then through the interventricular septum to reenter the left bundle *(32)* (Fig. 3). Because the ventricle is depolarized from the right bundle, the tachycardia has a LBBB configuration. Occasionally, the circuit revolves in the opposite direction, giving rise to tachycardia that has a RBBB configuration. Rarely, reentry occurs solely through fascicles of the LBB *(33,34)*. Sustained bundle-branch reentry usually requires abnormal, slowed conduction through the bundle branches. The surface ECG during sinus rhythm often displays incomplete LBBB, or occasionally a pattern of complete bundle-branch block (BBB). In the latter case, conduction through the left bundle is actually possible, but is so slow that conduction over the right bundle alone depolarizes the ventricles during sinus rhythm.

Bundle-branch reentry is a relatively rare arrhythmia, accounting for approx 5% of all sustained monomorphic VTs evaluated at electrophysiology study *(32,35)*. It should

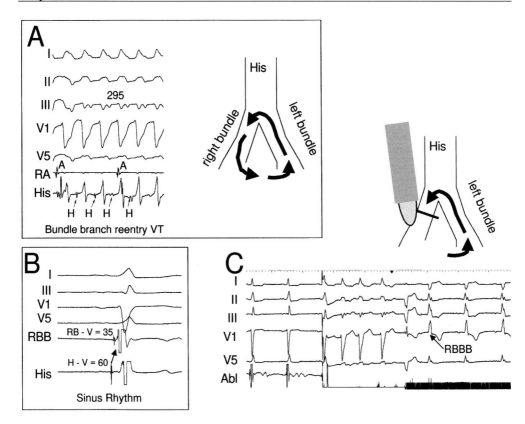

Fig. 3. Diagnosis and ablation of bundle-branch reentrant tachycardia is shown. In panel A, bundle-branch reentry tachycardia initiated in the electrophysiology laboratory is shown. Tachycardia has a LBBB configuration and cycle length of 295 ms. AV dissociation is evident in the right atrial recording (RA). A His bundle deflection (H) precedes each QRS, indicating that the His-Purkinje system is closely linked to the tachycardia. The mechanism is illustrated in the schematic at the right. In panel B, the ablation catheter has been placed distal to the His bundle, where the RBB potential is recorded. The H-V interval is 60 ms and the right bundle-V interval is 35 ms. In panel C, RF ablation of the RBB is performed. Radiofrequency current application causes transient accelerated automaticity of the RBB, inscribing three PVCs with a LBBB pattern. Then, RBBB is present (arrow). This interrupts the reentry circuit as illustrated in the schematic above the tracing. RBBB = right bundle branch.

be particularly suspected in patients who have sustained monomorphic VT associated with valvular heart disease *(36)*, cardiomyopathy, or muscular dystrophy *(37,38)*, in which a discrete region of myocardial scarring that could be an arrhythmia focus is absent. Most patients have severely depressed left ventricular function accompanying the His-Purkinje system disease. The tachycardia is often rapid (average rate of approx 215 beats per minute (BPM)), often causing syncope or cardiac arrest.

Bundle-branch reentrant tachycardia is easily cured by radiofrequency ablation of the RBB, which interrupts the circuit *(32,39)* (Fig. 3). The right bundle can be located by placing the catheter at the His bundle position, and then advancing the catheter distally from that point to the location where the potential from the RBB is recorded. Although curative, ablation of the RBB may further compromise atrioventricular (AV) conduction. A permanent pacemaker is recommended if the HV interval is markedly prolonged (>90 ms) after ablation of the RBB, and is required in up to 20–30%. Some patients, particularly those with prior MI, have scar-related VTs in addition to bundle-branch reentry; implantation of a defibrillator is usually considered. Patients with bundle-branch reentry associated with severely impaired ventricular dysfunction have a high mortality because of death from progressive heart failure *(32,35)*.

VT RELATED TO REGIONS OF SCAR

The Reentry Substrate

The most common cause of VT is reentry through regions of scar, most commonly an old MI (Fig. 4). Other scar-related VTs occur because of arrhythmogenic right ventricular dysplasia, sarcoidosis, Chagas' disease, and other nonischemic cardiomyopathies. Two features of ventricular scarring lead to reentrant VT *(40–42)*. First, dense scarring creates regions of anatomic conduction block. Second, the "scar" is not comprised completely of dense fibrotic tissue, but also contains surviving myocyte bundles *(43,44)*. Fibrosis between myocytes and myocyte bundles decreases cell-to-cell connections. The excitation wavefront propagates in a zig-zag manner from myocyte bundle to myocyte bundle, increasing the time for depolarization to procede through the region and thereby causing slow conduction *(44)*. Circulation of an excitation wavefront around an area of block leads to reentry. With slow conduction, each cell in the circuit has sufficient time to recover after each depolarization.

Most scar-related reentry circuits that allow catheter mapping can be modeled as shown in Fig. 4 *(45–48)*. Depolarization of myocytes in or near the scar or infarct generates only low-amplitude electrical signals that are not detectable from the body surface. The QRS complex occurs after the circulating wavefront reaches the border of the infarct and propagates across the ventricles. The site where the wavefront leaves the tachycardia focus is known as the exit. The location of the exit around the border of the scar is a major determinant of the QRS morphology. Often, the region of the scar that contains the exit can be inferred from the QRS morphology. The region proximal to the exit often forms a relatively narrow isthmus, which is a good target for catheter ablation. After the circulating wavefront leaves the exit, the wavefront travels through a broad outer loop along the margin of the scar or a loop within the scar (inner loop) to return to the isthmus. Circuits can consist of multiple loops or single loops. In some cases reentry results from circulation of a single broad reentry path around a region of block; i.e. a single outer loop. Radiofrequency catheter ablation lesions are usually small in relation to the entire circuit and outer loops *(3)*. Thus, the approach to ablation is to identify a narrow isthmus or channel in the circuit where a small number of radiofrequency lesions can interrupt reentry. Once a single channel is interrupted, there may be other channels that cause other tachycardias *(49)* (Fig. 4, panels B and C). Multiple morphologies of sustained monomorphic tachycardia, indicating multiple potential reentry circuits, are common (Fig. 4, panels B and C). Multiple morphologies of tachycardia make mapping and ablation more difficult, but do not preclude success. Often multiple morphologies of tachycardia originate from one general region of abnormal conduction *(50)*.

Reentry circuits can occur in any region around the scar. In most cases, a portion of the reentry circuit is located in the subendocardium, where it can be ablated. However, portions of the circuit are often deep within the endocardium and cannot be identified

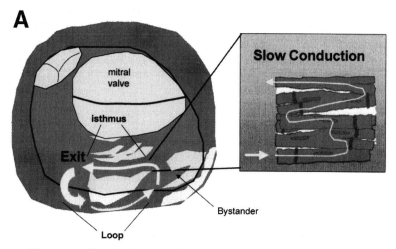

Reentry circuit in an infarct scar

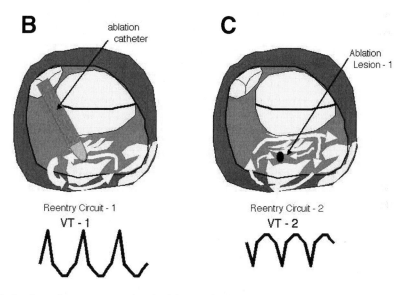

Fig. 4. Mechanism of reentry associated with ventricular scar is illustrated. The schematics show a view of the left ventricle from the apex looking into the ventricle toward the mitral and aortic valves. A region of heterogeneous scar is present in the inferior wall. In **(A)**, the reentry wavefront circulates counterclockwise around and through the scar. Regions of dense scar create an isthmus in the circuit. The QRS onset occurs when the wavefront emerges from the isthmus at the Exit. It then circulates around the border of the scar, returning to the isthmus. Slow conduction through some regions in the scar is caused by discontinuities between myocyte bundles, as illustrated in the magnified image at the right. A wavefront that enters the bottom left myocyte bundles takes a circuitous course to emerge at the superior left bundle. In **(B)**, an ablation catheter has been introduced through the aortic valve and positioned in the reentry circuit isthmus. In **(C)**, following ablation of the isthmus for VT-1, a second VT is still possible because of reentry through an isthmus beneath the mitral valve. This circuit revolves in the opposite direction from the first circuit; the resulting VT has a different QRS morphology. (*See* color plate 5 appearing in the insert following p. 208.)

or ablated using a catheter at the endocardium *(51)*. In some cases, the reentry circuit is epicardial in location. Some regions appear to give rise to endocardial portions of reentry circuit with disproportional frequency *(50,52)*. In patients with prior inferior-wall infarction, the mitral annulus forms a barrier to conduction that often delineates a portion of the reentry circuit. In some cases, a surviving rim of myocardium beneath the mitral annulus creates a long isthmus for reentry. The resulting VT has a RBBB configuration when reentry occurs with the circulating wavefront propagating from septal to lateral in the isthmus, and a LBB configuration when the circuit revolves in the opposite direction *(50)*.

Mapping Scar-Related Tachycardias

The first step in mapping is to identify the abnormal region. The region of scar is usually evident from an assessment of the ventricular-wall motion as an area of akinesis or dyskinesis. Regions of scar are also be identified during catheter-mapping as areas with low-amplitude electrograms *(53,54)*. Fig. 5 shows a voltage map of the left ventricle in a patient with an old anterior-wall MI. The scar can thereby be identified during stable sinus rhythm. In addition, the region that contains the reentry-circuit exit can often be located by pace-mapping, although this is less reliable than for the idiopathic tachycardias discussed previously *(1)*. Pacing from the mapping catheter during sinus rhythm can also identify regions of slow conduction in the scar, indicated by long conduction delays between the stimulus and the QRS onset *(55)*. Thus, during stable sinus rhythm, it is often possible to locate the scar, the likely quadrant of the scar that contains the reentry circuit exit, and the regions of slow conduction. To determine whether these areas are in the reentry circuit rather than a bystander region, further evaluation is performed during tachycardia.

By plotting the local activation at each site in the ventricle during VT, the entire reentry circuit can occasionally be delineated (Fig. 5, panel C). In most patients, portions of the reentry circuit are deep within the endocardium, and are inaccessible to endocardial electrode catheters. In addition, VT is often not tolerated sufficiently to allow enough time to move a mapping catheter to all regions of the ventricle. Therefore the approach is focused on rapidly identifying a critical isthmus, which is often proximal to the exit *(45)*. At these sites, depolarization precedes the QRS onset; the electrogram timing is referred to as "presystolic" or diastolic (Fig. 5), often with short-duration, low-amplitude signals referred to as "isolated diastolic potentials" *(56–59)*. To confirm that such a site is in the circuit and is not a bystander, the effect of pacing at the site is evaluated. Pacing stimuli that capture have a predictable effect on the tachycardia, depending on whether the pacing site is in the reentry circuit at a narrow isthmus or is at a bystander region. This is known as entrainment mapping *(45,57,59)*. Entrainment is continuous resetting of the reentry circuit by pacing at a rate faster than the circuit. At sites in a reentry circuit isthmus, the circuit can be reset without altering the QRS morphology (known as entrainment with concealed fusion or concealed entrainment) (Fig. 5, panel D), indicating that excitation wavefronts are capturing a relatively small region before interacting with the reentry circuit. This finding, in conjunction with other features of entrainment, allows a circuit isthmus to be identified without sampling sites throughout the ventricle. Radiofrequency current can then be applied during tachycardia; tachycardia termination provides further evidence that the site is critical to the reentry circuit. Additional radiofrequency lesions may be applied to enlarge the ablation lesion. Programmed stimulation is then repeated to attempt to reinitiate VT.

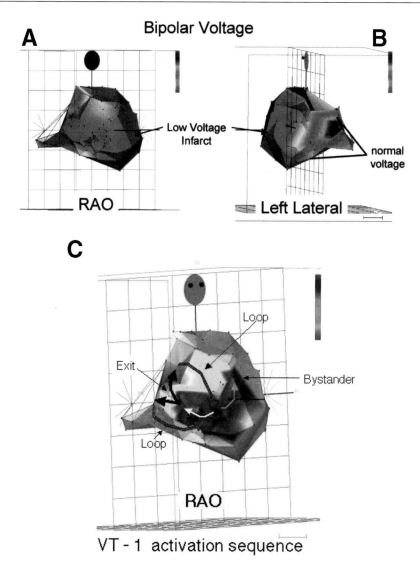

Fig. 5. Findings during catheter mapping in a patient with recurrent VT late after anterior-wall MI are shown. Left ventricular mapping was performed with an electroanatomic mapping system that records and displays catheter position along with the electrograms recorded. In **(A)** and **(B)** are shown the right anterior oblique (RAO) and left lateral views, respectively. Electrogram voltage is designated by colors with the lowest voltage shown in red, progressing to greater voltage regions of yellow, green, blue, and purple. The large anteroapical infarction is indicated by the extensive red region. In **(C)**, the activation sequence of induced VT is shown in the RAO view of the left ventricle. The colors now indicate the activation sequence, with red being the earliest activation (identifying the re-entry circuit exit), progressing to yellow, green, blue, and purple. The reentry circuit has a figure-eight configuration, consisting of two reentrant loops (marked by the red arrows) circulating clockwise and counterclockwise and sharing a common central path. A bystander region of abnormal conduction that is outside of the reentry circuit is marked by the pink arrow. **(D)** Shows the effect of pacing during tachycardia (entrainment) in the central common pathway ischmus. From the top are surface ECG leads I, II, III, V_1, and V_6 and an intracardiac recording from the ablation catheter. Pacing accelerates the QRS complexes to the pacing rate, but without changing the QRS morphology compared to that of tachycardia. Furthermore, there is a delay of 160 ms from the

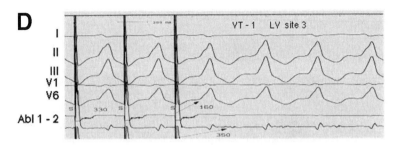

Fig. 5. *(Continued)*
stimulus to the following QRS onset, indicating slow conduction from the pacing site, through the
common path to the exit (red area in **C**). These findings indicate that the pacing site is in an isthmus
in the reentry circuit. Radiofrequency ablation at this site abolished tachycardia. (*See* color plate 6
appearing in the insert following p. 208.)

Ablation of Ventricular Tachycardia After MI

The common occurrence of multiple tachycardias in an individual patient, and the
various approaches to ablation, makes the interpretation of catheter ablation results
somewhat confusing. When VT is observed to occur spontaneously, this tachycardia
is often referred to as a "clinical tachycardia." Tachycardias induced in the electrophysiology laboratory that have not been previously documented to occur spontaneously are
sometimes referred to as "nonclinical tachycardias." This situation is complicated
because the 12-lead ECG is often not recorded when VT is terminated by an implantable
cardioverter defibrillator or by emergency medical technicians. Some centers select
patients who exhibit only one predominant morphology of "clinical" VT documented
with an ECG. If other tachycardias are induced at the time of study, these may be
ignored if they have not been observed to occur spontaneously. This approach reduces
the number of radiofrequency lesions required, but is more likely to leave potentially
important reentry circuits intact. A second approach targets all tachycardias that can
be induced and mapped. Some patients who have a "clinical tachycardia" that is no
longer inducible at the end of the procedure may be referred to as "not inducible"
despite the fact that other tachycardias are inducible. If tachycardias that were inducible
at the beginning of the procedure have been eliminated, but other tachycardias are
inducible, we designate this result as "modified." The reentry substrate has been altered,
but some reentry circuits remain. These issues also confuse the interpretation of reported
long-term outcomes. If a single tachycardia is targeted and ablated, but other tachycardias
that were not targeted occur during follow-up, this may be reported as a successful
outcome. In some cases, episodes of recurrent tachycardia are markedly reduced but
not abolished—a result designated as a "clinical success."

Radiofrequency catheter ablation that targets a single "clinical" morphology of VT
in selected patients was reported by Gonska and colleagues in 72 patients *(60)*. The
targeted tachycardia was no longer inducible at the end of the procedure in 74% of
patients. During a follow-up, 60% of the group were free from recurrent tachycardia.
Stevenson, Rothman, Strickberger, and colleagues targeted multiple tachycardias for
ablation in 108 patients with recurrent episodes of sustained monomorphic tachycardia
(61–63) (Fig. 6). Average left ventricular ejection fraction (LVEF) in these series
ranged from 0.22–0.33; amiodarone therapy had been ineffective in 14–76% of patients.
During the ablation procedure, an average of 3.6–4.7 different VTs were inducible per

A

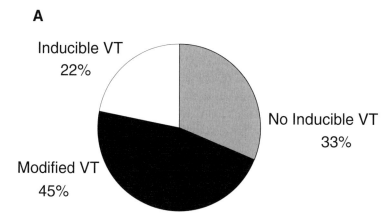

Acute Effect of VT ablation in 108 patients

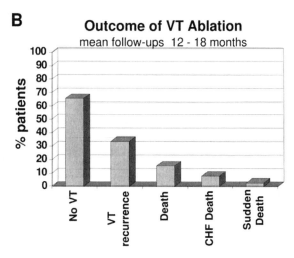

Fig. 6. The efficacy of catheter ablation in 108 patients with prior MI from three different centers targeting multiple VTs is shown *(61–63)*. Results are shown as assessed by inducible tachycardia early after ablation **(A)** and outcome during follow-up **(B).**

patient. Ablation abolished all inducible monomorphic tachycardias in 33% patients, tachycardias were inducible but modified in 45% of patients, and the procedure failed to abolish targeted, inducible tachycardias in 22% of patients (Fig. 6). During mean follow-ups ranging from 12–18 mo, 66% of patients remained free of recurrent tachycardia and 34% suffered one or more tachycardia recurrences. Spontaneous tachycardia recurred more frequently in patients whose arrhythmia substrate was modified, as opposed to those with no inducible tachycardia at the end of the procedure—but less often than in patients whose tachycardia was not altered by ablation. Sudden death occurred in 2.8% of patients—the majority of patients in all three series had implantable cardioverter defibrillators (ICDs).

Of the 180 patients reported in these four series, complications occurred in 10%; the most frequent were: atrioventricular (AV) block caused by ablation in the region of the conduction system, complications of arterial access, and pericardial effusion without tamponade *(60–63)* (Fig. 6). Procedure-related mortality was 1%. In a recent multicenter trial of catheter ablation using a saline-cooled ablation catheter in 146 patients (82% with prior MI), procedural mortality was 2.7% and the risk of stroke was 2.7% (64). When extensive lesions have been created in ventricular scar, anticoagulation with warfarin is recommended, although the efficacy and optimal duration of this therapy has not been established (65). Chronic warfarin therapy is a reasonable consideration for many of these patients because of associated severe ventricular dysfunction. These procedures are relatively difficult, as indicated by the average procedure duration of 4.8 h and fluoroscopy time of 56 min in the multicenter study (64). During follow-up, the major cause of mortality is heart failure, with a mortality of approx 10% over the following 12–18 mo (60–64). The high risk of heart failure is not unexpected, given the antecedent history of heart failure and depressed ventricular function in this patient population. However, damage to the adjacent contracting myocardium outside the infarct, or injury to the aortic or mitral valves, are procedural complications that could exacerbate heart failure. Attention to restriction of ablation lesions to regions of the infarct is prudent. As noted previously, sudden death is rare, but the majority of patients have ICDs.

Control of frequent, symptomatic shocks from an ICD has emerged as a major reason for catheter ablation in patients with VT after MI (63,66). In the year following defibrillator implantation, 60% of patients will be hospitalized again, usually for control of recurrent arrhythmias. Addition of an antiarrhythmic drug is required in more than 25% of patients. Catheter ablation can allow control of recurrent arrhythmias, avoiding drug toxicity and the adverse impact of many drugs—particularly amiodarone, on defibrillation threshold. Antiarrhythmic drugs can also slow the rate of spontaneous VT, making discrimination of VT from sinus tachycardia more difficult and leading to inappropriate defibrillator therapies. Because VT is usually associated with depressed ventricular function and a risk of sudden death, catheter ablation does not replace the need for an ICD in most patients. In some patient populations, the risk of sudden death may be acceptably low, and successful ablation may be adequate therapy (60). Ablation should be considered reasonable initial therapy for incessant VT, and can be life-saving in this situation (67,68).

Right Ventricular Dysplasia

In right ventricular dysplasia, portions of the right ventricle are replaced by fibrous or fatty tissue (69). Scar-related reentry circuits occur, giving rise to tachycardias that usually have a LBBB-like configuration. When involvement is sufficient to produce detectably depressed right ventricular function, the success of ablation is variable (70,71). Individual tachycardias can often be targeted and ablated, but other tachycardias can recur later, possibly related to progression of the disease process. We usually reserve ablation as a palliative therapy to control frequent episodes of tachycardia. Although the right ventricle can be quite thinned, the risk of perforation during mapping does not appear to be substantially increased, but reported series are small.

VT Caused by Non-Ischemic Cardiomyopathy

In patients with idiopathic nonischemic causes of cardiomyopathy, the mechanisms of sustained monomorphic VT are more diverse. Scar-related reentry is most common, but bundle-branch reentry and focal automaticity also occur (10,68). Discrete regions of scarring are often identified based on electrograms. Scar-related VT also occurs in patients with cardiac sarcoidosis *(5)*, sclerodema *(72)*, Chagas' disease *(73)*, and late after repair of tetralogy of Fallot *(74–76)*. Experience with ablation is confined to small series and case reports. Results are somewhat similar to those for patients with prior MI; multiple tachycardias are not rare, but reduction in number of episodes and termination of incessant tachycardia can often be achieved.

PROBLEMS AND EMERGING SOLUTIONS FOR SCAR-RELATED TACHYCARDIAS

Intramural and Epicardial Circuits

In some idiopathic and scar-related tachycardias the ablation target is not located on the endocardium, but is intramural or epicardial in location. In these cases, epicardial mapping can be attempted in one of two ways. Electrode catheters can be introduced into the cardiac venous system via the coronary sinus (CS). Small, 2 French multielectrode catheters are available that allow extensive epicardial mapping over regions of the left ventricle by canulating the branches of the CS and great cardiac vein *(77)*. The utility of this method is being evaluated.

A second approach developed by Sosa and colleagues involves percutaneous entry into the pericardial space in the manner used for pericardiocentesis, followed by insertion of an introducer and mapping catheter *(73,78,79)*. Epicardial foci have been identified and ablated. The risk of damage to adjacent lung and epicardial coronary vessels requires further evaluation. This method cannot be employed in patients who have had prior cardiac surgery with resulting scarring of the pericardial space. Initially primarily applied to patients with VT caused by Chagasic cardiomyopathy *(73,78,79)*, Sosa and colleagues have recently published their experience with epicardial mapping and ablation in 14 patients with VT related to remote inferior MI *(79a)*. However, the applicability and utility of this technique remain unclear *(79b)*.

When critical portions of scar-related reentry circuits are intramural or epicardial, the ablation lesion that can be created with a standard radiofrequency catheter may not penetrate sufficiently deep to interrupt reentry. As current is increased, the temperature at the tissue interface and the electrode touching the surface reaches 100°C *(80)*. Denatured protein adheres to the electrode and forms a high impedance barrier, reducing current delivery and lesion expansion. The catheter must be withdrawn and cleaned. To prevent coagulum formation, the electrode can be cooled by irrigating the catheter tip with room-temperature saline *(81)*. The first saline-irrigated catheter system approved for ablation circulates saline through the electrode and returns it through the catheter to be discarded, rather than infusing it into the circulation *(5,64)*. This system was evaluated in a multicenter trial that enrolled 146 patients who had an average 25 ± 31 episodes of VT in the 2 mo prior to ablation, and who had failed an average of 2.5 antiarrhythmic drugs, including amiodarone therapy in 40% of patients. VT was caused by MI in 82% of patients, and the average LVEF was $31 \pm 13\%$. Ablation eliminated all "mappable ventricular tachycardias" at EPS in 75% of patients *(64)*. During the initial 2 mo after ablation, 81% of patients experienced a reduction in number of VT episodes of more than 75% compared to that which had occurred in the preceding 2 mo. During follow-up of 243 ± 153 d (mean $\pm$ standard deviation), 54% of patients remained free of any spontaneous VT. Total mortality during follow-up was 17%, and 60% of deaths were caused by heart failure, consistent with prior reports in this patient population. Major procedural complications occurred in 8% of patients including stroke or transient ischemic event in 2.7%, tamponade in 2.7%, MI in 0.7% and unintentional AV block in 1% of patients. Procedural mortality was 2.7%. Direct comparison with standard radiofrequency catheters has not been performed.

Saline-irrigated catheters in which the saline flows out of small holes at the tip of the catheter are also being tested. An alternative means of cooling the electrode tip is to use a larger electrode, which therefore has a greater surface area exposed to the circulating blood pool *(82)*. With these methods that increase lesion size comes the risk of myocardial damage that could further depress ventricular function. Cooling the catheter displaces the maximal tissue temperature below the tissue surface. If temperature reaches 100°C, a steam pocket can form and explode either through the endocardium or epicardium. Thus, the risk of perforation may also be increased. It is important that lesion be confined to regions of scar. Risks will require careful assessment with each new advance.

Unmappable VT

For many patients, mapping during VT is not possible because of hemodynamic intolerance *(83,84)*. Several approaches to the problem are being evaluated. One approach is to define the scar and the likely quadrant containing the exit based on sinus-rhythm electrograms and pace-mapping, then to place radiofrequency lesions across that region of the scar. In an initial series, this approach was successful in abolishing recurrent episodes of VT in 3 of 5 patients *(84)*.

Another approach is to attempt to record electrical activity from multiple regions simultaneously with the use of a basket catheter *(85,86)*. These catheters can be deployed through a long sheath into the ventricle, where the splines of the basket catheter spread out against the endocardium. There are some regions of the ventricle that are not sampled. The risks and benefits of these catheters are under investigation.

A third approach involves the use of a system that mathematically calculates the electrical potentials at the endocardial surface based on the potentials recorded some distance away by a balloon electrode array inserted into the ventricle *(87–89)*. An isopotential map calculated from this "inverse solution" is displayed on the ventricular geometry constructed by sweeping a roving catheter around the ventricle. This system offers the potential for assessing the sequence of ventricular activation over the entire endocardial surface from a single tachycardia beat. Detailed mapping of unstable arrhythmias may be possible. Promising initial results have been reported; further evaluation and technical improvements are likely to be forthcoming.

CONCLUSION

Catheter ablation has emerged as a useful therapy for VTs. For patients with recurrent, symptomatic idiopathic VT ablation should be considered if therapy with calcium-channel blockers or beta-blockers is not effective, tolerated, or desired. Catheter ablation is the first-line therapy for patients with VT caused by bundle-branch reentry, although a substantial number of these patients will require an implantable defibrillator or pacemaker because of other associated VTs or impaired AV conduction. In patients with scar-related VT, ablation is more difficult, but plays an important role in controlling incessant VT, and frequent symptomatic episodes of VT terminated by an ICD.

REFERENCES

1. Josephson ME, Waxman HL, Cain ME, et al. Ventricular activation during ventricular endocardial pacing. II. Role of pace-mapping to localize origin of ventricular tachycardia. Am J Cardiol 1982;50(1):11–22.
2. Simmers TA, De Bakker JM, Wittkampf FFH, et al. Effects of heating on impulse propagation in superfused canine myocardium. J Am Coll Cardiol 1995;55(6):1457–1464.
3. Bartlett TG, Mitchell R, Friedman PL, et al. Histologic evolution of radiofrequency lesions in an old human myocardial infarct causing ventricular tachycardia. J Cardiovasc Electrophysiol 1995;6(8):625–629.
4. Grubman E, Pauri BB, Lyle S, et al. Histopathologic effects of radiofrequency catheter ablation in previously infarcted human myocardium. J Cardiovasc Electrophysiol 1999;10(3):336–342.
5. Delacretaz E, Stevenson WG, Winters GL, et al. Ablation of ventricular tachycardia with a saline-cooled radiofrequency catheter: anatomic and histologic characteristics of the lesions in humans. J Cardiovasc Electrophysiol 1999;10(6):860–865.
6. Varma N, Josephson ME. Therapy of "idiopathic" ventricular tachycardia. J Cardiovasc Electrophysiol 1997;8(1):104–116.
7. Rodriguez LM, Smeets JL, Timmermans C, et al. Predictors for successful ablation of right- and left-sided idiopathic ventricular tachycardia. Am J Cardiol 1997;79(3):309–314.
8. Ohe T, Aihara N, Kamakura S, et al. Long-term outcome of verapamil-sensitive sustained left ventricular tachycardia in patients without structural heart disease. J Am Coll Cardiol 1995;25(1):54–58.
9. Shinbane JS, Wood MA, Jensen DN, et al. Tachycardia-induced cardiomyopathy: a review of animal models and clinical studies. J Am Coll Cardiol 1997;29(4):709–715.
10. Delacretaz ESW, Ellison KE, Maisel WM, Friedman PL. Mapping and radiofrequency catheter ablation of the three types of sustained monomorphic ventricular tachycardia in nonischemic heart disease. J Cardiovasc Electrophys 2000;11(1):7–11.
11. Movsowitz C, Schwartzman D, Callans DJ, et al. Idiopathic right ventricular outflow tract tachycardia: narrowing the anatomic location for successful ablation. Am Heart J 1996;131(5):930–936.
12. Chinushi M, Aizawa Y, Ohhiva K, et al. Radiofrequency catheter ablation for idiopathic right ventricular tachycardia with special reference to morphological variation and long-term outcome. Heart 1997;78(3):255–261.
13. Wilber DJ, Baerman J, Olshansky B, et al. Adenosine-sensitive ventricular tachycardia. Clinical characteristics and response to catheter ablation. Circulation 1993;87(1):126–134.
14. Lerman BB, Stein K, Engelstein EV, et al. Mechanism of repetitive monomorphic ventricular tachycardia. Circulation 1995;92(3):421–429.
15. Zhu DW, Maloney JD, Timmons TW, et al. Radiofrequency catheter ablation for management of symptomatic ventricular ectopic activity. J Am Coll Cardiol 1995;26(4):843–849.
16. Markowitz SM, Litvak BL, Ramirez de Arellano EA, et al. Adenosine-sensitive ventricular tachycardia: right ventricular abnormalities delineated by magnetic resonance imaging. Circulation 1997;96(4):1192–2000.
17. O'Connor BK, Case CL, Sokoloski MC, et al. Radiofrequency catheter ablation of right ventricular outflow tachycardia in children and adolescents. J Am Coll Cardiol 1996;27(4):869–874.
18. Coggins DL, Lee RJ, Sweeney J, et al. Radiofrequency catheter ablation as a cure for idiopathic tachycardia of both left and right ventricular origin. J Am Coll Cardiol 1994;23(6):1333–1341.
19. Lee SH, Chen SA, Tai CT, et al. Electropharmacologic characteristics and radiofrequency catheter ablation of sustained ventricular tachycardia in patients without structural heart disease. Cardiology 1996;87(1):33–41.
20. Wen MS, et al. Determinants of tachycardia recurrences after radiofrequency ablation of idiopathic ventricular tachycardia. Am J Cardiol 1998;81(4):500–503.
21. Shimoike E, Ohba Y, Yanagi N, et al. Radiofrequency catheter ablation of left ventricular outflow tract tachycardia: report of two cases. J Cardiovasc Electrophysiol 1998;9(2):196–202.
22. Friedman PL, Bittl JA, Simon DI, Kay GN, Lerman BB, et al. Left main coronary artery occlusion during radiofrequency catheter ablation of idiopathic outflow tract ventricular tachycardia. PACE 1997;20:1123A.
23. Nakagawa H, Beckman KJ, McClelland JH, et al. Radiofrequency catheter ablation of idiopathic left ventricular tachycardia guided by a Purkinje potential. Circulation 1993;88(6):2607–2617.
24. Lin FC, Wen MS, Wang CC, et al. Left ventricular fibromuscular band is not a specific substrate for idiopathic left ventricular tachycardia. Circulation 1996;93(3):525–528.

25. Damle RS, et al. Radiofrequency catheter ablation of idiopathic left ventricular tachycardia originating in the left anterior fascicle. PACE 1998;21(5):1155–1158.

26. Thakur RK, Klein GJ, Sivavam CA, et al. Anatomic substrate for idiopathic left ventricular tachycardia. Circulation 1996;93(3):497–501.

27. Merliss AD, Seifert MJ, Collins RF, et al. Catheter ablation of idiopathic left ventricular tachycardia associated with a false tendon. PACE 1996;19(12 Pt 1):2144–2146.

28. Bogun F, et al. Radiofrequency ablation of idiopathic left anterior fascicular tachycardia. J Cardiovac Electrophysiol 1995;6(12):1113–1116.

29. Vohra J, Shah A, Hua W, et al. Radiofrequency ablation of idiopathic ventricular tachycardia. Aust N Z J Med 1996;26(2):186–194.

30. Tsuchiya T, Okumura K, Hondu T, et al. Significance of late diastolic potential preceding Purkinje potential in verapamil-sensitive idiopathic left ventricular tachycardia. Circulation 1999;99(18):2408–2413.

31. Callans DJ, Menz V, Schwartzman D, et al. Repetitive monomorphic tachycardia from the left ventricular outflow tract: electrocardiographic patterns consistent with a left ventricular site of origin. J Am Coll Cardiol 1997;29(5):1023–1027.

32. Blanck Z, Dhala A, Veshyande S, et al. Bundle branch reentrant ventricular tachycardia: cumulative experience in 48 patients. J Cardiovasc Electrophysiol 1993;4(3):253–262.

33. Simons GR, Sorrentino RA, Zimerman LI, et al. Bundle branch reentry tachycardia and possible sustained interfascicular reentry tachycardia with a shared unusual induction pattern. J Cardiovasc Electrophysiol 1996;7(1):44–50.

34. Berger RD, Orios P, Kasper EK, et al. Catheter ablation of coexistent bundle branch and interfascicular reentrant ventricular tachycardia. J Cardiovasc Electrophysiol 1996;7(4):341–347.

35. Caceres J, Jazayeri M, McKinnie J, et al. Sustained bundle branch reentry as a mechanism of clinical tachycardia. Circulation 1989;79(2):256–270.

36. Narasimhan C, Jazayeri M, Sra J, et al. Ventricular tachycardia in valvular heart disease: facilitation of sustained bundle-branch reentry by valve surgery. Circulation 1997;96(12):4307–4313.

37. Negri SM, Cowan MD. Becker muscular dystrophy with bundle branch reentry ventricular tachycardia (In Process Citation). J Cardiovasc Electrophysiol 1998;9(6):652–654.

38. Merino JL, Caumona JK, Fernandez-Lozano I, et al. Mechanisms of sustained ventricular tachycardia in myotonic dystrophy: implications for catheter ablation. Circulation 1998;98(6):541–546.

39. Mehdirad AA, Kaim S, Rist K, et al. Long-term clinical outcome of right bundle branch radiofrequency catheter ablation for treatment of bundle branch reentrant ventricular tachycardia. PACE 1995;18(12 Pt 1):2135–2143.

40. de Bakker JM, Coronel R, Tasseron S, et al. Ventricular tachycardia in the infarcted, Langendorff-perfused human heart: role of the arrangement of surviving cardiac fibers. J Am Coll Cardiol 1990;15(7):1594–1607.

41. de Bakker JM, van Capelle FJ, Janse MJ, et al. Reentry as a cause of ventricular tachycardia in patients with chronic ischemic heart disease: electrophysiologic and anatomic correlation. Circulation 1988;77(3):589–606.

42. Pogwizd SM, Saffitz JE, Hoyt RH, et al. Reentrant and focal mechanisms underlying ventricular tachycardia in the human heart. Circulation 1991;86:1872–1887.

43. de Bakker JM, van Capelle FJ, Janse MJ, et al. Fractionated electrograms in dilated cardiomyopathy: origin and relation to abnormal conduction. J Am Coll Cardiol 1996;27(5):1071–1078.

44. de Bakker JM, van Capelle FJ, Janse MJ, et al. Slow conduction in the infarcted human heart. 'Zigzag' course of activation. Circulation 1993;88(3):915–926.

45. Stevenson WG, Friedman PL, Sager PT, et al. Exploring postinfarction reentrant ventricular tachycardia with entrainment mapping. J Am Coll Cardiol 1997;29(6):1180–1189.

46. de Bakker JM, van Capelle FJ, Janse MJ, et al. Macroreentry in the infarcted human heart: the mechanism of ventricular tachycardias with a "focal" activation pattern. J Am Coll Cardiol 1991;18(4):1005–1014.

47. Littman L, Gallagher JJ, et al. Functional role of the epicardium in post-infarction ventricular tachycardia: observations derived from computerized epicardial activation mapping, entrainment, and epicardial laser photoablation. Circulation 1991;83:1577–1591.

48. Kaltenbrunner W, Cardinal R, Dubuc M, et al. Epicardial and endocardial mapping of ventricular tachycardia in patients with myocardial infarction. Is the origin of the tachycardia always subendocardially localized? Circulation 1991;84:1058–1071.

49. Downar E, Saito J, Doig JC, et al. Endocardial mapping of ventricular tachycardia in the intact human

ventricle. III. Evidence of multiuse reentry with spontaneous and induced block in portions of reentrant path complex. J Am Coll Cardiol 1995;25(7):1591–1600.

50. Wilber DJ, Kopp DE, Glascock DN, et al. Catheter ablation of the mitral isthmus for ventricular tachycardia associated with inferior infarction. Circulation 1995;92(12):3481–3489.

51. Svenson RH, Littman L, Gallagher JJ, et al. Termination of ventricular tachycardia with epicardial laser photocoagulation: a clinical comparison with patients undergoing successful endocardial photocoagulation alone. J Am Coll Cardiol 1990;15(1):163–170.

52. Hadjis TA, Stevenson WG, Harada T, et al. Preferential locations for critical reentry circuit sites causing ventricular tachycardia after inferior wall myocardial infarction. J Cardiovasc Electrophysiol 1997;8(4):363–370.

53. Callans DJ, Ken JF, Michele J, et al. Electroanatomic left ventricular mapping in the porcine model of healed anterior myocardial infarction: correlation with intracardiac echocardiography and pathological analysis (In Process Citation). Circulation 1999;100(16):1744–1750.

54. Harada T, Stevenson WG, Kocovic DZ, et al. Catheter ablation of ventricular tachycardia after myocardial infarction: relation of endocardial sinus rhythm late potentials to the reentry circuit. J Am Coll Cardiol 1997;30(4):1015–1023.

55. Stevenson WG, Sager PT, Watterson PD, et al. Relation of pace mapping QRS configuration and conduction delay to ventricular tachycardia reentry circuits in human infarct scars. J Am Coll Cardiol 1995;26(2):481–488.

56. Bogun F, Bahu M, Knight BP, et al. Response to pacing at sites of isolated diastolic potentials during ventricular trachycardia in patients with previous myocardial infarction. J Am Coll Cardiol 1997;30(2):505–513.

57. Bogun F, Bahu M, Knight BP, et al. Comparison of effective and ineffective target sites that demonstrate concealed entrainment in patients with coronary artery disease undergoing radiofrequency ablation of ventricular tachycardia. Circulation 1997;95(1):183–190.

58. Kocovic DZ, Harada T, Friedman PL, et al. Characteristics of electrograms recorded at reentry circuit sites and bystanders during ventricular tachycardia after myocardial infarction. J Am Coll Cardiol 1999;34(2):381–388.

59. El-Shalakany A, Hadjis T, Papageorgiou P, et al. Entrainment/mapping criteria for the prediction of termination of ventricular tachycardia by single radiofrequency lesion in patients with coronary artery disease. Circulation 1999;99(17):2283–2289.

60. Gonska BD, Cao K, Schaumann A, et al. Catheter ablation of ventricular tachycardia in 136 patients with coronary artery disease: results and long-term follow-up. J Am Coll Cardiol 1994;24(6):1506–1514.

61. Stevenson WG, Friedman PL, Ganz LI, et al. Radiofrequency catheter ablation of ventricular tachycardia after myocardial infarction. Circulation 1998;98(4):308–314.

62. Rothman SA, Hsia HH, Cossu SF, et al. Radiofrequency catheter ablation of postinfarction ventricular tachycardia: long-term success and the significance of inducible nonclinical arrhythmias. Circulation 1997;96(10):3499–3508.

63. Strickberger SA, Man KC, Daoud EG, et al. A prospective evaluation of catheter ablation of ventricular tachycardia as adjuvant therapy in patients with coronary artery disease and an implantable cardioverter-defibrillator. Circulation 1997;96(5):1525–1531.

64. Calkins H, Epstein A, Packer D, et al. Catheter ablation of ventricular tachycardia in patients with structural heart disease using cooled RF energy: reseults of a prospective multicenter study. Circulation 2000;35(7):1905–1914.

65. Zhou L, Keane D, Reed G, et al. Thromboembolic complications of cardiac radiofrequency catheter ablation: a review of the reported incidence, pathogenesis and current research directions. J Cardiovasc Electrophysiol 1999;10(4):611–620.

66. Stevenson WG, Friedman PL, Sweeney LM. Catheter ablation as an adjunct to ICD therapy [editorial; comment]. Circulation 1997;96(5):1378–1380.

67. Cao K, Gonska BD. Catheter ablation of incessant ventricular tachycardia: acute and long-term results. Eur Heart J 1996;17(5):756–763.

68. Kottkamp H, Hindricks G, Chen X, et al. Radiofrequency catheter ablation of sustained ventricular tachycardia in idiopathic dilated cardiomyopathy. Circulation 1995;92(5):1159–1168.

69. Marcus FI, Fontaine G. Arrhythmogenic right ventricular dysplasia/cardiomyopathy: a review. Pacing Clin Electrophysiol 1995;18(6):1298–1314.

70. Harada T, Aonuma K, Yarnauchi Y, et al. Catheter ablation of ventricular tachycardia in patients with right ventricular dysplasia: identification of target sites by entrainment mapping techniques. Pacing Clin Electrophysiol 1998;21(11 Pt 2):2547–2550.

71. Ellison KE, Friedman PL, Ganz LI, et al. Entrainment mapping and radiofrequency catheter ablation of ventricular tachycardia in right ventricular dysplasia. J Am Coll Cardiol 1998;32(3):724–728.

72. Rankin AC, Osswald S, McGovern BA, et al. Mechanism of sustained monomorphic ventricular tachycardia in systemic sclerosis. Am J Cardiol 1999;83(4):633–636, A11.

73. Sosa E, Scanavacca M, D'Avila A, et al. Endocardial and epicardial ablation guided by nonsurgical transthoracic epicardial mapping to treat recurrent ventricular tachycardia. J Cardiovasc Electrophysiol 1998;9(3):229–239.

74. Harrison DA, Harris L, Siu SC, et al. Sustained ventricular tachycardia in adult patients late after repair of tetralogy of Fallot. J Am Coll Cardiol 1997;30(5):1368–1373.

75. Gonska BD, Cao K, Raab J, et al. Radiofrequency catheter ablation of right ventricular tachycardia late after repair of congenital heart defects. Circulation 1996;94(8):1902–1908.

76. Stevenson WG, Delacretaz E, Friedman PL, et al. Identification and ablation of macroreentrant ventricular tachycardia with the CARTO electroanatomical mapping system. PACE 1998;21(7):1448–1456.

77. Cappato R, Schluter M, Weiss C, et al. Mapping of the coronary sinus and great cardiac vein using a 2-French electrode catheter and a right femoral approach. J Cardiovasc Electrophysiol 1997;8(4):371–376.

78. Sosa E, Scanavacca M, D'Avila A, et al. A new technique to perform epicardial mapping in the electrophysiology laboratory. J Cardiovasc Electrophysiol 1996;7(6):531–536.

79. Sosa E, Scanavacca M, D'Avila A, et al. Radiofrequency catheter ablation of ventricular tachycardia guided by nonsurgical epicardial mapping in chronic Chagasic heart disease. PACE 1999;22(1 Pt 1):128–130.

79a. Sosa E, Scanavacca M, d'Avila A, et al. Nonsurgical transthoracic epicardial catheter ablation to treat recurrent ventricular tachycardia occurring late after myocardial infarction. J Am Coll Cardiol 2000;35(6):1442–1449.

79b. Josephson ME. Epicardial approach to the ablation of ventricular tachycardia in coronary artery disease: An alternative or ancillary approach. J Am Coll Cardiol 2000;35(6):1450–1452.

80. Avitall B, Khan M, Krum D, et al. Physics and engineering of transcatheter cardiac tissue ablation. J Am Coll Cardiol 1993;22(3):921–932.

81. Nakagawa H, Yamanashi WS, Pitha JV, et al. Comparison of in vivo tissue temperature profile and lesion geometry for radiofrequency ablation with a saline-irrigated electrode versus temperature control in a canine thigh muscle preparation. Circulation 1995;91(8):2264–2273.

82. Hogh Petersen H, Chen X, Pietersen A, et al. Lesion dimensions during temperature-controlled radiofrequency catheter ablation of left ventricular porcine myocardium: impact of ablation site, electrode size, and convective cooling. Circulation 1999;99(2):319–325.

83. Callans DJ, Zado E, Sauter BH, et al. Efficacy of radiofrequency catheter ablation for ventricular tachycardia in healed myocardial infarction. Am J Cardiol 1998;82(4):429–432.

84. Ellison KE, Sweeney MO, LeFroy DC, Delacretaz F, Friedman PL. Catheter ablation for hemodynamically unstable monomorphic ventricular tachycardia. J Cardiovasc Electrophysiol 2000;11(1):41–44.

85. Greenspon AJ, Hsu SS, Datorre S. Successful radiofrequency catheter ablation of sustained ventricular tachycardia postmyocardial infarction in man guided by a multielectrode "basket" catheter. J Cardiovasc Electrophysiol 1997;8(5):565–570.

86. Schalij MJ, van Kugge FP, Siezenga M, et al. Endocardial activation mapping of ventricular tachycardia in patients: first application of a 32-site bipolar mapping electrode catheter. Circulation 1998;98(20):2168–2179.

87. Schilling RJ, Peters NS, Davies DW. Simultaneous endocardial mapping in the human left ventricle using a noncontact catheter: comparison of contact and reconstructed electrograms during sinus rhythm. Circulation 1998;98(9):887–898.

88. Schilling RJ, Peters NS, Davies DW. Mapping and ablation of ventricular tachycardia with the aid of a non-contact mapping system. Heart 1999;81(6):570–575.

89. Schilling RJ, Peters NS, Davies DW. Feasibility of a noncontact catheter for endocardial mapping of human ventricular tachycardia. Circulation 1999;19:2543–2552.

18

Long QT Syndrome, Brugada Syndrome, Right Ventricular Cardiomyopathy, Hypertrophic Cardiomyopathy, and Commotio Cordis

Eric J. Rashba, MD, Mark S. Link, MD, and N.A. Mark Estes III, MD

CONTENTS

CONGENITAL LONG QT SYNDROME

The hereditary long QT syndrome (LQTS) is a rare disorder characterized by prolongation of the QT interval on the electrocardiogram (ECG) and a propensity for syncope, torsades de pointes, ventricular arrhythmias, and sudden death. One form of LQTS, described by Jervell and Lange-Nielsen in 1957, is characterized by deafness and autosomal recessive inheritance *(1)*. The most common form of LQTS was initially described by Romano *(2)* and Ward *(3)*, and is characterized by autosomal dominant inheritance and normal hearing. Remarkable progress has been made in the last several years in our understanding of the pathogenesis of LQTS. It is now clear that LQTS is a heterogeneous disorder caused by mutations in specific ion channels that play a critical role in the control of cardiac repolarization *(4)*. These findings have revolutionized our understanding of LQTS, and may yield new insights into other conditions characterized by ventricular arrhythmias in the absence of ischemia or structural heart disease. Recent work has also identified LQTS as an important cause of sudden infant death syndrome (SIDS) *(5,6)*.

From: *Contemporary Cardiology: Management of Cardiac Arrhythmias*
Edited by: L. I. Ganz © Humana Press Inc., Totowa, NJ

Molecular Genetics of LQTS

At present, mutations in four cardiac ion-channel genes have been identified which cause the clinical manifestations of LQTS (LQT1, 2, 3, and 5) *(7)*. An additional LQTS gene has bee mapped to chromosome 4, but the mutant gene has not yet been identified (LQT4) *(8)*. These mutations account for only 50% of the known families with LQTS, which has important implications for molecular diagnosis *(9)*. In most instances, multiple mutations have been identified in each gene, which vary in their functional consequences (degree of current alteration and QT prolongation) *(10)*. This genetic heterogeneity contributes to a marked variability in clinical manifestations of the disorder. In addition, substantial variability in the clinical severity of the disorder exists among unrelated kindreds with identical mutations. These data suggest that "modifier genes" may exist, which also influence the prognosis.

The mutations that have been identified to date fall into two general categories. One type of mutation results in reduced function of the outward potassium currents that govern the repolarization process (I_{Kr} and I_{Ks}). The LQT1 gene (KvLQT1) on chromosome 11 encodes an abnormal α-subunit of I_{Ks} *(11)*. The LQT2 gene on chromosome 7 (also known as HERG) encodes an abnormal I_{Kr} protein, resulting in the clinical Romano-Ward syndrome *(12)*. The LQT5 gene (KCNE1) on chromosome 21 encodes the minK protein, which is the β-subunit of I_{Ks} *(13)*. The minK protein also complexes with HERG to regulate I_{Kr} *(14)*. LQT1 and LQT5 patients share an interesting clinical feature: some mutations cause Romano-Ward syndrome (autosomal dominant inheritance, normal hearing), and other distinct mutations are associated with Jervell and Lange-Neilsen syndrome (autosomal recessive inheritance, deafness) *(15)*. Many of the potassium-channel mutations that cause Romano-Ward syndrome exert a "dominant negative" effect, in that the degree of current reduction is greater than the expected 50% (2 mutant-channel proteins, 2 normal-channel protein incorporated in the channel tetramer) *(16)*. This property may result from a conformational change in the overall channel structure induced by a single mutant subunit. The second general class of mutations involves a "gain of function" of inward depolarizing sodium currents. The LQT3 gene on chromosome 3 (also known as SCN5A) encodes an abnormal Na^+ channel protein with alteration in rapid inactivation, leading to continued leakage of depolarizating Na^+ current into the cell and prolonged repolarization *(17)*.

A rapidly growing body of literature has emerged to support the hypothesis that the LQTS genotype influences the clinical phenotype that is observed. This correlation was first reported by Moss et al., who observed distinctive T-wave patterns that were characteristic of the LQT1, LQT2, and LQT3 genotypes (Fig. 1) *(18)*. Schwartz *(19)* and others *(20)* subsequently reported that the precipitants of arrhythmic events differ markedly among patients with the various genotypes. Auditory stimuli precipitate cardiac events more commonly in LQT2 patients than LQT1 patients *(20);* LQT3 patients are more prone to cardiac events during rest or sleep, which are rare among LQT1 patients *(19)*. Interestingly, LQT3 patients exhibit an exaggerated shortening of the QT interval during exercise, which may be protective against exertional events *(9)*. A mutation in the LQT3 (SCN5A) gene was recently identified in an infant who survived SIDS *(6)*. It must be emphasized that considerable overlap in phenotype exists among patients with the various genotypes, which prohibits definitive classification of patients based on the ECG T-wave pattern or the clinical presentation. The characteriza-

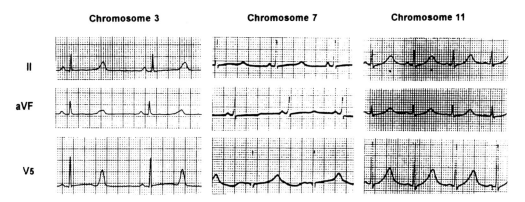

Fig. 1. ECG recordings from three patients from families with long QT syndrome (LQTS) linked to genes on chromosomes 3, 7, and 11. (Reproduced with permission from: Moss et al. ECG T-wave patterns in genetically distinct forms of the hereditary long QT syndrome. Circulation 1995;92:2933.)

tion of the precise abnormality in ion channel function that is associated with specific genotypes may ultimately yield novel pharmacologic therapies designed to improve ion-channel function ("gene-specific therapy").

Criteria for Diagnosis

The criteria developed to assist in the diagnosis of hereditary LQTS incorporate clinical features, electrocardiographic findings, and family history *(21)* (Table 1). The initial work-up should consist of a resting 12-lead ECG, a 24-h Holter monitor, and an exercise ECG. The baseline ECG is evaluated for the degree of QT prolongation (corrected for heart rate using the method of Bazett) as well as morphologic abnormalities of the T wave, such as notched T waves, TU complexes, or T-wave alternans (TWA). The morphologic T-wave abnormalities are believed to reflect increased dispersion of repolarization, which may have prognostic significance *(22,23)*. Rarely, visible TWA or episodes of torsades de pointes are observed during exercise stress testing or ambulatory monitoring, which can assist in diagnosis *(24)*. In rare cases, exercise stress testing can evoke QT prolongation and morphologic T-wave abnormalities that were not present in the resting state. Additional diagnostic criteria derived from the ECG and Holter monitoring have been proposed, but they remain investigational at present *(25,26)*. An echocardiogram should be performed in all cases to exclude underlying structural heart disease with secondary QT prolongation. It should be noted that some LQTS patients exhibit a characteristic wall-motion abnormality that can be eliminated by verapamil, and is believed to be another manifestation of repolarization heterogeneity *(27)*.

Only a few research laboratories worldwide now perform molecular diagnostic screening for all mutations that have been identified. Although a positive result establishes a definitive diagnosis for patients with borderline QT prolongation, a negative result does not exclude LQTS, since only 40–50% of LQT1 and LQT2 families have been genetically characterized *(9)*. In fact, it appears that every kindred has its own "private" mutation in the case of LQT2 *(28)*. The process of molecular diagnosis is time-consuming and expensive, and is not usually covered by insurance reimbursements; the cost of screening is presently covered by research funds in most instances *(9)*. Despite these limitations, molecular screening should be performed whenever possible

Table 1
Diagnostic Criteria for Congenital Long QT Syndrome

		Points
ECG findings*		
A.	QT$_c$†	
	≥480 msec$^{1/2}$	3
	460-470 msec$^{1/2}$	2
	450 msec$^{1/2}$ (in males)	1
B.	Torsade de pointes‡	2
C.	T-Wave alternans	1
D.	Notched T wave in three leads	1
E.	Low heart rate for age§	0.5
Clinical history		
A.	Syncope‡	
	With stress	2
	Without stress	1
B.	Congenital deafness	0.5
Family history‖		
A.	Family members with definite LQTS#	1
B.	Unexplained sudden cardiac death below age 30 among immediate family members	0.5

* In the absence of medications or disorders known to affect these electrocardiographic features.
† Calculated by Bazett's formula.
‡ Mutually exclusive.
§ Resting heart rate below second percentile for age.
‖ The same family member cannot be counted in both A and B.
Definite LQTS is defined by a LQTS score ≥4. Scoring: ≤1 point, low probability of LQTS; 2 to 3 points, intermediate probability of LQTS; ≥4 points, high probability of LQTS. (Reproduced with permission from: Schwartz et al. Diagnostic criteria for long QT syndrome. Circulation 1993;88[2]:783.)

in order to establish a definitive diagnosis and enable screening of the entire kindred to identify asymptomatic gene carriers. After a patient has been definitively diagnosed with LQTS by conventional or molecular criteria, all family members should be screened for LQTS, so that prophylactic beta-blocker treatment can be initiated in affected individuals. It is now established that up to 5% of asymptomatic gene carriers have normal QT intervals (29). Identification of these individuals using molecular diagnostic techniques is required because they may generate affected offspring and remain at risk for serious arrhythmic events, which can be prevented in some instances by prophylactic beta-blocker therapy. Molecular diagnostic techniques have also changed the approach to the so-called "sporadic cases." In these kindreds, the proband is the only individual diagnosed with LQTS on clinical grounds. Priori et al. recently reported that 33% of family members of "sporadic cases" who were previously considered normal were found to be asymptomatic gene carriers (30). These individuals must be identified if they are to receive appropriate genetic counseling, instruction regarding avoidance of QT-prolonging drugs, and consideration of prophylactic therapy.

Mechanism of Torsades de Pointes

Congenital and acquired LQTS are both characterized by an increased proclivity for torsades de pointes, which is the arrhythmia responsible for clinical events in this syndrome. Numerous in vitro experiments and mapping studies in animal models of torsades de pointes have yielded important clues as to the mechanism of this arrhythmia. The beat that initiates torsades de pointes is likely triggered from an early after-depolarization *(31)*. The prolongation of repolarization that is characteristic of both forms of LQTS is a known precipitant of early after-depolarizations. Two competing hypotheses have been proposed to explain the maintenance of torsades de pointes. The first theory posits that several competing foci of triggered activity exist, which originate from different regions of the ventricle. Alternatively, dispersion of ventricular repolarization may create the substrate for reentrant scroll waves that wander across the ventricular myocardium. The motion of these reentrant circuits creates a Doppler effect, which causes the polymorphic ECG appearance *(32)*. These new insights into the mechanism of torsades de pointes have stimulated the development of novel strategies to identify individuals who are at the greatest risk for this arrhythmia.

Risk Stratification For Arrhythmic Events

Once an individual has been definitively diagnosed with LQTS, the risk of subsequent cardiac events can be estimated using clinical and electrocardiographic criteria. The proband, defined as the first individual identified in a given kindred, is at greater risk for subsequent cardiac events than affected family members *(33)*. Patients with a prior history of cardiac events are at increased risk compared to individuals with asymptomatic QT prolongation. The length of the QT interval also bears a direct relation to the risk for subsequent events *(33)*. Among family members, relative bradycardia or tachycardia and female gender are associated with increased risk *(34)*. The association of female gender with cardiac events is unexpected in an autosomal dominant disorder, and may relate to the effects of female hormones on potassium-channel expression *(35)*. The specific genotype also appears to provide some prognostic information. Zareba et al. recently reported that the risk of cardiac events is significantly higher among subjects with mutations at the LQT1 or LQT2 locus than among those with mutations at the LQT3 locus *(36)*. Although cumulative mortality is similar regardless of the genotype, the percentage of lethal cardiac events is significantly higher in families with mutations at the LQT3 locus. Invasive electrophysiologic studies (EPS) do not appear to be useful for risk stratification of patients with LQTS *(37)*.

Therapeutic Options

Beta-adrenergic blockers should be instituted in all symptomatic patients (syncope and aborted cardiac arrest) and in asymptomatic affected individuals who are members of high-risk families *(4)*. Recent data indicates that the chance of having a recurrent cardiac event within 5 yr after starting beta-blockers is 32% in probands; 14% of patients who had aborted sudden cardiac death prior to taking beta-blockers had recurrent cardiac arrest within 5 yr despite beta-blocker therapy. Among affected family members, beta-blocker therapy reduced the event rate during follow-up, but cardiac events did occur *(38)*. These findings highlight the limitations of beta-blocker therapy, and the importance of identifying those individuals who are likely not to respond to beta-blockers. There is some data to suggest that patients who are likely to respond to beta-blockers are more likely to manifest a decrease in QT dispersion than nonresponders after therapy is initiated (39); however, the significance and reproducibility of QT dispersion remains controversial. A major focus of future research will be to develop automated electrocardiographic methods that can be employed to identify individuals at particularly high risk, and to assess the response to therapy. The adequacy of the beta-blocker dose should be assessed in all patients by determining the heart rate response to treadmill exercise, aiming for a heart rate of <130 beats per minute (BPM) (4). Concomitant pacemaker therapy may be required in individuals with resting or drug-induced sinus bradycardia. Beta-blockers would be expected to be most effective in LQT1 and LQT2 patients, who appear to have an adrenergic trigger for cardiac events in many instances. The benefit of beta-blockade may be less in LQT3 patients, who are more likely to experience cardiac events at rest or during sleep (9). It is now clear that women with LQTS who become pregnant are at increased risk for cardiac events during the postpartum interval; beta-blockers should therefore be continued during and after pregnancy in all affected individuals (40).

It is often difficult to decide how aggressively to treat LQTS patients at the time of their initial presentation. Implantable cardioverter defibrillator (ICD) implantation should be strongly considered in individuals who present with aborted cardiac arrest; the approach to patients who present with syncope should be individualized based on the severity of the disorder in a given kindred and the presence of other high-risk features. The management of asymptomatic affected members of high-risk families is also difficult. The choice of therapy must be based upon clinical judgment, as no comparative clinical trials have been conducted. Combination therapy with beta-blockers and a permanent pacemaker is highly effective in high-risk individuals (41,42). The mechanism of the benefit of pacing probably relates to the prevention of arrhythmogenic pauses; in addition, beta-blockers can often be titrated to higher doses. The advent of dual-chamber ICDs is likely to change the approach to pacing in LQTS, as these devices provide dual-chamber pacing capabilities as well as definitive sudden death protection. At present, it is reasonable to proceed to ICD implantation in individuals who initially present with aborted cardiac arrest or syncope with high-risk clinical features. Patients who have recurrent syncope on beta-blockers should also undergo ICD implantation. The effectiveness of left cervicothoracic sympathetic denervation remains controversial (43,44); this procedure should be reserved for patients who remain symptomatic despite treatment with beta-blockers and pacing.

The recognition that LQTS is caused by mutations in specific ion channels has stimulated the development of novel pharmacologic therapies designed to improve the function of the mutant ion channels ("gene-specific therapy"). In the case of LQT3, which is caused by persistent inward leakage of sodium current, class IB agents (e.g., lidocaine, mexilitene) appear to produce dramatic shortening of the QT interval. Some LQT2 patients also appear to exhibit shortening of the QT interval with mexilitene (19). It is also well-known that increases in the extracellular potassium-ion concentration result in activation of I_{Kr}. Compton et al. recently demonstrated that increases in the extracellular potassium concentration produce normalization of the length and morphology of the repolarization interval in LQT2 patients (45) (Fig. 2). Although these preliminary data are encouraging, none of these novel therapies have yet been demonstrated to decrease the risk for cardiac events.

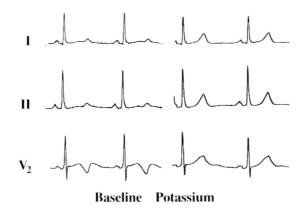

Baseline   Potassium

Fig. 2. Effect of potassium administration on resting QT morphology. (Reproduced with permission from: Compton et al. Genetically defined therapy of inherited long QT syndrome. Correction of abnormal repolarization by potassium. Circulation 1996;94:1021.)

Table 2
List of Drugs That Cause QT Prolongation and Torsades de Pointes

Category of drug	Specific drugs
Antiarrhythmic	Quinidine, procainamide, disopyramide d-sotalol, d,l-sotalol,
Class IA	ibutilide, amiodarone, bretylium, almokalant, sematilide,
Class III	dofetilide
Antimicrobial	Erythromycin, clarithromycin, trimethoprim-sulfamethoxazole
Antihistamine	Astemizole, terfenadine
Antimalarial/protozoal	Chloroquine, halofantrine, mefloquine, pentamidine, quinine
Gastrointestinal prokinetic	Cisapride
Psychoactive	Chloral hydrate, haloperidol, lithium, phenothiazines, pimozide,
	tricyclic antidepressants
Miscellaneous	Amantadine, probucol, tacrolimus, vasopressin

Adapted from: Roden DM. Taking the "idio" out of "idiosyncratic": predicting torsades de pointes. PACE 1998;21:1031.

ACQUIRED LQTS

The explosion in knowledge regarding the ionic mechanisms of the congenital LQTS has also generated new insights into the pathogenesis of various forms of acquired LQTS. It is now clear that many of the drugs that precipitate acquired LQTS are potent blockers of I_{Kr} (HERG), the same protein that is mutated in patients with the LQT2 form of congenital LQTS (46). Most cases of acquired LQTS occur in patients with no identifiable ion-channel mutations, although there have been occasional reports of patients with subclinical LQTS mutations that were revealed during treatment with an I_{Kr} blocker (47).

Drugs Associated With Acquired LQTS

Quinidine and other class IA drugs (e.g., procainamide, disopyramide) exert a number of electrophysiologic effects, including Na⁺ channel blockade and blockade of a number

Table 3
Drugs That Cause Torsades de Pointes by Inhibiting
the Metabolism of QT-Prolonging Drugs

Category of drug	Specific drugs
Antifungals	Ketoconazole, itraconazole, metronidazole
Serotonin re-uptake inhibitors	Fluoxetine, fluvoxamine, sertraline
Antidepressants	Nefazodone
HIV protease inhibitors	Indinavir, ritonavir, saquinavir
Dihydropyridine calcium-channel blockers	Nifedipine, felodipine, nicardipine
Miscellaneous	Grapefruit juice

of potassium channels (I_{Ks}, I_{TO}, I_{K1}, and I_{Kr}) (Table 2). Interestingly, the concentration required for blockade of I_{Kr} is an order of magnitude lower than that required for blockade of other potassium channels (48). Significant I_{Kr} block can be observed with quinidine at concentrations beneath the "therapeutic range," which may explain why some individuals develop torsades de pointes at low plasma concentrations of quinidine. In contrast, high drug doses or concentrations appear to predispose to torsades de pointes with other I_{Kr} blockers (e.g., the class III drug sotalol) (49). The newer class III agents ibutilide and dofetilide also pose a risk of torsades de pointes. In some instances, concomitant treatment with another agent that inhibits the biotransformation of the drug to a noncardioactive metabolite appears to pose a particular risk (e.g., terfenadine or cisapride administered with pyrrole antimycotics or macrolides) (50,51) (Table 3). In addition to its effects on terfenadine metabolism, erythromycin appears to possess I_{Kr}-blocking activity as well (52). Torsades de pointes is rarely observed with amiodarone administration, despite its activity against I_{Kr}; it is possible that the drug's activity against other ion channels exerts a protective effect (53).

Clinical Risk Factors For Torsades de Pointes

A number of clinical features associated with an increased risk for torsades de pointes have been identified (Table 4). Female gender has been associated with an increased risk for torsades de pointes in several studies (54–57). The effect appears to be independent of the degree of baseline QT prolongation, which is greater in women. The risk associated with female gender may be attributable to downregulation of I_{Kr} by female hormones (35), or by alteration of the affinity between I_{Kr}-blocking drugs and the HERG protein. Cardiac hypertrophy and overt congestive heart failure (CHF) are also associated with increased risk, probably as a consequence of baseline action-potential prolongation induced by potassium-current downregulation (predominantly I_{to}) (58–60). The period immediately following conversion of atrial fibrillation (AF) to sinus rhythm has been implicated in some reports; the mechanism may be withdrawal of neurohormonal activation following conversion, which is known to stimulate I_{Ks} (61,62). Other risk factors include bradycardia, electrolyte abnormalities, and diuretic use (48). Hypokalemia appears to exert its effect because of an inverse relationship between serum potassium levels and the magnitude of the I_{Kr} current (63). Interestingly, diuretic use has been identified as a risk factor in some studies, even in the absence of low serum potassium levels (64,65). These data suggest that depletion of total body potassium

Table 4
Risk Factors for Drug-Induced Torsades de Pointes

Female gender
Hypokalemia
Hypomagnesemia
Bradycardia
Diuretic use
High drug doses or concentrations (exception: quinidine)
Recent conversion from AF
Congestive heart failure or cardiac hypertrophy
Rapid iv infusion
Congenital LQTS
Baseline ECG: QT prolongation, T-wave lability
ECG during drug: marked QT prolongation, T-wave lability, T-wave morphology changes

Adapted from: Roden DM. Taking the "idio" out of "idiosyncratic": predicting torsades de pointes. PACE 1998;21:1031.

reserves may be important, or that some diuretic agents may have a direct effect on the ion channels responsible for ventricular repolarization. After treatment is initiated, excessive QT prolongation and the development of marked morphologic abnormalities in the T wave may identify individuals at risk (66).

Clinical Implications

The ever-expanding list of drugs associated with acquired LQTS presents the practitioner with several dilemmas. In the case of "non-cardiac" drugs that possess I_{Kr}-blocking activity, meticulous attention is required to avoid drug interactions that may result in QT prolongation. It is also reasonable to avoid these drugs in individuals with baseline QT prolongation, and to ensure that electrolyte levels are normal. The approach to these patients is complicated by the fact that these drugs are most commonly prescribed by non-cardiologists, who are less likely to screen patients in this manner.

A similar approach to the prevention of torsades de pointes is required for patients who are considered for treatment with class I or class III drugs for cardiac arrhythmias. In particular, avoidance of class I and class III drugs (other than amiodarone) is the best approach in patients with structural heart disease, CHF, baseline QT prolongation, or electrolyte abnormalities. When treatment with these agents is initiated or the dose is escalated, close monitoring is needed to detect excessive QT prolongation or morphologic T-wave abnormalities. In the case of sotalol, avoidance of higher doses and adjustment of the dose in patients with reduced renal function are particularly important. It is important to recognize that only 50% of cases of torsades occur during initiation of therapy (67); continued vigilance is required during follow-up to prevent arrhythmic complications. Although the absolute risk of torsades during initiation of class I or class III drug therapy for AF is low, the most prudent course is to initiate therapy in the inpatient setting, especially in individuals with risk factors for torsades (68). The labeling information for sotalol and dofetilide specifies that these agents should be initiated in the inpatient setting.

Treatment of Torsades de Pointes

Withdrawal of the offending agent and correction of any electrolyte abnormalities are usually sufficient to prevent recurrent torsades de pointes. In some instances, repetitive episodes occur that require immediate intervention. Intravenous (iv) magnesium, overdrive pacing, lidocaine, or isoproterenol administration may be efficacious in this situation *(69–71)*. When an individual develops symptomatic acquired LQTS, treatment with other agents that are known to predispose to torsades de pointes should also be avoided in the future.

THE BRUGADA SYNDROME

During the past decade, the Brugada syndrome has gained increasing recognition as an important cause of ventricular fibrillation (VF) among patients with structurally normal hearts ("primary electrical disease," "idiopathic VF"). This disorder may account for as many as 40–60% of all cases of idiopathic VF in some regions, such as Southeast Asia and Japan *(72)*. Recent evidence indicates that Brugada syndrome and congenital LQTS both represent primary disorders of cardiac ion channels *(73)*. Animal models have yielded important clues regarding the mechanisms responsible for the cardinal ECG manifestation of Brugada syndrome and its relation to arrhythmogenesis. At the same time, sufficient worldwide clinical experience has been gained to develop preliminary recommendations for the diagnosis and treatment of this disorder.

Diagnostic Criteria

The diagnostic criteria for Brugada syndrome incorporate three key elements: 1) ≥ 1 mm of ST segment elevation in leads V1, V2, and V3, in the absence of QT prolongation; 2) no structural heart disease, despite extensive investigation; 3) a personal or family history of unexplained syncope or sudden cardiac death *(74)*. When a family history is present, the mode of inheritance is consistent with autosomal dominant transmission with variable penetrance *(73)*. Men appear to be disproportionately affected, for unclear reasons (>90% male predominance). In some individuals, particularly Southeast Asian men, a marked predisposition for nocturnal cardiac events has been described *(72)*. This finding may be a manifestation of the deleterious influence of heightened vagal tone in this disorder.

Particular care is needed when attempting to distinguish the Brugada ECG from common normal variants. Right bundle-branch block (RBBB) has been described in association with ST segment elevation in Brugada syndrome; however, arrhythmic events appear to be related to the magnitude of ST-segment elevation and not to the presence or absence of RBBB *(75)*. In many instances, the expanded S wave in the left lateral leads is absent, indicating that true RBBB is not present (Fig. 3). The morphology of the ST segment in Brugada syndrome has been classified as either "coved" or "saddle-back" (Fig. 4). These patterns can be differentiated from the benign early repolarization variant by the localization and morphology of the ST-segment changes. Patients with the early repolarization variant characteristically have elevated ST segments in leads V2–V4, with an upward concavity and positive T-wave polarity accompanied by a notched J point (Fig. 5). In contrast, the ST elevation of Brugada syndrome is limited to leads V1–V3, is slowly down-sloping, and is accompanied by a negative T wave. It is important to recognize that right precordial ST-segment elevation

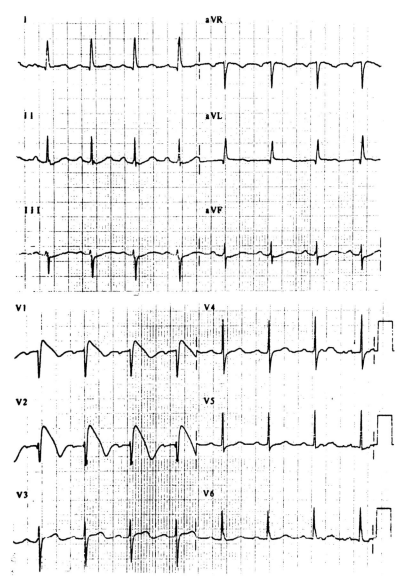

Fig. 3. Twelve-lead ECG of a patient with Brugada syndrome. (Reproduced with permission from Brugada et al. Right bundle-branch block (RBBB) and ST-segment elevation in leads V1 through V3: a marker for sudden death in patients without demonstrable structural heart disease. Circulation 1998;97:458.)

can be observed in a variety of other disorders (Table 5), which must be excluded before the diagnosis of Brugada syndrome is made *(75)*.

Mechanism of ST Segment Elevation

The mechanism of the characteristic ST segment elevation of Brugada syndrome can be best understood with reference to the ionic currents that are active during phases 1 and 2 of the cardiac action potential (Fig. 6). In normal individuals, the ST segment is isoelectric. This is because the voltage during the early portion of phase 2 of the

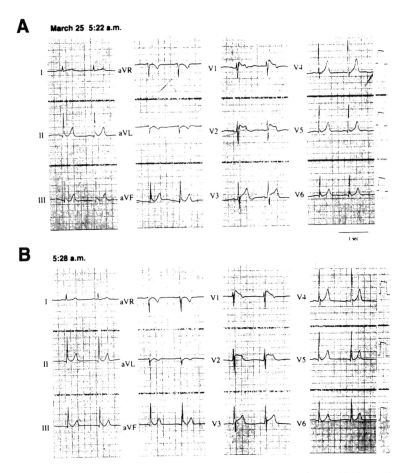

Fig. 4. Dynamic changes in the morphology of the ST segment in a patient with Brugada syndrome. (A) "Saddle-back" configuration of the ST segment in leads V1–V2. (B) "Coved" configuration of the ST segment in leads V1–V2. (Reproduced with permission from Matsuo et al. Dynamic changes of 12-lead electrocardiograms in a patient with Brugada syndrome. JCE 1998;9[5]:510.)

action potential is similar throughout the myocardium, because of the development of a prominent calcium current (I_{Ca})-mediated action-potential plateau *(75)*. The development of a normal plateau phase is critically dependent on the balance of ionic currents active at the end of phase 1—inward I_{Ca} and outward I_{to} (Fig. 6). It is noteworthy that the distribution of I_{to} is heterogeneous throughout the myocardium, with a greater concentration in the epicardium than the endocardium *(76)*. In addition, the right ventricular epicardium appears to have a greater concentration of I_{to} than the left ventricular epicardium *(77)*. Loss of the action-potential dome can occur when the net balance of current shifts outward at the end of phase 1. Conditions that can precipitate loss of the action-potential dome include genetic mutations in ion channels, such as SCN5A, ischemia, metabolic abnormalities, and pharmacologic interventions (I_{Na} and I_{Ca} blockers, $I_{K\text{-}ATP}$ activators). When these conditions are present, loss of the action-potential dome occurs preferentially in the epicardium because of the predominance of I_{to} in this layer, leading to a net flow of current from endocardium to epicardium and the ECG manifestation of ST-segment elevation. This phenomenon is most likely

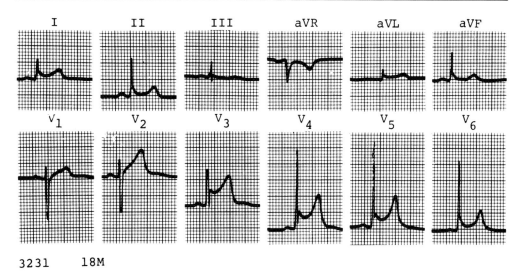

3231   18M

Fig. 5. Twelve-lead electrocardiogram with early repolarization pattern. Note the upward concavity of the ST segment in leads V3–V5, positive T-wave polarity, and notched J point.

Table 5
Abnormalities That Can Lead to ST Segment Elevation in the Right Precordial Leads

Right or left bundle-branch block, left ventricular hypertrophy
Acute MI
Left ventricular aneurysm
Exercise test-induced
Acute myocarditis
Right ventricular infarction
Aortic dissection
Acute pulmonary thromboemboli
Central nervous system and autonomic nervous system abnormalities
Heterocyclic antidepressant overdose
Duchenne muscular dystrophy
Friedrich ataxia
Thiamine deficiency
Hypercalcemia
Hyperkalemia
Compression of RVOT by metastatic tumor
Cocaine intoxication

Adapted with permission from: the American College of Cardiology (Gussak et al. The Brugada syndrome: clinical, electrophysiologic and genetic aspects. JACC 33[1]:8.)

to occur in the right precordial leads, because of the greater concentration of I_{to} in the right ventricular epicardium.

Candidate genes for the Brugada syndrome include mutations that increase I_{to} or I_{K-ATP}, decrease I_{Ca} or I_{Na}, or autonomic receptors that modulate the activity of these channels. The first gene linked to the Brugada syndrome was SCN5A, the same sodium-channel gene that is abnormal in the LQT3 form of congenital LQTS *(73)*. The mutations

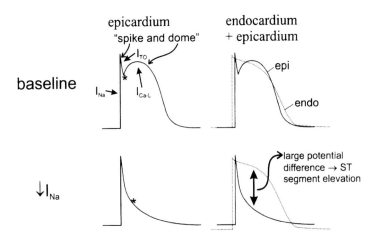

Fig. 6. Stylized epicardial (left) and epicardial + endocardial action potentials at baseline (top) and with sodium-channel block (bottom). The end of phase I (indicated by *) is determined by the balance between repolarizing I_{to} and depolarizing I_{Na} and I_{Ca-L}. With a decrease in I_{Na} (e.g. with flecainide), the resulting predominance of L_{to} moves the end of phase I sufficiently negative that I_{Ca-L} will not generate the phase 2 dome. Since this loss of the dome does not occur in the endocardium, there is a marked increase in heterogeneity of action-potential durations across the wall of the heart, which is believed to account for ST segment elevation and for reentrant excitation. (Reproduced with permission from: Roden et al. Drug-induced J point elevation: a marker for genetic risk of sudden death or ECG curiosity? JCE 1999;10:220.)

that were identified in the Brugada patients were at different loci than the LQT3 mutations and produce different functional consequences (reduced sodium current rather than the persistent leakage of sodium current that is characteristic of LQT3). SCN5A was excluded as a candidate gene in at least one family, indicating that significant genetic heterogeneity is likely to exist in Brugada syndrome as well.

The reported effects of various pharmacologic interventions on the magnitude of ST-segment elevation in experimental models and in Brugada syndrome patients are consistent with the ionic specificity of the individual agents. Autonomic neurotransmitters like acetylcholine facilitate loss of the action-potential dome by suppressing calcium current and augmenting potassium current, and beta-adrenergic agonists restore the dome by augmenting I_{Ca} *(78,79)*. Class I agents that block I_{Na} to a much greater extent than I_{to} (procainamide, ajmaline, flecainide) accentuate or unmask the syndrome (Fig. 7), but agents that block both channels (quinidine) diminish the ST segment elevation *(78,80)*.

Mechanisms of Arrhythmogenesis in Brugada Syndrome

Experimental models have yielded new insights into potential mechanisms of arrhythmogenesis in the Brugada syndrome. It appears that I_{to} is distributed heterogeneously throughout the epicardium, in addition to the transmural and regional differences that were previously described *(75)*. Conditions that favor loss of the action-potential dome are therefore likely to create dispersion of repolarization within the epicardium, as well as transmural and regional dispersion of repolarization. Local dispersion of repolarization within the epicardium gives rise to current fluxes that can cause local re-excitation of the areas that lack the action-potential dome, a phenomenon that has

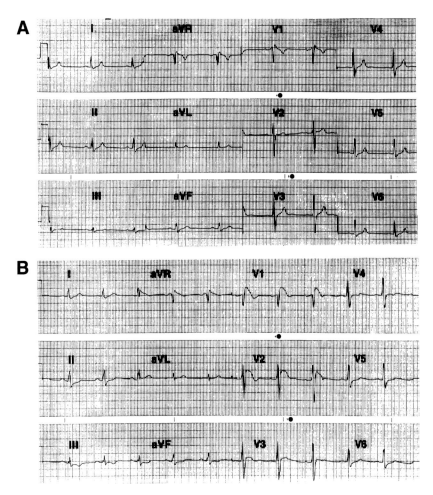

Fig. 7. (A) ECG tracing showing transient normalization of ST segments in a patient with Brugada syndrome. **(B)** ECG from the same patient after flecainide administration. (Reproduced with permission from: Alings et al. "Brugada" syndrome. Clinical data and suggested pathophysiologic mechanism. Circulation 1999;99:671.)

been called phase 2 reentry *(81)*. Phase 2 reentry produces the closely coupled premature ventricular beats that initiate ventricular arrhythmias. When these premature beats propagate to other regions of the myocardium, the transmural and regional dispersion of repolarization creates the substrate for circus movement reentry, which is believed to be the mechanism by which polymorphic ventricular tachycardia (PVT)/VF are perpetuated.

Diagnostic Workup and Treatment

When a patient presents with a clinical history of syncope/pre-syncope or aborted cardiac arrest and ECG findings that suggest Brugada syndrome, several additional diagnostic measures are required. Conditions that can mimic the ECG manifestations of the disorder should be excluded (Table 5). Occult coronary-artery disease (CAD) should be ruled out by cardiac catheterization or exercise stress testing with adjunctive imaging. Echocardiography is usually sufficient to exclude cardiomyopathy with secondary ECG changes, although magnetic resonance imaging (MRI) may be required in some instances to distinguish between Brugada syndrome and subtle presentations of right ventricular dysplasia. It is now well-recognized that the ECG findings in Brugada syndrome can be dynamic *(82)*. In some instances, ST-segment elevation may completely resolve, which can contribute to underdiagnosis of the disorder. For this reason, when symptomatic individuals with nondiagnostic ECG findings are encountered, pharmacologic challenge with procainamide or flecainide may reveal the typical ECG findings *(80)* (Fig. 7). All first-degree relatives of patients with proven Brugada syndrome should undergo ECG screening, with pharmacologic provocation if the resting ECG is nondiagnostic.

EPS reveals a prolonged HV interval in the majority of instances *(74)*. VF is inducible in 66% of patients, and an additional 11% of patients have induced nonsustained PVT *(74)*. The inducibility rates appear to be similar in symptomatic and asymptomatic patients. At present, the value of the EPS for risk-stratification of patients with Brugada syndrome is unclear. Specifically, insufficient information is available regarding the comparative prognosis of patients with sustained VF, nonsustained VT (NSVT), or no inducible arrhythmias. In the absence of definitive evidence that noninducible patients have a favorable prognosis, a "negative" study cannot be currently used to justify withholding therapy, considering the high incidence of serious arrhythmias during follow-up.

The available data indicate that the risk of serious arrhythmic events during follow-up is similar in symptomatic patients (14 of 41, or 34%) and asymptomatic patients (6 of 22, or 27%) *(83)*. Although no randomized comparative trials have been performed, it appears that the risk of arrhythmia recurrence is similar in patients treated with ICDs, antiarrhythmic drugs, or no therapy; however, these events are almost always fatal in drug-treated or untreated patients, and no patients treated with ICDs have died during follow-up *(83)*. In this study, treatment with beta-blockers, amiodarone, or both agents were all ineffective. In fact, there is some evidence that beta-blockers may actually be contraindicated *(78)*. At present, the preferred treatment for symptomatic patients with Brugada syndrome as well as asymptomatic relatives with definite evidence of the disorder is ICD implantation—the only treatment with demonstrated efficacy *(83)*. Quinidine, which has some activity against I_{to}, may be useful in some patients who sustain frequent ICD shocks. Anecdotal reports indicate that quinidine or other drugs guided by electrophysiology testing may be efficacious for patients with idiopathic VF, although it is unclear whether these patients in fact had Brugada syndrome *(84,85)*. At present, no drugs are clinically available that possess selective activity against I_{to}. There have been occasional reports of patients who developed the Brugada ECG pattern during treatment with class IC drugs for atrial arrhythmias *(86)*. As these patients do not appear to have an adverse prognosis, the most prudent approach is to simply discontinue the drug. It is possible that these patients have mutations in ion-channel genes that do not have severe functional consequences in the absence of class IC drugs; a similar phenomenon has been described in the case of LQTS. It is presently unclear whether treatment is warranted for asymptomatic individuals who have the Brugada ECG pattern noted incidentally on a screening ECG and have no family history of syncope or sudden cardiac death, although avoidance of class IC drugs would also be prudent in this situation.

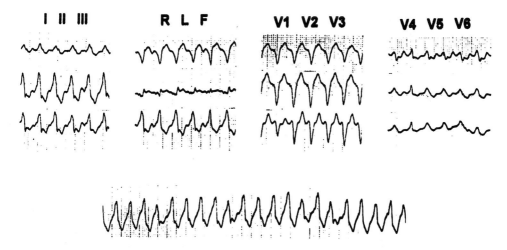

Fig. 8. ECG during VT in a patient with arrhythmogenic right ventricular dysplasia. Note the left bundle-branch-block (LBBB) configuration. (Reproduced with permission from: Marcus et al. Arrhythmogenic right ventricular dysplasia/cardiomyopathy. PACE 1995;18:1300.)

ARRHYTHMOGENIC RIGHT VENTRICULAR CARDIOMYOPATHY

Arrhythmogenic right ventricular cardiomyopathy (ARVC) is a disorder characterized by distinctive pathologic findings, abnormalities of impulse conduction and repolarization, and a propensity for life-threatening ventricular arrhythmias. In the past several years, new findings have yielded a greater understanding of the clinical spectrum of this disorder, and has provided important insights into the disease etiology. The 1995 World Health Organization/International Society and Federation of Cardiology (WHO/ISFC) task force classified this disorder as a unique form of cardiomyopathy; the term "dysplasia" was abandoned, because it wrongly implies that a congenital anomaly is present *(87)*.

Clinical Presentation

ARVC is a disease of young adults, with 80% of cases diagnosed before the age of 40 yr *(88)*. There is a marked male predominance (3:1). The prevalence of ARVC has been estimated at 1:5000, which may be an underestimate because of difficulties in diagnosis *(89)*. Most patients request medical attention because of symptoms related to ventricular arrhythmias (such as pre-syncope/syncope, palpitations, aborted cardiac arrest, or sudden death), which are commonly provoked by exercise. The ventricular tachycardia (VT) is monomorphic with a left bundle-branch block (LBBB) morphology, which is consistent with the right ventricular origin of the arrhythmia *(88)* (Fig. 8). Occasionally, sudden death is the first manifestation of the disorder. There appears to be a marked geographic variation in the prevalence of ARVC. In Italy, ARVC is the most common cause of sudden death in athletes, accounting for 25% of cases *(90)*; in the rest of the world, ARVC is implicated in <5% of athletic field deaths *(91)*. Approximately 25% of ARVC patients who are referred for treatment of VT have concomitant supraventricular arrhythmias (AF, atrial tachycardia, and atrial flutter, in descending order of frequency) *(92)*.

Pathology

It is now well-recognized that ARVC can present with a spectrum of clinical and pathologic manifestations. The "pure form" of ARVC consists of dilatation and thinning of the right ventricle, with aneurysms and fissures located in the infundibular, apical, and subtricuspid areas ("the triangle of dysplasia") *(93)*. The typical histologic pattern consists of replacement of midmural and/or external layers of myocardium by fatty tissue and fibrosis ("fibrofatty replacement") *(94)*. The abnormal areas are embedded within strands or sheets of normal myocardium. ARVC is distinguished pathologically from benign fatty infiltration of the heart by the presence of right ventricular myocardial thinning, associated fibrosis, and histologic evidence of inflammation *(94)*. The fatty infiltration of ARVC is preferentially distributed in the triangle of dysplasia, whereas benign fatty infiltration occurs uniformly throughout the heart. In the "pure form" of ARVC, minimal pathologic changes are observed in the left ventricle *(95)*.

Right ventricular outflow tract (RVOT) tachycardia has traditionally been regarded as an "idiopathic" VT, which occurs in the absence of structural abnormalities of the right ventricle. Recent evidence indicates that some patients with RVOT VT have structural abnormalities typical of ARVC that are confined to the infundibulum *(96)*. The localized nature of these changes probably accounts for the low incidence of sudden death among patients with RVOT VT, as monomorphic VT is less likely to degenerate into VF when the anatomic substrate for reentry is absent.

In patients with longstanding ARVC, the disease can progress to involve the left ventricle (biventricular dysplasia). Biventricular dysplasia more commonly presents with CHF, and can be mistaken for idiopathic dilated cardiomyopathy. The identification of fatty infiltration within the left and right ventricular myocardium should lead to the correct diagnosis. A recent autopsy study compared patients with biventricular dysplasia with patients who had isolated right ventricular involvement *(97)*. Patients with biventricular dysplasia more commonly had longstanding disease, clinical heart failure, warning symptoms, and clinical ventricular arrhythmias. Severe right ventricular thinning and inflammatory infiltrates were also more common among patients with concomitant left ventricular involvement. Notably, sudden cardiac death was the first manifestation of ARVC in 70% of the cases with isolated right ventricular involvement.

Etiology

Familial ARVC has been recognized since the initial descriptions of this disorder *(98)*. Previous estimates of the prevalence of familial ARVC were based on the identification of a living family member with overt ARVC or a family history of premature sudden cardiac death. Using these clinical criteria, ARVC had been classified as familial in 30% of cases *(87)*. Although no gene has yet been identified, five loci have been mapped in families demonstrating autosomal dominant transmission: 1q42 *(89)*, 2q32 *(99)*, 3p23 *(100)*, 14q12 *(101)*, 14q23 *(89)*. In addition, a form of the disease (Naxos disease) is coinherited with a skin disorder as an autosomal recessive trait and maps to 17q21 *(102)*. When the causative genes are identified and genetic screening is available, it is likely that a greater proportion of ARVC cases will be classified as familial. In one recent study, signal-averaged electrocardiograms (SAECGs) and ECGs were performed in asymptomatic family members of ARVC patients in order to screen for occult ARVC *(103)*. In 7 of the 12 families examined, the ARVC case had been classified as sporadic. The combined incidence of late potentials or abnormal ECG

Table 6
Diagnostic Criteria for Right Ventricular Dysplasia/Cardiomyopathy

I. Global and/or Regional Dysfunction and Structural Alterations*
- Major

Severe dilatation and reduction of right ventricular ejection fraction with no (or only mild) LV impairment.

Localized right ventricular aneurysms (akinetic or dyskinetic areas with diastolic bulging).

Severe segmental dilatation of the right ventricle.
- Minor

Mild global right ventricular dilatation and/or ejection fraction reduction with normal left ventricle.

Mild segmental dilatation of the right ventricle.

Regional right ventricular hypokinesia.

II. Tissue Characterization of Walls
- Major

Fibrofatty replacement of myocardium on endomyocardial biopsy.

III. Repolarization Abnormalities
- Minor

Inverted T waves in right precordial leads (V_2 and V_3) (people aged >12 years, in absence of right bundle branch block).

IV. Depolarization/Conduction Abnormalities
- Major

Epsilon waves or localized prolongation (>110 ms) of the QRS complex in right precordial leads (V_1–V_3).
- Minor

Late potentials (signal-averaged ECG).

V. Arrhythmias
- Minor

Left bundle branch block type ventricular tachycardia (sustained and nonsustained) (ECG, Holter, exercise testing).

Frequent ventricular extrasystoles (>1000/24 hours) (Holter).

VI. Family History
- Major

Familial disease confirmed at necropsy or surgery.
- Minor

Familial history of premature sudden death (< 35 years) due to suspected right ventricular dysplasia.

Familial history (clinical diagnosis based on present criteria).

* Detected by echocardiography, angiography, magnetic resonance imaging, or radionuclide scintigraphy. ECG = electrocardiogram; LV = left ventricle.

(Reproduced with permission from: Marcus et al. Arrhythmogenic right ventricular dysplasia/cardiomyopathy. PACE 1995;18:1306.)

findings in asymptomatic family members was 38%. One or more family members with abnormal ECG/SAECG findings were detected for all seven of the "sporadic" cases. Although definitive imaging studies were not performed to confirm the diagnosis of ARVC in the family members with abnormal ECG/SAECG findings, this study supports the hypothesis that many cases of ARVC currently classified as sporadic may actually be familial.

Other etiologic factors must be considered to explain cases of ARVC that are truly sporadic and to account for the marked variability in the severity of the clinical presentation that exists among affected family members with ARVC. The severity of the clinical phenotype appears to be significantly influenced by the magnitude of inflammation that is present (95). The presence of acute inflammation is synonymous with myocarditis, which may be the result of multiple causes (infectious or autoimmune). Although genetic factors may also contribute to an autoimmune response, it is likely that the degree of inflammation is determined in part by environmental factors. Recent evidence also indicates that myocardial atrophy in ARVC may be mediated by apoptosis, or programmed cell death (104).

Diagnosis

The criteria for the diagnosis of ARVC are based on the demonstration of the structural alterations, ECG manifestations, arrhythmias, and family history that are characteristic of the disorder (88) (Table 6). Numerous imaging techniques have been evaluated for their utility in the detection of ARVC, including echocardiography,

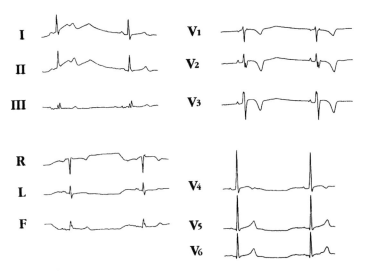

Fig. 9. ECG during sinus rhythm in a patient with arrhythmogenic right ventricular dysplasia. There is a small upright deflection in lead V1 just after the QRS complex (epsilon wave). Also note the T-wave inversion in leads V1–V3. (Reproduced with permission from: Marcus et al. Arrhythmogenic right ventricular dysplasia/cardiomyopathy. PACE 1995;18:1301.)

electron-beam CT, MRI, and right ventricular contrast angiography. A "routine" echo-cardiographic study may lack sufficient sensitivity to detect subtle right ventricular abnormalities, although experienced laboratories have reported satisfactory results *(105)*. MRI is uniquely suited to detect fatty infiltration, but caution is needed when attempting to distinguish between benign fatty infiltration and ARVC *(106)*. The "gold standard" for diagnosis remains contrast right ventricular angiography, which is useful to demonstrate right ventricular size and function, wall bulgings, and deep fissures *(107,108)*. The choice of imaging modality should ultimately be determined by the experience of the individual laboratories with the diagnosis of ARVC. Right-ventricular endomyocardial biopsy lacks sufficient sensitivity to detect the histological findings of ARVC, which are localized to the right ventricular free wall rather than the septum *(88)*. Biopsy of the right ventricular free wall is not recommended because of an increased risk of perforation. In one report, plasma brain natriuretic peptide levels were significantly increased among ARVC patients who presented with sustained VT compared to patients with RVOT VT or normal controls *(109)*; however, these results must be confirmed in a larger population of patients with ARVC before this test is used for diagnostic purposes.

The ECG findings in ARVC consist of epsilon waves (Fig. 9), localized prolongation of the QRS in leads V1–V3 (>100 ms), and right precordial T-wave inversion *(87)*. Although many patients with ARVC have positive time-domain signal-SAECGs, almost one-third of ARVC patients with spontaneous or inducible sustained monomorphic VT (SMVT) have normal tracings *(110)*. In one study, the combination of time- and frequency-domain analyses of the SAECG yielded improved sensitivity (100%) and specificity (94%) for the diagnosis of ARVC *(111)*. A major limitation of this study is that ARVC patients with SMVT were compared with normal controls; the results of this test among patients with ARVC but without VT are unknown.

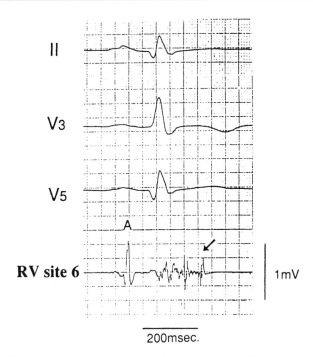

Fig. 10. Fractionated intracardiac right ventricular electrograms recorded from a patient with arrhythmogenic right ventricular dysplasia. (Reproduced with permission from: Tada et al. Usefulness of electron-beam computed tomography in arrhythmogenic right ventricular dysplasia. Relation to electrophysiologic abnormalities and left ventricular involvement. Circulation 1996;94(3):440.)

Electrophysiologic Findings

When endocardial electrograms are recorded from the right ventricles of patients with ARVC during sinus rhythm, significant fractionation is observed *(112)* (Fig. 10). This finding is consistent with slow conduction, which is an important substrate for reentrant ventricular arrhythmias. This substrate can be detected noninvasively by the presence of epsilon waves and QRS prolongation on the standard ECG and by SAECG *(88,111)*. VT is usually induced using programmed stimulation, which is characteristic of a reentrant mechanism. In contrast to RVOT VT, multiple morphologies of monomorphic VT are often induced in patients with ARVC. The presence of fibrofatty infiltration in many regions of the right ventricle is believed to create the substrate for multiple reentrant circuits, which accounts for the presence of multiple VT morphologies. Repolarization abnormalities have also been demonstrated in patients with ARVC using body-surface mapping, which may reflect local prolongation of repolarization in the regions affected by ARVC *(113)*. Others have demonstrated that ARVC is characterized by an increase in repolarization dispersion, which favors the occurrence of unidirectional block and reentrant ventricular arrhythmias *(114)*.

Risk Stratification

Several clinical features have been identified that are associated with an adverse prognosis among patients with ARVC. These include a history of syncope *(115)*, sustained ventricular arrhythmias *(116)*, the presence of left ventricular involvement

(97), and right ventricular failure *(117)*. It appears that late potentials are more closely related to the extent of right ventricular disease than with the occurrence of ventricular arrhythmias *(114)*. No data is presently available regarding the utility of invasive electrophysiologic studies for risk stratification. The occurrence of sudden cardiac death during follow-up remains unpredictable in many instances. In particular, patients with isolated right ventricular involvement, which is believed to represent an early form of the disease, are more likely to present with sudden cardiac death as the first manifestation of their disease *(97)*.

Management

Because of the rarity of this disorder, no controlled studies have been performed to compare the efficacy of treatment with antiarrhythmic drugs or nonpharmacologic therapies. In one retrospective study, 81 patients with ARVC and documented sustained VT or NSVT were examined *(118)*. The 42 patients who had inducible sustained VT during EPS were treated with a variety of antiarrhythmic drugs in a nonrandom fashion. A response to a drug was considered to be present if there was no spontaneous arrhythmia recurrence and if the VT was no longer inducible or rendered more difficult to induce during follow-up EPS. Using these criteria, sotalol had a higher efficacy rate (68.4%) than class I drugs, amiodarone, beta-blockers, or verapamil (0–15%). Different criteria were used to determine drug efficacy for the 39 patients who had NSVT induced at EPS. Arrhythmia recurrence was determined using a combination of 48-h Holter monitoring and exercise stress testing. A drug response was defined as the abolition of sustained VT and NSVT, and a >70% reduction in the frequency of ventricular runs (3–10 consecutive beats). Sotalol had the highest efficacy rate (82.8%), followed by verapamil (50%), beta-blockers (28.6%), amiodarone (25%), and other agents (0–17%). Follow-up data was available on 33 patients who were discharged on antiarrhythmic drugs (14 ± 13 mo); 4 (12%) had nonfatal relapses of their clinical ventricular arrhythmia. The determination of drug efficacy in this study is obviously limited by nonrandom treatment assignment, as well as spontaneous variability in the prevalence of arrhythmias during serial EPS, Holter monitors, or exercise tests. Other investigators have reported favorable results with empiric treatment with amiodarone, sotalol, or beta-blockers. The arrhythmic death rate among patients treated with empiric antiarrhythmic drugs in 1–2% per yr *(95)*. It is unclear whether this relatively low sudden-death rate is related to drug efficacy or an intrinsically more benign clinical course among patients with ARVC compared to other forms of heart-muscle disease.

Limited data is available regarding the use of implantable cardioverter defibrillators (ICDs) for patients with ARVC. Link et al. reported on a series of 12 patients who were treated with ICDs *(119)*. Three patients presented with cardiac arrest, four patients presented with syncope, and five patients presented with presyncope. Nine of the 12 patients had inducible sustained VT, and antiarrhythmic drug testing was unsuccessful in all 8 patients for whom it was attempted. During an average of 22 mo of follow-up, 8 of 12 patients had appropriate therapy delivered by the ICD. One sudden death occurred in a patient who depleted therapy following multiple successful cardioversions for VT, because of prompt reinitiation of VT each time that sinus rhythm was reestablished. Although pacing and sensing parameters were less desirable compared to patients with other disorders who underwent ICD implantation at the same institution, defibrillation thresholds were not significantly different. Adjunctive treatment with sotalol may have slowed the rate of recurrent VTs sufficiently to allow termination of the arrhythmia with anti-tachycardia pacing rather than cardioversion in some instances.

In the absence of definitive data, treatment recommendations for ARVC are necessarily arbitrary. All ARVC patients should be prohibited from engaging in strenuous exercise, which provoke arrhythmias in a significant proportion of patients. It is our practice to treat patients who present with aborted cardiac arrest, syncope, or presyncope with ICD implantation in order to provide definitive sudden-death protection. Adjunctive treatment with beta-blockers, sotalol, or amiodarone may be required to decrease the frequency of ICD shocks. Radiofrequency ablation of VT may be useful in selected patients who receive frequent shocks and do not respond adequately to antiarrhythmic drugs (120). Therapy should be individualized for patients who present with palpitations or who are asymptomatic. Screening of asymptomatic family members can be justified as long as the limitations of available diagnostic techniques are discussed. The potential benefits of identifying an asymptomatic family member are that these individuals can be provided with genetic counseling, and the risk for sudden death may be decreased by restriction of physical activity and treatment with beta-blockers. A reasonable approach to screening would include a standard ECG, SAECG, Holter monitoring, and exercise stress testing to detect ventricular arrhythmias (103). If abnormalities are detected, the diagnosis should be confirmed with an imaging study.

HYPERTROPHIC CARDIOMYOPATHY

Hypertrophic cardiomyopathy (HCM) is defined by the presence of a hypertrophied, nondilated left ventricle in the absence of secondary causes of hypertrophy (e.g., systemic hypertension or aortic-valve stenosis) (121). Although hypertrophic cardiomyopathy was previously considered a rare disorder, recent evidence indicates that the prevalence of hypertrophic cardiomyopathy in the general population is about 0.2% (1 in 500) (122,123). Patient with hypertrophic cardiomyopathy are frequently referred to electrophysiologists for management of several important complications of the disease: primary and secondary prevention of sudden cardiac death, AF, and consideration of pacemaker implantation in patients with hypertrophic obstructive cardiomyopathy (HOCM) who have symptoms that are refractory to medical management.

Sudden Cardiac Death in Hypertrophic Cardiomyopathy

Sudden cardiac death is an important clinical problem in patients with HCM. A substantial proportion of patients with hypertrophic cardiomyopathy who die prematurely collapse during or immediately following vigorous physical activity. In the United States, hypertrophic cardiomyopathy is the most common cause of sudden death on the athletic field in young competitive athletes (91). Many patients who die suddenly have previously been asymptomatic; in these individuals, sudden death is the first manifestation of the disease. The annual incidence of sudden cardiac death is 2–4% in studies conducted at tertiary referral centers (124), but appears to be substantially lower in community-based populations (<1%) (125,126). These data have important implications for the development of strategies for the primary prevention of sudden cardiac death. Although numerous risk factors for sudden death have been described in patients with HCM (Table 7), the positive predictive value of abnormal findings is low because of the relatively low incidence of this catastrophic complication.

Table 7
Risk Factors for Sudden Cardiac Death in Patients with Hypertrophic Cardiomyopathy

Aborted cardiac arrest
Sustained ventricular tachycardia
Family history of sudden cardiac death*
High-risk genotype
Young age (<14 years)
Repetitive, prolonged episodes of NSVT on Holter
Massive left ventricular hypertrophy (≥35-mm septal thickness)
Recurrent syncope
Myocardial ischemia (particularly in young patients)
Impaired blood-pressure response to treadmill exercise
LVOT gradient >30 mmHg.

* 2 or more unexpected sudden deaths in young family members.

The development of an effective risk-stratification strategy is critically dependent on a thorough understanding of the mechanisms of sudden cardiac death in patients with HCM. The myocardial structure in HCM is characterized by myocyte disarray, hypertrophy, and fibrosis *(127)*. All of these features contribute to nonhomogeneity of electrical conduction and dispersion of repolarization, which form the substrate for reentrant ventricular arrhythmias. The available data suggest that ventricular tachyarrhythmias are the cause of sudden death in most patients with HCM, either as a primary event related to an arrhythmogenic substrate or as a secondary phenomenon triggered by myocardial ischemia, diastolic dysfunction, abnormal vascular control, outflow-tract obstruction, or supraventricular arrhythmias *(128)*.

There is little doubt that the highest-risk patients with HCM are those who survive a cardiac arrest with documented VF or who have spontaneous episodes of sustained VT *(128)*. In addition, young patients with a substantial family history of sudden cardiac death (defined as a cluster of two or more sudden deaths in young family members) or a high-risk genetic mutation are also at extremely high risk *(128)*. Hypertrophic cardiomyopathy is now recognized to be a genetic disorder with autosomal dominant inheritance *(129)*. All of the genes that have been identified encode proteins of the cardiac sarcomere: the β-myosin heavy chain *(130)*, cardiac troponins T *(131)*, and I *(132)*, α-tropomyosin *(131)*, myosin light chains *(133)*, and myosin-binding protein C *(134)*. In addition, a locus in chromosome 7q3 has been linked to hypertrophic cardiomyopathy associated with Wolff-Parkinson-White syndrome (WPW) *(135)*. Multiple distinct mutations in each gene have been identified, which have varying penetrance, functional consequences, and prognostic significance *(129)* (Fig. 11). In the case of troponin T-mutations, outflow obstruction is absent and symptoms are typically mild, but a substantial risk for sudden cardiac death is present *(131)*. It is estimated that less than 50% of hypertrophic cardiomyopathy cases are accounted for by these genes *(129)*. Genetic screening is presently performed by only a few specialized centers worldwide, and is therefore seldom obtained for many kindreds; however, when this information is available and the prognostic consequences of the mutation in question have been previously characterized, the results can be used to guide management.

The prognostic significance of NSVT in patients with hypertrophic cardiomyopathy

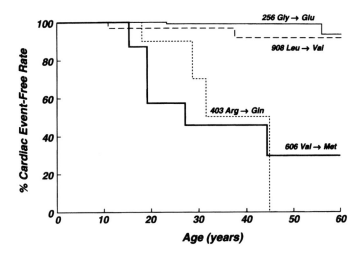

Fig. 11. Figure comparing survival rates in hypertrophic cardiomyopathy patients in which the disease is caused by distinct β-myosin heavy chain mutations. (Reproduced with permission from: Fananapazir et al. Genotype-phenotype correlations in hypertrophic cardiomyopathy. Circulation 1994;89:25.)

has been the subject of much debate. Early reports by two groups indicated that the presence of NSVT was associated with a 7–8% annual mortality rate *(136,137)*. These data prompted the widespread use of prophylactic amiodarone in patients with hypertrophic cardiomyopathy and NSVT. Recent evidence indicates that NSVT is not associated with an adverse prognosis in asymptomatic patients *(138)*. In addition, short, isolated runs of NSVT do not appear to be a marker of high risk (only one burst in 24 h, <5 beats in duration) *(138)*. Repetitive, more prolonged runs of NSVT are of greater concern, especially in patients who present with pre-syncope/syncope.

The utility of invasive EPS for risk stratification has been investigated by a number of groups. The induction of sustained monomorphic tachycardia is unusual in hypertrophic cardiomyopathy patients, and much controversy has centered on the significance of induced PVT/VF. Some authors have postulated that the induction of sustained PVT with two extrastimuli is a specific marker of an adverse prognosis; however, this finding is infrequent (10–15% of patients) *(139)*. In several small studies, induced PVT with three extrastimuli was not associated with an adverse prognosis *(140,141)*. In contrast, Fananapazir et al. reported in a large series that sustained PVT induced with three extrastimuli was a specific marker of an adverse prognosis in patients with or without symptoms of impaired consciousness *(139)*. It is possible that the adverse prognosis of induced PVT was partially attributable to patient selection, as many of the patients who were inducible also had high-risk clinical features (such as prior cardiac arrest or syncope). Other authors have raised concerns regarding the safety of programmed stimulation in patients with HCM *(142,143)*. Given these safety concerns and the lack of consensus regarding the interpretation of the results of testing, EPS is not currently recommended for risk stratification of patients with HCM.

Other factors associated with an increased risk for SCD include recurrent syncope *(128)*, an impaired blood-pressure response to exercise *(144)*, inducible myocardial ischemia *(145)*, left ventricular outflow-tract pressure gradient >30 mmHg *(146)*, marked left ventricular hypertrophy (LVH) (≥35 mm) *(128)*, and young age (<14 yr) *(129)*. In children, ischemia provoked by myocardial bridging of the left anterior descending coronary artery appears to be associated with VT and SCD *(147,148)*.

Treatment

HIGH-RISK PATIENTS

Patients with aborted cardiac arrest or spontaneous sustained ventricular arrhythmias, a strong family history of premature cardiac arrest, or a "high-risk" genetic mutation constitute the highest-risk subset of patients with HCM. There is general agreement that prophylactic treatment is warranted for patients who meet these criteria *(128)*. The available data indicate that amiodarone does not provide complete protection from sudden cardiac death and may in fact be proarrhythmic at higher doses *(149)*. Although no randomized comparative studies have been performed, ICD implantation appears to offer superior sudden-death protection *(150,151)*. The reported incidence of appropriate shocks during follow-up among cardiac arrest survivors with HCM who underwent ICD implantation is 15–50% *(150,152,153)*. Every effort should be made to address other factors that may contribute to recurrent ventricular arrhythmias, such as myocardial ischemia, severe outflow-tract obstruction, or supraventricular arrhythmias. Pediatric patients who have demonstrable myocardial bridging may benefit from surgical unroofing of the left anterior descending coronary artery. Similarly, cardiac-arrest survivors with severe outflow-tract obstruction should be considered for procedures that reduce the gradient (septal myectomy, permanent pacemaker, ethanol ablation).

LOW-RISK PATIENTS

Patients who are asymptomatic and who do not have any high-risk clinical features (Table 7) do not warrant specific treatment for the primary prevention of sudden cardiac death *(154)*. It is important to stress that this subset comprises a sizeable proportion of the patients with HCM, especially in community settings. All patients who are diagnosed with HCM should avoid strenuous physical activity such as competitive athletics *(155)*.

INTERMEDIATE-RISK PATIENTS

It is often difficult to decide whether to recommend aggressive prophylactic treatment for patients who have one or more high-risk clinical features. This is particularly true of patients who present with syncope. Many patients with HCM report isolated or remote episodes of syncope *(126,138)*. These patients should generally be managed conservatively with noninvasive tests such as Holter monitoring to quantify ambient ectopy and patient-activated event recorders. Therapy should be individualized for patients with recurrent syncope and one or more additional high-risk features; our practice has been to recommend ICD implantation in these instances.

Atrial Fibrillation

AF is a common clinical problem in patients with hypertrophic cardiomyopathy. In community-based series of patients with hypertrophic cardiomyopathy, up to 28% of patients have chronic or paroxysmal AF *(126)*. AF has been associated with a significant increase in cardiovascular mortality in patients with hypertrophic cardiomyopathy. In one recent series, AF was present in 70% of the study patients who died during follow-

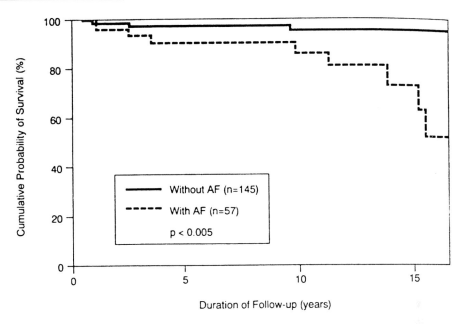

Duration of Follow-up (years)

Fig. 12. Cumulative survival of hypertrophic cardiomyopathy patients with and without AF. (Reproduced with permission from: the American College of Cardiology. Cecchi et al. Hypertrophic cardiomyopathy in Tuscany: clinical course and outcome in an unselected regional population. JACC 1995;26[6]:1532.)

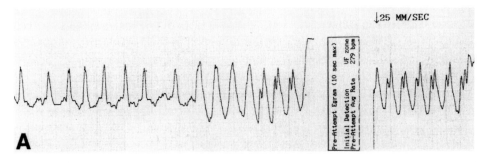

Fig. 13. Electrograms retrieved from an implanted cardioverter-defibrillator implanted in a patient with hypertrophic cardiomyopathy. The initial rhythm is AF, followed by PVT. The episode was successfully terminated by the device. (Reproduced with permission from: the American College of Cardiology, Elliott et al. Sudden death in hypertrophic cardiomyopathy. Journal of the American College of Cardiology 1999;33[6]:1599.)

up; in addition, >50% of patients with this arrhythmia experienced disease progression or died during the study period (Fig. 12) *(126)*. In rare instances, rapid AF can provoke malignant ventricular arrhythmias and sudden cardiac death, either by a triggered mechanism, the induction of myocardial ischemia, or by causing prolonged hypotension (Fig. 13) *(150)*. In the majority of patients with hypertrophic cardiomyopathy, the adverse prognosis associated with AF is more closely related to exacerbation of CHF, systemic embolism, and stroke *(156)*. Paroxysmal episodes of AF often cause rapid clinical deterioration by reducing diastolic filling and cardiac output, usually as a consequence of the high ventricular rate. When the ventricular rate is well-controlled patients may remain asymptomatic, particularly when outflow-tract obstruction is absent.

Several risk factors for AF have been identified in patients with hypertrophic cardiomyopathy, including age, increased left atrial size, marked hypertrophy, and the presence of outflow-tract obstruction with concomitant mitral regurgitation (136). Management consists of control of the ventricular rate using either verapamil or beta-blockers, anticoagulation to prevent systemic embolism, and administration of agents to maintain sinus rhythm. Amiodarone is the most effective agent for the maintenance of sinus rhythm (157); however, in young patients, consideration may be given to an initial trial of sotalol because of the toxicity associated with long-term amiodarone administration (127). Some individuals with obstructive HCM and AF may be candidates for septal myectomy, which may reduce left atrial size and restore sinus rhythm by this mechanism (158).

Permanent Pacemaker Implantation

Dual-chamber (DDD) pacing, with the right ventricular lead positioned in the right ventricular apex, has been proposed as a therapeutic alternative for patients with HCM who have outflow-tract obstruction, and who are symptomatic despite maximal medical treatment with beta-blockers or verapamil. It is important to emphasize that patients who meet these criteria comprise only 5% of all patients with HCM (128). Results from several uncontrolled studies indicated that pacing produced a dramatic reduction in the magnitude of the left ventricular outflow-tract gradient and sustained symptomatic improvement (159,160). These data have led to a widespread enthusiasm in the cardiology community for pacing as a treatment for HCM. The recent publication of three randomized, crossover trials (DDD pacing vs inactive pacemaker) has prompted a reevaluation of the utility of pacing for the treatment of HCM patients with refractory symptoms (161–163). In particular, it appears that much of the apparent benefit of pacing in HOCM is caused by placebo effect (164).

The theoretical basis for the use of pacing for the treatment of patients with HOCM is derived from the results of acute hemodynamic studies. Atrial synchronous right ventricular apical pacing, with a short atrioventricular delay produces preexcitation of the interventricular septum, which causes the septum to move away from the left ventricular wall during systole, resulting in an increase in left ventricular outflow-tract dimensions and relief of outflow-tract obstruction (159). Although the atrioventricular interval must be short enough to maintain complete ventricular capture, pacing at extremely short atrioventricular intervals may also have adverse hemodynamic consequences, such as increased filling pressures and diastolic dysfunction (165). For these reasons, an acute hemodynamic study is performed to select the longest atrioventricular interval that maintains complete ventricular capture without a detrimental effect on blood pressure, cardiac output, or left atrial pressure (165).

In 1997, Nishimura et al. reported the results of a randomized, double-blind crossover trial involving 21 patients with HOCM (162). The patients were selected on the basis of symptoms refractory to medical therapy (predominantly NYHA class III), and a resting LVOT gradient >30 mmHg at rest. Sixteen patients had resting gradients of >50 mHg at rest; five patients had resting gradients between 30 and 50 mmHg at rest and augmentation to >100 mmHg with isoproterenol infusion. Pacemakers were implanted in all patients, who were then randomly assigned to receive either DDD pacing or AAI pacing at 30 BPM (inactive pacemaker). After 3 mo, the pacing mode was reversed. The LVOT gradient was modestly decreased with DDD pacing (55 ± 38 mmHg) compared to either AAI pacing (83 ± 59 mmHg) or baseline (76 ± 61 mmHg). The Minnesota quality-of-life score and exercise duration were significantly improved with DDD spacing compared to baseline but were not significantly different from AAI DDD pacing. Overall, 63% of patients had symptomatic improvement with DDD pacing, but 31% had no change and 5% had deterioration of symptoms. Strikingly, 42% of patients had symptomatic improvement with backup AAI pacing, which indicates that placebo effect may account for most of the apparent symptomatic benefit associated with pacemaker implantation. These data were subsequently confirmed in the M-PATHY trial, which enrolled 48 symptomatic hypertrophic cardiomyopathy patients (77% class III or IV) with resting gradients >50 mmHg *(163)*. One potential flaw of this study was that a decrease in the gradient during the acute catheterization study was not required for study entry; however, others have reported that patients who do not manifest an acute drop in gradient also respond to chronic DDD pacing *(166)*. The study design was similar, with randomization to either DDD or backup AAI pacing for 3 mo followed by a crossover phase. A modest decrease in outflow-tract gradient was noted in 57% of patients, but 43% of patients had either no change or an increase. No differences were found between pacing and no pacing for any subjective or objective measure of symptoms or exercise capacity. A post-hoc analysis indicated that elderly patients (age >65 yrs) showed a clinical response to DDD pacing, but these data require prospective confirmation. The results of the M-PATHY trial were also corroborated by the Pacing In Cardiomyopathy (PIC) Study Group *(161)*. This trial enrolled 83 patients with class II/III symptoms and LVOT gradientsss of >30 mmHg with or without provocation. This study also had a randomized crossover design, with consecutive 3-mo follow-up intervals. In this study, a similar improvement in angina and dyspnea was noted with DDD pacing and AAI pacing compared to baseline, and no difference in objective measures of exercise capacity was found.

At present, DDD pacing cannot be recommended for the routine treatment of patients with HOCM who have symptoms that are refractory to medical therapy. In experienced centers, septal myectomy can be performed with minimal complications, greater relief of outflow-tract obstruction, and more profound symptomatic benefit *(167)*. Ethanol ablation of the septum may also provide effective relief of outflow-tract obstruction, although the procedure can be complicated by heart block and concerns persist regarding late development of ventricular arrhythmias *(168)*. DDD pacing should be reserved for those patients who are judged to be unable to tolerate surgery. Further studies are required to determine if the elderly patients with HOCM derive a benefit from DDD pacing.

COMMOTIO CORDIS

Commotio cordis, or cardiac concussion, refers to sudden death caused by a relatively low-energy chest-wall impact. Although a rare syndrome, it has been reported with increasing frequency in young individuals participating in athletic activities *(169–176)*. Commotio cordis typically occurs in youths age 5–16, who are participating in athletic activities in which there is blunt impact to the chest. Commotio cordis has usually been described with baseball, but has also been reported with hockey, lacrosse, fistfights, soccer, and other athletic activities. In all instances, a chest-wall impact results in rapid loss of consciousness, cardiac arrest, and usually death. The most common initial reported rhythm is VF. Tragically, resuscitation is ultimately successful in less than 10% of victims *(165–177)*. Victims of commotio cordis do not appear to have any predisposing cardiac abnormalities or cardiac pathology—such as contusion or damaged coronary arteries—that would give an anatomic basis for sudden cardiac death *(176)*.

In the commotio cordis registry *(174)*, the mean age of occurrence is 12 yr, and 70% of individuals are less than 16 yr of age. It has been hypothesized that the increased occurrence of commotio cordis in young athletes is caused by a more flexible chest wall, which permits transmission of energy more efficiently to the myocardium. With maturation of the chest wall and loss of cartilage tissue, the thoracic cage stiffens, and the chest wall may absorb more of the impact energy rather than transmitting it directly to the myocardium. With commotio cordis, collapse occurs instantaneously in most of the victims. In some cases, there is a period of presyncope which precedes the loss of consciousness. In the rare instances where a cardiac rhythm has been immediately documented, it is usually VF. There have been case reports of idioventricular rhythm and complete heart block documented as the initial rhythm *(170,172)*. However, in these instances, a substantial time interval elapsed between the actual collapse and documentation of the rhythm. In a recent report of resuscitation after commotio cordis, an immediate 12-lead ECG showed marked ST-segment elevation *(175)*. Unfortunately, survival is rare with commotio cordis. Of the 70 cases reported in the Commotio Registry, only 11 patients survived until arrival at the hospital *(174)*. Of these 11 patients, 4 ultimately died while hospitalized. Of the seven patients who survived to the point of hospital discharge, five had complete neurologic recovery.

Mechanism of Commotio Cordis

Experimental models of high-energy chest-wall trauma have shown that bradyarrhythmias (sinus bradycardia, heart block) and tachyarrhythmias (VT, VF) could result from myocardial contusion *(178–180)*. However, these models of chest-wall trauma did not accurately reproduce commotio cordis, in which the force of chest-wall impact does not result in any cardiac pathology. To study the pathophysiology of commotio cordis, a swine model of low-energy chest-wall impact was developed *(181)*. With this model, a wood sphere and regulation baseballs were propelled at 30 mph at anesthetized juvenile swine. The impact was aimed at the papillary muscle in the left ventricle using transthoracic echocardiographic guidance and gated to the cardiac cycle using an electrophysiologic stimulator. Transthoracic echocardiography was performed to detect wall-motion abnormalities, and myocardial blood flow was evaluated with tectnecium-99m sestamibi imaging and coronary angiography. The electrophysiologic consequences of chest-wall impact were found to be critically dependent on the timing of the impact within the cardiac cycle. Impacts that occurred during the vulnerable period of repolarization, defined as a 15–30 ms window prior to the peak of the T wave, caused immediate VF. Impact during other portions of cardiac cycle did not produce VF, but caused ST-segment elevations and occasionally complete heart block. Despite the absence of cardiac pathology, transient wall-motion abnormalities were observed at the apex of the heart over the papillary muscle (distant from the area of impact). In addition, mild apical perfusion defects were found in approx 25% of animals with sestamibi imaging. Coronary angiography revealed no epicardial coronary-artery abnormalities.

More recent observations have indicated that mechanical activation of the K^+-adenosine triphosphate (ATP) channel may be responsible for the ST segment elevation and VF that is characteristic of commotio cordis *(182)*. The K^+-ATP channel is normally inactivated by physiologic concentrations of ATP. When the concentration of ATP decreases and the concentration of ADP increases, the channel is open and potassium exits the cell. In experimental models of acute ischemia, activation of the K^+-ATP channel is associated with ST-segment elevation and an increased risk of VF *(183)*. These observations led Link et al. to hypothesize that a similar mechanism may be responsible for the ST-segment elevation and VF observed in commotio cordis. Indeed, when glibenclamide (a specific K^+-ATP-channel blocker) was administered prior to chest-wall impact, a decrease in the magnitude of ST-segment elevation and the incidence of VF was observed.

Prevention and Treatment of Commotio Cordis

Clinical and experimental evidence indicates that early defibrillation is critical to survival from commotio cordis. Accordingly, use of defibrillators and strategies for early employment of cardiopulmonary resuscitation (CPR) are likely to have a favorable impact on survival. Availability of automatic external defibrillators (AED) at sporting events and training of coaches, trainers and other sporting personnel in basic life support and AED use would probably improve survival.

In addition, it is likely that strategies for the primary prevention of commotio cordis would also help to decrease the tragic deaths from this syndrome. In this respect, of the 25 victims of commotio cordis originally reported by Maron *(176)*, seven were wearing a commercially available chest protector. However, in many instances, it appears that the victims lifted their arms prior to the impact, thereby exposing the chest. It is evident that more research needs to be done on materials and designs for chest-wall protectors for high-risk athletic activities.

Recent evidence indicates that the use of softer "safety" baseballs may decrease the frequency of commotio cordis. In our experimental model, the incidence of VF was significantly reduced when safety baseballs were used. The softest balls (reduced injury factor-RIF 1, Worth, Inc, Tullahoma, TN), which are marketed for use in T-ball for children aged 5–7, are similar to a tennis ball in consistency. In our experimental model, the ball had an incidence of VF of 8% at 30 mph and 8% at 40 mph. This contrasts with a medium-soft ball, marketed for children aged 8–10, which had an incidence of VF of 22% at 30 mph and 23% at 40 BPM. Balls with a hardness slightly less than regulation baseballs (RIF 10) had an incidence of VF of 29% at 30 mph and 20% at 40 mph. The incidence of VF with standard regulation baseballs was 35% at 30 mph, and 69% at 40 mph. Thus, at all velocities, the incidence of VF was significantly less with safety baseballs as compared to regulation baseballs.

REFERENCES

1. Jervell A, Lange-Neilsen F. Congenital deaf-mutism, functional heart disease with prolongation of the QT interval and sudden death. Am Heart J 1957;54:59–68.
2. Romano C, Gemme G, Pongiglione R. Artimie cardiac rare dell'eta pediatrica. Clin Pediatr 1963,45:656–683.
3. Ward OC. A new familial cardiac syndrome in children. J Irish Med Assoc 1964;54:103–106.
4. Moss AJ. Management of patients with the hereditary long QT syndrome. J Cardiovasc Electrophysiol 1998;9(6):668–674.

5. Schwartz PJ, Stramba-Badiale M, Segantini A, et al. Prolongation of the QT interval and the sudden infant death syndrome. N Engl J Med 1998;338(24):1709–1714.

6. Schwartz PJ, Priori SG, Dumaine R, et al. A molecular link between the sudden infant death syndrome and the long-QT syndrome. N Engl J Med 2000;343(4):262–267.

7. Vincent GM. The molecular genetics of the long QT syndrome: genes causing fainting and sudden death. Annu Rev Med 1998;49:263–274.

8. Schott JJ, Charpentier F, Peltier S, Foley P, Drouin E, Bouhour JB, et al. Mapping of a gene for long QT syndrome to chromosome 4q25–4q27. Am J Hum Genet 1995;57(5):1114–1122.

9. Schwartz PJ, Priori SG. The long QT syndrome. ANE 1998;3(1):63–73.

10. Dumaine R, Wang Q, Keating MT, Hartmann HA, Schwartz PJ, Brown AM, et al. Multiple mechanisms of Na+ channel-linked long-QT syndrome. Circ Res 1996;78(5):916–924.

11. Sanguinetti MC, Curran ME, Zou A, Shen J, Spector PS, Atkinson DL, et al. Coassembly of K(V)LQT1 and minK (IsK) proteins to form cardiac I(Ks) potassium channel. Nature 1996;384(6604):80–83.

12. Sanguinetti MC, Jiang C, Curran ME, Keating MT. A mechanistic link between an inherited and an acquired cardiac arrhythmia: HERG encodes the Ikr potassium channel. Cell 1995;81(2):299–307.

13. Schulze-Bahr E, Wang Q, Wedekind H, Haverkamp W, Chen Q, Sun Y, et al. KCNE1 mutations cause Jervell and Lange-Nielsen syndrome. Nat Genet 1997;17(3):267–268.

14. Abbott GW, Sesti F, Splawski I, Buck ME, Lehmann MH, Timothy KW, et al. MiRP1 forms IKr potassium channels with HERG and is associated with cardiac arrhythmia. Cell 1999;97(2):175–187.

15. Tyson J, Tranebjaerg L, Bellman S, Wren C, Taylor JF, Bathen J, et al. IsK and KvLQT1: mutation in either of the two subunits of the slow component of the delayed rectifier potassium channel can cause Jervell and Lange-Nielsen syndrome. Hum Mol Genet 1997;6(12):2179–2185.

16. Demolombe S, Baro I, Pereon V, Bliek J, Mohammad-Panah R, Pollard H, et al. A dominant negative isoform of the long QT syndrome 1 gene product. J Biol Chem 1998;273(12):6837–6843.

17. Wang Q, Shen J, Li Z, Timothy K, Vincent GM, Priori SG, et al Cardiac sodium channel mutations in patients with long QT syndrome, an inherited cardiac arrhythmia. Hum Mol Genet 1995;4(9):1603–1607.

18. Moss AJ, Zareba W, Benhorin J, Locati EH, Hall WJ, Robinson JL, et al. ECG T-wave patterns in genetically distinct forms of the hereditary long QT syndrome. Circulation 1995;92(10):2929–2934.

19. Schwartz PJ, Priori SG, Locati EH, Napolitano C, Cantu F, Towbin JA, et al. Long QT syndrome patients with mutations of the SCN5A and HERG genes have differential responses to Na+ channel blockade and to increases in heart rate. Implications for gene-specific therapy. Circulation 1995;92(12):3381–3386.

20. Wilde AA, Jongbloed RJ, Doevendans PA, Duren DR, Hauer RN, van Langen IM, et al. Auditory stimuli as a trigger for arrhythmic events differentiate HERG-related (LQTS2) patients from KVLQT1-related patients (LQTS1). J Am Coll Cardiol 1999;33(2):327–332.

21. Schwartz PJ, Moss AJ, Vincent GM, Crampton RS. Diagnostic criteria for the long QT syndrome. An update. Circulation 1993;88(2):782–784.

22. Lehmann MH, Suzuki F, Fromm BS, Frankovich D, Elko P, Steinman RT, et al. T wave "humps" as a potential electrocardiographic marker of the long QT syndrome. J Am Coll Cardiol 1994;24(3):746–754.

23. Malfatto G, Beria G, Sala S, Bonazzi O, Schwartz PJ. Quantitative analysis of T wave abnormalities and their prognostic implications in the idiopathic long QT syndrome. J Am Coll Cardiol 1994;23(2):296–301.

24. Zareba W, Moss AJ, le Cessie S, Hall WJ. T wave alternans in idopathic long QT syndrome. J Am Coll Cardiol 1994;23(7):1541–1546.

25. Linker NJ, Colonna P, Kekwick CA, Till J, Camm AJ, Ward DE. Assessment of QT dispersion in symptomatic patients with congenital long QT syndromes. Am J Cardiol 1992;69(6):634–638.

26. Priori SG, Mortara DW, Napolitano C, Diehl L, Paganini V, Cantu F, et al. Evaluation of the spatial aspects of T-wave complexity in the long-QT syndrome. Circulation 1997;96(9):3006–3012.

27. De Ferrari GM, Nador F, Beria G, Sala S, Lotto A, Schwartz PJ. Effect of calcium channel block on the wall motion abnormality of the idiopathic long QT syndrome. Circulation 1994;89(5):2126–2132.

28. Priori SG, Barhanin J, Hauer RN, Haverkamp W, Jongsma HJ, Kleber AG, et al. Genetic and molecular basis of cardiac arrhythmias: impact on clinical management parts I and II. Circulation 1999;99(4):518–528.

29. Vincent GM, Timothy KW, Leppert M, Keating M. The spectrum of symptoms and QT intervals in carriers of the gene for the long-QT syndrome. N Engl J Med 1992;327(12):846–852.

30. Priori SG, Napolitano C, Schwartz PJ. Low penetrance in the long-QT syndrome: clinical impact. Circulation 1999;99(4):529–533.

31. El-Sherif N, Chinushi M, Caref EB, Restivo M. Electrophysiological mechanism of the characteristic electrocardiographic morphology of torsade de pointes tachyarrhythmias in the long-QT syndrome: detailed analysis of ventricular tridimensional activation patterns. Circulation 1997;96(12):4392–4399.

32. Pertsov AM, Davidenko JM, Salomonsz R, Baxter WT, Jalife J. Spiral waves of excitation underlie reentrant activity in isolated cardiac muscle. Circ Res 1993;72(3):631–650.

33. Moss AJ, Schwartz PJ, Crampton RS, Tzivoni D, Locati EH, MacCluer J, et al. The long QT syndrome. Prospective longitudinal study of 328 families. Circulation 1991;84(3):1136–1144.

34. Zareba W, Moss AJ, le Cessie S, Locati EH, Robinson JL, Hall WJ, et al. Risk of cardiac events in family members of patients with long QT syndrome. J Am Coll Cardiol 1995;26(7):1685–1691.

35. Drici MD, Burklow TR, Haridasse V, Glazer RI, Woosley RL. Sex hormones prolong the QT interval and downregulate potassium channel expression in the rabbit heart. Circulation 1996;94(6):1471–1474.

36. Zareba W, Moss AJ, Schwartz PJ, Vincent GM, Robinson JL, Priori SG, et al. Influence of genotype on the clinical course of the long-QT syndrome. International Long-QT Syndrome Registry Research Group. N Engl J Med 1998;339(14):960–965.

37. Bhandari AK, Shapiro WA, Morady F, Shen EN, Mason J, Scheinman MM. Electrophysiologic testing in patients with the long QT syndrome. Circulation 1985;71(1):63–71.

38. Moss AJ, Zareba W, Hall WJ, Robinson JL, Benhorin J, Locati-Heilbrun E, et al. Effectiveness and limitations of β-blocker therapy in long QT syndrome. Circulation 2000;101(6):616–623.

39. Priori SG, Napolitano C, Diehl L, Schwartz PJ. Dispersion of the QT interval. A marker of therapeutic efficacy in the idiopathic long QT syndrome. Circulation 1994;89(4):1681–1689.

40. Rashba EJ, Zareba W, Moss AJ, Hall WJ, Robinson J, Locati EH, et al. Influence of pregnancy on the risk for cardiac events in patients with hereditary long QT syndrome. LQTS Investigators. Circulation 1998;97(5):451–456.

41. Moss AJ, Liu JE, Gottlieb S, Locati EH, Schwartz PJ, Robinson JL. Efficacy of permanent pacing in the management of high-risk patients with long QT syndrome. Circulation 1991;84(4):1524–1529.

42. Eldar M, Griffin JC, Van Hare GF, Witherell C, Bhandari A, Benditt D, et al. Combined use of beta-adrenergic blocking agents and long-term cardiac pacing for patients with the long QT syndrome. J Am Coll Cardiol 1992;20(4):830–837.

43. Schwartz PJ, Locati EH, Moss AJ, Crampton RS, Trazzi R, Ruberti U. Left cardiac sympathetic denervation in the therapy of congenital long QT syndrome. A worldwide report. Circulation 1991;84(2):503–511.

44. De Ferrari GM, Locati EH, Priori SG, Schwartz PJ. Left cardiac sympathetic denervation in long QT syndrome patients. J Interv Cardiol 1995;8(6 Suppl):776–781.

45. Compton SJ, Lux RL, Ramsey MR, Strelich KR, Sanguinetti MC, Green LS, et al. Genetically defined therapy of inherited long-QT syndrome. Correction of abnormal repolarization by potassium. Circulation 1996;94(5):1018–1022.

46. Roy M, Dumaine R, Brown AM. HERG, a primary human ventricular target of the nonsedating antihistamine terfenadine. Circulation 1996;94(4):817–823.

47. Donger C, Denjoy I, Berthet M, Neyroud N, Cruaud C, Bennaceur M, et al. KVLQT1 C-terminal missense mutation causes a forme fruste long-QT syndrome. Circulation 1997;96(9):2778–2781.

48. Roden DM. Taking the "idio" out of "idiosyncratic": predicting torsades de pointes. Pacing Clin Electrophysiol 1998;21(5):1029–1034.

49. Chung MK, Schweikert RA, Wilkoff BL, Niebauer MJ, Pinski SL, Trohman RG, et al. Is hospital admission for initiation of antiarrhythmic therapy with sotalol for atrial arrhythmias required? Yield of in-hospital monitoring and prediction of risk for significant arrhythmia complications. J Am Coll Cardiol 1998;32(1):169–176.

50. Zimmermann M, Duruz H, Guinand O, Broccard O, Levy P, Lacatis D, et al. Torsades de pointes after treatment with terfenadine and ketoconazole. Eur Heart J 1992;13(7):1002–1003.

51. van Haarst AD, van't Klooster GA, van Gerven JM, Schoemaker RC, van Oene JC, Burggraaf J. The influence of cisapride and clarithromycin on QT intervals in healthy volunteers. Clin Pharmacol Ther 1998;64(5):542–546.

52. Antzelevitch C, Sun ZQ, Zhang ZQ, Yan GX. Cellular and ionic mechanisms underlying erythromycin-induced long QT intervals and torsade de pointes. J Am Coll Cardiol 1996;28(7):1836–1848.

53. Lazzara R. Amiodarone and torsade de pointes. Ann Intern Med 1989;111(7):549–551.

54. Drici MD, Knollmann BC, Wang WX, Woosley RL. Cardiac actions of erythromycin: influence of female sex. JAMA 1998;280(20):1774–1776.

55. Makkar RR, Fromm BS, Steinman RT, Meissner MD, Lehmann MH. Female gender as a risk factor for torsades de pointes associated with cardiovascular drugs. JAMA 1993;270(21):2590–2597.

56. Lehmann MH, Hardy S, Archibald D, Quart B, MacNeil DJ. Sex difference in risk of torsade de pointes with d,1-sotalol. Circulation 1996;94(10):2535–2541.

57. Reinoehl J, Frankovich D, Machado C, Kawasaki R, Baga JJ, Pires LA, et al. Probucol-associated tachyarrhythmic events and QT prolongation: importance of gender. Am Heart J 1996;131(6):1184–1191.

58. Nabauer M, Kaab S. Potassium channel down-regulation in heart failure. Cardiovasc Res 1998;37(2):324–334.

59. Kaab S, Nuss HB, Chiamvimonvat N, O'Rourke B, Pak PH, Kass DA, et al. Ionic mechanism of action potential prolongation in ventricular myocytes from dogs with pacing-induced heart failure. Circ Res 1996;78(2):262–273.

60. Kaab S, Dixon J, Duc J, Ashen D, Nabauer M, Beuckelmann DJ, et al. Molecular basis of transient outward potassium current downregulation in human heart failure: a decrease in Kv4.3 mRNA correlates with a reduction in current density. Circulation 1998;98(14):1383–1393.

61. Choy AM, Darbar D, Dell'Orto S, Roden DM. Exaggerated QT prolongation after cardioversion of atrial fibrillation. J Am Coll Cardiol 1999;34(2):396–401.

62. Prystowsky EN. Proarrhythmia during drug treatment of supraventricular tachycardia: paradoxical risk of sinus rhythm for sudden death. Am J Cardiol 1996;78(8A):35–41.

63. Yang T, Roden DM. Extracellular potassium modulation of drug block of IKr. Implications for torsade de pointes and reverse use-dependence. Circulation 1996;93(3):407–411.

64. Daleau P, Turgeon J. Triamterene inhibits the delayed rectifier potassium current (IK) in guinea pig ventricular myocytes. Circ Res 1994;74(6):1114–1120.

65. Fiset C, Drolet B, Hamelin BA, Turgeon J. Block of Iks by the diuretic agent indapamide modulates cardiac electrophysiological effects of the class III antiarrhythmic drug dl-sotalol. J Pharmacol Exp Ther 1997;283(1):148–156.

66. Houltz B, Darpo B, Edvardsson N, Blomstrom P, Brachmann J, Crijns HJ, et al. Electrocardiographic and clinical predictors of torsades de pointes induced by almokalant infusion in patients with chronic atrial fibrillation or flutter: a prospective study. Pacing Clin Electrophysiol 1998;21(5):1044–1057.

67. Thibault B, Nattel S. Optimal management with Class I and Class III antiarrhythmic drugs should be done in the outpatient setting: protagonist. J Cardiovasc Electrophysiol 1999;10(3):472–481.

68. Myerburg RJ, Kloosterman M, Yamamura K, Mitrani R, Interian A, Jr, Castellanos A. The case for inpatient initiation of antiarrhythmic therapy. J Cardiovasc Electrophysiol 1999;10(3):482–487.

69. Roden DM. A practical approach to torsade de pointes. Clin Cardiol 1997;20(3):285–290.

70. Assimes TL, Malcolm I. Torsade de pointes with sotalol overdose treated successfully with lidocaine. Can J Cardiol 1998;14(5):753–756.

71. Kurita T. Antiarrhythmic effect of parenteral magnesium on ventricular tachycardia associated with long QT syndrome. Magnes Res 1994;7(2):155–157.

72. Nademanee K, Veerakul G, Nimmannit S, Chaowakul V, Bhuripanyo K, Likittanasombat K, et al. Arrhythmogenic marker for the sudden unexplained death syndrome in Thai men. Circulation 1997;96(8):2595–2600.

73. Chen Q, Kirsch GE, Zhang D, Brugada R, Brugada J, Brugada P, et al. Genetic basis and molecular mechanism for idiopathic ventricular fibrillation. Nature 1998;392(6673):293–296.

74. Alings M, Wilde A. "Brugada" syndrome: clinical data and suggested pathophysiological mechanism. Circulation 1999;99(5):666–673.

75. Gussak I, Antzelevitch C, Bjerregaard P, Towbin JA, Chaitman BR. The Brugada syndrome: clinical, electrophysiologic and genetic aspects. J Am Coll Cardiol 1999;33(1):5–15.

76. Litovsky SH, Antzelevitch C. Transient outward current prominent in canine ventricular epicardium but not endocardium. Circ Res 1988;62(1):116–126.

77. Di Diego JM, Sun ZQ, Antzelevitch C. I(to) and action potential notch are smaller in left vs. right canine ventricular epicardium. Am J Physiol 1996;271(2 Pt 2):H548–61.

78. Miyazaki T, Mitamura H, Miyoshi S, Soejima K, Aizawa Y, Ogawa S. Autonomic and antiarrhythmic drug modulation of ST segment elevation in patients with Brugada syndrome. J Am Coll Cardiol 1996;27(5):1061–1070.

79. Kasanuki H, Ohnishi S, Ohtuka M, Matsuda N, Nirei T, Isogai R, et al. Idiopathic ventricular fibrillation induced with vagal activity in patients without obvious heart disease. Circulation 1997;95(9):2277–2285.

80. Brugada J, Brugada P. Further characterization of the syndrome of right bundle branch block, ST segment elevation, and sudden cardiac death. J Cardiovasc Electrophysiol 1997;8(3):325–331.

81. Lukas A, Antzelevitch C. Phase 2 reentry as a mechanism of initiation of circus movement reentry in canine epicardium exposed to simulated ischemia. Cardiovasc Res 1996;32(3):593–603.

82. Matsuo K, Shimizu W, Kurita T, Inagaki M, Aihara N, Kamakura S. Dynamic changes of 12-lead electrocardiograms in a patient with Brugada syndrome. J Cardiovasc Electrophysiol 1998;9(5):508–512.

83. Brugada J, Brugada R, Brugada P. Right bundle-branch block and ST-segment elevation in leads V1 through V3: a marker for sudden death in patients without demonstrable structural heart disease. Circulation 1998;97(5):457–460.

84. Belhassen B, Shapira I, Shoshani D, Paredes A, Miller H, Laniado S. Idiopathic ventricular fibrillation: inducibility and beneficial effects of class I antiarrhythmic agents. Circulation 1987;75(4):809–816.

85. Belhassen B, Viskin S, Fish R, Glick A, Setbon I, Eldar M. Effects of electrophysiologic-guided therapy with class IA antiarrhythmic drugs on the long-term outcome of patients with idiopathic ventricular fibrillation with or without the Brugada syndrome. J Cardiovasc Electrophysiol 1999;10(10):1301–1312.

86. Krishnan SC, Josephson ME. ST segment elevation induced by class IC antiarrhythmic agents: underlying electrophysiologic mechanisms and insights into drug-induced proarrhythmia. J Cardiovasc Electrophysiol 1998;9(11):1167–1172.

87. McKenna WJ, Thiene G, Nava A, Fontaliran F, Blomstrom-Lundqvist C, Fontaine G, et al. Diagnosis of arrhythmogenic right ventricular dysplasia/cardiomyopathy. Task Force of the Working Group Myocardial and Pericardial Disease of the European Society of Cardiology and of the Scientific Council on Cardiomyopathies of the International Society and Federation of Cardiology. Br Heart J 1994;71(3):215–218.

88. Marcus FI, Fontaine G. Arrhythmogenic right ventricular dysplasia/cardiomyopathy: a review. Pacing Clin Electrophysiol 1995;18(6):1298–1314.

89. Thiene G, Basso C, Danieli G, Rampazzo A, Corrado D, Nava A. Arrhythmogenic right ventricular cardiomyopathy. Trends Cardiovasc Med 1997;7:84–90.

90. Furlanello F, Bertoldi A, Dallago M, Furlanello C, Fernando F, Inama G, et al. Cardiac arrest and sudden death in competitive athletes with arrhythmogenic right ventricular dysplasia. Pacing Clin Electrophysiol 1998;21(1 Pt 2):331–335.

91. Maron BJ, Shirani J, Poliac LC, Mathenge R, Roberts WC, Mueller FO. Sudden death in young competitive athletes. Clinical, demographic, and pathological profiles. JAMA 1996;276(3):199–204.

92. Tonet JL, Castro-Miranda R, Iwa T, Poulain F, Frank R, Fontaine GH. Frequency of supraventricular tachyarrhythmias in arrhythmogenic right ventricular dysplasia. Am J Cardiol 1991;67(13):1153.

93. Marcus FI, Fontaine GH, Guiraudon G, Frank R, Laurenceau JL, Malergue C, Grosgogeat Y. Right ventricular dysplasia: a report of 24 adult cases. Circulation 1982;65(2):384–398.

94. Burke AP, Farb A, Tashko G, Virmani R. Arrhythmogenic right ventricular cardiomyopathy and fatty replacement of the right ventricular myocardium: are they different diseases? Circulation 1998;97(16):1571–1580.

95. Fontaine G, Fontaliran F, Frank R. Arrhythmogenic right ventricular cardiomyopathies: clinical forms and main differential diagnoses. Circulation 1998;97(16):1532–1535.

96. Globits S, Kreiner G, Frank H, Heinz G, Klaar U, Frey B, et al. Significance of morphological abnormalities detected by MRI in patients undergoing successful ablation of right ventricular outflow tract tachycardia. Circulation 1997;96(8):2633–2640.

97. Corrado D, Basso C, Thiene G, McKenna WJ, Davies MJ, Fontaliran F, et al. Spectrum of clinicopathologic manifestations of arrhythmogenic right ventricular cardiomyopathy/dysplasia: a multicenter study. J Am Coll Cardiol 1997;30(6):1512–1520.

98. Nava A, Thiene G, Canciani B, Scognamiglio R, Daliento L, Buja G, et al. Familial occurrence of right ventricular dysplasia: a study involving nine families. J Am Coll Cardiol 1988;12(5):1222–1228.

99. Rampazzo A, Nava A, Miorin M, Fonderico P, Pope B, Tiso N, et al. ARVD4, a new locus for arrhythmogenic right ventricular cardiomyopathy, maps to chromosome 2 long arm. Genomics 1997;45(2):259–263.

100. Ahmad F, Li D, Karibe A, Gonzalez O, Tapscott T, Hill R, et al. Localization of a gene responsible for arrhythmogenic right ventricular dysplasia to chromosome 3p23. Circulation 1998;98(25):2791–2795.

101. Severini GM, Krajinovic M, Pinamonti B, Sinagra G, Fioretti P, Brunazzi MC, et al. A new locus for arrhythmogenic right ventricular dysplasia on the long arm of chromosome 14. Genomics 1996;31(2):193–200.

102. Coonar AS, Protonotarios N, Tsatsopoulou A, Needham EW, Houlston RS, Cliff S, et al. Gene for arrhythmogenic right ventricular cardiomyopathy with diffuse nonepidermolytic palmoplantar keratoderma and woolly hair (Naxos disease) maps to 17q21. Circulation 1998;97(20):2049–2058.

103. Hermida JS, Minassian A, Jarry G, Delonca J, Rey JL, Quiret JC, et al. Familial incidence of late ventricular potentials and electrocardiographic abnormalities in arrhythmogenic right ventricular dysplasia. Am J Cardiol 1997;79(10):1375–1380.

104. Mallat Z, Tedgui A, Fontaliran F, Frank R, Durigon M, Fontaine G. Evidence of apoptosis in arrhythmogenic right ventricular dysplasia. N Engl J Med 1996;335(16):1190–1196.

105. Foale RA, Nihoyannopoulos P, Ribeiro P, McKenna WJ, Oakley CM, Krikler DM, et al. Right ventricular abnormalities in ventricular tachycardia of right ventricular origin: relation to electrophysiological abnormalities. Br Heart J 1986;56(1):45–54.

106. Blake LM, Scheinman MM, Higgins CB. MR features of arrhythmogenic right ventricular dysplasia. AJR Am J Roentgenol 1994;162(4):809–812.

107. Daubert C, Descaves C, Foulgoc JL, Bourdonnec C, Laurent M, Gouffault J. Critical analysis of cineangiographic criteria for diagnosis of arrhythmogenic right ventricular dysplasia. Am Heart J 1988;115(2):448–459.

108. Daubert C, Mabo P, Druelles P, Foulgoc JL, De Place C, Paillard F. Benefits and limits of selective right ventricular cineangiography in arrhythmogenic right ventricular dysplasia. Eur Heart J 1989;10 Suppl D:46–8.

109. Matsuo K, Nishikimi T, Yutani C, Kurita T, Shimizu W, Taguchi A, et al. Diagnostic value of plasma levels of brain natriuretic peptide in arrhythmogenic right ventricular dysplasia. Circulation 1998;98(22):2433–2440.

110. Turrini P, Angelini A, Thiene G, Buja G, Daliento L, Rizzoli G et al. Late potentials and ventricular arrhythmias in arrhythmogenic right ventricular cardiomyopathy. Am J Cardiol 1999;83(8):1214–1219.

111. Kinoshita O, Fontaine G, Rosas F, Elias J, Iwa T, Tonet J, et al. Time- and frequency-domain analyses of the signal-averaged ECG in patients with arrhythmogenic right ventricular dysplasia. Circulation 1995;91(3):715–721.

112. Tada H, Shimizu W, Ohe T, Hamada S, Kurita T, Aihara N, et al. Usefulness of electron-beam computed tomography in arrhythmogenic right ventricular dysplasia. Relationship to electrophysiological abnormalities and left ventricular involvement. Circulation 1996;94(3):437–444.

113. Peeters HA, SippensGroenewegen A, Schoonderwoerd BA, Wever EF, Grimbergen CA, Hauer RN, et al. Body-surface QRST integral mapping. Arrhythmogenic right ventricular dysplasia versus idiopathic right ventricular tachycardia. Circulation 1997;95(12):2668–2676.

114. De Ambroggi L, Aime E, Ceriotti C, Rovida M, Negroni S. Mapping of ventricular repolarization potentials in patients with arrhythmogenic right ventricular dysplasia: principal component analysis of the ST-T waves. Circulation 1997;96(12):4314–4318.

115. Marcus FI, Fontaine GH, Frank R, Gallagher JJ, Reiter MJ. Long-term follow-up in patients with arrhythmogenic right ventricular disease. Eur Heart J 1989;10 (Suppl D):68–73.

116. Canu G, Atallah G, Claudel JP, Champagnac D, Desseigne D, Chevalier P, et al. [Prognosis and long-term development of arrhythmogenic dysplasia of the right ventricle]. Arch Mal Coeur Vaiss 1993;86(1):41–48.

117. Pinamonti B, Di Lenarda A, Sinagra G, Silvestri F, Bussani R, Camerini F. Long-term evolution of right ventricular dysplasia-cardiomyopathy. The Heart Muscle Disease Study Group. Am Heart J 1995;129(2):412–415.

118. Wichter T, Borggrefe M, Haverkamp W, Chen X, Breithardt G. Efficacy of antiarrhythmic drugs in patients with arrhythmogenic right ventricular disease. Results in patients with inducible and noninducible ventricular tachycardia. Circulation 1992;86(1):29–37.

119. Link MS, Wang PJ, Haugh CI, Homoud MK, Foote CB, et al. Arrhythmogenic right ventricular dysplasia: clinical results with implantable cardioverter defibrillators. J Interv Card Electrophysiol 1997;1(1):41–48.

120. Ellison KE, Friedman PL, Ganz LI, Stevenson WG. Entrainment mapping and radiofrequency catheter ablation of ventricular tachycardia in right ventricular dysplasia. J Am Coll Cardiol 1998;32(3):724–728.

121. Richardson P, McKenna W, Bristow M, Maisch B, Mautner B, O'Connell J, et al. Report of the 1995 World Health Organization/International Society and Federation of Cardiology Task Force on the Definition and Classification of cardiomyopathies. Circulation 1996;93(5):841–842.

122. Maron BJ, Gardin JM, Flack JM, Gidding SS, Kurosaki TT, Bild DE. Prevalence of hypertrophic cardiomyopathy in a general population of young adults. Echocardiographic analysis of 4111 subjects in the CARDIA Study. Coronary Artery Risk Development in (Young) Adults. Circulation 1995;92(4):785–789.

123. Fananapazir L, Epstein ND. Prevalence of hypertrophic cardiomyopathy and limitations of screening methods. Circulation 1995;92(4):700–704.

124. Maron BJ, Spirito P. Impact of patient selection biases on the perception of hypertrophic cardiomyopathy and its natural history. Am J Cardiol 1993;72(12):970–972.

125. Maron BJ, Mathenge R, Casey SA, Poliac LC, Longe TF. Clinical profile of hypertrophic cardiomyopathy identified de novo in rural communities. J Am Coll Cardiol 1999;33(6):1590–1595.

126. Cecchi F, Olivotto I, Montereggi A, Santoro G, Dolara A, Maron BJ. Hypertrophic cardiomyopathy in Tuscany: clinical course and outcome in an unselected regional population. J Am Coll Cardiol 1995;26(6):1529–1536.

127. Wigle ED, Rakowski H, Kimball BP, Williams WG. Hypertrophic cardiomyopathy. Clinical spectrum and treatment. Circulation 1995;92(7):1680–1692.

128. Spirito P, Seidman CE, McKenna WJ, Maron BJ. The management of hypertrophic cardiomyopathy. N Engl J Med 1997;336(11):775–785.

129. Fananapazir L. Advances in molecular genetics and management of hypertrophic cardiomyopathy. JAMA 1999;281(18):1746–1752.

130. Geisterfer-Lowrance AA, Kass S, Tanigawa G, Vosberg HP, McKenna W, Seidman CE, et al. A molecular basis for familial hypertrophic cardiomyopathy: a beta cardiac myosin heavy chain gene missense mutation. Cell 1990;62(5):999–1006.

131. Thierfelder L, Watkins H, MacRae C, Lamas R, McKenna W, Vosberg HP, et al. Alpha-tropomyosin and cardiac troponin T mutations cause familial hypertrophic cardiomyopathy: a disease of the sarcomere. Cell 1994;77(5):701–712.

132. Kimura A, Harada H, Park JE, Nishi H, Satoh M, Takahashi M, et al. Mutations in the cardiac troponin I gene associated with hypertrophic cardiomyopathy. Nat Genet 1997;16(4):379–382.

133. Poetter K, Jiang H, Hassanzadeh S, Master SR, Chang A, Dalakas MC, et al. Mutations in either the essential or regulatory light chains of myosin are associated with a rare myopathy in human heart and skeletal muscle. Nat Genet 1996;13(1):63–69.

134. Bonne G, Carrier L, Bercovici J, Cruaud C, Richard P, Hainque B, et al. Cardiac myosin binding protein-C gene splice acceptor site mutation is associated with familial hypertrophic cardiomyopathy. Nat Genet 1995;11(4):438–440.

135. MacRae CA, Ghaisas N, Kass S, Donnelly S, Basson CT, Watkins HC, et al. Familial hypertrophic cardiomyopathy with Wolff-Parkinson-White syndrome maps to a locus on chromosome 7q3. J Clin Invest 1995;96(3):1216–1220.

136. Maron BJ, Savage DD, Wolfson JK, Epstein SE. Prognostic significance of 24 hour ambulatory electrocardiographic monitoring in patients with hypertrophic cardiomyopathy: a prospective study. Am J Cardiol 1981;48(2):252–257.

137. McKenna WJ, England D, Doi YL, Deanfield JE, Oakley C, Goodwin JF. Arrhythmia in hypertrophic cardiomyopathy. I: Influence on prognosis. Br Heart J. 1981;46(2):168–172.

138. Spirito P, Rapezzi C, Autore C, Bruzzi P, Bellone P, Ortolani P, et al. Prognosis of asymptomatic patients with hypertrophic cardiomyopathy and nonsustained ventricular tachycardia. Circulation 1994;90(6):2743–2747.

139. Fananapazir I, McAreavey D. Hypertrophic cardiomyopathy: evaluation and treatment of patients at high risk for sudden death. Pacing Clin Electrophysiol 1997;20(2 Pt 2):478–501.

140. Geibel A, Brugada P, Zehender M, Stevenson W, Waldecker B, Wellens HJ. Value of programmed

electrical stimulation using a standardized ventricular stimulation protocol in hypertrophic cardiomy-opathy. Am J Cardiol 1987;60(8):738–739.

141. Anderson KP, Stinson EB, Derby GC, Oyer PE, Mason JW. Vulnerability of patients with obstructuve hypertrophic cardiomyopathy to ventricular arrhythmia induction in the operating room. Analysis of 17 patients. Am J Cardiol 1983;51(5):811–816.

142. Krikler DM, Davies MJ, Rowland E, Goodwin JF, Evans RC, Shaw DB. Sudden death in hyper-trophic cardiomyopathy: associated accessory atrioventricular pathways. Br Heart J 1980;43(3):245–251.

143. Wellens HJ, Barr FW, Vanagt EJ. Death after ajmaline administration. Am J Cardiol 1980;45(4):905.

144. Sadoul N, Prasad K, Elliott PM, Bannerjee S, Frenneaux MP, McKenna WJ. Prospective prognostic assessment of blood pressure response during exercise in patients with hypertrophic cardiomyopathy. Circulation 1997;96(9):2987–2991.

145. Lazzeroni E, Picano E, Morozzi L, Maurizio AR, Palma G, Ceriati R, et al. Dipyridamole-induced ischemia as a prognostic marker of future adverse cardiac events in adult patients with hypertrophic cardiomyopathy. Echo Persantine Italian Cooperative (EPIC) Study Group, Subproject Hypertrophic Cardiomyopathy. Circulation 1997;96(12):4268–4272.

146. Maki S, Ikeda H, Muro A, Yoshida N, Shibata A, Koga Y, et al. Predictors of sudden cardiac death in hypertrophic cardiomyopathy. Am J Cardiol 1998;82(6):774–778.

147. Yetman AT, Hamilton RM, Benson LN, McCrindle BW. Long-term outcome and prognostic determi-nants in children with hypertrophic cardiomyopathy. J Am Coll Cardiol 1998;32(7):1943–1950.

148. Yetman AT, McCrindle BW, MacDonald C, Freedom RM, Gow R. Myocardial bridging in children with hypertrophic cardiomyopathy—a risk factor for sudden death. N Engl J Med 1998;339(17):1201–1209.

149. Fananapazir L, Leon MB, Bonow RO, Tracy CM, Cannon RO, 3d, Epstein SE. Sudden death during empiric amiodarone therapy in symptomatic hypertrophic cardiomyopathy. Am J Cardiol 1991;67(2):169–174.

150. Elliott PM, Sharma S, Varnava A, Poloniecki J, Rowland E, McKenna WJ. Survival after cardiac arrest or sustained ventricular tachycardia in patients with hypertrophic cardiomyopathy. J Am Coll Cardiol 1999;33(6):1596–1601.

151. Maron BJ, Shen WK, Link MS, et al. Efficacy of implantable cardioverter-defibrillators for the prevention of sudden death in patients with hypertrophic cardiomyopathy. N Engl J Med 2000;342(6):365–373.

152. Primo J, Geelen P, Brugada J, Filho AL, Mont L, Wellens F, et al. Hypertrophic cardiomyopathy: role of the implantable cardioverter-defibrillator. J Am Coll Cardiol 1998;31(5):1081–1085.

153. Zhu DW, Sun H, Hill R, Roberts R. The value of electrophysiology study and prophylactic implanta-tion of cardioverter defibrillator in patients with hypertrophic cardiomyopathy. Pacing Clin Electro-physiol 1998,21(1 Pt 2):299–302.

154. Takagi E, Yamakado T, Nakano T. Prognosis of completely asymptomatic adult patients with hypertrophic cardiomyopathy. J Am Coll Cardiol 1999;33(1):206–211.

155. Maron BJ, Isner JM, McKenna WJ. 26th Bethesda conference: recommendations for determining eligibility for competition in athletes with cardiovascular abnormalities. Task Force 3: hypertrophic cardiomyopathy, myocarditis and other myopericardial diseases and mitral valve prolapse. J Am Coll Cardiol 1994;24(4):880–885.

156. Glancy DL, O'Brien KP, Gold HK, Epstein SE. Atrial fibrillation in patients with idiopathic hypertro-phic subaortic stenosis. Br Heart J 1970;32(5):652–659.

157. McKenna WJ, Harris L, Rowland E, Kleinebenne A, Krikler DM, Oakley CM, et al. Amiodarone for long-term management of patients with hypertrophic cardiomyopathy. Am J Cardiol 1984;54:802–810.

158. Watson DC, Henry WL, Epstein SE, Morrow AG. Effects of operation on left atrial size and the occurrence of atrial fibrillation in patients wiht hypertrophic subaortic stenosis. Circulation 1977;55:178–181.

159. Fananapazir L, Cannon RO 3d, Tripodi D, Panza JA. Impact of dual-chamber permanent pacing in patients with obstructuve hypertrophic cardiomyopathy with symptoms refractory to verapamil and beta-adrenergic blocker therapy. Circulation 1992;85:2149–2161.

160. Fananapazir L, Epstein ND, Curiel RV, Panza JA, Tripodi D, McAreavey D. Long-term results of dual-chamber (DDD) pacing in obstructuve hypertrophic cardiomyopathy. Evidence for progressive

symptomatic and hemodynamic improvement and reduction of left ventricular hypertrophy. Circulation 1994;90:2731–2742.

161. Gadler F, Linde C, Daubert C, McKenna W, Meisel E, Aliot E, et al. Significant improvement of quality of life following atrioventricular synchronous pacing in patients with hypertrophic obstructive cardiomyopathy. Data from 1 year of follow-up. PIC study group. Pacing In Cardiomyopathy. Eur Heart J 1999;20:1044–1050.

162. Nishimura RA, Trusty JM, Hayes DL, Ilstrup DM, Larson DR, Hayes SN, et al. Dual-chamber pacing for hypertrophic cardiomyopathy: a randomized, double-blind, crossover trial. J Am Coll Cardiol 1997;29:435–441.

163. Maron BJ, Nishimura RA, McKenna WJ, Rakowski H, Josephson ME, Kieval RS. Assessment of permanent dual-chamber pacing as a treatment for drug-refractory symptomatic patients with obstructive hypertrophic cardiomyopathy. A randomized, double-blind, crossover study (M-PATHY). Circulation 1999;99:2927–2933.

164. Linde C, Gadler F, Kappenberger L, Ryden L. Placebo effect of pacemaker implantation in obstructive hypertrophic cardiomyopathy. PIC Study Group. Pacing In Cardiomyopathy. Am J Cardiol 1999;83:903–907.

165. Nishimura RA, Symanski JD, Hurrell DG, Trusty JM, Hayes DL, Tajik AJ. Dual-chamber pacing for cardiomyopathies: a 1996 clinical perspective. Mayo Clin Proc 1996;71:1077–1087.

166. Kappenberger L, Linde C, Daubert C, McKenna W, Meisel E, Sadoul N, et al. Pacing in hypertrophic obstructive cardiomyopathy. A randomized crossover study. PIC Study Group. Eur Heart J 1997;18:1249–1256.

167. Ommen SR, Nishimura RA, Squires RW, Schaff HV, Danielson GK, Tajik AJ. Comparison of dual-chamber pacing versus septal myectomy for the treatment of patients with hypertrophic obstructive cardiomyopathy: a comparison of objective hemodynamic and exercise end points. J Am Coll Cardiol 1999;34:191–196.

168. Seggewiss H, Gleichmann U, Faber L, Fassbender D, Schmidt HK, Strick S. Percutaneous transluminal septal myocardial ablation in hypertrophic obstructive cardiomyopathy: acute results and 3-month follow-up in 25 patients. J Am Coll Cardiol 1998;31(2):252–258.

169. Dickman GL, Hassan A, Luckstead EF. Ventricular fibrillation following baseball injury. Physician Sportsmed 1978;6:85–86.

170. Green ED, Simson LR, Kellerman HH, Horowitz RN. Cardiac concussion following softball blow to the chest. Ann Emerg Med 1980;9:155–157.

171. Abrunzio TJ. Commotio cordis: the single, most common cause of traumatic death in youth baseball. Am J Dis Child 1991;145:1279–1282.

172. Kaplan JA, Karofsky PS, Volturo GA. Commotio cordis in two amateur ice hockey players despite the use of commercial chest protectors: case reports. J Trauma 1993;34:151–153.

173. Maron BJ, Strasburger JF, Kugler JD, Bell BM, Brodkey FD, Poliac LC. Survival following blunt chest impact induced cardiac arrest during sports activities in young athletes. Am J Cardiol 1997;79:840–841.

174. Maron BJ, Link MS, Wang PJ, Estes NAM. Clinical profile of commotio cordis: an under-appreciated cause of sudden death in the young during sports and other activities. J Cardiovasc Electrophysiol 1999;10:114–120.

175. Link MS, Ginsburg SH, Wang PJ, Kirchhoffer JB, Estes NAM, Parris YM. Commotio cordis: cardiovascular manifestations of a rare survivor. Chest 1998;114:326–328.

176. Maron BJ, Poliac LC, Kaplan JA, Mueller FO. Blunt impact to the chest leading to sudden death from cardiac arrest during sports activities. N Engl J Med 1995;333:337–342.

177. Adler P, Monticone RCJ. Injuries and deaths related to baseball. In: Kyle SB, ed. Youth Baseball Protective Equipment Project Final Report. Washington, DC: United States Consumer Product Safety Commission, 1996;1–43.

178. Viano DC, Artinion CG. Myocardial conducting system dysfunctions from thoracic impact. J Trauma 1978;18:452–459.

179. Liedtke AJ, Gault JH, Demuth WE. Electrographic and hemodynamic changes following nonpenetrating chest trauma in the experimental animal. Am J Physiol 1974;226:377–382.

180. Cooper GJ, Pearce BP, Stainer MC, Maynard RL. The biomechanical response of the thorax to nonpenetrating impact with particular reference to cardiac injuries. J Trauma 1982;22:994–1008.

181. Link MS, Wang PJ, Pandian NG, et al. An experimental model of sudden death due to low energy chest wall impact (commotio cordis). N Engl J Med 1998;338:1805–1811.
182. Link MS, Wang PJ, VanderBrink BA, et al. Selective activation of the K+ATP channel is a mechanism by which sudden death is produced by low-energy chest-wall impact (commotio cordis). Circulation 1999;100:413–418.
183. Kubota I, Yamaki M, Shibata T, Ikeno E, Hosoya Y, Tomoike H. Role of ATP-sensitive K$^+$ channel on ECG ST segment elevation during a bout of myocardial ischemia. Circulation 1993;88:1845–1851.

19 Cardiac Arrhythmias During Acute Myocardial Infarction

Leonard I. Ganz, MD,
and Elliott M. Antman, MD

CONTENTS

INTRODUCTION

Dysrhythmias are common during acute myocardial infarction (AMI); these range from benign premature beats to ventricular fibrillation (VF). Reports from the early coronary-care unit (CCU) era suggested that the majority of patients with AMI have some abnormality of heart rhythm *(1)*. In recent years, the management of arrhythmias associated with AMI has evolved significantly, along with other elements of CCU care. Malignant ventricular arrhythmias remain the cause of most prehospital sudden deaths as a result of AMI.

Tachyarrhythmias during AMI may be caused by reentry, enhanced automaticity, and perhaps triggered activity. Bradyarrhythmias may be caused by conduction block or diminished automaticity. Ischemia, heart failure, metabolic derangements, and fluctuations in autonomic tone may have important effects on arrhythmogenesis during AMI. Recently, an American College of Cardiology/American Heart Association (ACC/AHA) task force issued updated recommendations for the management of AMI and complications including arrhythmias *(2)*. Table 1 outlines the treatment objectives and therapeutic options for the various arrhythmias that occur during AMI.

From: *Contemporary Cardiology: Management of Cardiac Arrhythmias*
Edited by: L. I. Ganz © Humana Press Inc., Totowa, NJ

Table 1
Arrhythmias during Acute MI

Category	Arrhythmia	Objective of therapy	Acute therapeutic options
Ventricular tachyarrhythmias	VF	Urgent reversion to sinus rhythm	Defibrillation; lidocaine; amiodarone; bretylium*
	VT	Restoration of hemodynamic stability	Cardioversion/defibrillation; lidocaine; amiodarone; procainamide
	Accelerated idioventricular rhythm	Observation unless hemodynamic compromise	Atropine; atrial pacing
	Ventricular premature beats	None	Observation
Supraventricular tachyarrhythmias	Sinus Tachycardia	Reduce heart rate to diminish myocardial work/oxygen demand	Identify and treat underlying cause: beta-blockers
	AF/atrial flutter	Reduce ventricular rate; restore sinus rhythm	Cardioversion if unstable; beta-blockers, calcium-blockers; digoxin; rapid atrial pacing (for flutter); anticoagulation; consider anti-arrhythmic therapy
	PSVT	Reduce ventricular rate; restore sinus rhythm	Vagal maneuvers; adenosine; beta-blockers, calcium-blockers; cardioversion if unstable
	NPJT	Search for precipitating cause (e.g., digitalis toxicity); observation unless hemodynamic compromise	Consider overdrive atrial pacing; consider suppressive anti-arrhythmic therapy; Digibind® if digitalis toxic
Bradyarrhythmias and conduction disturbances	Sinus bradycardia	Increase heart rate only if hemodynamic compromise	Atropine; temporary pacing
	Junctional bradycardia	Increase heart rate only if hemodynamic compromise	Atropine; temporary pacing
	Atrioventricular block or intraventricular conduction block	Increase heart rate; prophylax against progression to high-grade A-V block	Atropine; aminophylline; ventricular pacing

*Currently unavailable.

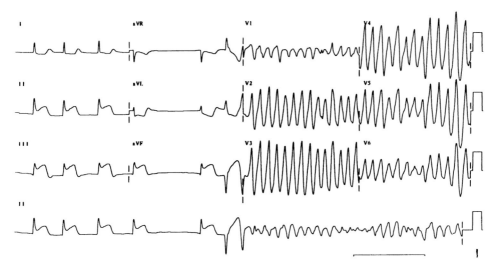

Fig. 1. This patient presented early in the course of an acute inferior MI. Note the marked inferior ST elevation. The initial rhythm is junctional. Following a pause, there is a junctional beat, followed by VF. She was promptly defibrillated, and then treated with primary angioplasty.

VENTRICULAR ARRHYTHMIAS DURING ACUTE MI

The metabolic sequelae of ischemia, including intracellular hypercalcemia and acidosis, anaerobic lipid metabolism, and free-radical production, may contribute to arrhythmogenesis during AMI *(3)*. Rapid efflux of intracellular potassium, leading to membrane depolarization, may be the most important of these effects. In addition, increased sympathetic tone augments electrical instability, provoking both ventricular and supraventricular tachyarrhythmias. Enhanced parasympathetic tone, usually occurring in the setting of acute inferior infarction, predisposes to bradyarrhythmias but may be protective against VF.

Ventricular arrhythmias may be temporarily divided into three phases: prehospital, CCU, and late. Prehospital (or early CCU phase) arrhythmias, most notably VF, probably result from chaotic reentry arising in the region of infarction. After several hours, progressive myocardial damage compromises intramyocardial conduction so that these reentrant arrhythmias occur less frequently *(4)*. Six to eight hours after the onset of infarction, Purkinje fibers in the infarct zone may develop abnormal automaticity, leading to the second phase of arrhythmogenesis *(5)*. This CCU phase lasts approx 48 h. When late ventricular arrhythmias—typically monomorphic ventricular tachycardia (VT) occur more than 24–48 h into the infarct, they may reflect the development of an anatomic substrate (scar) which supports reentry, suggesting a risk of recurrent ventricular arrhythmias after discharge.

Ventricular Fibrillation

Untreated VF (*see* Fig. 1) is generally lethal, and is the cause of most prehospital deaths in AMI. Rare cases of spontaneous reversion of VF have been reported, however. *Primary VF* is distinguished from *secondary VF,* which occurs in the setting of significant congestive heart failure (CHF) or cardiogenic shock. *Late VF* occurs more than 48 h after the onset of an acute MI.

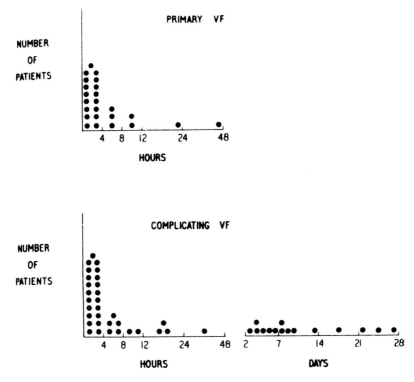

Fig. 2. These graphs show the timing of VF after symptom onset in patients admitted with AMI early in the CCU era. The top graph reflects primary VF, and the bottom reflects complicating, or secondary, VF. Note the clustering of events in the first few hours after onset of symptoms. (Reprinted from Lawrie DM, Higgins MR, Godman MJ, et al. Ventricular fibrillation complicating acute myocardial infarction. Lancet 1968;2:525.)

INCIDENCE

The incidence of VF is highest in the first few hours of an AMI, and declines sharply thereafter *(5)* *(see* Fig. 2). In GISSI-2, the incidence of primary VF in the first 4 h after presentation was 3.1%, and in hours 4–48 the incident was only 0.6% *(6)*. Clinical studies have shown that the incidence of both primary *(7–9)* and secondary *(10)* VF are proportional to the extent of infarction, measured either enzymatically or in terms of left ventricular ejection fraction (LVEF). VF occurs rarely in the setting of non-Q-wave MI (NQMI) *(11)*. In inferior MI, VF occurs more frequently with concomitant right ventricular infarction *(12,13)*. In GISSI-1, the incidences of primary and secondary VF were 2.8% *(14)* and 2.7% *(15)*, respectively; thrombolytic therapy with streptokinase reduced the frequency of secondary but not primary VF. A meta-analysis *(16)* suggested that the incidence of primary VF has been decreasing since 1970 *(see* Fig. 3), probably because of improvements in the overall management of AMI. In contrast, a retrospective review of patients with AMI admitted to community hospitals between 1975 and 1990 suggested that the rate of primary VF remained constant at 5.1% during this period *(17)*. Late VF—occurring more than 48 h into the infarct—is rare, but tends to occur following large anterior MI, particularly when complicated by CHF and/or bundle-branch block (BBB) *(18)*.

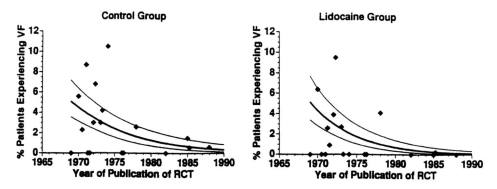

Fig. 3. Patients in randomized clinical trials of lidocaine in AMI who experienced VF as a function of the year the study was published. In both the control and lidocaine groups, the incidence of VF appears to be decreasing with time. (Reprinted from Antman EM, Berlin JA. Declining incidence of ventricular fibrillation in myocardial infarction: Implications for the prophylactic use of lidocaine. Circulation 1992;86:770.)

Prognosis

Traditionally, it has been taught that patients successfully resuscitated from primary VF have a good short-term prognosis. Recent studies *(14,19)*, however, suggest that primary VF is associated with a significantly increased in-hospital mortality, which may be as high as 10–20%. It remains unclear whether the episode of VF is a significant cause of, or is simply a marker for, the high mortality. Notably, patients with primary VF who survive until hospital discharge have the same medium-term prognosis as patients who do not experience VF *(6–9,19,20)*. Compared with primary VF, patients who have secondary VF have a much higher (38–56%) in-hospital mortality *(10,15)*. Survivors of secondary VF appear to have the same medium-term prognosis as patients with similar degrees of left ventricular impairment who did not have VF *(10,15)*.

Prophylaxis

Lidocaine had traditionally been used prophylactically to prevent primary VF. Early randomized trials *(21,22)* demonstrated a significant reduction in primary VF in patients treated with lidocaine. Overviews *(23,24)* of randomized trials documented a reduction in VF by about one-third, as well as an increased mortality in lidocaine-treated patients with suspected AMI. These meta-analyses included trials conducted largely in the pre-reperfusion therapy era. A more recent study, in which patients were randomized to prophylactic lidocaine and thrombolytic therapy in factorial design, yielded similar results *(25)*. The mechanism of this excess mortality is not entirely clear; asystole, bradyarrhythmias, heart failure, and proarrhythmic effects may all play contributing roles. Of note, lidocaine was not associated with an increased mortality in GUSTO-I and II-b, although lidocaine use in these trials was by physician preference and not randomized *(26)*.

Prophylactic lidocaine administered via intramuscular (im) injection prior to hospital arrival has also been considered. Some randomized trials have shown efficacy in reducing VF *(27,28)*, and others have not *(29–31)*. Inability to achieve therapeutic serum levels after im injection may have led to the lack of efficacy in these trials.

Meta-analyses have suggested a trend toward less VF *(23)* in patients who received prehospital im lidocaine, but no mortality advantage or disadvantage *(23,24)*.

Efforts to define a high-risk population who might benefit from lidocaine prophylaxis have been unsuccessful. Initial enthusiasm regarding "warning arrhythmias" (>5 ventricular premature beats (VPBs) per minute, R on T (early phase) VPBs, multifocal VPBs, couplets, and salvos) waned when careful studies *(32,33)* revealed poor sensitivity (58–60%), specificity (41–45%), and positive predictive value (4–8%) for VF. Not surprisingly, a randomized study comparing "selective" and "broad" lidocaine prophylaxis showed no significant difference in the incidence of VF. Thus, prophylactic lidocaine should not be used routinely in AMI *(34)*.

Fewer data are available regarding prophylactic amiodarone. The GEMICA trial in Argentina randomized patients within the first few hours of AMI to either intravenous (iv) and oral amiodarone or placebo *(35)*. Treatment continued for 6 mo. Total mortality with the original "high-dose" regimen was higher than with placebo, although it is not clear how much of this excess mortality occurred during the index hospitalization compared with during follow-up. The protocol was modified, and there was no significant difference in mortality between the "lower-dose" regimen and placebo. Amiodarone was not associated with a significant decrease in the risk of sudden death. Amiodarone-treated patients had more adverse effects than placebo patients, including hypotension in the "high-dose" group. Thus, there is no indication for amiodarone prophylaxis with AMI.

Studies in the pre-thrombolytic era consistently documented that early iv beta-blockade reduced mortality in AMI *(36)*; a portion of this benefit is attributable to an antifibrillatory effect. A single iv dose of propranolol, followed by oral therapy, markedly reduced the incidence of VF in a randomized trial of 735 patients *(37)*. In the Göteburg metoprolol trial, a double-blind, randomized study, 15 mg of iv metoprolol (administered 5 mg every 2 min for three doses) reduced the incidence of VF from 2.4%–0.9% *(38)*. Atenolol, administered intravenously (5 mg) and then orally, reduced the incidence of cardiac arrest in a randomized study involving 477 patients *(39)*. An overview of 28 randomized trials, including ISIS-1, revealed a significant decrease in VF or cardiac arrest in patients treated with iv beta-blockade *(40)*. It remains unclear whether this effect of beta-blockers is directly antifibrillatory, anti-ischemic, anti-adrenergic, or caused by infarct-size limitation or another factor.

There are fewer data for patients treated with thrombolytic therapy *(41)* or direct angioplasty. In fact, the routine use of iv beta-blockade seems to be decreasing in AMI as well as in other settings *(42)*. In the Fourth International Study of Infarct Survival (ISIS-4), only 9% of the 58,050 received iv beta-blockers *(43)*. The National Registry of MI confirmed a low utilization of iv beta-blockade in the United States, particularly in patients receiving thrombolytic therapy *(44)*. The Thrombolysis in Myocardial Infarction (TIMI) II trial evaluated early iv metoprolol vs delayed oral therapy following treatment with recombinant tissue-type plasminogen activator (rt-PA) for AMI *(45)*. Although there was no reduction of VF in the patients treated early, this therapy was safe, and conferred a mortality benefit in low-risk patients. A subsequent study revealed no excess of clinically significant bradyarrhythmias or tachyarrhythmias in patients who received both iv atenolol and rt-PA *(46)*. In a nonrandomized analysis from the GUSTO study, patients treated with early iv atenolol had more complications, despite more favorable baseline characteristics than the group treated with later oral atenolol *(47)*.

Although further investigation is needed, early aggressive beta-blockade is still recommended in patients treated with thrombolytic therapy or direct angioplasty *(41,48)*.

Hypokalemia, commonly observed upon admission to the CCU, has been associated with increased frequency of ventricular ectopy *(49)*, VF *(50)*, ventricular tachycardia (VT) *(51)*, and cardiac arrest *(7)* (*see* Fig. 4). Although no data exist confirming that potassium supplementation lowers the risk of ventricular arrhythmias, vigorous repletion to maintain a serum level of at least 4.5 meq/L is recommended in patients with AMI.

Magnesium metabolism may also be important in the AMI setting *(52)*. A number of studies *(53)*, including LIMIT-2, suggested a striking mortality reduction in patients given iv magnesium supplementation, although the effect on ventricular arrhythmia has not been consistent *(54)*. This benefit seemed attributable to a protective effect on the myocardium rather than a primary reduction in VT and VF. Accordingly, in LIMIT-2, the magnesium-treated patients had an improved long-term *(55)* as well as short-term prognosis. The ISIS-4 megatrial, however, showed no advantage with respect to ventricular arrhythmias or mortality in AMI patients randomized to high-dose magnesium supplementation *(43)*. This lack of effect may be attributed to the late administration of magnesium in this relatively low-risk cohort of patients *(56)*. A more recent trial conducted in high-risk patients who were considered unsuitable for thrombolysis revealed a significant mortality advantage with aggressive iv magnesium supplementation *(57)*. Early magnesium supplementation in high-risk AMI patients is currently being studied in the MAGIC trial.

Although they improve the long-term survival in AMI patients, angiotensin-converting enzyme (ACE) inhibitors have not been proven to reduce the incidence of ventricular arrhythmias during the acute phase of MI. In ISIS-4, there was no significant difference in the rates of VF or cardiac arrest in patients randomized to early captopril or placebo *(43)*. However, there was a reduction in sudden death in long-term follow-up in MI survivors with left ventricular dysfunction treated with captopril in the SAVE study *(58)*. A similar effect was noted in a meta-analysis of studies utilizing ACE inhibitors post-infarct *(59)*. This may be mediated by the salutory effect of ACE inhibitors on left ventricular remodeling *(60)*.

Although the widespread use of thrombolytic therapy has raised concerns of "reperfusion arrhythmias," clinical studies have not confirmed the dramatic increase in VF and VT following reperfusion in animal models *(61)*. In fact, GISSI-1 *(62)* and ISIS-2 *(63)* demonstrated a slight reduction of VF in patients given thrombolytic therapy. A recent meta-analysis *(64)* of these and other randomized controlled trials showed no increased risk of early VF—in fact, there was a lower incidence of late VF in patients who received thrombolytic therapy. In the EMIP trial, however, a temporal relationship was noted between the infusion of thrombolytic therapy and VF *(65)*. Finally, in the PAMI trial *(66)*, there was a higher incidence of VF in patients treated with angioplasty compared with thrombolytic therapy. Thus, it remains possible that malignant reperfusion arrhythmias may follow revascularization therapy—particularly primary angioplasty.

Early beta-blockade and potassium repletion may reduce the risk of VF in patients with AMI. Lidocaine should not be administered prophylactically to all patients admitted to the CCU with AMI, but rather reserved as treatment for those who manifest VF or sustained VT. Short-term lidocaine prophylaxis may be a good choice for patients for whom prompt defibrillation would not be possible, but this has not been studied

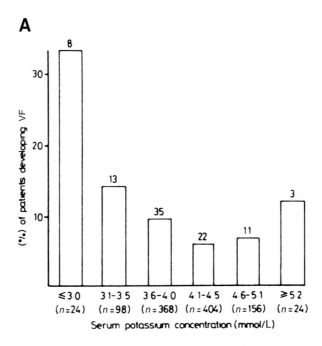

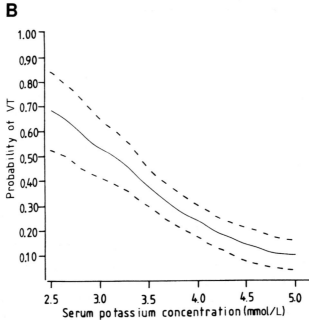

Fig. 4. Risk of developing VF (**A**) and VT (**B**) as a function of serum potassium level. (Reprinted from Nordrehaug JE, von der Lippe G. Hypokalemia and ventricular fibrillation in acute myocardial infarction. Br Heart J 1983;50:526 and Nordrehaug JE, Johannessen K-A, von der Lippe G. Serum potassium concentration as a risk factor of ventricular arrhythmia early in acute myocardial infarction. Circulation 1985;71:647.)

Table 2
Antiarrhythmic Agents for use in Ventricular Arrhythmias

Drug	Loading dose	Infusion rate	Comments
Lidocaine	1.0–1.5 mg/kg	2–4 mg/min	Rebolus with 0.5–0.75 mg/kg every 5–10 min as needed, maximum load 3 mg/kg.
Amiodarone	150 mg	1 mg/min for 6 h, then 0.5 mg/min	Load over 10 min; monitoring blood pressure. Rebolus with 50–100 mg as needed.
Bretylium tosylate*			
Standard regimen	5 mg/kg	1–2 mg/min	If refractory, rebolus with 10 mg/kg every 10 min to a maximal dose of 30–35 mg/kg.
Alternative regimen	500–750 mg	500–750 mg/kg every 6 h	Compared with standard regimen, may cause less hypotension, but ventricular ectopy may worsen transiently after each dose.
Procainamide	17 mg/kg	1–4 mg/min	Administer load at 20 mg/min unless patient develops hypotension or excessive widening of QRS.

*Currently unavailable.

(16,67). The efficacy of prophylactic magnesium infusion requires further investigation. Aggressive measures to ensure reperfusion, limit infarct size, prevent recurrent ischemia, and treat heart failure probably act synergistically to further reduce the incidence of malignant ventricular arrhythmias. Finally, continuous electrocardiographic (ECG) monitoring, coupled with an efficient plan for prompt defibrillation if needed, is a cornerstone of CCU care.

TREATMENT

Treatment of VF requires a well-rehearsed, orderly, rapid resuscitation effort. Because the likelihood of successful resuscitation decreases with time *(68),* immediate electrical defibrillation with a nonsynchronized discharge should be performed. For monophasic defibrillators, an initial energy setting of 200 J is appropriate; up to 360 J can be used if necessary *(69).* Energy requirements for newer, biphasic defibrillators tend to be lower. Lidocaine and bretylium tosylate are equally effective in preventing recurrences of VF *(70);* however, bretylium more frequently causes significant hypotension *(71).* Epinepherine and amiodarone may be beneficial in refractory VF.

Patients who are successfully resuscitated should generally receive iv lidocaine; Table 2 reviews dosing information. The optimal duration of therapy is unknown; lidocaine may generally be discontinued after 6–24 h in patients whose post-VF course is uncomplicated. Careful attention should be paid to metabolic (hypoxia, acidemia, or hypokalemia) and hemodynamic (e.g., ongoing ischemia or heart failure) derangements that may have contributed to the episode of VF. Lidocaine toxicity is common in elderly patients and in those with hepatic and/or left ventricular dysfunction. Signs of lidocaine toxicity include confusion, lethargy, slurred speech, and seizures. Therefore,

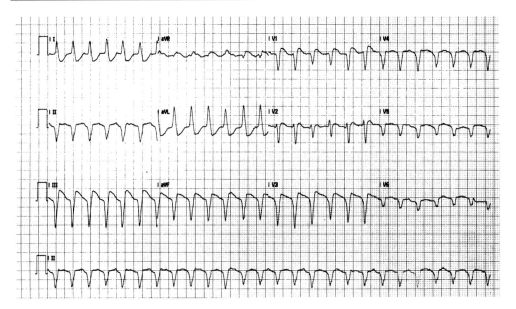

Fig. 5. This patient presented with an acute anterior MI and presumed new LBBB. Minutes after arrival in the emergency room, this sustained wide-complex tachycardia was recorded. Note the A-V dissociation in the lead II rhythm, indicative of VT.

the patient's clinical status and serum lidocaine levels should be carefully monitored. During prolonged infusion of lidocaine (greater than 24–48 h), the terminal half-life of elimination may increase, necessitating a reduction in dose. Cimetidine *(72)* and propranolol *(73)* have been noted to increase the serum level of lidocaine.

Patients who suffer from recurrent VF despite lidocaine therapy should be treated with amiodarone. Bretylium is not presently available in the United States; it is unclear whether it will become available again in the future. Bretylium increases the VF threshold in normal tissue and averts the decrease in VF threshold usually caused by ischemia *(74,75)*. Standard and alternative dosing regimens are reviewed in Table 2. Although iv amiodarone is of proven benefit in refractory or recurrent VF *(76,77)*, fewer data exist regarding its use in the setting of AMI. In a canine model of acute infarction, iv amiodarone facilitated defibrillation in cases of refractory VF *(78)*.

Ventricular Tachycardia

Ventricular tachycardia (VT) (*see* Fig. 5, 6) is a potentially fatal arrhythmia in the setting of AMI. The frequently employed broad definition of VT—three or more consecutive ventricular complexes at a rate of at least 100–120 beats per minute (BPM)—encompasses benign as well as life-threatening arrhythmias, and is therefore of limited clinical utility. Several definitions, are useful from a practical perspective. *Sustained VT* lasts more than 30 s and/or causes hemodynamic collapse requiring countershock; *nonsustained VT* (NSVT) lasts less than 30 seconds. *Primary* VT occurs in the absence of significant CHF; *secondary VT* occurs in the setting of profound pump failure. Finally, VT may be *monomorphic* or *polymorphic (79)*. Relatively narrow fascicular tachycardias, likely reflecting reentry or abnormal automaticity in Purkinje fibers, have occasionally been noted early in the course of anterior MI (*see* Fig. 7).

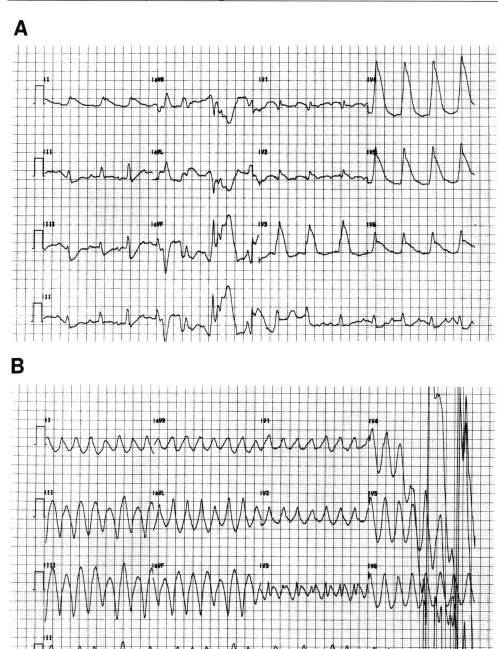

Fig. 6. This patient presented with extensive anterolateral infarction. Note the massive ST elevation in the anterolateral leads, frequently called "tombstones." **(A)** Thirty-five minutes later, he developed VT, with hemodynamic collapse. **(B)** Although a countershock restored sinus rhythm, the patient developed cardiogenic shock and died.

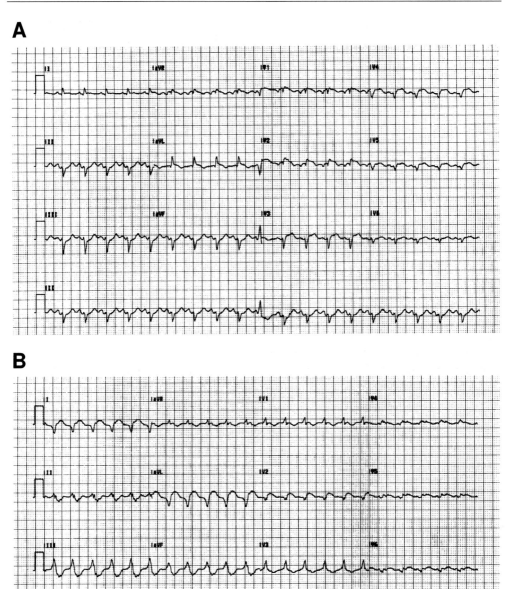

Fig. 7. This 80-yr-old woman suffered an anterior MI, presenting with sinus tachycardia, an incomplete RBBB, and left anterior fascicular block (**A**). Note the precordial ST elevation. Minutes later, this relatively narrow wide-complex tachycardia (**B**) was recorded. Note the incomplete RBBB and right axis deviation, consistent with a fascicular tachycardia originating from the left anterior fascicle. The mechanism is likely abnormal automaticity caused by ischemia/injury to the anterior fascicle. Note the retrograde P waves. This tachycardia terminated spontaneously, and did not recur.

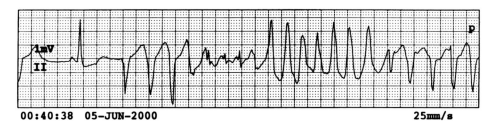

Fig. 8. This patient presented with an anterior MI and had recurrent episodes of nonsustained polymorphic VT. Primary angioplasty and stenting of a subtotally occluded LAD was performed, and no further VT occurred.

PROGNOSIS AND INCIDENCE

Using the standard, broad definition of VT, the SPRINT investigators found the incidence of primary VT to be 3.7% *(80)*. Seventeen percent of these patients, or 0.6% of the entire cohort, had sustained primary VT; 50% of these episodes were polymorphic. Patients with sustained VT had a substantially higher in-hospital cardiac mortality than patients with NSVT or no VT, but there was no difference in survival at 1 yr among patients who survived until hospital discharge. Mont and colleagues *(81)* reviewed 1120 consecutive AMI patients; 1.9% had early (<48 h) sustained monomorphic VT (SMVT). These patients had larger infarcts, and were more likely to have antecedent BBB than patients who did not have VT. Patients with early SMVT had a much higher mortality in-hospital (43% vs 11%) and after discharge than patients without VT. Patients with VT had larger infarcts, worse Killip class, and a higher risk of recurrent ventricular arrhythmias than patients who had VF.

As with VF, so-called "warning arrhythmias" do not accurately predict VT *(82)*. One study conducted in the pre-thrombolytic era suggested a connection between accelerated idiioventricular rhythm (AIVR) and VT *(83)*. In a recent meta-analysis *(16)*, thrombolytic therapy was associated with an increased incidence of VT compared with conventional therapy, but "VT" was broadly defined, including clinically insignificant short salvos as well as sustained VT. As with VT, hypokalemia predisposes to VT *(see* Fig. 4) *(50,51)*.

Extremely rapid monomorphic VT may be seen in acutely ischemic or infarcted ventricles and has been labeled ventricular flutter. Polymorphic VT (PVT) *(see* Fig. 8) rarely occurs in the setting of an acute MI, but is often preceded by symptoms or electrocardiographic signs of ischemia *(79)*. These episodes are usually not consistently related to a long QT interval, sinus pauses, or electrolyte abnormalities, as in other forms of PVT, and connote a high mortality. Lidocaine may be used initially; if ineffective, iv amiodarone may suppress the arrhythmia. Intraortic balloon counterpulsation may be of benefit, but revascularization seems to provide the most definitive therapy for this arrhythmia *(79)*.

Few data are available regarding nonsustained VT (NSVT) in the setting of AMI *(see* Fig. 9). In one series, patients with NSVT had a higher incidence of VF than control patients, but overall did not have a higher in-hospital mortality. The timing of the NSVT may be important. Patients with NSVT within the first few hours of presentation with AMI did not have an increased mortality. Patients with NSVT occurring more

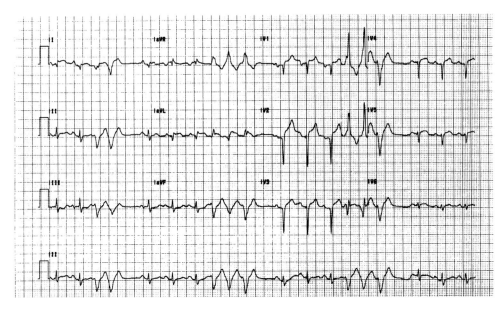

Fig. 9. This patient presented with recurrent nonsustained VT early in the setting of an acute anterior MI. The patient was treated with primary angioplasty, beta-blocker, and an ACE inhibitor, and VT did not recur after 36 h from symptom onset.

than 12 h after presentation, however, did have a substantially higher mortality than control patients *(84)*.

TREATMENT

Management of VT depends on the degree of hemodynamic compromise associated with the arrhythmia. For purposes of management, pulseless VT and sustained PVT should be considered like VF and treated with an unsynchronized discharge of 200 J as quickly as possible. Monomorphic VT is often highly sensitive to electrical energy; some cases can be reverted to sinus rhythm with a discharge of 25 J or less. This sensitivity explains the occasional reversion to sinus rhythm following a "chest thump" (that delivers approx 0.5–1.0 J). Although a chest thump can occasionally convert VT (or rarely VF), a thump can also cause VT to deteriorate to VF. Thus, "thump-version" should be attempted with caution. After successful resuscitation from sustained VT, patients should receive iv lidocaine, amiodarone, or procainamide (*see* Table 2).

If a pulse is present, but VT is accompanied by hypotension, ischemia, or significant heart failure, immediate cardioversion should be considered. If the tachycardia is hemo-dynamically tolerated, a synchronized cardioversion (50–200 J) should be performed following administration of sedation/anesthesia. Frequently, several different leads must be checked in order to find one in which synchronization is possible. If a rapid rate or the particular QRS morphology during VT makes synchronization impossible, an unsynchronized discharge should be delivered.

VT that is tolerated hemodynamically may be treated initially with iv antiarrhythmic drugs. Lidocaine, amiodarone, or procainamide may be administered intravenously as previously mentioned (*see* Table 2). Following acute management of the VT, a continu-ous infusion of the effective agent may be continued for 6–24 h. If pharmacologic

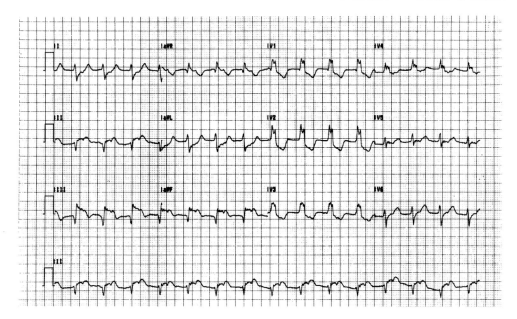

Fig. 10. This 61-yr-old female presented with an acute inferoposterior MI, and had episodes of AIVR lasting minutes. Note the retrograde atrial activation. Interestingly, there is clearly ST elevation in the inferior leads.

therapy is unsuccessful, synchronized cardioversion should be performed (following anesthesia/sedation), as the increased heart rate and myocardial oxygen demand, as well as propensity of VT to degenerate into VF, may be harmful. As with VF, a diligent search should be made for reversible causes of ventricular irritability, such as sympathomimetic drugs, CHF, hypoxemia, ischemia, hypokalemia, or an intracardiac catheter that could be irritating the ventricle. Refractory or recurrent cases of VT may respond to iv amiodarone (*see* Table 2).

Late VT (occurring more than 24–48 h into the infarct) often connotes an anatomic substrate from which reentrant ventricular tachyarrhythmias may recur, and thus warrants specific electrophysiologic evaluation *(85)*. Such recurrent arrhythmias occur most commonly following large anterior MIs, particularly when complicated by CHF and BBB. Occasionally, refractory recurrent VT occurring in the acute phase of AMI responds favorably to percutaneous revascularization *(86)*.

Accelerated Idioventricular Rhythm

AIVR (*see* Figs. 10, 11), or "slow VT," is defined as a ventricular rhythm at a rate of 60–100 (or 120) BPM. Slow idioventricular rhythms may serve as escape rhythms during periods of profound sinus bradycardia; at other times, AIVR suggests abnormal automaticity in the Purkinje fibers. AIVR is frequently nonsustained and well tolerated; occasionally, however, the loss of atrioventricular (AV) synchrony may be important clinically. In such rare instances, treatment options include atropine or atrial pacing to increase the sinus rate or antiarrhythmic therapy to suppress the abnormal automaticity.

The prognostic implication of AIVR has not been rigorously evaluated. Although one study *(83)* suggested an association between AIVR and VT, AIVR has never been convincingly linked to sustained VT, VF, or a poor prognosis. In fact, the incidence

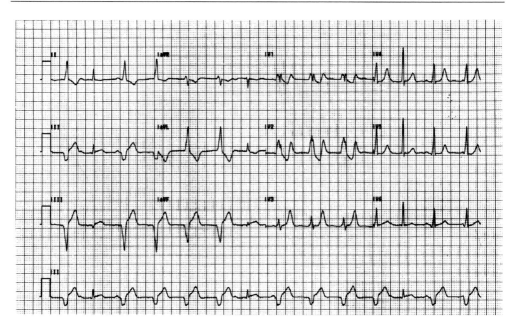

Fig. 11. This 44-yr-old male presented with prolonged chest pain. In this AIVR, there is no retrograde conduction; rather, there are occasional sinus capture beats which conduct with first-degree AV block and inferior ST elevation.

of AIVR may actually increase with successful reperfusion therapy, which generally connotes a better prognosis. Thus, AIVR that is well-tolerated hemodynamically is typically not treated.

Ventricular Premature Beats

Ventricular premature beats (VPBs) are extremely common in both the AMI and non-AMI settings. As described above, VPBs and so-called "warning arrhythmias" have not been reliably linked with malignant ventricular arrhythmias. In fact, in the post-MI setting, suppression of asymptomatic VPBs with various antiarrhythmic drugs has been associated with a higher mortality (*see* CAST Trial). Thus, specific anti-arrhythmic therapy for VPBs other than beta-blockade and aggressive electrolyte reple-tion is not recommended.

Reperfusion Arrhythmias

As alluded to previously, efforts to identify clinically significant dysrhythmias follow-ing reperfusion therapy have been largely unrewarding. In animal models of infarction using coronary ligation, reperfusion is accompanied by a high incidence of VT and VF. Some thrombolytic trials such as ISAM *(87)* and ASSET *(88)* have documented a high incidence of low-grade ventricular ectopic activity (VEA), but no significant difference in the likelihood of life-threatening arrhythmias compared with conventional therapy. Several hypotheses for the discrepancy between the animal models and human clinical experience have been offered. One potential explanation is that coronary occlu-sion in animal models typically lasts less than 1 h, unlike in typical AMI, when treatment may not occur for 6–12 h after the onset of symptoms. The recent EMIP study *(65)*, in which thrombolytic therapy was delivered extremely early, documented a relatively

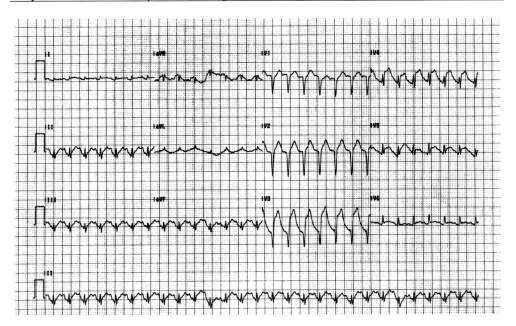

Fig. 12. This 64-yr-old female presented with acute antolateral MI, CHF, and marked sinus tachycardia. Despite aggressive treatment, sinus tachycardia persisted and the patient succumbed to cardiogenic shock and recurrent ventricular arrhythmias.

high incidence of VF. However, there was a high incidence of cardiogenic shock in the group receiving prehospital thrombolytic therapy, suggesting that much of this VF was secondary rather than primary *(89)*. A second potential explanation for the lower incidence of VF in humans compared with experimental models is that more rapid reperfusion in animals without residual stenoses may predispose to malignant arrhythmias *(90)*. Although some clinical studies have suggested that AIVR and low-grade ventricular ectopy are indicative of reperfusion *(91)*, in the TAMI trial *(92)*, these arrhythmias were not unreliable markers of successful reperfusion.

SUPRAVENTRICULAR ARRHYTHMIAS DURING ACUTE MI

Supraventricular arrhythmias complicating AMI are commonly associated with increased sympathetic tone. Many factors in the AMI setting can cause a hyperadrenergic state, including fear, anxiety, fever, pain, ongoing ischemia, hypoxia, dyspnea, and pericarditis *(93)*. Management of these arrhythmias requires careful attention to such provocative influences.

Sinus Tachycardia

Persistent sinus tachycardia (*see* Fig. 12) is deleterious during AMI because of the increased oxygen demands imposed by the rapid heart rate. Refractory sinus tachycardia portends a poor prognosis, since it is usually associated with a large area of infarction *(94)*.

Treatment of sinus tachycardia includes a search for and correction of precipitating factors. Fever should be suppressed with aspirin or acetaminophen. Anxiety and chest discomfort may be relieved with sedation and iv morphine. If present, CHF should be

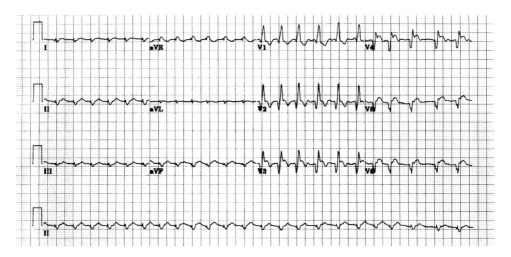

Fig. 13. This 73-yr-old female presented with massive anterolateral infarction, bifascicular block, and pulmonary edema. AF with a rapid ventricular rate developed a few hours after admission.

treated with diuretics, oxygen, nitrates, and morphine. If no specific cause of sinus tachycardia is found, careful administration of beta-blockers may be helpful unless significant heart failure or hypotension is present.

Atrial Fibrillation and Flutter

Atrial fibrillation (AF, *see* Fig. 13) and flutter (*see* Fig. 14) occur in 10–20% of AMI *(95–96)*. The prevalence of AF with AMI probably increases with age. In a Medicare dataset, 22% of patients greater than 65 yr of age with AMI either had AF at presentation (11%) or developed AF during hospitalization (11%) *(97)*. In the SPRINT study, the mortality in AMI patients with AF was 25.5% *(95)*. Patients with chronic AF who experience AMI do not seem to have a higher mortality than their counterparts without chronic AF. Conversely, patients who develop AF in the setting of AMI have high rates of complications and in-hospital mortality *(97)*. AF occurs more commonly in the setting of pump failure, perhaps because of left atrial distension related to high filling pressures. In multivariate analysis, this excess mortality in patients with AF was attributable entirely to CHF *(95)*. The association between AF, CHF, and high mortality is even more pronounced in patients in whom AF occurs relatively late (>12 h) after the onset of MI *(98)*. Thus, AF developing during AMI seems to be a marker for rather than a direct cause of poor outcome. Notably, AF tends to occur earlier in the course of IMI (within 12 h), than anterior MI (12 h–4 d) *(98)*. In addition to heart failure and high sympathetic tone, atrial infarction, elevated right atrial pressure, pericarditis, right ventricular infarction *(13,99)* and pulmonary embolus have been specifically linked with paroxysms of AF during AMI. Both electrocardiographic *(100)* and angiographic *(101)* stigmata of atrial infarction may occur in patients who develop AF. Early beta-blockade reduces the incidence of AF complicating AMI *(39)*. In GUSTO-1, AF was associated with a higher rate of stroke and in-hospital mortality, suggesting AF remains a significant risk factor even in the setting of thrombolytic therapy. Thrombolytic therapy may, however, reduce the incidence of AF during AMI *(102)*.

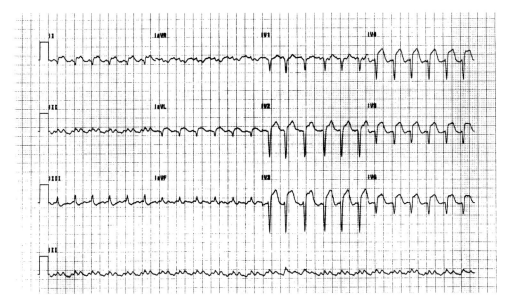

Fig. 14. This patient presented late in the course of an anterolateral infarct. Atrial flutter with 2:1 A:V conduction led to recurrent ischemia.

Acceleration of the ventricular rate with the onset of AF or atrial flutter increases myocardial oxygen demand and reduces the time available for diastolic perfusion of the coronary arteries. With loss of the contribution of atrial contraction to left ventricular filling, cardiac output may decrease. As with sinus tachycardia, these rhythm disturbances may have an identifiable underlying cause, may persist if not treated correctly, and may cause infarct extension and clinical deterioration.

Specific measures used to treat AF or atrial flutter depend upon the degree of hemodynamic compromise present in association with the arrhythmia. The potential risk of thromboembolic complications with cardioversion should also be considered in patients with AF or atrial flutter of unknown duration who are not chronically anticoagulated. If significant hypotension, heart failure, or angina ensues, urgent electrical cardioversion may be required. The patient should be sedated with a short-acting agent if possible, and a synchronized electrical discharge should be delivered. An initial discharge of 200 J for AF and 50–100 J for atrial flutter is reasonable; subsequent shocks titrated to higher energy levels may be delivered if necessary. Lower energies are typically required for atrial flutter than for AF. Biphasic waveforms may increase the success of external cardioversion compared with traditional monophasic waveforms. After cardioversion, the potential benefits and risks of antiarrhythmic therapy to suppress further episodes of AF must be carefully considered.

Patients who develop AF but maintain hemodynamic stability should be treated medically. Therapy should focus initially on control of the ventricular response to AF. Because of the probable contributions of ischemia and adrenergic tone to the initiation of AF, beta-blockade is the preferred first-line therapy for AF in the setting of AMI. If it is unclear whether a beta-blocker will be tolerated, a trial of esmolol, an ultra-short-acting beta-blocker, may be employed. Other pharmacologic alternatives include diltiazem and verapamil. Digoxin may be employed, but generally takes several hours before slowing AV nodal conduction by increasing vagal tone; in contrast, beta-blockers and calcium-channel blockers act directly at the AV node.

The role of antiarrhythmic therapy for suppression of recurrences of AF has not been critically evaluated in AMI patients. Sotalol and amiodarone are frequently used in patients with coronary disease and AF, although there is little data in the AMI setting. In one small study, iv amiodarone appeared to be relatively effective in converting AF to SR in patients with AMI *(103)*. Data are similarly scant with the IA agents, although proarrhythmic risks may be higher in the setting of acute ischemia and/or infarction. Although dofetilide appears to be relatively safe in post-infarct patients *(104)*, no data exists for AF in the AMI setting. Nevertheless, in patients who experience recurrent symptomatic AF despite beta-blocker or other AV-nodal-blocking therapy, a course of an antiarrhythmic agent may be reasonable.

Atrial flutter, in which atrial activity is organized into a single macro-reentrant right atrial circuit, is much less common than AF during AMI *(98)*. Pharmacologic options are the same as for AF, although ventricular rate control is typically more difficult to achieve in atrial flutter. In addition, atrial flutter may be terminated by overdrive atrial pacing. Catheter ablation for atrial flutter, although extremely effective in the non-AMI setting, has not been reported in AMI patients.

Initiating anticoagulation should also be considered in patients with AF and atrial flutter. Intravenous heparin is frequently used adjunctively in patients managed with thrombolytic therapy and primary angioplasty/stent, as well as in patients managed conservatively. No data exist with respect to the efficacy of low molecular weight heparins and the newer antiplatelet agents in preventing thromboembolic complications related to AF.

Finally, consideration should be given to the need for long-term oral antiarrhythmic therapy and anticoagulation if AF or atrial flutter recur or if conditions likely to precipitate these arrhythmias persist. Although such a decision must be individualized, a conservative approach with anticoagulation for at least 6 wk following restoration of sinus rhythm is reasonable. The long-term need for suppressive antiarrhythmic therapy should frequently be reassessed.

Paroxysmal Supraventricular Tachycardia

Paroxysmal supraventricular tachycardia *(105)* (PSVT, *see* Fig. 15) is a rare rhythm disturbance that occurs during acute MI *(98)*. When PSVT does occur, it is often both transient and recurrent *(93)*. Left ventricular failure and increased sympathetic tone may be precipitating factors, but this has not been firmly established.

The most common forms of PSVT, AV-nodal reentrant tachycardia (AVNRT) and AV reentrant tachycardia (AVRT) using an accessory pathway, are reentrant rhythms that utilize the AV node as one limb of the circuit. Vagal maneuvers will often terminate these tachycardias *(106)*. If vagal maneuvers are ineffective, iv adenosine is the drug of choice in non-AMI patients *(105)*; iv verapamil is also extremely effective. Unfortunately, few data exist in the AMI setting. Adenosine frequently causes transient anginal chest discomfort, dyspnea, and flushing. Clinically significant hypotension is more commonly a side-effect of iv verapamil than adenosine. Verapamil may be contraindicated if there is significant left ventricular dysfunction. Intravenous metoprolol may be effective in terminating PSVT *(107)*, and oral beta-blockers may prevent recurrences.

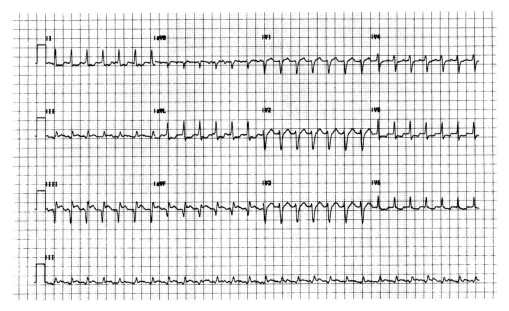

Fig. 15. This 62-yr-old male presented with inferior MI and recurrent SVT. Following aggressive beta blockade, no further SVT recurred. Notably, the patient had complained of paroxysmal palpitations in the years preceding his AMI.

Diltiazem may also be effective. Synchronized cardioversion is rarely necessary, but is usually effective in patients with PSVT.

Atrial tachycardias are relatively unusual during AMI. Atrial tachycardias may respond to treatment with beta-blockers or calcium-channel blockers, but are often refractory to medical therapy.

Junctional Rhythms

Several types of junctional rhythms have been described in the context of AMI. As with AIVR, a junctional escape rhythm (rate 35–60 BPM, *see* Fig. 16) may occur at times of sinus slowing. This is relatively common in cases of inferior MI (IMI) and probably is not indicative of poor prognosis. If this bradycardia causes hypotension, the heart rate may be accelerated with atropine or temporary pacing. Accelerated junctional rhythms (*see* Fig. 17), also called nonparoxysmal junctional tachycardia (NPJT, *see* Fig. 18) when rates are rapid, reflect abnormal automaticity of the AV-nodal tissue. In pre-thrombolytic era studies, the incidence was about 10% *(108)*, with a poor prognosis when it accompanies anterior but not inferior MI *(109)*.

BRADYARRHYTHMIAS AND CONDUCTION DISTURBANCES

Bradyarrhythmias and conduction disturbances during AMI vary in etiology, prognosis, and management according to the site of infarction. The blood supply to the conducting system determines the pathophysiology of conduction defects observed in AMI. The sinoatrial (SA)-nodal artery originates from the right coronary artery (RCA) in 65% of patients and the left circumflex coronary artery (LCA) in 25%; in 10% of patients, there is a dual supply *(10)*. The AV-nodal artery is a tributary of the posterior

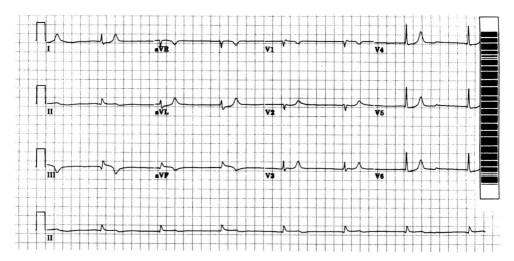

Fig. 16. This 56-yr-old female with acute inferior MI had sustained junctional bradycardia. Because of hypotension, atropine was administered, with acceleration of the ventricular rate.

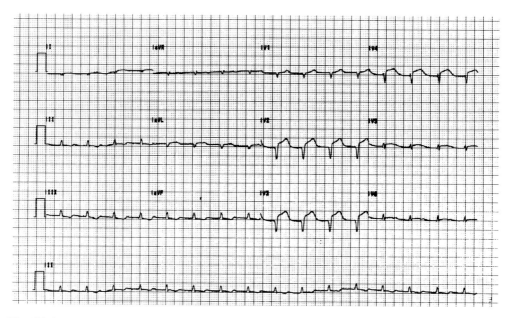

Fig. 17. An accelerated junctional rhythm was noted in this patient, who presented with anterior MI.

descending artery (PDA), which is a branch of the RCA in 80% of patients. In addition, the left anterior descending artery (LAD) provides some collateral flow to the AV node. The bundle of His and proximal right bundle branch (RBB) are supplied by the AV-nodal artery and septal branches of the LAD. Most of the RBB and the anterior fascicle of the left bundle branch (LBB) are perfused by septal perforators of the LAD, and the posterior fascicle of the LBB receives blood from the LAD and PDA *(111)*.

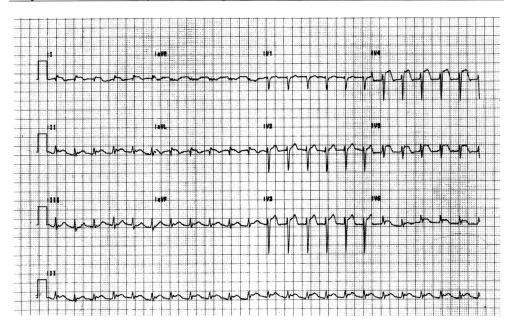

Fig. 18. In this patient with anterolateral infarction, persistent SVT was noted. Although AVNRT could not be excluded, the clinical syndrome appeared consistent with nonparoxysmal junctional tachycardia (NPJT).

Sinus Bradycardia

Sinus bradycardia (*see* Fig. 19) occurs in 10–41% of cases of AMI *(112–115),* and is especially common within the first hours of infarction *(113).* Sinus bradycardia and junctional bradycardia (*see* Fig. 16) are more common with IMI and inferoposterior infarction (IPMI) than anterior MI *(113).* The incidence of bradycardia and hypotension is higher in patients treated with early iv beta-blockers *(39,85)* although the need for treatment with atropine or temporary pacing because of hemodynamic compromise is not more frequent. In IMI, the mechanism of bradycardia with or without associated hypotension is generally believed to be a manifestation of the Bezold-Jarisch or vaso-vagal reflex, which accompanies both ischemia and reperfusion of the inferior wall *(116).* Cardiac receptors—more numerous in the inferoposterior than in the anterior portion of the left ventricle—transmit impulses via nonmyelinated (C-fiber) vagal afferents. A brainstem reflex results in efferent vagal stimulation of the heart *(117).* Teleologically, this reflex may be protective in the setting of AMI; experimental and clinical evidence suggests that vagal stimulation within the first few hours of infarction may enhance electrical stability, thus reducing the likelihood of VF. In addition, sinus bradycardia may occasionally develop as a result of ischemia or infarction of the sinus node or surrounding tissue.

Management of sinus and junctional bradycardia depends upon whether symptoms, hypotension, angina, heart failure, or ventricular arrhythmias accompany the reduced sinus rate. Isolated bradycardia without hemodynamic compromise should simply be observed, since the prognosis is generally excellent and not affected by atropine *(118).* In fact, asymptomatic sinus bradycardia with rates of 50–60 BPM caused by beta-

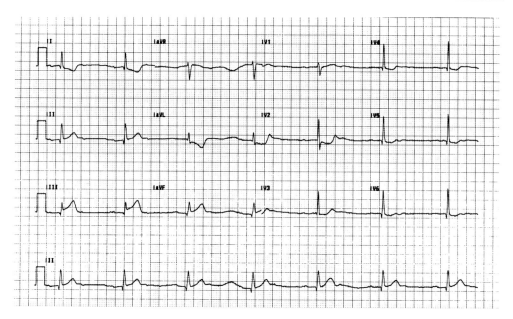

Fig. 19. This 82-yr-old male presented with acute inferoposterior MI. Note the profound sinus brady-cardia and first-degree A-V block.

blocker therapy might be optimal in AMI. For profound asymptomatic sinus bradycardia, beta-blocker therapy should be held. Pain, nausea, and medications such as morphine and nitroglycerin have also been associated with vasovagal-type decreases in blood pressure and heart rate *(119)*.

When sinus bradycardia is associated with symptoms and/or hemodynamic compromise, atropine should be administered intravenously, initially in small doses (0.5–1.0 mg). A paradoxical increase in vagal tone, and therefore more profound bradycardia, is rarely seen after small doses of atropine *(120)*. Sequential iv boluses may then be given to a total dose of 2.0–2.5 mg *(2)*. If administered in the first 4–6 h after infarction, atropine is frequently effective in treating bradycardia and accompanying hypotension, particularly if hypervagotonia is the cause. It should also be noted that several cases of atropine-induced VF have been reported in the literature *(121,122)*.

Sinus bradycardia that occurs more than 6 h after the onset of chest pain is often transient. It may be caused by sinus-node dysfunction, infarction, or ischemia rather than vagal hyperactivity, and tends to be less responsive to atropine. If atropine is unsuccessful in abolishing symptomatic bradycardia, a temporary transvenous pacemaker may be inserted into the right atrium or right ventricle to accelerate the heart rate. Isoproterenol, which is a positive chronotropic and inotropic agent, should be avoided except under extreme circumstances, because this agent markedly augments myocardial oxygen demand.

Atrioventricular (AV) Block

AV block occurs frequently in the setting of AMI, and is especially common in IMI (*see* Tables 3, 4). The pathophysiology, prognostic significance, and management depend both on the degree of block and the location of the infarct. An overview of randomized trials by Yusuf *(36)* did not suggest excess AV block in appropriately selected AMI

Table 3
AV Block During Acute MI

	Approximate incidence	Risk of CHB	Anterior MI	Inferior MI
Sinus bradycardia	up to 40%		observe*	observe*
First-degree AV block	5–13%	low	observe	observe
Second-degree AV block				
Mobitz I	5–10%	high		treat if symptomatic#
Mobitz II	1%	high	temporary pacemaker	
Third-degree AV block	11–13% (IMI) 5% (ASMI)		temporary pacemaker	treat if symptomatic#

* If symptomatic, treat with atropine and temporary pacing if necessary.
# If symptomatic, treat with atropine and temporary pacing if necessary. Late AV block in IMI may respond to iv aminophylline.

Table 4
Intraventricular Block during Acute MI

	Incidence	Progression to CHB	Management
LAHB	3–5%	low	observe
LPHB	1–2%	low	observe
LBBB	2–7%	moderate	observe*
RBBB	2–5%	moderate	observe*
1° AVB and RBBB		moderate	observe*
1° AVB and LBBB		moderate–high	consider temporary pacemaker*
RBBB/LAHB	1–6%	high	temporary pacemaker
RBBB/LPHB	0–1%	high	temporary pacemaker
Trifascicular block		high	temporary pacemaker
Alternating BBB		high	temporary pacemaker

*Optimal management in these patients remains unclear.

patients treated with beta-blockers, but this complication was not specifically reported in many of the studies. Trials of thrombolytic therapy have suggested that the frequency of clinically significant AV block may be somewhat lower than in the pre-reperfusion therapy era.

FIRST-DEGREE AND MOBITZ I (WENKEBACH) SECOND-DEGREE AV BLOCK

First-degree AV block (*see* Fig. 19) occurs in 7–13% of patients with AMI; Mobitz I block (*see* Fig. 20) occurs slightly less frequently *(123)*. More common in IMI than anterior MI, these conduction abnormalities frequently reflect increased vagal activity at the AV node. Marked first-degree AV block (PR interval >0.24 s) is a relative contraindication to beta-blocker therapy; in less severe cases, the PR interval should be monitored and the dose of beta-blocker therapy held or reduced if progressive PR prolongation occurs. Mobitz I block (*see* Fig. 20) is generally-well tolerated in the setting of IMI; patients with hemodynamic compromise generally respond to atropine. The presence of low-grade AV block does not seem to affect prognosis.

A

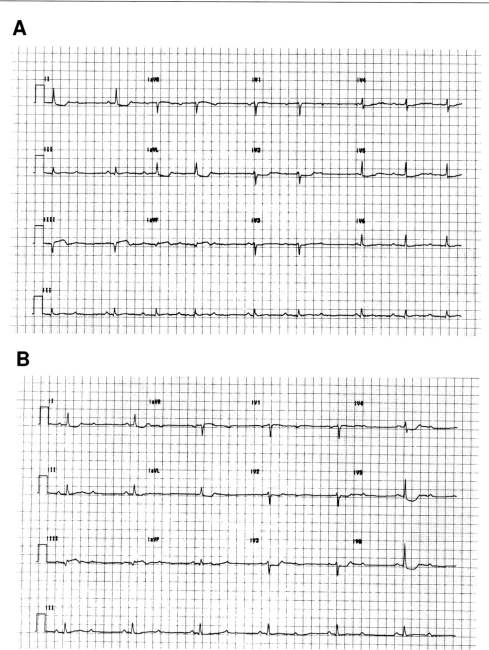

B

Fig. 20. Mobitz 1 2nd degree A-V block **(A)**, 2:1 A-V block **(B)**, and third-degree A-V block **(C)** in this patient with acute IMI. The ventricular escape rate in this case is relatively low for heart block related to IMI, but the QRS complex is narrow. Atropine improved A-V conduction.

MOBITZ II SECOND-DEGREE AND THIRD-DEGREE AV BLOCK

High-grade AV block is a more ominous sign in the setting of AMI. Mobitz II heart block occurs in less than 1% of patients with AMI *(124)*. Complete heart block (CHB, *see* Fig. 20, 21) complicated 11% of IMIs managed conservatively in the SPRINT study *(125)* and 13% of IMIs managed with thrombolytic therapy in the TAMI database

C

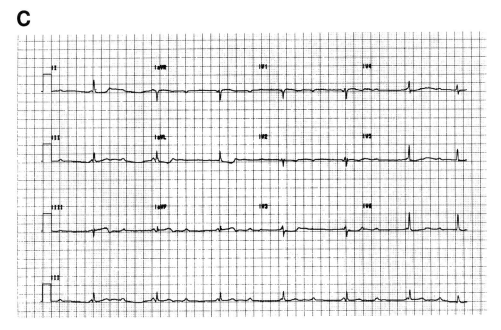

Fig. 20. (*Continued.*)

(126). The prevalence is likely higher when IMI is complicated by right ventricular infarction *(13,127,128)*. CHB in IMI is frequently transient; the median duration in the TAMI cohort was 2.5 h *(126)*. In the TIMI II study, there was a trend toward more second- and third-degree heart block in IMI patients who received iv beta-blockade *(129)*. Although patients with CHB had a higher in-hospital mortality, there was no difference in long-term follow-up in patients who survived until discharge. The incidence of CHB in anterior MI is approx 3.9%, although the in-hospital mortality is much higher than when CHB complicates IMI *(130)*. The long-term prognosis of hospital survivors remains unaffected. For both inferior and anterior MIs, it remains unclear whether CHB is an independent cause of poor in-hospital outcome or simply a marker for a large infarction. In IMI, in-hospital mortality is considerably higher in the setting of concomitant CHB and right ventricular infarction *(131)*.

The GUSTO experience with AV block was recently reported. The frequency of second- and third-degree AV block was 11.6% and 3.8% in patients with IMI and AMI, respectively. Patients with AV block had more AF, ventricular arrhythmias, and a substantially higher in-hospital mortality than patients without heart block. Only 2.1% of patients with second- or third-degree AV block received permanent pacemakers, confirming that AV block complicating AMI is usually transient *(132)*.

The pathophysiology and management of CHB differs in inferior and anterior MI (*see* Table 3). In IMI, block is typically intranodal; patients characteristically progress from first-degree to Mobitz I second-degree AV block before developing CHB (*see* Fig. 20). The escape rhythm is usually narrow, suggesting a focus in the proximal portion of the specialized conducting system. During the first 24 h of infarction, this is likely a manifestation of the Bezold-Jarisch reflex and therefore responds to atropine. CHB later in the course of an IMI usually may be caused by AV nodal ischemia, which

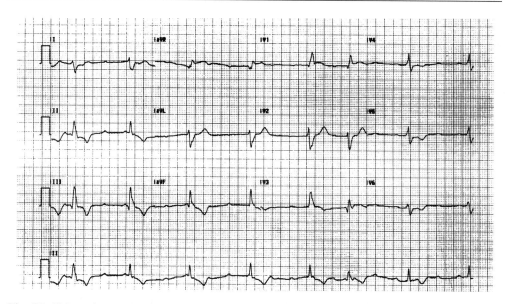

Fig. 21. This patient presented with antolateral MI, and bifascicular block. Complete heart block occurred; note that the escape focus has a wide QRS complex. A temporary transvenous pacer and eventually a permanent pacemaker were placed.

typically does not respond to atropine. Recent experimental evidence suggests that this late block may be mediated by adenosine at the cellular level; iv aminophylline, an adenosine antagonist, may improve such conduction disturbances *(133,134)*. Several series have been published in which iv aminophylline at doses of 5–7 mg/kg infused over 15–20 min has improved AV block late in the course of IMI *(133,134)*.

In anterior MI, block is usually within or below the bundle of His rather than within the AV node. The escape complex is generally wide, undependable, and poorly responsive to atropine. CHB usually develops in anterior MI patients who have previously displayed BBB rather than lower-grade AV block, as in IMI (*see* Fig. 21). In anterior MI, CHB usually results from proximal LAD occlusion, which causes ischemia/infarction in the infranodal conducting system. Thus, CHB is a marker of extensive infarction in the setting of anterior MI. Beta-blocker therapy should be discontinued in patients with high-grade AV block. If a pacemaker (temporary or permanent) is placed, however, beta-blocker therapy may be resumed, as the benefits of beta-blockade extend beyond the negative chronotropic effects and continuation of these protective effects is desirable.

Intraventricular Conduction Disturbances

Like AV block, intraventricular conduction disturbances (IVCDs) occur frequently during AMI *(135)*. More common in anterior than inferior MI, these defects reflect large infarctions, typically caused by proximal occlusions of the LAD coronary artery, and are associated with high in-hospital mortality *(136–138)*. The incidence of the various IVCDs and approximate rates of progression to CHB are noted in Table 4. Prethrombolytic-era studies suggest that left anterior fascicular block (LAFB) and left posterior fascicular block (LPFB) occur in 3–5% and 1–2% of AMI patients, respectively, and if isolated do not progress at high rates to CHB *(139)*. Right bundle-branch block (RBBB) occurs in approx 2–5% of cases of AMI *(136)*; approx 14–23% develop high-grade AV block *(136,140)*. In anterior but not inferior MI patients, RBBB is associated with CHF, CHB, and a high in-hospital mortality, although this excess mortality is present only in patients with RBBB who also manifest CHF *(141,142)*. There is also a high incidence of late VF in these patients *(18)*. More common than RBBB during AMI, left bundle-branch block (LBBB) progresses less frequently to CHB, but also connotes a high in-hospital mortality *(136)*. Patients with BBB and first-degree AV block are at higher risk *(140)*, and patients with alternating BBB (*see* Fig. 22) extremely high risk of progressing to CHB *(136)*. Finally, up to 50% of BBBs may actually be chronic and precede the index MI *(136)*. In this case, there is a greater chance of developing CHB in anterior but not inferior MI *(137)*.

Bifascicular block (RBBB with LAFB or LPFB, *see* Fig. 23) progresses at very high rates (27–34%) to CHB in the setting of anterior MI *(136,140)* and is associated with a very high in-hospital mortality. Bifascicular block with a prolonged PR interval is called "trifascicular block," because the prolonged PR interval may reflect delayed conduction in the "healthy" fascicle rather than in the AV node (*see* Fig. 24). Trifascicular block progresses in CHB in approx 38% of patients *(140)*. Beta-blocker therapy should be suspended in patients with bifascicular or trifascicular block pending temporary pacemaker placement.

More recent data from the National Registry of Myocardial Infarction 2 suggests that newer therapies of AMI may have modified these findings. The prevalence of RBBB and LBBB with AMI were 6.2% and 6.7%, respectively. Patients with BBB were older and were more likely to develop CHF than patients without BBB. In-hospital mortality was almost double in patients with BBB compared without BBB, but the rate of progression to second- or third-degree AV block was relatively low—6.1% and 4.4%—with RBBB and LBBB, respectively *(143)*.

Fewer data are available in patients treated with thrombolytic therapy. In GUSTO-I, the prevalence of RBBB and LBBB were 1.1% and 0.7%, respectively *(144)*. Patients with BBB had a higher incidence of VT/VF, AV block, and cardiogenic shock than patients without BBB; mortality was also substantially higher in these patients *(132)*. This probably reflects the fact that BBB occurs primarily in patients with large anterior MIs. In this trial, mortality was substantially higher with isolated RBBB or RBBB/LAFB than with LBBB. Permanent BBB was associated with a higher mortality than transient BBB.

Indications for Temporary Pacemaker During Acute MI

Indications for temporary pacemaker placement during AMI depend on the particular rhythm disturbance, hemodynamic consequence, and site of infarction (*see* Tables 3, 4). The availability of reliable temporary transcutaneous pacing has obviated the need for prophylactic transvenous pacing in some patients; in low-risk patients, a prophylactic transcutaneous system may be appropriate. Once a patient demonstrates a pacemaker dependence, however, a transvenous system should be placed. The risk of right ventricular perforation, infection, vascular complications, and bleeding must be carefully considered, especially in patients who have received thrombolytic and/or antithrombotic therapy.

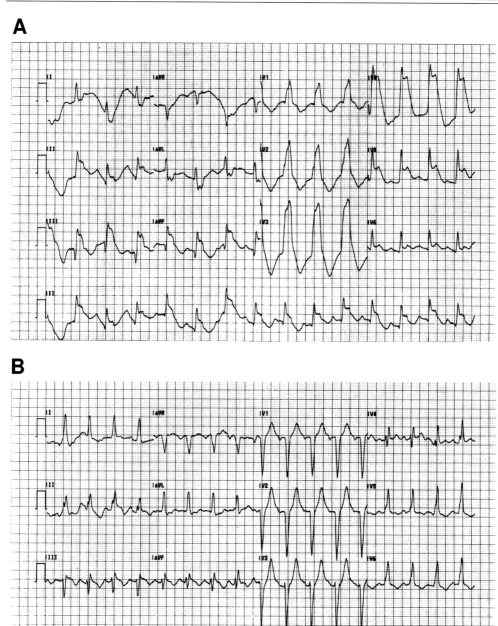

Fig. 22. This 71-yr-old female presented with massive anterolateral infarction. In panel A, there is RBBB and massive ST elevation ("tombstones"). After 2 h, a LBBB pattern was noted. The patient received a permanent pacemaker for alternating BBB.

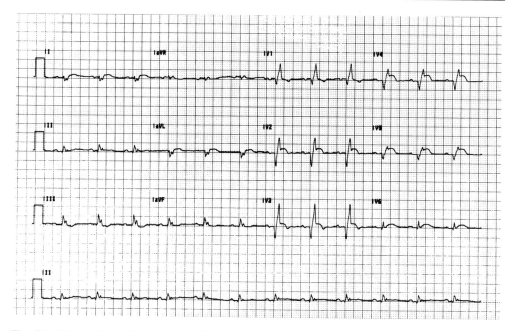

Fig. 23. This patient with anterolateral MI developed RBBB and LPFB. A temporary pacemaker was placed. Because of intermittent second-degree A-V block, a permanent pacemaker was implanted.

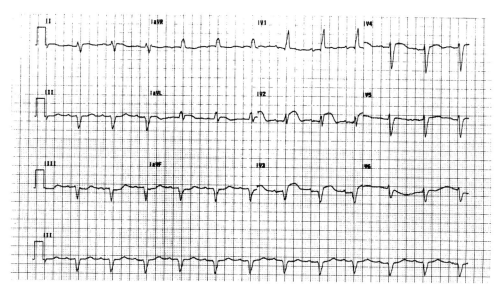

Fig. 24. This 75-yr-old male with anteroseptal MI developed RBBB, LAFB, and first-degree A-V block—so-called trifascicular block. Because the patient had received thrombolytic therapy, transcutaneous pacing pads were placed. No pacing was required over the next 72 h. Sustained monomorphic VT occurred 5 d post-MI, and a dual-chamber ICD was placed.

Indications for Permanent Pacemaker After MI

Clinical trial data are few regarding indications for permanent pacemaker implantation in patients with AMI *(145)*. A retrospective, nonrandomized multicenter study *(140)* suggested a better outcome when permanent pacemakers were placed in patients who have transient high-grade AV block and permanent BBB. The recently updated ACC/AHA task force AMI guidelines discuss indications for permanent pacing after AMI in detail *(2)*. Any patient with persistent, symptomatic sinus bradycardia or AV block should receive a permanent pacemaker (or ICD, if indicated) prior to discharge. The same is true of any patient with permanent second- or third-degree block at the level of the His-Purkinje system, as well as patients with permanent BBB and transient Mobitz II second-degree AV block or third-degree AV block. The utility of permanent pacing in asymptomatic patients with persistent second- or third-degree block at the AV nodal level (following IMI) has not been demonstrated, although there is frequently a reluctance to discharge patients in CHB without permanent pacemakers. In general, patients with evidence of tenuous infranodal conduction will probably benefit from permanent pacing. A limited electrophysiologic study (EPS) is reasonable if the level of conduction block is unclear from the clinical scenario.

POST-INFARCTION ARRHYTHMIA MANAGEMENT

VF and sustained VT occurring late (>48 h) in the course of an AMI suggest an ominous prognosis. Among 390 patients in a multicenter Dutch study, 49% had recurrent VT or VF over a mean follow-up period of 1.9 yr. Nineteen percent died because of recurrent VT or VF, and the total mortality during this period was 34% *(146)*. Thus, late ventricular arrhythmias during AMI suggest a high risk for arrhythmia recurrence.

As with VT and VF not temporarily related to AMI, the therapeutic approaches are the implantable cardioverter defibrillator (ICD) and antiarrhythmic therapy, primarily with amiodarone. No randomized studies comparing these treatment strategies have been performed in patients recovering from AMI. Nevertheless, extrapolation from the AVID *(147)*, CIDS *(148)*, and CASH *(149)* trials has led to increased ICD use in patients recovering from AMI. Few data exist to guide clinicians in the management of NSVT in the early post-MI setting. Two recent trials, MADIT *(150)* and MUSTT *(151)* showed a significant survival benefit in patients with prior infarct, decreased left ventricular function, NSVT, and inducible VT or VF at EPS when treated with ICDs. AMI patients were excluded from MADIT. Although 17% of the patients in MUSTT were enrolled within 1 mo of AMI, it is not known how many of these patients were enrolled during the AMI admission. Nevertheless, extrapolation from these clinical trials will probably make electrophysiology testing available to AMI patients with late NSVT, with ICD implantation if inducible. The results of the CABG Patch trial *(152)* suggest that revascularization may also be an important component in preventing sudden cardiac death in coronary patients.

Rigorous, placebo-controlled double-blind studies have been performed in patients with relatively low-grade VEA following AMI. Because asymptomatic VEA is associated with increased mortality following AMI *(153,154)*, the Cardiac Arrhythmia Suppression Trials (CAST) I and II were designed to determine whether expression of asymptomatic VEA would improve survival. Although encainide, flecainide *(155)*, and ethmozine *(156)* effectively suppressed VPBs, the trials were terminated prematurely because of excess mortality in the encainide and flecainide treatment arms and no possibility of reduced mortality in the ethmozine group. Several smaller studies using other type I drugs have shown either no benefit or an adverse effect *(157,158)*.

Amiodarone, on the other hand, may be of some benefit in post-infarct patients. In CAMIAT, patients with ventricular ectopy 6–45 d post-infarct were randomized to amiodarone or placebo. Amiodarone reduced the likelihood of SCD or resuscitated cardiac arrest, but had no effect on total mortality *(159)*. EMIAT, which enrolled infarct survivors with LVEF <40%, yielded similar results *(160)*. In a meta-analysis of these two trials and other studies of post-infarct and heart-failure patients, amiodarone was associated with a lower mortality than control patients *(161)*. In a randomized, placebo-controlled study involving 1456 post-infarct patients completed in 1980, there was a trend toward lower mortality in patients assigned to racemic sotalol *(162)*. More recently, however, enthusiasm has been dampened by the premature termination of the SWORD trial *(163)*. Post-MI patients randomized to D-sotalol, a pure type III agent, had a higher mortality than patients treated with placebo. Data are beginning to emerge regarding newer class III agents. Preliminary data suggests that dofetilide is mortality-neutral in post-MI patients (DIAMOND-MD) *(104)*, and a similar study utilizing azimilide is in progress (ALIVE) *(164)*.

The results of these trials have been transmitted quickly into clinical practice. The GISSI investigators noted that the use of antiarrhythmic agents in patients after AMI decreased by approx 50% between 1984 and 1994. Throughout this period, amiodarone was the most frequently prescribed agent, although its use diminished significantly during this period *(165)*.

POST-INFARCT ARRHYTHMIC RISK STRATIFICATION

Even patients whose MI course is unremarkable have a finite risk of malignant ventricular arrhythmias after hospital discharge. This risk is highest in the first year after MI. Thrombolytic therapy seems to reduce this risk; the rate of sudden cardiac death was only 1% at 6 mo in the GISSI-2 study *(166)* compared with a 5.4% rate of sudden cardiac death in the MILIS study *(167)*. Left ventricular dysfunction remains an important predictor of sudden cardiac death following AMI.

A number of strategies have been employed to identify patients at high risk for arrhythmic events. Sustained monomorphic VT (SMVT) induced at EPS is associated with a high arrhythmic event rate. In a study of 1209 survivors of uncomplicated AMI, Bourke and colleagues *(168)* noted that inducible VT carried a relative risk of 15-fold. The low event rate, however, made the positive predictive value only 30%, limiting the use of invasive EPS as a screening test. In the same study, LVEF < 40% carried a relative risk of 4.8-fold. Frequent VPBs and higher-grade ventricular ectopy on a predischarge Holter monitor also have been associated with a higher mortality among MI survivors, both in the prethrombolytic *(153)* and thrombolytic *(166)* eras. Patients with NSVT early post-MI and inducibility at EPS may benefit from ICD implantation, as in the MADIT and MUSTT trials. Finally, techniques including signal-averaged electrocardiography (SAECG), heart-rate variability (HRV), baroreflex sensitivity, and T-wave alternans (TWA) have been used to assess risk. Although thrombolytic therapy reduces the incidence of late potentials *(169)*, an abnormal SAECG remains associated with a higher incidence of arrhythmic events *(170,171)*. HRV reflects the relative contributions of sympathetic and parasympathetic tone *(172,173)*. Low HRV, indicative of decreased vagal tone, is a predictor of increased mortality in patients after MI *(174)*. A nonrandomized trial suggested that patients treated with thrombolytic therapy have higher HRV and a lower incidence of ventricular arrhythmia during follow-up than patients managed conservatively *(175)*. Baroceptor sensitivity also measures parasympathetic tone *(173)*. QT dispersion (QT_D), an index of regional heterogeneity of ventricular repolarization, may also help predict which patients are at risk for VT or VF after MI *(176)*. Detection of microvolt TWA may also reflect electrical instability and risk of ventricular arrhythmias in MI survivors *(177)*. Finally, an occluded infarct-related artery (IRA) may be associated with an increased risk of ventricular arrhythmias during follow-up *(178)*. Although these techniques need further investigation, it remains possible that a combination of these methods will be able to effectively identify a high-risk population *(179,180)*. The ongoing MADIT-2 study will assess whether severe left ventricular dysfunction alone is enough of a discriminant to select MI survivors who will benefit from an ICD *(181)*.

SUMMARY AND RECOMMENDATIONS

Currently, the only routine antiarrhythmic prophylaxis generally recommended is beta-blockade. In an overview of randomized trials evaluating oral beta-blocker therapy after MI, Yusuf and colleagues estimated a 30% reduction in the risk of sudden cardiac death *(36)*. This has been documented most definitively for timolol *(182)* and propranalol *(183)*. Thus, oral beta-blocker therapy is strongly recommended indefinitely in survivors of MI unless a contraindication exists *(184)*. Assessment for residual ischemia and, if warranted, coronary revascularization should be performed. While no relationship has been rigorously documented between long-term aspirin therapy after MI and recurrent arrhythmic events, aspirin or other antiplatelet therapy is recommended to all patients post-MI for its proven role in secondary prevention. ACE-inhibitors are recommended to any patients with significant left ventricular dysfunction, even if asymptomatic *(58,59)*. Aggressive use of HMG CoA reductase inhibitors is also recommended, given their proven role in preventing future coronary events. The results of MADIT and MUSTT suggest that routine Holter monitoring of AMI survivors with significant left ventricular dysfunction may be a reasonable strategy, with EPS if NSVT is detected. Finally, routine performance of EPS, SAECG, baroreflex sensitivity, or HRV in survivors of uncomplicated MIs is not recommended at this time unless part of a research protocol, as it remains unclear how best to use the results of these studies.

REFERENCES

1. Spann JF, Moellering RC, Haber E, Wheeler EO. Arrhythmias in acute myocardial infarction: a study utilizing an electrocardiographic monitor for automatic detection and recording arrhythmias. N Engl J Med 1964;271:427–431.
2. Ryan TJ, Antman EM, Brooks NH, et al. ACC/AHA guidelines for the management of patients with acute myocardial infarction: 1999 update: a report of the American College of Cardiology/American Heart Association Task Force on practice guidelines (Committee on management of acute myocardial infarction). Available at http://www.acc.org/clinical/guidelines and http://americanheart.org.
3. Weiss JN, Nademanee K, Stevenson WG, Singh B. Ventricular arrhythmias in ischemic heart disease. Ann Int Med 1991;114:784–797.
4. Clayton RH, Murray A, Higham PD, Campbell RWF. Self-terminating ventricular arrhythmias—a diagnostic dilemma. Lancet 1993;341:93–95.

5. Lawrie DM, Higgins MR, Godman MJ, et al. Ventricular fibrillation complicating acute myocardial infarction. Lancet 1968;2:523–528.

6. Volpi A, Cavalli A, Santoro L, et al. Incidence and prognosis of early primary ventricular fibrillation in acute myocardial infarction—results of the gruppo italiano per lo studio della sopravvivenza nell'infarcto miocardico (GISSI-2) database. Am J Cardiol 1998;82:265–271.

7. Tofler GH, Stone PH, Muller JE, et al. Prognosis after cardiac arrest due to ventricular tachycardia or ventricular fibrillation associated with acute myocardial infarction (The MILIS Study). Am J Cardiol 1987;60:755–761.

8. Goldberg RJ, Gore JM, Haffajee CI, Alpert JS, Dalen JE. Outcome after cardiac arrest during acute myocardial infarction. Am J Cardiol 1987;59:251–255.

9. Nicod P, Gilpin E, Dittrich, et al. Late clinical outcome in patients with early ventricular fibrillation after myocardial infarction. J Am Coll Cardiol 1988;11:464–470.

10. Behar S, Reicher-Riess H, Shecter M, et al. Frequency and prognostic significance of secondary ventricular fibrillation complicating acute myocardial infarction. Am J Cardiol 1993;71:152–156.

11. Brezens M, Elyassov S, Elimelech I, Raguin N. Comparison of patients with acute myocardial infarction with and without ventricular fibrillation. Am J Cardiol 1996;78:948–950.

12. Zehender M, Kasper W, Kauder E, et al. Right ventricular infarction as an independent predictor of prognosis after acute inferior myocardial infarction. N Engl J Med 1993;328:981–988.

13. Kinch JW, Ryan TJ. Right ventricular infarction. N Engl J Med 1994;330:1211–1217.

14. Volpi A, Maggioni A, Franziosi MG, Pampallona S, Mauri F, Tognoni G. In-hospital prognosis of patients with acute myocardial infarction complicated by primary ventricular fibrillation. N Engl J Med 1987;317:257–261.

15. Volpi A, Cavalli A, Santoro E, Tognoni G, and GISSI Investigators. Incidence and prognosis of secondary ventricular fibrillation in acute myocardial infarction. Circulation 1990;82:1279–1288.

16. Antman EM, Berlin JA. Declining incidence of ventricular fibrillation in myocardial infarction: implications for the prophylactic use of lidocaine. Circulation 1992;86:764–773.

17. Chiriboga D, Yarzebski J, Goldberg RJ, Gore JM, Alpert JS. Temporal trends (1975 through 1990) in the incidence and case-fatality rate of primary ventricular fibrillation complicating acute myocardial infarction—A communitywide perspective. Circulation 1994;89:998–1003.

18. Lie KI, Liem KL, Schuilenberg RM. Early identification of patients developing late in-hospital ventricular fibrillation after discharge from the coronary care unit: a 5.5 year retrospective study of 1897 patients. Am J Cardiol 1978;41:674–677.

19. Behar S, Goldbourt U, Reicher-Reiss H, Kaplinsky E, and the Principal Investigators of the SPRINT Study. Prognosis of acute myocardial infarction complicated by primary ventricular fibrillation. Am J Cardiol 1990;66:1208–1211.

20. Volpi A, Cavali A, Franzosi MG, et al. One year prognosis of primary ventricular fibrillation complicating acute myocardial infarction. Am J Cardiol 1989;63:1174–1178.

21. Lie KI, Wellens HJ, van Capelle FJ, Durrer D. Lidocaine in the prevention of primary ventricular fibrillation. N Engl J Med 1974;291:1324–1326.

22. DeSilva RA, Lown B, Hennekens CH, Casscells W. Lignocaine prophylaxis in acute myocardial infarction: an evaluation of randomised trials. Lancet 1981;2:855–858.

23. MacMahon S, Collins R, Peto R, Koster RW, Yusuf S. Effects of prophylactic lidocaine in suspected acute myocardial infarction: an overview of results from the randomized controlled trials. JAMA 1988;260:1910–1916.

24. Hine LK, Laird N, Hewitt P, Chalmers TC. Meta-analytic evidence against prophylactic use of lidocaine in acute myocardial infarction. Arch Int Med 1989;149:2694–2698.

25. Sadowski ZP, Alexander JH, Skrabucha B, et al. Multicenter randomized trial and a systematic overview of lidocaine in acute myocardial infarction. Am Heart J 1999;137:792–798.

26. Alexander JH, Granger CB, Sadowski Z, et al. Prophylactic lidocaine in use in acute myocardial infarction: incidence and outcomes from two international trials. Am Heart J 1999;137:799–805.

27. Koster RW, Dunning AJ. Intramuscular lidocaine for prevention of lethal arrhythmias in the prehospital phase of acute myocardial infarction. N Engl J Med 1985;313:1105–1110.

28. Velentine PA, Frew JL, Mashford ML, Sloman JG. Lidocaine in the prevention of sudden death in the pre-hospital phase of acute myocardial infarction: a double-blind study. N Engl J Med 1974; 291:1327–1331.

29. Bernsten RF, Rasmussen K. Lidocaine to prevent ventricular fibrillation in the prehospital phase of

suspected acute myocardial infarction: the North-Norwegian Lidocaine Intervention Trial. Am Heart J 1992;124:1478–1483.

30. Dunn HM, McComb JM, Kinney CD, et al. Prophylactic lidocaine in the early phase of suspected myocardial infarction. Am Heart J 1985;110:353–362.

31. Lie KI, Liem KL, Louridtz WJ, Janse MJ, Willebrands AF, Durrer D. Efficacy of lidocaine in preventing primary ventricular fibrillation within 1 hour after a 300 mg intramuscular injection. Am J Cardiol 1978;42:486–488.

32. Lie KI, Wellens HJJ, Downar E, Durrer D. Observations on patients with primary ventricular fibrillation complicating acute myocardial infarction. Circulation 1975;52:755–759.

33. El-Sharif N, Myerburg RJ, Scherlag BJ, et al. Electrocardiographic antecedents of primary ventricular fibrillation: value of the R-on-T phenomenon in myocardial infarction. Br Heart J 1976;38:415–422.

34. Ayanian JZ, Hauptman PJ, Guadagnoli E, et al. Knowledge and practice of generalist and specialist physicians regarding drug therapy for acute myocardial infarction. N Engl J Med 1994;331:1136–1142.

35. Elizari MV, Martinez JM, Belziti, et al. Morbidity and mortality following early administration of amiodarone in acute myocardial infarction. Eur Heart J 2000;21:198–205.

36. Yusuf S, Peto R, Lewis J, Collins R, Sleight P. Beta-blockade during and after myocardial infarction: an overview of the randomized trials. Prog Cardiovasc Dis 1985;27:335–371.

37. Norris RM, Brown MA, Clark ED, Barnaby PF, Geary GG, Logan RL. Prevention of ventricular fibrillation during acute myocardial infarction by intravenous propranalol. Lancet 1984;2:883–886.

38. Rydén L, Ariniego R, Arnman K, et al. A double-blind trial of metoprolol in acute myocardial infarction: effects on ventricular tachyarrhythmias. N Engl J Med 1983;308:614–618.

39. Yusuf S, Sleight P, Rossi P, et al. Reduction in infarct size, arrhythmias and chest pain by early intravenous beta blockade in suspected acute myocardial infarction. Circulation 1983;67(Suppl I): I-32–I-41.

40. ISIS-1 Collaborative Group. Randomised trial of intravenous atenolol among 16,027 cases of suspected acute myocardial infarction: ISIS-1. Lancet 1986;2:57–66.

41. Rapaport E. Should β-blockers be given immediately and concomitantly with thrombolytic therapy in acute myocardial infarction? Circulation 1991;83:695–697.

42. Kennedy HL, Rosenson RS. Physician use of beta-adrenergic blocking therapy: a changing perspective. J Am Coll Cardiol 1995;26:547–552.

43. ISIS-4 Collaborative Group. ISIS-4: A randomized factorial trial assessing early oral captopril, oral mononitrate, and intravenous magnesium sulphate in 58 050 patients with suspected acute myocardial infarction. Lancet 1995;345:669–685.

44. Rogers WJ, Bowlby LJ, Chandra NC, et al. Treatment of myocardial infarction in the United States (1990 to 1993): Observations from the National Registry of Myocardial Infarction. Circulation 1994;90:2103–2114.

45. Roberts R, Rogers WJ, Mueller HS, et al. Immediate versus deferred β-blockade following thrombolytic therapy in patients with acute myocardial infarction: results of the thrombolysis in myocardial infarction (TIMI) II-B Study. Circulation 1991;83:422–437.

46. Van de Werf F, Janssens L, Brzostek T, et al. Short-term effects of early intravenous treatment with a beta-adrenergic blocker or a specific bradycardic agent in patients with acute myocardial infarction receiving thrombolytic therapy. J Am Coll Cardiol 1993;22:407–416.

47. Pfisterer ME, Cox JL, Granger CB, et al. Atenolol use and clinical outcomes after thrombolysis for acute myocardial infarction: the GUSTO-I Experience. J Am Coll Cardiol 1998;32:634–640.

48. Becker RC. Beta-adrenergic blockade following thrombolytic therapy: is it harmful or helpful? Clin Cardiol 1994;17:171–174.

49. Kafka H, Langeuin L, Armstrong PW. Serum magnesium and potassium in acute myocardial infarction: influence on ventricular arrhythmias. Arch Intern Med 1987;147:465–469.

50. Nordrehaug JE, von der Lippe G. Hypokalemia and ventricular fibrillation in acute myocardial infarction. Br Heart J 1983;50:525–529.

51. Nordrehaug JE, Johannessen K-A, von der Lippe G. Serum potassium concentration as a risk factor of ventricular arrhythmias early in acute myocardial infarction. Circulation 1985;71:645–649.

52. Higham PD. Serum magnesium and ventricular fibrillation after myocardial infarction. Cardiovasc Res Rev 1994;11:15–16, 18–19.

53. Horner SM. Efficacy of intravenous magnesium in acute myocardial infarction in reducing arrhythmias

and morbidity: meta-analysis of magnesium in acute myocardial infarction. Circulation 1992;86:774–779.

54. Woods KL, Fletcher S, Roffe C, Haider Y. Intravenous magnesium sulphate in suspected acute myocardial infarction: results of the second Leicester Intravenous Magnesium Intervention Trial (LIMIT-2). Lancet 1992;339:1553–1558.

55. Woods KL, Fletcher S. Long-term outcome after intravenous magnesium sulphate in suspected acute myocardial infarction: the second Leicester Intravenous Magnesium Intervention Trial (LIMIT-2). Lancet 1994;343:816–819.

56. Antman EM. Randomized trials of magnesium in acute myocardial infarction: big numbers do not tell the whole story. Am J Cardiol 1995;75:391–393.

57. Shechter M, Hod H, Kaplinsky E, Chouraqui P, Rabinowitz B. Magnesium as alternate therapy in patients with acute myocardial infarction who are not candidates for thrombolytic therapy. Am J Cardiol 1995;75:321–323.

58. Pfeffer MA, Braunwald E, Moye LA, et al. Effects of captopril on mortality and morbidity in patients with left ventricular dysfunction after myocardial infarction. N Engl J Med 1992;327:669–677.

59. Domanski MJ, Exner DV, Borkowf CB, et al. Effect of angiotensin converting enzyme inhibition on sudden cardiac death in patients following acute myocardial infarction: a meta-analysis of randomized clinical trials. J Am Coll Cardiol 1999;33:598–604.

60. Sogaard P, Gotzsche C-O, Ravkilde J, Norgaard A, Thygesen K. Ventricular arrhythmias in the acute and chronic phases after acute myocardial infarction: effect of intervention with captopril. Circulation 1994;90:101–107.

61. Kloner RA. Does reperfusion injury exist in humans? J Amer Coll Cardiol 1993;21:537–545.

62. GISSI Investigators. Effectiveness of intravenous thrombolytic treatment in acute myocardial infarction. Lancet 1986;1:397–402.

63. ISIS-2 Collaborative Group. Randomised trial of intravenous streptokinase, oral aspirin, both, or neither among 17,187 cases of suspected acute myocardial infarction: ISIS-2. Lancet 1988;2:249–360.

64. Solomon SD, Ridker PM, Antman EM. Ventricular arrhythmias in trials of thrombolytic therapy for acute myocardial infarction: a meta-analysis. Circulation 1993;88:2575–2581.

65. Boissel J-P, Castaigne A, Mercier C, et al. Ventricular fibrillation following administration of thrombolytic treatment: The EMIP experience. Eur Heart J 1996;17:213–221.

66. Grines CL, Browne KF, Marco J, et al. A comparison of immediate angioplasty with thrombolytic therapy for acute myocardial infarction. N Engl J Med 1993;328:673–679.

67. Singh BN. Routine prophylactic lidocaine administration in acute myocardial infarction: an idea whose time has come and gone? Circulation 1992;86:1033–1035.

68. Hargarten KM, Stueven HA, Waite EM, et al. Prehospital experience with defibrillation of coarse ventricular fibrillation: a ten-year review. Ann Emery Med 1990;19:157–162.

69. Guidelines 2000 for cardiopulmonary resuscitation and emergency cardiac care. Circulation 2000;102(Suppl I): I1–I384.

70. Haynes RE, Chinn TL, Copass MK, Cobb LA. Comparison of bretylium tosylate and lidocaine in management of out of hospital ventricular fibrillation: a randomized clinical trial. Am J Cardiol 1981;48:353–356.

71. Olson DW, Thompson BM, Darin JC, Milbrath MH. A randomised comparison study of bretylium tosylate and lidocaine in resuscitation of patients from out-of-hospital ventricular fibrillation in a paramedic system. Ann Emerg Med 1984;13:807–810.

72. Feely J, Wilkinson GR, McAllister CB, Wood AJJ. Increased toxicity and reduced clearance of lidocaine by cimetidine. Ann Int Med 1982;96:592–594.

73. Branch RA, Shand DG, Wilkinson GR, Nies AS. The reduction of lidocaine clearance by DL-propranolol: an example of haemodynamic drug interaction. J Pharmacol Exp Ther 1973;184:515–519.

74. Bacaner MB. Treatment of ventricular fibrillation and other acute arrhythmias with bretylium tosylate. Am J Cardiol 1968;21:530–543.

75. Heissenbuttel RH, Bigger TJ. Bretylium tosylate: a newly available antiarrhythmic drug for ventricular arrhythmias. Ann Int Med 1979;91:229–238.

76. Desai AD, Chun S, Sung RJ. The role of intravenous amiodarone in the management of cardiac arrhythmias. Ann Intern Med 1997;127:294–303.

77. Kudenchuk PJ, Cobb LA, Copass MK, et al. Amiodarone for resuscitation after out-of-hospital cardiac arrest due to ventricular fibrillation. N Engl J Med 1999;341:871–878.

78. Anastasiou-Nana MI, Nanas JN, Nanas SN, et al. Effects of amiodarone on refractory ventricular fibrillation in myocardial infarction: experimental study. J Am Coll Cardiol 1994;23:253–258.

79. Wolfe CL, Nibley C, Bhandari A, Chatterjee K, Scheinman M. Polymorphous ventricular tachycardia associated with acute myocardial infarction. Circulation 1991;84:1543–1551.

80. Eldar M, Sievner Z, Goldbourt U, et al. Primary ventricular tachycardia in acute myocardial infarction: clinical characteristics and mortality. Ann Int Med 1992;117:31–36.

81. Mont L, Cinca J, Blanch P, et al. Predisposing factors and prognostic value of sustained monomorphic ventricular tachycardia in the early phase of acute myocardial infarction. J Am Coll Cardiol 1996; 28:1670–1676.

82. de Soyza N, Meacham D, Murphy ML, Kane JJ, Doherty JE, Bissett. Evaluation of warning arrhythmias before paroxysmal ventricular tachycardia during acute myocardial infarction in man. Circulation 1979;60:814–818.

83. de Soyza N, Bissett JK, Kane JJ, Murphy ML, Doherty JE. Association of accelerated idioventricular rhythm and paroxysmal ventricular tachycardia in acute myocardial infarction. Am J Cardiol 1974; 34:667–670.

84. Cheema AN, Shehu K, Parker M, Kadish AH, Goldberger JL. Nonsustained ventricular tachycardia in the setting of acute myocardial infarction: tachycardia characteristics and their prognostic significance. Circulation 1998;98:2030–2036.

85. Josephson ME. Clin Cardiac Electrophysiol. Lea & Febiger, Philadelphia, PA 1993, 622–623.

86. Bhaskaran A, Seth A, Kumar A, et al. Coronary angioplasty for the control of intractable ventricular arrhythmia. Clin Cardiol 1995;18:480–483.

87. The ISAM Study Group. A prospective trial of Intravenous Streptokinase in Acute Myocardial infarction (ISAM): Mortality, morbidity, and infarct size at 21 days. N Engl J Med 1986;314:1465–1471.

88. Wilcox RG, Eastgate J, Harrison E, Skene AM. Ventricular arrhythmia during treatment with alteplase (recombinant tissue plasminogen activator) in suspected acute myocardial infarction. Br Heart J 1991;65:4–8.

89. Solomon SD, Antman EM. Prehospital thrombolytic therapy in patients with suspected myocardial infarction (letter). N Engl J Med 1994;330:291.

90. Krumholz HM, Goldberger AL. Reperfusion arrhythmias after thrombolysis: electrophysiologic tempest, or much ado about nothing. Chest 1991;99(Suppl):135S–140S.

91. Gorgels APM, Vos MA, Letsch IS, et al. Usefulness of the accelerated idioventricular rhythm as a marker for myocardial necrosis and reperfusion during thrombolytic therapy in acute myocardial infarction. Am J Cardiol 1988;61:231–235.

92. Califf RM, O'Neill W, Stack RS, et al. Failure of simple clinical measurements to predict perfusion status after intravenous thrombolysis. Ann Int Med 1988;108:658–662.

93. DeSanctis RW, Block P, Hunter AM. Tachyarrhythmias in myocardial infarction. Circulation 1972;45:681–702.

94. Crimm A, Severance HW, Coffey K, McKinnis R, Wagner GS, Califf RM. Prognostic significance of isolated sinus tachycardia during the first three days of acute myocardial infarction. Am J Med 1984;76:983–988.

95. Behar S, Zahavi Z, Goldbourt U, Reicher-Reiss H, and the SPRINT Study Group. Long-term prognosis of patients with paroxysmal atrial fibrillation complicating acute myocardial infarction. Eur Heart J 1992;13:45–50.

96. Goldberg RJ, Seeley D, Becker RC, et al. Impact of atrial fibrillation on the in-hospital and long-term survival of patients with acute myocardial infarction: a community-wide perspective. Am Heart J 1990;119:996–1001.

97. Rathore SS, Berger AK, Weinfurt KP, et al. Acute myocardial infarction complicated by atrial fibrillation in the elderly: prevalence and outcomes. Circulation 2000;101:969–974.

98. Serrano CV, Ramires JAF, Mansur AP, Pileggi F. Importance of the time of onset of supraventricular tachyarrhythmias on prognosis of patients with acute myocardial infarction. Clin Cardiol 1995; 18:84–90.

99. Sugiura T, Takahashi N, Nakamura S, et al. Atrial fibrillation in inferior Q-wave acute myocardial infarction. Am J Cardiol 1991;67:1135–1136.

100. Nielsen FE, Andersen HH, Gram-Hansen P, Sørensen HT, Klausen IC. The relationships between ECG signs of atrial infarction and the development of supraventricular arrhythmias in patients with acute myocardial infarction. Am Heart J 1992;123:69–72.

101. Hod H, Lew AS, Keltai M, et al. Early atrial fibrillation during evolving myocardial infarction: a consequence of impaired left atrial perfusion. Circulation 1987;75:146–150.

102. Crenshaw BS, Ward SR, Granger CB, et al. Atrial fibrillation in the setting of acute myocardial infarction: the GUSTO-I experience. J Am Coll Cardiol 1997;30:406–413.

103. Cowan JC, Gardiner P, Reid DS, Newell DJ, Campbell RWF. A comparison of amiodarone and digoxin in the treatment of atrial fibrillation complicating acute myocardiovasc infarction. J Cardiac Pharmacol 1986;8:252–256.

104. Kober L, the Diamond Study Group. A clinical trial of dofetilide in patients with acute myocardial infarction and left ventricular dysfunction. The Diamond MI study. Circulation 1998;98:1–93.

105. Ganz LI, Friedman PL. Supraventricular tachycardia. N Engl J Med 1995;332:162–173.

106. Mehta D, Ward DE, Wafa S, Camm AJ. Relative efficacy of various physical manoeuvres in the termination of junctional tachycardia. Lancet 1988;1:1181–1185.

107. Möller B, Ringqvist C. Metoprolol in the treatment of supraventricular tachyarrhythmias. Ann Clin Res 1979;11:34–41.

108. Konecke LL, Knoebel SB. Nonparoxysmal junctional tachycardia complicating acute myocardial infarction. Circulation 1972;45:367–374.

109. Fishenfeld J, Desser KB, Benchimol A. Non-paroxysmal A-V junctional tachycardia associated with acute myocardial infarction. Am Heart J 1973;86:754–758.

110. Mangrum JM, DiMarco JP. The evaluation and management of bradycardia. N Engl J Med 2000; 342:703–709.

111. Scheinman MM, Gonzalez RP. Fascicular block in acute myocardial infarction. JAMA 1980; 244:2646–2649.

112. Lown B, Klein MD, Hershberg PI. Coronary and precoronary care. Am J Med 1969;46:705–724.

113. Adgey AAJ, Mulholland HC, Geddes JS, Keegan DAJ, Pantridge JF. Incidence, significance, and management of early bradyarrhythmia complicating acute myocardial infarction. Lancet 1968;2:1097–1101.

114. Rotman M, Wagner GS, Wallace AG. Bradyarrhythmias in acute myocardial infarction. Circulation 1972;45:703–722.

115. Webb S, Adgey AAJ, Pantridge JF. Autonomic dysfunction at onset of acute myocardial infarction. Br Med J 1972;3:89–92.

116. Koren G, Weiss AT, Ben-David J, Hasin Y, Luria MH, Gotsman MS. Bradycardia and hypotension following reperfusion with streptokinase (Bezold-Jarisch reflex): a sign of coronary thrombolysis and myocardial salvage. Am Heart J 1986;112:468–471.

117. Thames MD, Klopfenstein HS, Abboud FM, Allyn ML, Walker JL. Preferential distribution of inhibitory cardiac receptors with vagal afferents to the inferoposterior wall of the left ventricle during coronary occlusion in the dog. Circ Res 1978;43:512–519.

118. Norris RM, Mercer CJ, Yeater SE. Sinus rate in acute myocardial infarction. Br Heart J 1972;34:901–904.

119. Come PC, Pitt B. Nitroglycerin-induced severe hypotension and bradycardia in patients with acute myocardial infarction. Circulation 1976;54:624–628.

120. Kottmeier CA, Gravenstein JS. The parasympathomimetic activity of atropine and atropine methylbromide. Anesthesiology 1968;29:1125–1133.

121. Massimi RA, Mason DT, Amsterdam EA, et al. Ventricular fibrillation after intravenous atropine for treatment of bradycardias. N Engl J Med 1972;287:336–338.

122. Cooper MJ, Abinader EG. Atropine-induced ventricular fibrillation: case report and review of the literature. Am Heart J 1979;97:225–228.

123. Johansson BW. Atrioventricular and bundle branch block in acute myocardial infarction: natural history and prognosis. In: Meltzer LE, Dunning AJ, eds. Textbook of Coronary Care. The Charles Press Publishers, Inc., MD, 1972, pp. 328–340.

124. Bhandari AK, Sager PT. Management of peri-infarctional ventricular arrhythmias and conduction disturbances. In: Naccarelli GV, ed. Cardiac Arrhythmias: A Practical Approach. Futura Publishing Company, Inc., Mount Kisco, N.Y., 1991, pp. 283–324.

125. Behar S, Zissman E, Zion M, et al. Complete atrioventricular block complicating inferior wall myocardial infarction: short and long-term prognosis. Am Heart J 1993;125:1622–1627.

126. Clemmensen P, Bates ER, Califf RM, et al. Complete atrioventricular block complicating inferior wall acute myocardial infarction treated with reperfusion therapy. Am J Cardiol 1991;67:225–230.

127. Braat SH, de Zwaan C, Brugada P, Loenegracht JM, Wellens HJJ. Right ventricular involvement

with acute inferior myocardial infarction identifies high risk of developing atrioventricular nodal conduction disturbances. Am Heart J 1984;107:1183–1187.

128. Zehender M, Kasper W, Kauder E, et al. Right ventricular infarction as an independent predictor of prognosis after acute inferior myocardial infarction. N Engl J Med 1993;328:981–988.

129. Berger PB, Ruoccona NA, Ryan TJ, et al. Incidence and prognostic implications of heart block complicating inferior myocardial infarction treated with thrombolytic therapy: results from TIMI II. J Am Coll Cardiol 1992;20:533–540.

130. Goldberg RJ, Zevallos JC, Yarzebski, et al. Prognosis of acute myocardial infarction complicated by complete heart block (the Worcester Heart Attack Study). Am J Cardiol 1992;69:1135–1141.

131. Mavric Z, Zaputovic L, Matana A, et al. Prognostic significance of complete atrioventricular block in patients with acute inferior myocardial infarction with and without right ventricular involvement. Am Heart J 1990;119:823–828.

132. Simons GR, Sgarbossa E, Wagner G, et al. Atrioventricular and intraventricular conduction disorders in acute myocardial infarction: a reappraisal in the thrombolytic era. PACE 1998;2651–2663.

133. Shah PK, Peter T. Atropine resistant post infarction complete AV block: Possible role of adenosine and improvement with aminophylline. Am Heart J 1987;113:194–195.

134. Strasgerg B, Bassevich R, Mager A, Kusniec J, Sagie A, Sclarovsky S. Effects of aminophylline on atrioventricular conduction in patients with late atrioventricular block during inferior wall acute myocardial infarction. Am J Cardiol 1991;67:527–528.

135. Ip JH. Intraventricular conduction disturbances in patients with acute myocardial infarction: indications for a temporary pacemaker. Cardiovasc Res Rev 1990;46–48.

136. Klein RC, Vera Z, Mason DT. Intraventricular conduction defects in acute myocardial infarction: incidence, prognosis, and therapy. Am Heart J 1984;108:1007–1013.

137. Hollander G, Nadiminti V, Lichstein E, Greengart A, Sanders M. Bundle branch block in acute myocardial infarction. Am Heart J 1983;105:738–743.

138. Hindman MC, Wagner GS, JaRo M, et al. The clinical significance of bundle branch block complicating acute myocardial infarction: 1. Clinical characteristics, hospital mortality, and one-year follow-up. Circulation 1978;58:679–688.

139. Antman EM, Braunwald E. Acute myocardial infarction. In: Braunwald E, Zipes DP, Libby P. eds. Heart Disease 6th ed. Philadelphia: W.B. Saunders, 2001, pp. 114–1231.

140. Hindman MC, Wagner GS, JaRo M, et al. The clinical significance of bundle branch block complicating acute myocardial infarction: 2. Indications for temporary and permanent pacemaker insertion. Circulation 1978;58:689–699.

141. Ricou F, Nicod P, Gilpin E, Henning H, Ross J. Influence of right bundle branch block on short- and long-term survival after acute anterior myocardial infarction. J Am Coll Cardiol 1991;17:858–863.

142. Ricou F, Nicod P, Gilpin E, Henning H, Ross J. Influence of right bundle branch block on short- and long-term survival after inferior Q-wave myocardial infarction. Am J Cardiol 1991;67:1143–1146.

143. Go AS, Barron HV, Rundle AC, et al. Bundle-branch block and in-hospital mortality in acute myocardial infarction. Ann Intern Med 1998;129:690–697.

144. Sgarbossa EB, Pinski SL, Topol EJ, et al. Acute myocardial infarction and complete bundle branch block at hospital admission: clinical characteristics and outcome in the thrombolytic era. J Am Coll Cardiol 1998;31:105–110.

145. Lieberman EH, Aude YW. Permanent cardiac pacing after acute myocardial infarction. Cardiovasc Electrophysiol Rev 1999;2:377–380.

146. Willems AR, Tijssen JG, van Capelle FJL, et al. Determinants of prognosis in symptomatic ventricular tachycardia or ventricular fibrillation late after myocardial infarction. J Am Coll Cardiol 1990;16:521–530.

147. The AVID Investigators. A comparison of antiarrhythmic-drug therapy with implantable defibrillators in patients resuscitated from near-fatal ventricular arrhythmias. N Engl J Med 1998;337:1576–1583.

148. Connolly SJ, Gent M, Roberts RS, et al. Canadian implantable defibrillator study (CIDS): A randomized trial of the implantable cardioverter defibrillator against amiodarone. Circulation 2000;101:1297–1302.

149. Kuck KH, Cappato R, Siebels J, et al. Randomized comparison of antiarrhythmic drug therapy with implantable defibrillators in patients resuscitated from cardiac arrest. The Cardiac Arrest Study Hamburg (CASH). Circulation 2000;102:748–754.

150. Moss AJ, Hall WJ, Cannom D, et al. Improved survival with an implanted defibrillator in patients with coronary disease at high risk for ventricular arrhythmias. N Engl J Med 1996;335:1933–1940.

151. Buxton AE, Fisher JD, Lee KL, et al. A randomized study of the prevention of sudden death in patients with coronary artery disease. N Engl J Med 1999;341:1882–1890.

152. Bigger JT. Prophylactic use of implanted cardiac defibrillators at high risk for ventricular arrhythmias after coronary-bypass graft surgery. N Engl J Med 1997;337:1569–1575.

153. Bigger JT, Fleiss JL, Kleiger R, Miller JP, Rolnitzky LM, and the Multicenter Post-Infarction Research Group. The relationships between ventricular arrhythmias, left ventricular dysfunction, and mortality in the 2 years after myocardial infarction. Circulation 1984;69:250–258.

154. Hallstrom AP, Bigger JT Jr, Roden D, et al. Prognostic significance of ventricular premature depolarizations measured one year after myocardial infarction in patients with early postinfarction ventricular arrhythmia. J Am Coll Cardiol 1992;20:259–264.

155. Echt DS, Liebson PR, Mitchell LB, et al. Mortality and morbidity in patients receiving encainide, flecainide, or placebo: The Cardiac Arrhythmia Suppression Trial. N Engl J Med 1991;324:782–788.

156. The Cardiac Arrhythmia Suppression Trial II Investigators. Effect of the antiarrhythmic agent moricizine on survival after myocardial infarction. N Engl J Med 1992;327:227–233.

157. Hine LK, Laird NM, Hewitt P, Chalmers TC. Meta-analysis of empirical long-term antiarrhythmic therapy after acute myocardial infarction. JAMA 1989;262:3037–3040.

158. Teo KT, Yusuf S, Furberg CD. Effects of prophylactic antiarrhythmic drug therapy in acute myocardial infarction: an overview of results from randomized controlled trials. JAMA 1993;270:1589–1595.

159. Cairns JA, Connolly SJ, Roberts R, Gent M. Randomised trial of outcome after myocardial infarction in patients with frequent or repetitive ventricular premature depolarisations: CAMIAT. Lancet 1997;349:675–682.

160. Julian DG, Camm AJ, Frangin G, et al. Randomised trial of effect of amiodarone on mortality in patients with left-ventricular dysfunction after recent myocardial infarction. EMIAT. Lancet 1997;349:667–674.

161. Amiodarone Trials Meta-Analysis Investigators. Effect of prophylactic amiodarone on mortality after acute myocardial infarction and in congestive heart failure: meta-analysis of individual data from 6500 patients in randomised trials. Lancet 1997;350:1417–1424.

162. Julian DG, Jackson FS, Prescott RJ, Szekely P. Controlled trial of sotalol for one year after myocardial infarction. Lancet 1982;1:1142–1147.

163. Waldo AL, Camm AJ, de Ruyter H, et al. Effect of d-sotalol on mortality in patients with left ventricular dysfunction after recent and remote myocardial infarction. Lancet 1996;348:7–12.

164. Camm AJ, Karam R, Pratt CM. The azimilide post-infarct survival trial evaluation (ALIVE). Am J Cardiol 1998;81:35D–39D.

165. Avanzini F, Latini R, Maggioni A, et al. Antiarrhythmic drug prescription in patients after myocardial infarction in the last decade: experience of the Gruppo Italiano per lo Studio della Sopravvivenza nell'Infarcto miocardio (GISSI). Arch Intern Med 1995;155:1041–1045.

166. Maggiona AP, Zuanetta G, Franzosi MG, et al. Prevalence and prognostic significance of ventricular arrhythmias after acute myocardial infarction in the thrombolytic era. Circulation 1993;87:312–322.

167. Mukharji J, Rude RE, Poole K, et al. Risk factors for sudden death after acute myocardial infarction: two year follow-up. Am J Cardiol 1984;54:31–36.

168. Bourke JP, Richards DAB, Ross DL, Wallace EM, McGuire MA, Other JB. Routine programmed electrical stimulation in survivors of acute myocardial infarction for prediction of spontaneous ventricular tachyarrhythmias during follow-up: results, optimal stimulation protocol, and cost-effective screening. J Am Coll Cardiol 1991;18:780–788.

169. Gang ES, Lew AS, Hong M, Wang F, Siebert CA, Peter T. Decreased incidence of ventricular late potentials after successful thrombolytic therapy for acute myocardial infarction. N Engl J Med 1989;321:712–716.

170. Pedretti R, Laporta A, Etro MD, et al. Influence of thrombolysis on signal-averaged electrocardiogram and late arrhythmic events after acute myocardial infarction. Am J Cardiol 1992;69:866–872.

171. McClements BM, Adgey AAJ. Value of signal-averaged electrocardiography, radionuclide ventriculography, Holter monitoring and clinical variables for prediction of arrhythmic events in survivors of acute myocardial infarction in the thrombolytic era. J Am Coll Cardiol 1993;21:1419–1427.

172. Hayano J, Sakakibara Y, Yamada M, et al. Accuracy of assessment of cardiac vagal tone by heart rate variability. Am J Cardiol 1991;67:199–204.

173. Kjellgren O, Gomes JA. Heart rate variability and baroreflex sensitivity in myocardial infarction. Am Heart J 1993;125:204–215.

174. Kleiger RE, Miller JP, Bigger JT, Moss AJ, and the Multicenter Post-Infarction Research Group.

Decreased heart rate variability and its association with increased mortality after acute myocardial infarction. Am J Cardiol 1987;59:256–262.

175. Pedretti RF, Colombo E, Braga SS, Caru B. Effect of thrombolysis on heart rate variability and life-threatening ventricular arrhythmias in survivors of acute myocardial infarction. J Am Coll Cardiol 1994;23:19–26.

176. Perkiomaki JS, Koistinen MJ, Yli-Mayry S, Huikuri HV. Dispersion of QT interval in patients with and without susceptibility to ventricular tachyarrhythmia after previous myocardial infarction. J Am Coll Cardiol 1995;26:174–179.

177. Rosenbaum DS, Jackson LE, Smith JM, Garan H, Ruskin JN, Cohen RJ. Electrical alternans and vulnerability to ventricular arrhythmias. N Engl J Med 1994;330:235–241.

178. Hohnloser SH, Franck P, Klingenheber T, Zabel M, Just H. Open infarct artery, late potentials, and other prognostic factors in patients after acute myocardial infarction in the thrombolytic era—A prospective trial. Circulation 1994;90:1747–1756.

179. Farrell TG, Bashir Y, Cripps T, et al. Risk stratification for arrhythmic events in postinfarction patients based on heart rate variability, ambulatory electrocardiographic variables and the signal-averaged electrocardiogram. J Am Coll Cardiol 1991;18:687–697.

180. La Rovere MT, Bigger JT Jr, Marcus FI, Mortara A, Schwartz PJ. Baroreflex sensitivity and heart-rate variability in prediction of total cardiac mortality after myocardial infarction: ATRAMI. Lancet 1998;351:478–484.

181. Moss AJ, Cannom DS, Daubert JP, et al. Multicenter automatic defibrillator implantation trial II (MADIT II): Design and clinical protocol. Ann Noninvasiv Electrocardiol 1999;4:83–91.

182. The Norwegian Multicenter Study Group. Timolol-induced reduction in mortality and reinfarction in patients surviving acute myocardial infarction. N Engl J Med 1981;304:801–807.

183. β-blocker Heart Attack Trial Research Group. A randomized trial of propranolol in patients with acute myocardial infarction. 1. Mortality results. JAMA 1982;247:1707–1714.

184. Kendall MJ, Lynch HP, Hjalmarson A, Kjekshus J. B-blockers and sudden cardiac death. Ann Intern Med 1995;123:358–367.

20   Arrhythmias in Pediatric Patients

Special Considerations

John K. Triedman, MD

CONTENTS

INTRODUCTION
SUPRAVENTRICULAR TACHYCARDIAS
VENTRICULAR ARRHYTHMIAS AND DEVICE THERAPY
BRADYARRHYTHMIAS
SPECIAL TOPICS IN PEDIATRIC ARRHYTHMIA
REFERENCES

INTRODUCTION

Most of the fundamental principles of adult cardiac electrophysiology describing cellular activation and repolarization and propagation of the action potential in cardiac tissue can be applied to the pediatric age group directly and with little alteration. However, the manifestations of arrhythmic disease and the clinical approach to their management are quite different in children compared to adults. Certain categories of arrhythmia that are of major interest to the adult electrophysiologist because of their associated risks of sudden death and other major adverse outcomes, such as atrial fibrillation (AF) and ventricular tachycardia (VT) occurring after myocardial infarction (MI), are rare in the pediatric age group. Conversely, supraventricular arrhythmias and especially atrioventricular (AV) reciprocating tachycardias are commonly identified in children, the majority of whom are otherwise healthy and free from abnormalities of cardiac structure or function. Thus, our understanding of the natural history of arrhythmias in children is more strongly based on the recording of symptoms reported by healthy patients with supraventricular tachycardia (SVT), an outcome that is rather difficult to measure. For this reason, it has often been difficult to apply to pediatric arrhythmia syndromes the same rigorous epidemiological tools that have been used to characterize the natural history and response to therapy of adult problems of greater prevalence and severity.

The diagnosis and therapy of arrhythmias in children must also be viewed in the more global context of pediatric developmental physiology and psychology. There are several general pediatric issues that have a significant impact on arrhythmia management in children. These include a generalized lack of knowledge regarding the age-specific

From: *Contemporary Cardiology: Management of Cardiac Arrhythmias*
Edited by: L. I. Ganz © Humana Press Inc., Totowa, NJ

pharmacology of antiarrhythmic medications, developmental changes in cellular metabolism, and growth which may affect the response of the child's heart both to therapy with antiarrhythmic drugs and tissue injury caused by biophysical means such as radiofrequency ablation. There are significant and as yet poorly understood developmental changes in cardiovascular function and its autonomic regulation that may affect the hemodynamic response to tachycardia and bradycardia. These issues are complicated further in the small but significant minority of children with congenital heart disease, who are clearly at significantly elevated risk for all varieties of arrhythmia and whose hemodynamics are often complex and fragile, giving them a reduced cardiac reserve to cope with acute changes in rhythm. On a practical level, the size of the patient often has major implications with regard to suitability of commercially available monitoring and therapeutic devices. Finally, there are important developmental issues of psychological responses to disease and clinical intervention that must be considered in the care of the whole patient, and the complex ethics of obtaining informed consent from parents and guardians for therapies on behalf of minors. The importance of these issues varies significantly with the specifics of age and size of the patient and their medical history and arrhythmia diagnosis and proposed therapy, and clearly creates a rich and challenging environment for clinical problem-solving.

This chapter examines aspects of the epidemiology, natural history, and current clinical management of SVT, VT, and complete heart block. Emphasis will be placed on those features which are of particular importance in the pediatric age group or which distinguish children in some way from adults with similar disease processes. Additionally, some of the arrhythmia issues specific to children and young adults with congenital heart disease and fetal tachycardias are briefly discussed.

SUPRAVENTRICULAR TACHYCARDIAS

Epidemiology and Natural History

Epidemiological studies have suggested that the prevevalence of SVT is 2–2.5 cases/1000 people, with an incidence of 35 cases/100,000 person-years (1). SVTs are as common among children as adults with otherwise anatomically normal hearts, and thus this pediatric problem is not uncommon. The types of SVT encountered in children and their underlying mechanisms are generally similar to those seen in adults, but the relative frequency of specific arrhythmia types differs. Common SVTs that may require diagnosis and treatment in these age groups include: accessory pathway-mediated tachycardias such as Wolff-Parkinson-White syndrome (WPW), concealed accessory pathway, Mahaim fiber tachycardia, and permanent junctional reciprocating tachycardia (PJRT), atrioventricular nodal reentrant tachycardia (AVNRT), and ectopic atrial tachycardias. Rarely, children with anatomically normal hearts may also present with atrial reentrant arrhythmias, such as atrial flutter and AF, but these are more commonly encountered in patients with underlying congenital or acquired heart disease.

Several features of the natural history of SVT in children affect clinical decision-making related to acute and chronic management of the tachycardia. Age-based changes in prevalence have been documented in WPW (2) and AVNRTs (3). Younger patients with supraventricular arrhythmia are more likely to have an accessory pathway-mediated tachycardia than either AVNRT or primary atrial tachycardia. AVNRT is particularly uncommon in infancy, and does not begin to increase in frequency until children reach

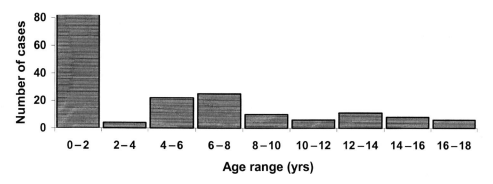

Fig. 1. Age at clinical presentation of SVT in children. (Data adapted from Perry and Garson *[2]*.)

school age. Age at clinical presentation of SVT in children has a bimodal distribution, with the first clinically apparent event usually occurring during early childhood, or even detected obstetrically during prenatal life, and a secondary peak occurring during the school-age years (Fig. 1). Among infants presenting with SVT, a significant fraction—possibly more than one-half of patients—will have no clinical tachycardias after initial presentation, may be noninducible during provocative electrophysiological study (EPS) or, in the case of children with WPW *(4)* may exhibit disappearance of pre-excitation. This apparent resolution of the tachycardia symptoms and substrate may reflect age-related increases in accessory-pathway refractoriness *(5)*. However, such patients may be vulnerable to recurrence later in childhood *(2)*. The natural histories of incessantly recurring tachycardias such as ectopic atrial tachycardia and PJRT are less well known, but there is some clinical evidence to suggest that these tachycardias may also resolve spontaneously in a significant number of cases *(6)*.

As with the adult population, the clinical and electrocardiographic presentations of SVTs are strongly influenced by the activities of the AV node and the specialized conduction systems. Sinus tachycardia may be frequently confused with SVT, especially in sick, febrile infants or children in respiratory distress, who may have sinus rates of 200–220 BPM. Mean resting heart rates and percentile ranges are presented by age in Fig. 2. Although orthodromic SVT associated with a narrow QRS complex is the most common electrocardiographic appearance of SVT in children, bundle-branch aberration—and occasionally, antidromic tachycardias—may result in a wide-complex tachycardia. It should be emphasized, however, that any wide-complex tachycardia should be considered to be a potentially hemodynamically unstable rhythm, and treated accordingly. An algorithm for the electrocardiographic diagnosis of narrow-complex paroxysmal tachycaridas in children is provided in Table 1.

In most cases, acute tachycardia events are well-tolerated by children who have otherwise normal cardiac anatomy and function, with syncope or other severe presentation very rare. Thus, the risks of SVT are low in this group, and clinical evolution is favorable. This suggests that it is preferable to avoid therapeutic choices with even a relatively small potential for major adverse side effects when treating infants and young children with clinically benign supraventricular arrhythmias. Thus, consideration of radiofrequency catheter ablation or treatment with certain classes of potent anti-arrhythmic agents, such as class IC and class III antiarrhythmic agents, would only be

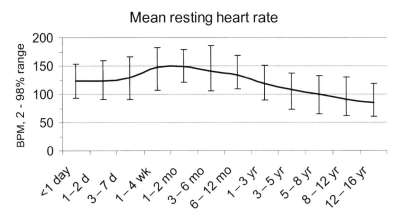

Fig. 2. Mean resting heart rate by age, with 2–98% range bars. Normal heart rate at rest increases slightly in the first weeks and months of life, and then slowly declines. Heart rates greater than 180 BPM are rare in healthy, quiet children, but maximum heart rate may be as high as 200–220 BPM under stress caused by extreme exertion, fever, hypovolemia, or medication with adrenergic agents.

considered suitable for children with unusually severe or unremitting tachycardia and for older children with established disease.

Although SVTs that occur in otherwise normal children are typically benign events, they may be associated with severe symptoms such as syncope and seizure under conditions of physiological stress, such as dehydration or intercurrent illness. Fatal outcomes associated with SVT are typically only seen in specific patient subpopulations: patients with severe structural congenital heart disease and hemodynamic derangement, patients with cardiomyopathies and significant abnormalities of ventricular function, and patients with WPW at risk for rapid conduction of atrial arrhythmias (Fig. 3). Of these groups, the latter is the most problematic from the perspective of clinical management, as patients with pre-excitation make up a relatively large proportion of the population of children with SVT and many are either minimally symptomatic or asymptomatic. The prevalence of cardiac arrest in patients with WPW may be similar to that observed in adult series (2.3%), with a mean age of this severe presentation of 11–12 yr *(7)*. This small but real risk of sudden death is present although the incidence of AF, the electrophysiological risk factor for this event, is low in children. The antegrade conduction characteristics of accessory pathways tend to manifest longer refractory periods with increasing patient age; thus, it might be expected that the potential for rapid antegrade conduction in young patients is higher than in adults. Many pediatric electrophysiologists elect to assess the "risk" associated with pre-excitation by assessing the antegrade conduction characteristics of the accessory pathway directly by induction of AF and/or rapid atrial pacing, or indirectly by observing the response of pre-excitation to sinus tachycardia induced by exercise. The presence or absence of pre-excitation below a given RR interval is implicitly related to studies which have demonstrated that WPW patients with the shortest RR interval in AF of ≤220 ms constitute a group at greater risk of cardiac arrest *(8)*. The presence of WPW also increases the likelihood of associated congenital heart disease, which may be clinically occult. The prevalence of pre-excitation has been particularly linked with Ebstein's malformation of the tricuspid valve *(4,9)*, as well as congenitally corrected transposition of the great arteries

Table 1
Electrocardiographic Diagnosis of Paroxysmal Narrow-Complex Tachycardias (SVT) in Children

	Sinus tachycardia	Ectopic atrial tachycardia	Atrial flutter	Atrial fibrillation	AV-nodal reentry	Orthodromic SVT (WPW)	Orthodromic SVT (concealed)	PJRT
Onset and termination	gradual	gradual	abrupt	abrupt	abrupt	abrupt	abrupt	incessant
SVT rate variation	variable	variable	fixed/abrupt changes		fixed	fixed	fixed	fixed (may vary slightly)
A-V ratio in SVT	1:1	≥1:1	≥1:1	>1:1	1:1 (rarely, 2:1 or 1:2)	1:1	1:1	1:1
P wave axis in SVT	normal	abnormal	abnormal	indeterminate	retrograde (QRS often hides P wave)	retrograde	retrograde	retrograde
V-A time for retrograde P-wave					<70 ms	>70 ms	>70 ms	>>70 ms (RP interval > PR interval)
Response to vagal stimulation or adenosine	mild ↓ atrial rate	AV block, may cause mild ↓ atrial rate	AV block	AV block	terminate, with antegrade or retrograde block	terminate, usually with antegrade block	terminate, usually with antegrade block	terminate, with antegrade or retrograde block
QRS complex in sinus rhythm	normal	normal	normal	normal	normal	preexcited	normal	normal
Prevalence (infants)	very common	rare	rare	rare	rare	common	common	rare
Prevalence (older children)	very common	rare	rare	rare	common	common	common	rare

Abbreviations: SVT = supraventricular tachycardia, WPW = Wolff-Parkinson-White syndrome, PJRT = permanent form of junctional reciprocating tachycardia.

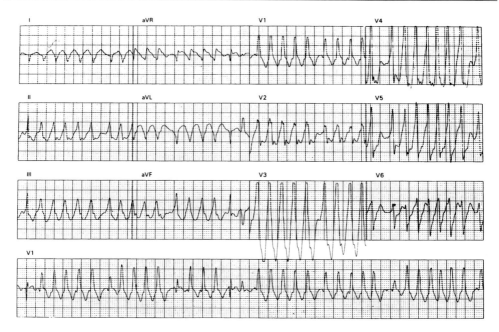

Fig. 3. Electrocardiographic presentation of AF with rapid, irregular pre-excited conduction in a patient with WPW.

(L-TGA), which has a frequent finding of Ebstein's malformation of the left-sided tricuspid valve. Other forms of congenital heart disease do not appear to be clearly associated with an increased prevalence of accessory pathways, but they may be present in some patients by chance and may significantly complicate the management of patients with significant abnormalities of hemodynamics and oxygenation. Other myocardial substrates for SVT are more frequent in congenital heart disease, particularly atrial flutter and other forms of intra-atrial reentrant tachycardia based on scars and abnormal atrial anatomy.

Patients with incessant tachycardias, such as ectopic atrial tachycardia, PJRT, and poorly controlled SVT or SVT of long duration, may develop ventricular dysfunction secondary to tachycardia-induced cardiomyopathy *(10)*. It appears that tachycardia-induced cardiomyopathy is reversible with treatment of the underlying tachycardia in almost all cases *(11)*. The presentation of congestive heart failure (CHF) in these patients may be severe, with cardiomegaly, hepatic congestion, and acidemia occasionally constituting presentation in an infant who has been in SVT for some time *(12)*. Prenatally, infants with sustained tachycardia are at significant risk for the development of hydrops fetalis (fetal CHF) and intrauterine fetal demise. The association of such adverse clinical outcomes with sustained tachycardia in very young children suggests that such patients' inability to report symptoms and obtain medical therapy may result in an increased risk of a poor outcome. In all patients presenting with ventricular dysfunction, the use of antiarrhythmic therapies with significant negative cardiac inotropic effects may be relatively contraindicated.

In summary, the natural history of most SVT occurring in children is favorable. Most patients who present with an accessory pathway-mediated tachycardia early in childhood are otherwise healthy. Some will have sporadic and occasionally frequent symptomatic recurrences, but many can expect complete and spontaneous resolution of their symptoms. Thus, any therapy proposed for such patients must have a very favorable safety profile. A minority of children will have more severe, high-risk disease because of the presence of manifest pre-excitation (WPW), severe symptoms, association with hemodynamically significant congenital heart disease, or tachycardia-mediated cardiomyopathy.

Acute Therapy of AV Reciprocating Tachycardia

VAGAL MANEUVERS

As in the adult population, acute termination of AV reciprocating tachycardia is most easily achieved by causing transient slowing or block of AV-nodal conduction. The AV node is heavily innervated by vagal and sympathetic efferent fibers, and children generally manifest a greater degree of vagal tone and modulation of cardiac electrical activity than adults. For this reason, it is often possible to eliminate tachycardias in children with maneuvers that decrease sympathetic tone and increase vagal activity, and many patients and their families teach themselves such maneuvers. The rebound phase of a Valsalva maneuver, which causes transient hypertension and engages the arterial baroreceptors, is the classic physiological maneuver resulting in AV block and termination of SVT. In infants, a different bradycardia reflex related to the mammalian diving response may be engaged by placing a bag of ice gently on the forehead and the bridge of the nose for 10–15 s. The efficacy of such maneuvers may be improved by increasing venous return to the heart by placing the patient in a supine position and elevating the legs (in infants, gentle pressure may be applied to the abdomen). This tends to increase atrial and arterial pressure and decrease sympathetic tone; among older children, just lying supine with legs elevated for several minutes often results in the spontaneous termination of the episode. The use of ocular pressure to engage a bradycardic reflex in infants and children is not recommended because of the risk of ophthalmic injury. A variety of other techniques have been anecdotally reported by patients, including standing on their heads or having their parents swing them by their ankles! Presumably, such activities transiently engage the arterial baroreflex and cause transient slowing at the AV node.

PHARMACOLOGICAL AGENTS

A variety of short-acting pharmacologic agents have been used acutely to terminate AV reciprocating tachycardias. Many of these, such as the hypertensive agents methoxamine and trimethaphan, and the vagomimetic agent neostigmine, cause AV slowing or blockade by transiently engaging the cardiac vagal mechanisms. Currently, the use of such agents has been supplanted by the availability of adenosine and the intravenous Ca^{++}-channel-blocking agents verapamil and diltiazem.

Adenosine. Adenosine has been demonstrated to be an effective drug for terminating AV reciprocating tachycardias in children, as in adults. Adenosine causes transient suppression of the AV node, typically resulting in AV block, which terminates the tachycardia. It is rapidly metabolized, with an effect on nodal tissue that lasts only 10–15 s. Adenosine must thus be administered through good iv access as a bolus, followed by an inert vehicle (e.g., normal saline) in sufficient quantity to rapidly convey the drug to the central circulation. Standard initial dosing of adenosine in children is 0.1–0.2 mg/kg body wt, which may be repeated as necessary. Adenosine should be given during continuous electrocardiographic (ECG) monitoring. Although the drug is generally considered to be safe *(13)*, transient sinus bradycardia, high-grade AV block, ventricular ectopy, and, rarely, AF may be seen after administration. These cardiac side effects represent predictable electrophysiological actions of the drug and generally resolve spontaneously over 10–30 s as the drug is metabolized. Occasionally, the catecholamine surge that typically follows adenosine therapy, along with ectopy and AV block of varying degree, may result in the immediate reinduction of SVT. Although generally considered quite safe because of its extremely short half-life, prolonged bradycardia and asystole have been reported to occur rarely with adenosine *(14)*. It is important to recognize that children, especially those with congenital heart disease, may be chronically treated with dipyridamole, which by blocking the metabolic pathway for degradation of adenosine may prolong the cardiac effects of adenosine. Fatal interactions of these two drugs have been observed. Unpleasant sensations of chest tightness, pressure, and dyspnea may also be reported. It has been speculated that adenosine may result in bronchospasm, and active asthma is a relative contraindication to the agent. Methylxanthine drugs, such as aminophylline and theophylline, may reduce the efficacy of adenosine at standard doses. Occasionally the efficacy of adenosine may also be reduced by slow venous return to the heart, as is the case in some forms of congenital heart disease or severe CHF.

Verapamil and diltiazem. Intravenous calcium-channel-blocking agents have been demonstrated to have the same efficacy as adenosine for the acute termination of AV reciprocating tachycardias. For verapamil, a standard initial iv bolus dose is 0.05–0.1 mg/kg. In contrast to adenosine, calcium-channel-blocking agents are more long-lasting in their acute effect and do not cause a rebound catecholamine surge and ectopy. They may also be used in some settings, such as those mentioned previously, in which the use of adenosine is contraindicated or ineffective. However, these agents also have negative inotropic effects and the potential to cause severe myocardial dysfunction. Close attention must be paid to monitoring of blood pressure and perfusion during their use. They are absolutely contraindicated for the routine therapy of SVT in infants and children under the age of 1, as profound, lethal ventricular dysfunction has been reported to occur with iv verapamil, presumably because of the immature developmental stage of intracellular calcium metabolism in children of this age *(15,16)*. Additionally, caution should be used when iv calcium-channel blockers are administered in conjunction with beta-blocking agents, because of the potential for synergism of negative inotropic effects.

PACE TERMINATION

AV reciprocating tachycardias—and atrial reentrant tachycardias in general, such as atrial flutter—can often be terminated by overdrive atrial pacing. This can be achieved using a transesophageal pacing catheter *(17)*, often with a high degree of patient acceptability. Again, the mechanism of termination of the tachycardia is generally observed to be an interval-dependent block in the AV node.

Chronic Antiarrhythmic Therapy of SVT

Antiarrhythmic drugs have served as the mainstay of therapy of SVT in children for years. Although no prospective controlled studies have been performed to test the efficacy of these agents for prophylaxis of SVTs in children, many retrospective reviews of institutional experience have firmly established the role of drug therapy in these patients. Digoxin and beta-blockers such as propranolol are generally well-tolerated and unlikely to provoke adverse side effects, and are thus commonly used as first-line agents in the absence of any specific contraindications. Therapy with one or both of these agents is associated with a high likelihood of freedom from supraventricular arrhythmia in early childhood (18). In the face of frequent recurrences despite digoxin and/or beta-blockade, second-line therapies that have been used with apparent efficacy in children with SVT include verapamil, sotalol, a variety of class IC agents such as flecainide, propafenone, and moricizine, and amiodarone. Multiple drug regimens have also been successfully used to treat refractory supraventricular arrhythmias in small series, such as amiodarone and flecainide (19).

Although liquid formulations of digoxin and propranolol in concentrations appropriate for pediatric dosing are available, calculating and making an appropriate, weight-based dose of antiarrhythmic medications is often problematic for pediatric patients. Few pharmacokinetic data are available to guide dosing schedules, although it is generally assumed that infants and very small children require more frequent dosing intervals than older patients. Specific adverse events of antiarrhythmic drug therapy have been reported for virtually every antiarrhythmic agent in association with pediatric use, including mortality (20–23). A partial list of examples includes the potential for aggravation of reactive airway disease with beta-blocker therapy, the general contraindication to verapamil therapy in infants and in other children with pre-excitation, the extracardiac morbidity associated with amiodarone therapy, and the propensity of sotalol to prolong the QT interval. Knowledge of these associations and others, and a plan for appropriate monitoring and follow-up, are necessary before embarking on a course of therapy.

Antiarrhythmic agents that are commonly used in pediatric patients are presented in Table 2.

Radiofrequency Catheter Ablation

Radiofrequency catheter ablation is performed in children using procedural techniques adapted from and largely similar to those applied in the adult population. The safety and efficacy of catheter ablation in children over the age of four is comparable to that observed in adults for treatment of recurrent SVTs mediated by an accessory pathway or AVNRT (24–26). The overall efficacy of catheter ablation of accessory pathways for these patients approaches 95% with increasing operator experience (27). The risk of complications attributable to the ablation procedure has been initially estimated to be 3.7% (28), a number that includes transient clinical events as well as major complications. About 5% of children successfully treated using ablation will have a recurrence, usually occurring within several months. As with adults, the likelihood of initial success and recurrence are related to the location of the accessory pathway, and the pathways on the free wall of the right atrium have a lower expected acute success rate (28). The presence of congenital malformation also significantly lowers the acute efficacy. This understanding of the risks and benefits of catheter ablation have allowed a reasonably broad consensus on the indications for the procedure in the pediatric population (29). These include symptomatic, frequently recurrent tachycardias not suppressed by chronic medical therapy, or SVT associated with severe symptoms (e.g., syncope), especially in the presence of pre-excitation. As patients grow older and became more capable of acting as informed participants in their own care, elective

Table 2
Antiarrhythmic Agents Commonly Used in Pediatric Practice

Drug	Primary metabolic route	Oral dosing	Intravenous dosing	Half-life	Comments	Drug levels
Digoxin	Renal	Load: 3 doses divided over 24 h, total doses— Premature—20 μg/kg Newborn—30 μg/kg Infant/child—40 μg/ kg Maintenance: ¼ loading dose divided bid	75–80% of oral dosing	Premature—61 h Newborn—35 h Infant—18 h Child—37 h	Nausea, heart block, automatic tachycardias Toxic effects increased in setting of hypocalcemia, hypokalemia	0.5–2.0 ng/mL Toxic: >2.2 ng/mL
Adenosine	RBC/endothelial metabolism	Not available	0.1–0.3 mg/kg by rapid iv bolus with flush, may repeat dose maximum dose: 12 mg	9 s	Dipyridamole, diltiazem, verapamil may accentuate effects Theophylline may antagonize effects May provoke wheezing and dyspnea	Not clinically used
Procainamide	Renal (hepatic transformation to N-acetylprocainamide	50–100 mg/kg/d Conventional: divided q4 h Slow release: divided q6 h—q12 h	Load: 7–15 mg/kg at 0.5mg/kg/min Infusion: 20–60 μg/kg/min, titrated to level and effect	Conventional: 2.5–4.7 h Slow release oral: 6–7 h	Rapid iv administration may provoke hypotension Chronic therapy associated with lupus-like syndrome	Procainamide: 4–12 μg/mL Procainamide + NAPA: 8–22 μg/mL
Lidocaine	Hepatic	Not available	Load: 1 mg/kg, may repeat q5 min × 2 Infusion: 20–50 μg/kg/min	Neonate: 3.2 h Infant–adult: 1.8 h	Nausea, seizures	1.5–5.0 μg/mL Toxic > 8 μg/mL
Propranolol	Hepatic	1–5 mg/kg/d, divided q6 h–q8 h	0.01–0.2 mg/kg over 5 min (0.1 mg/kg typical dose)	iv: 2.3 h po: 3.2 h	Negative inotrope. Avoid concurrent iv verapamil	Not clinically used
Atenolol	Renal	1–2 mg/kg/d, divided q12 h–q24 h	Not available	5–9 h Renal failure: 16–30 h	Negative inotrope	Not clinically used

470

Esmolol	RBC esterases	Not available	Load: 250–500 μg/kg Infusion: 50–20 μg/kg/min	9 min	Negative inotrope. Avoid concurrent iv verapamil	Not clinically used
Sotalol	Renal	80–240 mg/M/d Infants: divided q8 h Children: divided q12 h	Not available in U.S.A.	6.3–13.6 h Renal failure: > 80 h	Worsening CHF Pro-arrhythmia (torsades de pointes)	Not clinically used
Amiodarone	?Biliary	Load: 10–20 mg/kg/d × 3–5 d Maintenance: 5 mg/kg/d	Load: 5 mg/kg over 30 min, may repeat × 1 Infusion: 10–20 mg/kg/d	8–107 d	Hypotension with iv use Multiple noncardiac toxicities with chronic oral dosing, incl. thyroid, pulmonary, ophthalmologic, hepatic	Amiodarone: 1–2.5 mg/mL Desethylamiodarone: 0.2–2.6 mg/mL reverse T3 × 4 normal implies therapeutic serum level
Verapamil	Hepatic	3–12 mg/kg/d	Load: 0.05 mg/kg, may repeat × 2 Infusion: 5–10 μg/kg/min	3–12 h	Hypotension Should not be used in infants <1 y/o, or in patients with pre-excited sinus rhythm	Not clinically used

ablation performed for troublesome symptoms or the desire to stop taking medicine begins to become a reasonable indication, as in adults. Although the technical aspects of the ablation procedure are similar in children and adults, several issues suggest the desirability of managing young patients referred for catheter ablation in a clinical environment skilled and experienced in meeting the special needs of the pediatric patient. These include the small body size and vascular caliber of the patient, the relative frequency of associated congenital heart defects and intercurrent pediatric medical issues, and nursing and anesthetic considerations.

In patients who do not fall into the group of otherwise healthy children ≥4 years old, the risk and benefits of ablation therapy are more poorly quantified, and the indications for ablation are less clear. Younger children, and especially infants, have been found to have a higher rate of adverse events associated with ablation and a lower likelihood of success (28). Although this may reflect a group of patients who are more ill before the catheterization procedure, catheterization generally poses a higher risk in infancy (30), and experimental studies have also shown that immature myocardium may have a less tolerant response to ablation injury. SVT itself is rarely associated with a poor clinical outcome when carefully managed medically, and many children resolve their clinical tachycardias spontaneously in the first year of life. Thus, it seems appropriate to defer ablation whenever possible for tachycardias which do not appear to be life-threatening. There are exceptions to this rule. These may include infants with severe and refractory tachycardia who manifest signs of tachycardia-mediated cardiomyopathy, and young children with an accessory pathway who will require surgery for complex congenital heart disease which would be complicated by perioperative SVT and/or which will limit postoperative ablative access to the pathway.

VENTRICULAR ARRHYTHMIAS AND DEVICE THERAPY

Epidemiology and Natural History

VT is considerably less common and generally carries a more serious prognosis in the pediatric age group than SVT. Coronary-artery disease (CAD) is extremely rare in this age group. When present, CAD is more likely to be associated with congenital anomaly of coronary anatomy and/or postoperative anomalies of coronary anatomy than with atherosclerotic heart disease, which in children is a marker of an inherited hyperlipidemia syndrome. Nevertheless, the occurrence of VT does suggest an increased likelihood of an abnormal, injured myocardial substrate (*see* Table 3). Patients who present with VT usually fit into one of three groups: those who have undergone prior surgery for a congenital heart defect, those with familial myopathies which can be characterized either electrocardiographically or by functional imaging (e.g., long QT syndrome (LQTS), Brugada syndrome, hypertrophic cardiomyopathy, dilated cardiomyopathy, arrhythmogenic right ventricular dysplasia), and those who have a truly idiopathic ventricular tachycardia (IVT) occurring in a heart which otherwise appears on comprehensive evaluation to be anatomically and functionally normal.

Clinical presentation of VT is variable in children. Not infrequently, VT may first be discovered in an asymptomatic patient noted to have an irregular pulse on routine examination. Symptomatic patients may complain of palpitation, dizziness, shortness of breath, or syncope. As with WPW, cardiac arrest may be the first presentation of severe ventricular arrhythmia substrates, such as prolonged QT syndrome (31). Infants

Table 3
Etiologies of VT in Young Patients

1. **Congenital myopathy**
   Hypertrophic cardiomyopathy
   Arrhythmogenic right ventricular dysplasia
   Carnitine deficiency
   Storage diseases
   Muscular dystrophy
   Histiocytoid cardiomyopathy
2. **Acquired myopathy**
   Myocarditis
   Idiopathic dilated cardiomyopathy
   Adriamycin cardiotoxicity
   Hemochromatosis
   HIV infection
3. **Anatomic defects**
   Tetralogy of Fallot/ventricular septal defect
   Aortic stenosis
   Transposition of the great arteries (TGA)
   Mitral-valve prolapse
   Cardiac tumors
4. **Primary electrical disorders**
   Congenital prolonged QT syndrome
   Idiopathic VT
   Catecholaminergic VT
   Brugada's syndrome
   Diffuse conduction system disease
5. **Coronary-artery abnormalities**
   Coronary vasculitis
   Kawasaki's syndrome
   Anomalous origin of left coronary from pulmonary artery
   Interarterial course of left coronary arising from right coronary cusp
   Hyperlipidemia and premature coronary atherosclerotic disease
6. **Intoxication/exposure**
   Digoxin toxicity
   Acquired prolonged QT syndrome
   Antiarrhythmic drugs (class I and III)
   Tricyclic antidepressant overdose
   Organophosphate exposure
   Substance abuse

and very young children may tolerate long periods of VT quite well; occasionally they may present with incessant VT and associated tachycardia-mediated cardiomyopathy.

LONG QT SYNDROME

As is the case with adults, children with a prolonged corrected QT interval are at risk of arrhythmic sudden death. LQTS in children may present in a variety of ways, including aborted sudden death, unexplained syncope, and 2:1 AV block, especially in infancy (32). In recent years, it has been increasingly common to discover this diagnosis as an asymptomatic observation made in the course of evaluating the family members of another patient diagnosed with long QT, or serendipitously on a random ECG obtained for an unrelated reason. Patients with deafness of undetermined etiology often have ECGs checked to assess whether they may have the associated recessive form of LQTS, Jervell-Lange-Nielsen syndrome. Patients may also be more likely to present at times when they are prescribed other medications which may increase QT interval, such as certain antibiotic, antifungal, and GI motility agents. In some patients, specific genetic diagnosis of a variety of point mutations affecting membrane-channel proteins for potassium and/or sodium transport is now possible. As the varied genetic picture of this disease becomes more fully understood and related to the phenotypic variability in clinical presentation *(33)*, it is likely that specific therapies may be developed and improved tools made available for risk assessment in individual patients.

VT Associated with Congenital Heart Disease

Late cardiac mortality caused by acute atrial tachycardios and VTs is seen in a significant number of children and young adults with tetralogy of Fallot *(34)*, transposition of the great arteries *(35)*, aortic stenosis *(36)*, and single ventricle *(37)*. Certain congenital anomalies, most notably tetralogy of Fallot and other malformations that result in chronic hypertrophy and/or surgical injury to the ventricles, seem to pose particular risk of ventricular arrhythmias. However, the overall mortality caused by sudden cardiac death even in these "high-risk" subgroups is still quite low—on the order of 3 of 1000 patient-years *(38)*. Simple formulas for predicting the specific risk of individual patients in this group do not exist at present, and several retrospective studies have come to sometimes conflicting conclusions with respect to factors associated with poor outcomes in this group. Associations which have been proposed and seem to have some relevance include: age *(39)*, occurrence of spontaneous VT *(39,40)*, positive ventricular stimulation study (i.e., EPS) *(39)*, and prolonged QRS duration on a 12-lead ECG *(41)*.

IVT in Childhood

Premature ventricular contractions (PVCs) are a frequent observation in childhood. Ambulatory ECG monitoring studies of children and young adults have demonstrated that higher grades of ventricular ectopy (such as ventricular bigeminy or couplets) may also be observed in children with normal hearts, recognizing that the more abnormal the monitoring study, the more a focused cardiac evaluation is needed before the heart is pronounced "normal." More problematic are those patients who present with sustained VT, either with symptoms (palpitations, dizziness and/or fainting) or without, and on evaluation have no other detectable abnormalities of cardiac structure or ventricular function. VT in the anatomically normal heart occurs in young patients in the same electrocardiographic patterns as the adult population: a common left bundle-branch block (LBBB) morphology which generally originates from a focus in the outflow tract of the right ventricle, and a less common right bundle-branch block (RBBB) morphology which originates in the ventricular septum (Fig. 4).

Concern has been expressed in the past that such VTs may be the initial signs of subtle underlying abnormalities of the ventricular myocardium. Although some forms of IVT that occur in an otherwise normal heart may be quite benign, in cases where overt clinical abnormalities are known or discovered in the course of diagnostic evalua-

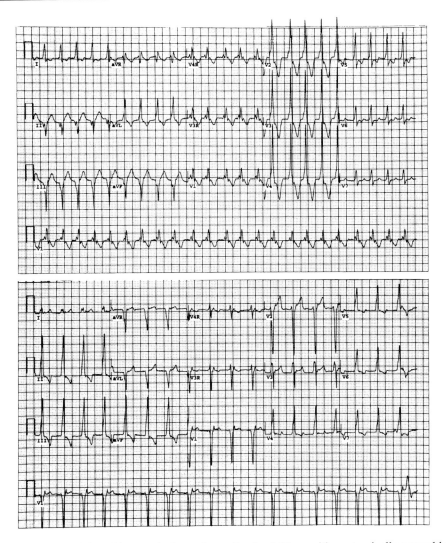

Fig. 4. Examples of idiopathic ventricular tachycardias in children with anatomically normal hearts. (Top frame) Superior axis and right BBB pattern consistent with origin from left ventricular septal surface. (Bottom frame) Inferior axis and left BBB pattern consistent with origin from right ventricular overflow tract area.

tion, patients may be at increased risk for cardiac sudden death *(42)*. More malignant etiologies of VT in an apparently normal heart include arrhythmogenic right ventricular dysplasia, acquired or congenital abnormalities of the coronary arteries, and catecholaminergic VT. Thus any child who presents with an episode of sustained VT of uncertain etiology should be subject to a comprehensive cardiac evaluation, which may sometimes include magnetic resonance imaging (MRI) imaging and endomyocardial biopsy to rule out more malignant causes of VT. Among patients with no evidence of myocardial abnormalities, these "idiopathic" VTs (IVTs) are generally considered to be benign because they appear to have a very low association with either progressive ventricular dysfunction or with cardiac arrest and sudden death, and have a high likelihood of spontaneous regression *(43)*. Nonetheless, they are often symptomatic enough to demand either pharmcological or ablative therapy.

Emergency Management of VTs

Emergency management of VT in children and young adults begins with the ABCs of basic life support, with immediate institution of cardiopulmonary resuscitation (CPR) and the advanced cardiac life-support/pediatric advanced life-support sequences in the event of cardiac arrest. Recommended initial drug doses and cardioversion energies for therapy of VT and VF are listed in Table 4.

A more difficult decision-making process must be applied for those patients who present in sustained, wide-complex tachycardias that are hemodynamically stable. In general, it is safest to make the presumption that all such rhythms represent VT until proven otherwise. However, as with adults, a wide-complex tachycardia in such patients will occasionally be revealed to be supraventricular in origin—either atrial, AV-nodal, or AV reciprocating—with aberrant ventricular conduction. Some patients in VT may spontaneously revert to sinus rhythm or break in response to interventions such as infusion of lidocaine, other antiarrhythmic agents, or, in the case of recurrent torsades des pointes, magnesium. If external cardioversion is necessary in these patients, it should be performed if possible under conditions that maximize patient safety and comfort, with adequate iv access and monitoring and an appropriate level of sedation monitored by an anesthesiologist. Extra care must be taken with these patients to monitor the evolution of their vascular status while they await cardioversion, and especially when they are sedated for cardioversion, as abrupt hemodynamic collapse may occur.

Chronic management of patients with VT is often problematic, although recent innovations in the design and utilization of implantable cardioverter defibrillators (ICDs) have allowed this therapy to be used with increasing freedom in the pediatric age group. As mentioned previously, a variety of retrospective studies have allowed identification of empiric approaches to risk stratification in certain categories of children with VT. However, with the exception of utilization of beta-blocker therapy for the prevention of sudden death in patients with LQTS, there are no available studies of pediatric patients, which clearly suggests a specific benefit of any antiarrhythmic agent in the prevention of VT and sudden death. Similarly, the value of serial testing of anti-arrhythmic agents for their ability to suppress inducible VT in pediatric patients has not been investigated. To a significant degree, the choice of antiarrhythmic agents in this special population has been extrapolated from the results of studies in adult popula-tions of VT occurring in patients with acquired cardiomyopathy with or without coronary atherosclerosis. At present, standard therapeutic choices include beta-blockers and class III agents, such as sotalol and amiodarone. As in the adult population, the chronic use of amiodarone has been associated with significant extracardiac morbidity.

Device Therapy in Children

ICD therapy for prophylaxis against cardiac sudden death is now being used with increasing frequency among patients in the pediatric age group who have recurrent, potentially lethal ventricular arrhythmias. In prospective, controlled adult studies, a clear survival benefit has been demonstrated, comparing ICD therapy to chronic therapy with antiarrhythmic medications. Although sudden cardiac death does occur in children,

Table 4
Initial Drug Doses and Cardioversion Energies for Therapy of VT and VF

Rhythm	Assessment	Drug sequence	Shock sequence	Comments
Bradycardia	Intervention appropriate if clinical evidence of cardiorespiratory compromise caused by bradycardia	1. Epinephrine 0.01 mg/kg of 1:10,000 solution, iv/io 2. Atropine 0.02 mg/kg iv/io (min dose—0.1 mg)		Consider transcutaneous pacing
Supraventricular tachycardia	Hemodynamically stable	Adenosine 0.1 mg/kg iv		Consider adenosine if stable and possible SVT with aberration
Ventricular tachycardia	Hemodynamically stable	Lidocaine 1.0 mg/kg iv/io		Use small (4.5-cm) paddles for infants <10 kg (~1 yr)
Hemodynamically unstable tachycardia	Evidence of cardiorespiratory compromise	See above	Synchronized cardioversion 1. 0.5–1.0 J/kg 2. 2.0 J/kg	
Ventricular fibrillation		1. Epinephrine 0.01 mg/kg of 1:10,000 solution, iv/io 2. Lidocaine 1.0 mg/kg iv/io 3. Epinephrine 0.1 mg/kg of 1:1,000 solution, iv/io 4. Bretylium 5 mg/kg iv/io	Asynchronous defibrillation 1. 2.0 J/kg 2. 3.0 J/kg 3. 4.0 J/kg	1. Administer initial 3 rescue shocks before medications! 2. Alternate medication doses with repeat 4J/kg shocks 3. Use small (4.5-cm) paddles for infants <10 kg (~1 yr)
Asystole	Confirm absence of cardiac rhythm in multiple leads	1. Epinephrine 0.01 mg/kg of 1:10,000 solution, iv/io 2. Epinephrine 0.1 mg/kg of 1:1,000 solution, iv/io 3. Repeat epinephrine q3–5 min		
Pulseless electrical activity		1. Epinephrine 0.01 mg/kg of 1:10,000 solution, iv/io 2. Epinephrine 0.1 mg/kg of 1:1,000 solution, iv/io 3. Repeat epinephrine q3–5 min		Rule out treatable causes: 1. Pneumothorax 2. Severe acidosis, hypoxemia, hypovolemia 3. Tamponade 4. Hypothermia

iv = intravenous; io = intraosseus.
Based on Pediatric Advanced Life Support algorithms.

it is rare, and when life-threatening arrhythmias do occur, they are usually caused by a variety of diseases that are individually and collectively rare in the adult population. Thus, an important question is whether the survival benefits of ICDs demonstrated in adult studies can be extrapolated to device therapy in children.

Follow-up of pediatric patients is not nearly as extensive and well-controlled, but it has also shown that these patients receive appropriate therapies for ventricular arrhythmias *(44,45)*. Innovations in ICD design and fabriation that have been important in the development of pediatric indications have included migration from epicardial patch electrodes to transvenous electrodes and the development of progressively smaller devices, suitable for implantation in children of small body size. Although the dimensions of ICDs and defibrillation leads is still not optimal for children, implantation of these systems in patients as young as 1 yr of age has been reported. Continued reductions in ICD volume and utilization of novel approaches to implantation may render it possible to provide such therapy to virtually any patient, regardless of size.

In contrast to the relatively well-established patient profiles for ICD implantation in adult populations with acquired heart disease, no prospective collected data exists to guide patient selection for ICD implantation in young patients. The most common indications considered to require ICD therapy in children include LQTS and ventricular arrhythmia complicating cardiomyopathy or congenital heart disease. Poor arrhythmia control, a prior history of cardiac arrest, and—in the case of familial arrhythmia syndromes—a malignant family history of sudden death are important cofactors in prescribing device therapy. Conversely, excessively small patient size and/or anatomic cardiovascular issues which make it impossible to obtain safe transvenous access to the ventricle may render device therapy less attractive for certain patients. As in patients with bradyarrhythmia devices, careful follow-up and attention to the interaction of device therapy and lifestyle are important.

BRADYARRHYTHMIAS

The indications for implantation of permanent cardiac pacemakers in children are generally similar to those applied to adults, and include symptomatic bradycardia, recurrent bradycardia-tachycardia syndromes, congenital AV block, and advanced second- or third-degree AV block, either surgical or acquired. Specific recommendations for classifying pediatric indications for pacing have been recently published by working groups of the American Heart Association (AHA) and the American College of Cardiology (ACC) *(46)*; these are summarized in Table 5.

Although pediatric pacing was formerly limited by the availability of leads and generators which were suitable with respect to size, heart-rate range, and longevity, technological development in all of these areas has rendered it possible to provide permanent transvenous or epicardial pacing to all but the smallest children (Fig. 5). Recent developments in epicardial leads are useful for children who are too small for transvenous systems, have persistent intracardiac shunts, or are undergoing lead-placement concomitant with other cardiac surgical procedures that expose the epicardium. Temporary pacing is occasionally necessary for transient heart block observed in the perioperative period, and in children may be accomplished by placement temporary transcutaneous pacing wires, for short periods of time, by utilization of a transcutaneous pacing system.

Table 5
Indications for Pacing in Pediatric Patients

Class I—Evidence and consensus on usefulness/efficacy:
- Advanced 2° or 3° AV block with symptomatic bradycardia/CHF/low cardiac output
- Symptomatic sinus node dysfunction with correlation during age-inappropriate bradycardia
- Postoperative advanced second- or third-degree AV block persists ≥ 7 d after cardiac surgery
- Congenital third-degree AV block with a wide QRS escape rhythm of ventricular dysfunction
- Congenital third-degree AV block in the infant with a ventricular rate <50 to 55 BPM or with congenital heart disease and a ventricular rate <70 BPM
- Sustained pause-dependent VT, with or without prolonged QT, in which the efficacy of pacing documented

Class IIa—Conflicting evidence and opinion, generally favoring usefulness/efficacy:
- Bradycardia-tachycardia syndrome with the need for long-term antiarrhythmic treatment other than digitalis
- Congenital third-degree AV block beyond the first year of life, with an average heart rate <50 BPM or abrupt pauses in ventricular rate two or three times the basic cycle length
- Long QT syndrome with advanced 2° or 3°AV block
- Asymptomatic sinus bradycardia in the child complex congenital heart disease with resting heart rate <35 BPM or pauses in ventricular rate >3 s

Class IIb—Conflicting evidence and opinion, usefulness/efficacy less well-established:
- Transient postoperative third-degree AV block that reverts to sinus rhythm with residual bifascicular block
- Congenital third-degree AV block, asymptomatic, with an acceptable rate, narrow QRS complex, and normal ventricular function
- Asymptomatic sinus bradycardia in the adolescent with congenital heart disease, with resting heart rate <35 BPM or passes in ventricular rate >3 s

(From: Gregoratos G, Cheitlin MD, Conill A, Epstein AE, Fellows C, Ferguson TB Jr, Freedman RA, Hlatky MA, Naccarelli GV, Saksena S, Schlant RC, Silka MJ, Ritchie JL, Gibbons RJ, Cheitlin MD, Eagle KA, Gardner TJ, Lewis RP, O'Rourke RA, Ryan TJ, Garson A Jr: ACC/AHA guidelines for implantation of cardiac pacemakers and antiarrhythmia devices. Journal of the American College of Cardiology 1998;31:1175–1209.)

Congenital Heart Block

Congenital heart block is typically diagnosed prenatally during routine obstetrical evaluation or in the newborn period. Ventricular function in complete congenital heart block is typically normal *(47)*, and as the problem is often asymptomatic, heart block may not be discovered until later in childhood. The ECG diagnosis is usually that of complete AV dissociation. More severe presentations include the occurrence of fetal CHF (hydrops fetalis), symptoms of CHF early in infancy or ventricular extrasystoles, and tachycardia. Mothers of children with congenital heart block are commonly observed to have high titers of the maternal lupus antibodies anti-Ro and anti-La, even in the absence of overt maternal systemic lupus erythematosus. The presence of these antibodies has been linked specifically to the pathogenesis of injury to the developing fetal AV node *(48)*, and this is recognized as the most significant underlying etiology to heart block occurring in an infant with normal cardiac anatomy. This common form of congenital heart block is most often identified in the late second trimester, carries a substantial mortality in the neonatal period, and frequently requires pacing *(49)*.

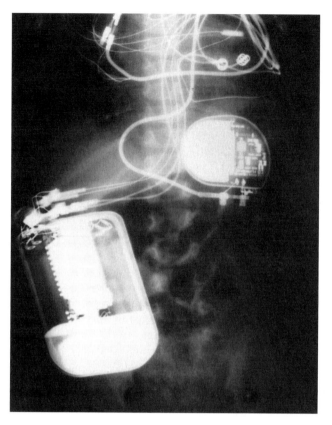

Fig. 5. Epicardial single-chamber atrial pacemaker and ICD implants in a child one year of age with refractory prolonged QT syndrome and a history of multiple cardiac arrests.

Complete AV canal and other endocardial cushion defects and L-transposition of the great arteries (L-TGA "congenitally corrected transposition") are congenital lesions which are also recognized to carry an elevated risk for the occurrence of heart block throughout life, independent of maternal antibody status. This clinical observation is believed to represent vulnerability of the specialized conduction system secondary to deformation associated with the underlying congenital defect *(50)*.

Indications for pacing of congenital heart block in infancy are debated, but have been suggested to include: signs of CHF, extreme bradycardia (e.g., ventricular rate <55/min in isolated block or <65/min when associated with other congenital defects), prolongation of the QT interval, syncope or seizure, and frequent ventricular ectopy. Less commonly, previously asymptomatic children may present with clinical symptoms that may be secondary to bradycardia, especially exercise intolerance and fatigue, and this may prompt pacemaker placement. Although the natural history of congenital heart block has not been completely elucidated, it would appear that even in its completely asymptomatic form, long-term survival may be enhanced by provision of pacing *(51)*. Thus, a typical recommendation for management of a patient who tolerates heart block well in infancy may be to defer pacemaker placement until symptoms occur, or until the patient has reached his or her expected adult body.

Postoperative Complete Heart Block

Postoperative heart block is most often associated with operations which involve resection, suturing, or another manipulation of the ventricular septum, such as repair of a VSD, although it may be seen after any type of cardiac procedure. Natural history studies (performed prior to the era of technically reliable and appropriate pediatric pacing systems) have demonstrated that medical management of these patients without pacemaker implantation is associated with very high mortality (52,53). Postoperative heart block is caused either by direct surgical injury to the AV node and the specialized conduction system or by indirect damage to those structures by stretch, swelling and/ or inflammatory response. Approximately two-thirds of patients who leave the operating room with newly acquired heart block will recover normal AV conduction in 7–10 d (54). Thus, it is appropriate to provide temporary pacing using transcutaneous wires over this period of time prior to implanting a permanent pacing system.

TECHNICAL ASPECTS OF PEDIATRIC PACING

Several issues must be considered when planning to provide permanent cardiac pacing for pediatric patients. First, vascular caliber and infraclavicular muscle and SC tissue mass will be roughly proportional to body size (55). These will affect the choice of lead as well as the placement of the generator pocket, with the smallest patients having placement of a single epicardial lead and a generator pocket on the abdominal wall. Second, it is likely that over the life of the patient, pacemaker generators may need to be replaced several times, as may the leads themselves in the event of failure. The presence of multiple, large pacing leads in the innominate vein is associated with thrombosis and occlusion of the vessel, which adds to the desirability of epicardial leads or single, low-profile transvenous leads in small children with AV block. Finally, in the case of patients with congenital heart disease, the patient's anatomy or the surgical procedures he or she has undergone may complicate, limit, or even preclude access to the right ventricle via the transvenous route. This necessitates a careful anatomical survey to be performed prior to implantation, and may result in the use of inventive approaches to lead placement (56). Comparisons of single- and dual-chamber pacing specific to the pediatric age group have not been performed. Based on studies performed in adults, who are generally elderly and have significant underlying acquired heart disease, it would seem desirable when possible to provide dual-chamber pacing for children as well. However, for young children with otherwise well-preserved myocardial function, even in the presence of congenital heart disease, single-chamber pacing is not commonly associated with pacemaker syndrome or evidence of depressed global cardiac output (57).

A frequent problem encountered in patients in whom atrial pacing is necessary—for instance, those with congenital heart disease, sinus-node dysfunction, and atrial tachycardias—is the difficulty in placing a lead which is reliably able to sense atrial electrical activity, and differentiate it from "far-field" ventricular activity. Recognition of this issue at the time of lead placement may demand use of a bipolar lead, whether endo- or epicardial, and requires a willingness to search diligently for an implantation site which allows clear discrimination of an atrial potential much larger than the ventricular.

Residual intracardiac shunts are an important consideration, and in many cases, an absolute contraindication to transvenous lead placement. In patients with cyanosis caused by a right-to-left shunt, such leads are associated with a significant risk of thromboembolic events, and are contraindicated. Among patients with small left-to-right shunts, especially at the ventricular level (e.g., a tiny residual VSD after surgical repair), it is less clear that the risk of thromboembolism from transvenous pacing leads is elevated.

Pacemaker Follow-Up and Lifestyle

Pacemaker and device therapy in children has different implications for long-term follow-up, both because of the significantly increased life expectancy of pediatric patients compared to the older adult populations and their physically active lifestyle. Higher programmed heart-rate ranges and the frequent use of unipolar ventricular epicardial leads may significantly reduce the expected longevity of the generator battery, especially in very young children. Somatic growth over time may also result in problems with lead length, especially in transvenous systems. Thus, routine clinical follow-up at a maximum interval of 6–12 mo and in combination with transtelephonic monitoring is mandatory.

Because many children have a strong desire to participate in sports, and because there may be considerable peer pressure for them to do so, reasonable judgment must be used in determining whether any constraints on physical activity are indicated. Factors which should be considered in this decision include the nature of the activity being considered; whether it is competitive or recreational, whether it likely to result in an impact injury to the pacemaker pocket in the event of a mishap, whether appropriate protective clothing or equipment can be worn, and whether the activity may interact in any adverse way with the patient's underlying hemodynamic and/or arrhythmia problems. Guidance for participation in physical activities for patients with cardiac disease in general is available *(58,59)*.

SPECIAL TOPICS IN PEDIATRIC ARRHYTHMIA

Fetal Arrhythmias

Irregular fetal heart sounds are often observed during prenatal care; less commonly, fetal tachycardia or bradycardia may present as a clinically significant arrhythmia. Either may result in fetal hydrops when severe, with a constellation of findings of CHF including polyhydramnios and effusions by fetal ultrasonography and an increased risk of fetal demise (Fig. 6). Although normal cardiac anatomy is likely, concomitant structural congenital heart disease has been observed, and necessitates echocardiograhic evaluation of these children at the time of diagnosis *(60)*.

Fetal tachycardia most commonly represents a SVT, and may be either an AV reciprocating tachycardia associated with an accessory pathway or atrial flutter. The presence of sustained tachycardia *(61)* and/or marked elevation of fetal heart rate *(62)* increases the risk of development of hydrops, particularly if the fetus is of early gestational age. Because these tachycardias are frequently characterized by incessant recurrence and spontaneous termination, techniques used postnatally for acute termination of arrhythmia are not likely to be useful in clinical management of these patients. Given the difficulties both of ECG monitoring and of drug delivery to the fetus, by the most effective method of management is to defer specific arrhythmia therapy until after the infant is delivered. A variety of different agents have been used to attempt

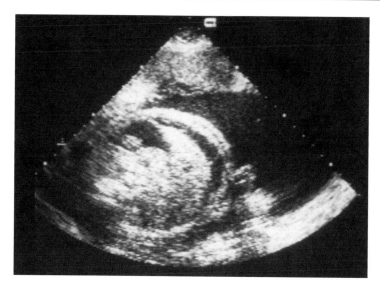

Fig. 6. Ultrasonographic appearance of fetal hydrops with effusions and polyhydramnios resulting from fetal SVT.

to establish chronic control of these tachycardias, with the goal being to allow the fetus to remain *in utero* for as much of its normal gestation as possible. The first intervention attempted is usually transplacental digoxin therapy administered to the mother. In refractory cases, various drugs have been administered to the mother. In the many case reports and short series which describe the outcomes of these drug trials, some response may be attributed to almost every agent which has been tried. It is clear that a major issue in drug therapy for these patients is the difficulty in achieving therapeutic levels of drug in the fetal circulation *(63),* which is presumably caused by both the buffering effects of the placental circulation and to the alteration of normal pharmacokinetics in pregnancy. Successful direct intraperitoneal (IP) and intravascular therapy, using long-acting antiarrhythmic agents such as amiodarone and guided by fetal ultrasonography, has also been reported *(64).*

Fetal bradycardia is usually associated with congenital complete heart block; this is typically, although not universally, associated with a maternal lupus syndrome and maternal positivity for SSA/Ro and SSA/La antibodies. Other associations of fetal complete heart block include anatomical malformations such as corrected transposition of the great arteries (L-TGA) and complete AV canal defects. Profound fetal bradycardia (<55 BPM) and observation of fetal hydrops are ominous prognostic signs. Although attempts have been made experimentally to develop intrauterine cardiac pacing as a surgical technique to rescue severely ill infants, at present this does not appear to be a viable clinical option. Similarly, maternal steroid and plasmapheresis therapy has been of uncertain benefit. Thus, bradycardic fetuses must be monitored closely, and delivered electively if signs of CHF evolve so that they may be paced.

Postoperative Acquired Atrial Arrhythmias

Atrial flutter in its common form or other atypical reentrant tachycardias are a common problem after repair of many forms of congenital heart disease *(65–67).*

Factors that predispose these patients to arrhythmia include atrial scarring and hypertrophy, abnormal atrial anatomy, and sinus-node dysfunction. These tachycardias are most prevalent in patients who have undergone procedures involving significant alterations of the atrium, especially the Mustard and Senning operations (68) and the Fontan procedure (67). These atrial tachycardias frequently recur, and are a cause of significant morbidity and even mortality in these patients (65,69).

Management of atrial tachycardias after repair of congenital heart disease is challenging and often problematic. The underlying congenital heart lesions are often associated with a marginal hemodynamic status, which not only exacerbates the effects of the tachycardia, but may also limit the options for arrhythmia management. Although the use of antiarrhythmic agents from every class has been reported, none have been clearly efficacious (18,65), and most agents carry the risk of pro-arrhythmia. Recent studies have suggested that radiofrequency ablation for the treatment of atrial reentrant tachycardia in the setting of postoperative congenital heart disease may be feasible (70–72). However, although early results using this approach have been encouraging, more extended follow-up of these patients has demonstrated recurrence rates of over 50% at 2 yr (72), only marginally better than the results of conventional therapy. Although discouraging, the results of both arrhythmia surgery and catheter ablation procedures for AF (73,74) suggest that a combination of more accurate identification of the reentry circuits and improved techniques for creation of radiofrequency lesions may successfully address this problem. Surgical modification of the atria—either as a curative procedure for patients with established arrhythmia or prophylactically performed at the time of congenital heart repair—has also been proposed, and studies of the safety and efficacy of those techniques are in progress.

Evaluation of Syncope in Pediatric Patients

Syncope is a frequent presenting complaint in the pediatric age range (75). Loss of consciousness as a primary complaint, with or without associated seizure activity, demands careful consideration of possible cardiac etiologies by the evaluating physician. The most common causes of syncopal and near-syncopal episodes in children are the various expressions of neurocardiogenic syncope (75–77). However, potentially malignant arrhythmic causes of syncope that must be carefully excluded include abnormalities of repolarization such as LQTS, Brugada syndrome, and metabolic, toxic or drug-induced abnormalities of repolarization, pre-excitation (WPW), idiopathic ventricular tachycardia and acquired heart block (e.g., secondary to infectious causes such as Lyme disease). Syncope may also be a presenting symptom of neurological syndromes, as well as several less serious arrhythmias, such as AV reciprocating tachycardias and breath-holding spells in toddlers (Fig. 7).

Basic outpatient evaluation of syncope in children includes several elements. A detailed history of the event is needed, including its associations with exercise, cardiovascular symptoms, and any witnessed objective cardiovascular signs. Past medical history must include prior occurrences of similar syncopal or presyncopal events, migraines and/or seizure disorders, prior cardiac evaluations, and current medications (including over-the-counter medicines). A family history should document occurrence of sudden death, syncope, seizure disorder, "named arrhythmia" such as LQTS or WPW, hypertrophic cardiomyopathy, use of pacemakers, ICDs, and antiarrhythmic medications in the extended as well as the immediate family. Complete cardiac and

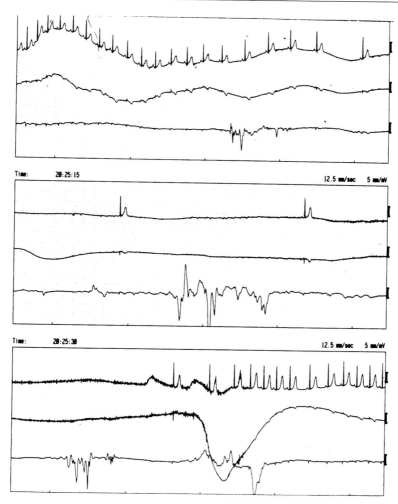

Fig. 7. Holter monitoring record of an 18-mo-old toddler experiencing a breath-holding spell.

neurological physical examination should be performed, and the ECG should be carefully examined for evidence of pre-excitation, LQTS, or other abnormalities.

If the screening evaluation is negative, certain historical characteristics of the syncopal event may allow the physician to assign a diagnosis of neurocardiogenic syncope with a high degree of certainty. A typical history for neurocardiogenic syncope in children notably includes an association with standing or sitting posture, presyncopal warmth, nausea and diaphoresis, brief duration of loss of consciousness, and an observation of pallor and fatigue after the event. The patient will often be able to draw a parallel with a similar and more frequent but less severe symptom complex experienced in association with presyncope.

When the clinical evaluation of a syncopal pediatric patient does not clearly lead to exclusion of malignant arrhythmia and a positive diagnosis of neurocardiogenic syncope by historical features, additional work-up may be needed. Evaluation of atypical syncope in the child is a significant diagnostic challenge, given the a priori low risk of major cardiac disease in this age group and the often low sensitivity and specificity of the diagnostic tests available. Tests often used to screen for occult cardiac and arrhythmic disease in greater depth include echocardiography, Holter and/or ambulatory event monitoring, and tilt-table testing. Neurological consultation and electroencephalography may also be indicated. Less commonly, and in response to specific positive findings on history, physical, or electrocardiography, it may be appropriate to consider exercise testing, cardiac catheterization, and programmed electrical stimulation, use of an implantable loop recorder (ILR), drug testing, and/or cardiac magnetic resonance imaging.

REFERENCES

1. Orejarena LA, Vidaillet HJ, DeStefano F, Nordstrom DL, Vierkant RA, Smith PN, et al. Paroxysmal supraventricular tachycardia in the general population. J Am Coll Cardiol 1998;31:150–157.
2. Perry JC, Garson A, Jr. Supraventricular tachycardia due to Wolff-Parkinson-White syndrome in children: early disappearance and late recurrence. J Am Coll Cardiol 1990;16:1215–1220.
3. Ko JK, Deal BJ, Strasburger JF, Benson DW, Jr. Supraventricular tachycardia mechanisms and their age distribution in pediatric patients. Am J Cardiol 1992;69:1028–1032.
4. Deal BJ, Keane JF, Gillette PC, Garson A, Jr. Wolff-Parkinson-White syndrome and supraventricular tachycardia during infancy: management and follow-up. J Am Coll Cardiol 1985;5:130–135.
5. Chang RK, Wetzel GT, Shannon KM, Stevenson WG, Klitzner TS. Age- and anesthesia-related changes in accessory pathway conduction in children with Wolff-Parkinson-White syndrome. Am J Cardiol 1995;76:1074–1076.
6. Naheed ZJ, Strasburger JF, Benson DWJ, Deal BJ. Natural history and management strategies of automatic atrial tachycardia in children. Am J Cardiol 1995;75:405–407.
7. Russell MW, Dorostkar PC, Dick M II. Incidence of catastrophic events associated with the Wolff-Parkinson-White syndrome in young patients: diagnostic and therapeutic dilemma. Circulation 1993; 88:I-484 (Abstract).
8. Bromberg BI, Lindsay BD, Cain ME, Cox JL. Impact of clinical history and electrophysiologic characterization of accessory pathways on management strategies to reduce sudden death among children with Wolff-Parkinson-White syndrome. J Am Coll Cardiol 1996;27:690–695.
9. Levine JC, Walsh EP, Saul JP. Radiofrequency ablation of accessory pathways associated with congenital heart disease including heterotaxy syndrome. Am J Cardiol 1993;72:689–693.
10. Fenelon G, Wijns W, Andries E, Brugada P. Tachycardiomyopathy: mechanisms and clinical implications. Pacing Clin Electrophysiol 1996;19:95–106.
11. Fishberger SB, Colan SD, Saul JP, Mayer JEJ, Walsh EP. Myocardial mechanics before and after ablation of chronic tachycardia. Pacing Clin Electrophysiol 1996;19:42–49.
12. Gikonyo BM, Dunnigan A, Benson DW, Jr. Cardiovascular collapse in infants: association with paroxysmal atrial tachycardia. Pediatrics 1985;76:922–926.
13. Losek JD, Endom E, Dietrich A, Stewart G, Zempsky W, Smith K. Adenosine and pediatric supraventricular tachycardia in the emergency department: multicenter study and review. Ann Emerg Med 1999;33:185–191.
14. Reed R, Falk JL, O'Brien J. Untoward reaction to adenosine therapy for supraventricular tachycardia. Am J Emerg Med 1991;9:566–570.
15. Radford D. Side effects of verapamil in infants. Arch Dis Child 1983;58:465–466.
16. Abinader E, Borochowitz Z, Berger A. A hemodynamic complication of verapamil therapy in a neonate. Helv Paediatr Acta 1981;36:451–455.
17. Rhodes LA, Walsh EP, Saul JP. Conversion of atrial flutter in pediatric patients by transesophageal atrial pacing: a safe, effective, minimally invasive procedure. Am Heart J 1995;130:323–327.
18. Weindling SN, Saul JP, Walsh EP. Efficacy and risks of medical therapy for supraventricular tachycardia in neonates and infants. Am Heart J 1996;131:66–72.
19. Fenrich ALJ, Perry JC, Friedman RA. Flecainide and amiodarone: combined therapy for refractory tachyarrhythmias in infancy. J Am Coll Cardiol 1995;25:1195–1198.
20. Sasse M, Paul T, Bergmann P, Kallfelz HC. Sotalol associated torsades de pointes tachycardia in a

15-month-old child: successful therapy with magnesium aspartate. Pacing Clin Electrophysiol 1998;21:1164–1166.

21. Mulla N, Karpawich PP. Ventricular fibrillation following adenosine therapy for supraventricular tachycardia in a neonate with concealed Wolff-Parkinson-White syndrome treated with digoxin. Pediatr Emerg Care 1995;11:238–239.

22. Pfammatter JP, Paul T, Lehmann C, Kallfelz HC. Efficacy and proarrhythmia of oral sotalol in pediatric patients. J Am Coll Cardiol 1995;26:1002–1007.

23. Fish FA, Gillette PC, Benson DW, Jr. Proarrhythmia, cardiac arrest and death in young patients receiving encainide and flecainide. The Pediatric Electrophysiology Group. J Am Coll Cardiol 1991;18:356–365.

24. Kugler JD, Danford DA, Deal BJ, Gillette PC, Perry JC, Silka MJ, et al. Radiofrequency catheter ablation for tachyarrhythmias in children and adolescents. The Pediatric Electrophysiology Society. N Engl J Med 1994;330:1481–1487.

25. Scheinman MM. NASPE Survey on Catheter Ablation. Pacing Clin Electrophysiol 1995;18:1474–1478.

26. Park JK, Halperin BD, McAnulty JH, Kron J, Silka MJ. Comparison of radiofrequency catheter ablation procedures in children, adolescents, and adults and the impact of accessory pathway location. Am J Cardiol 1994;74:786–789.

27. Danford DA, Kugler JD, Deal B, Case C, Friedman RA, Saul JP. The learning curve for radiofrequency ablation of tachyarrhythmias in pediatric patients. Participating members of the Pediatric Electrophysiology Society. Am J Cardiol 1995;75:587–590.

28. Kugler JD, Danford DA, Houston K, Felix G. Radiofrequency catheter ablation for paroxysmal supraventricular tachycardia in children and adolescents without structural heart disease. Pediatric EP Society, Radiofrequency Catheter Ablation Registry. Am J Cardiol 1997;80:1438–1443.

29. Van Hare GF. Indications for radiofrequency ablation in the pediatric population. J Cardiovasc Electrophysiol 1997;8:952–962.

30. Erickson CC, Walsh EP, Triedman JK, Saul JP. Efficacy and safety of radiofrequency ablation in infants and young children <18 months of age. Am J Cardiol 1994;74:944–947.

31. Vincent GM, Timothy KW, Leppert M, Keating M. The spectrum of symptoms and QT intervals in carriers of the gene for the long-QT syndrome. N Engl J Med 1992;327:846–852.

32. Tanel RE, Triedman JK, Walsh EP, Epstein MR, DeLucca JM, Mayer JEJ, et al. High-rate atrial pacing as an innovative bridging therapy in a neonate with congenital long QT syndrome. J Cardiovasc Electrophysiol 1997;8:812–817.

33. Moss AJ, Zareba W, Benhorin J, Locati EH, Hall WJ, Robinson JL, et al. ECG T-wave patterns in genetically distinct forms of the hereditary long QT syndrome. Circulation 1995;92:2929–2934.

34. Silka MJ, Park JK. Mechanisms in current management of ventricular tachycardia in children. Heart Disease & Stroke 1994;3:372–376.

35. Gelatt M, Hamilton RM, McCrindle BW, Connelly M, Haris L, et al. Arrhythmia and mortality after the Mustard procedure: a 30-year single-center experience. J Am Coll Cardiol 1997;29:194–201.

36. Wolfe RR, Driscoll DJ, Gersony WM, Hayes CJ, Keane JF, Kidd L, et al. Arrhythmias in patients with valvar aortic stenosis, valvar pulmonary stenosis, and ventricular septal defect. Results of 24-hour ECG monitoring. Circulation 1993;87:I89–I101.

37. Gentles TL, Gauvreau K, Mayer JEJ, Fishberger SB, Burnett J, Colan SD, et al. Functional outcome after the Fontan operation: factors influencing late morbidity. J Thorac Cardiovasc Surg 1997;114:392–403.

38. Nollert G, Fischlein T, Bouterwek S, Bohmer C, Klinner W, Reichart B. Long-term survival in patients with repair of tetralogy of Fallot: 36-year follow-up of 490 survivors of the first year after surgical repair. J Am Coll Cardiol 1997;30:1374–1383.

39. Alexander ME, Walsh EP, Saul JP, Epstein MR, Triedman JK. Value of programmed ventricular stimulation in patients with congenital heart disease. J Cardiovasc Electrophysiol 1999;10:1033–1044.

40. Chandar JS, Wolff GS, Garson AJ, Bell TJ, Beder SD, Bink B, et al. Ventricular arrhythmias in postoperative tetralogy of Fallot. Am J Cardiol 1990;65:655–661.

41. Gatzoulis MA, Till JA, Somerville J, Redington AN. Mechanoelectrical interaction in tetralogy of Fallot. QRS prolongation relates to right ventricular size and predicts malignant ventricular arrhythmias and sudden death. Circulation 1995;92:231–237.

42. Deal BJ, Miller SM, Scagliotti D, Prechel D, Gallastegui JL, Hariman RJ. Ventricular tachycardia in a young population without overt heart disease. Circulation 1986;73:1111–1118.

43. Pfammatter JP, Paul T. Idiopathic ventricular tachycardia in infancy and childhood: a multicenter

study on clinical profile and outcome. Working Group on Dysrhythmias and Electrophysiology of the Association for European. J Am Coll Cardiol 1999;33:2067–2072.

44. Silka MJ. Implantable cardioverter-defibrillators in children. A perspective on current and future uses. J Electrocardiol 1996;(29 Suppl):223–225.

45. Epstein MR, Alexander ME, Saul JP, Triedman JK, Tanel RE, Walsh EP. Automatic implantable cardioverter defibrillators in the very young: has the technology not gone for enough? Circulation 1999;100:I–803(Abstract).

46. Gregoratos G, Cheitlin MD, Conill A, Epstein AE, Fellows C, Ferguson TB, Jr., et al. ACC/AHA guidelines for implantation of cardiac pacemakers and antiarrhythmia devices. J Am Coll Cardiol 1998;31:1175–1209.

47. Kertesz NJ, Friedman RA, Colan SD, Walsh EP, Gajarski RJ, Gray PS, et al. Left ventricular mechanics and geometry in patients with congenital complete atrioventricular block. Circulation 1997;96:3430–3435.

48. Mazel JA, El-Sherif N, Buyon J, Boutjdir M. Electrocardiographic abnormalities in a murine model injected with IgG from mothers of children with congenital heart block. Circulation 1999;99:1914–1918.

49. Buyon JP, Hiebert R, Copel J, Craft J, Friedman D, Katholi M, et al. Autoimmune-associated congenital heart block: demographics, mortality, morbidity and recurrence rates obtained from a national neonatal lupus registry. J Am Coll Cardiol 1998;31:1658–1666.

50. Bharati S, McCue CM, Tingelstad JB, Mantakas M, Shiel F, Lev M. Lack of connection between the atria and the peripheral conduction system in a case of corrected transposition with congenital atrioventricular block. Am J Cardiol 1978;42:147–153.

51. Michaelsson M, Jonzon A, Riesenfeld T. Isolated congenital complete atrioventricular block in adult life. A prospective study. Circulation 1995;92:442–449.

52. Hofschire PJ, Nicoloff DM, Moller JH. Postoperative complete heart block in 64 children treated with and without cardiac pacing. Am J Cardiol 1977;39:559–562.

53. Hoffman JL. Heart block in congenital heart disease. Bull NY Acad Med 1971;47:885–904.

54. Weindling SN, Saul JP, Gamble WJ, Mayer JE, Wessel D, Walsh EP. Duration of complete atrioventricular block after congenital heart disease surgery. Am J Cardiol 1998;82:525–527.

55. Molina JE, Dunnigan AC, Crosson JE. Implantation of transvenous pacemakers in infants and small children. Ann Thorac Surg 1995;59:689–694.

56. Spotnitz HM. Transvenous pacing in infants and children with congenital heart disease. Ann Thorac Surg 1990;49:495–496.

57. Ragonese P, Guccione P, Drago F, Turchetta A, Calzolari A, Formigari R. Efficacy and safety of ventricular rate responsive pacing in children with complete atrioventricular block. Pacing Clin Electrophysiol 1994;17:603–610.

58. Graham TPJ, Bricker JT, James FW, Strong WB. 26th Bethesday conference: recommendations for determining eligibility for competition in athletes with cardiovascular abnormalities. Task Force 1: congenital heart disease. J Am Coll Cardiol 1994;24:867–873.

59. Maron BJ, Thompson PD, Puffer JC, McGrew CA, Strong WB, Douglas PS, et al. Cardiovascular preparticipation screening of competitive athletes. A statement for health professionals from the Sudden Death Committee (clinical cardiology) and Congenital Cardiac Defects Committee (cardiovascular disease in the young), American Heart Association. Circulation 1996;94:850–856.

60. Dunnigan A, Benson W Jr, Benditt DG. Atrial flutter in infancy: diagnosis, clinical features, and treatment. Pediatrics 1985;75:725–729.

61. Naheed ZJ, Strasburger JF, Deal BJ, Benson DWJ, Gidding SS. Fetal tachycardia: mechanisms and predictors of hydrops fetalis. J Am Coll Cardiol 1996;27:1736–1740.

62. Guntheroth WG, Cyr DR, Shields LE, Nghiem HV. Rate-based management of fetal supraventricular tachycardia. Journal of Ultrasound in Medicine 1996;15:453–458.

63. Triedman JK, Walsh EP, Saul JP. Response of fetal tachycardia to transplacental procainamide therapy. Cardiol in the Young 1996;6:235–238.

64. Mangione R, Guyon F, Vergnaud A, Jimenez M, Saura R, Horovitz J. Successful treatment of refractory supraventricular tachycardia by repeat intravascular injection of amiodarone in a fetus with hydrops. Eur J Obstet Gynecol & Reprod Biol 1999;86:105–107.

65. Garson A Jr, Bink-Boelkens MTE, Hesslein PS, Hordorf AJ, Keane JF, Neches WH, et al. Atrial flutter in the young: a collaborative study in 380 cases. J Am Coll Cardiol 1985;6:871–878.

66. Roos-Hesselink J, Perlroth MG, McGhie J, Spitaels S. Atrial arrhythmias in adults after repair of

tetralogy of Fallot. Correlation with clinical, exercise, and echocardiographic findings. Circulation 1995;91:2214–2219.

67. Fishberger SB, Wernovsky G, Gentles TL, Gauvreau K, Burnett J, Mayer JE J, et al. Factors that influence the development of atrial flutter after the Fontan operation. J Thorac Cardiovasc Surg 1997;113:80–86.

68. Gelatt M, Hamilton RM, McCrindle BW, Gow RM, Williams WG, Trusler GA, et al. Risk factors for atrial tachyarrhythmias after the Fontan operation. J Am Coll Cardiol 1994;24:1735–1741.

69. Feltes TF, Friedman RA. Transesophageal echocardiographic detection of atrial thrombi in patients with nonfibrillation atrial tachyarrhythmias and congenital heart disease. J Am Coll Cardiol 1994;24:1365–1370.

70. Kalman JM, VanHare GF, Olgin JE, Saxon LA, Stark SI, Lesh MD. Ablation of 'incisional' reentrant atrial tachycardia complicating surgery for congenital heart disease. Use of entrainment to define a critical isthmus of conduction. Circulation 1996;93:502–512.

71. Baker BM, Lindsay BD, Bromberg B, Frazier DW, Cain ME, Smith JM. Catheter ablation of intraatrial reentrant tachycardias resulting from previous atrial surgery: locating and transecting the critical isthmus. J Am Coll Cardiol 1996;28:411–417.

72. Triedman JK, Bergau DM, Saul JP, Epstein MR, Walsh EP. Efficacy of radiofrequency ablation for control of intraatrial reentrant tachycardia in patients with congenital heart disease. J Am Coll Cardiol 1997;30:1032–1038.

73. Cox JL, Sundt TM. The surgical management of atrial fibrillation. Am Rev Med 1997;48:511–523.

74. Haissaguerre M, Shah DC, Jais P, Clementy J. Role of catheter ablation for atrial fibrillation. Curr Opin Cardiol 1997;12:18–23.

75. Driscoll DJ, Jacobsen SJ, Porter CJ, Wollan PC. Syncope in children and adolescents. J Am Coll Cardiol 1997;29:1039–1045.

76. McHarg ML, Shinnar S, Rascoff H, Walsh CA. Syncope in childhood. Pediatr Cardiol 1997;18:367–371.

77. Tanel RE, Walsh EP. Syncope in the pediatric patient. Cardiol Clin 1997;15:277–294.

21 Arrhythmias During Pregnancy

Special Considerations

José A. Joglar, MD and Richard L. Page, MD

INTRODUCTION

Cardiac arrhythmias that occur during pregnancy represent a unique problem, since two lives may be in jeopardy. Most arrhythmias originate in the mother, but occasionally fetal arrhythmias require therapy through maternal administration of drugs. When considering therapeutic interventions, pro-arrhythmia and other adverse effects to both the mother and fetus must be considered. There are also unique risks to the fetus, such as congenital malformations.

Although arrhythmias and conduction disturbances can occur in both the mother and fetus, this chapter focuses mainly on problems that affect the mother. When there is a clear understanding of the maternal hemodynamic changes associated with pregnancy, as well as the appropriate antiarrhythmic therapies available and their potential risks, most cases can be treated successfully. The full spectrum of cardiac arrhythmias and conduction disturbances can occur during pregnancy. In the setting of a structurally normal heart and asymptomatic or minimally symptomatic arrhythmias (such as premature ventricular or atrial beats), reassurance is the only treatment necessary. Antiarrhythmic drug therapy and invasive procedures should be reserved for cases that cause significant symptoms or are life-threatening.

PHYSIOLOGIC CHANGES DURING PREGNANCY

The changes observed in the maternal-fetal circulatory system during pregnancy complicate the administration of antiarrhythmic agents, and may affect the clinical

From: *Contemporary Cardiology: Management of Cardiac Arrhythmias*
Edited by: L. I. Ganz © Humana Press Inc., Totowa, NJ

response of the mother to various agents. Drug absorption and bioavailability may be altered because of changes in gastric secretions and gut motility. Increases in cardiac output by 30–50% augment renal blood flow and the glomerular filtration rate, resulting in increased clearance of renally excreted drugs. Progesterone-induced hepatic stimulation may also increase the clearance of some hepatically metabolized drugs. Increases in blood volume by 40–50% may make it necessary to raise the loading dose needed to achieve therapeutic drug concentrations. Since most of the increase in blood volume is a result of higher plasma volume, there is an associated drop in serum protein concentration. This change in serum protein concentration can lead to decreased drug protein binding, which may result in increased drug clearance and lower total drug concentrations despite adequate free levels. Since a lower total drug level is required to provide a desired effect, therapeutic drug serum levels are usually lower than during the nonpregnant state; this can lead to unnecessary—and potentially dangerous—dose adjustments if this phenomenon is not considered (1–4).

Since the magnitude of these changes can vary, depending on the stage of pregnancy, closer drug monitoring and more frequent dose adjustment are needed in comparison to the nonpregnant condition. In addition, it is important to closely monitor the clinical and electrophysiologic response of the patient to the particular agent, rather than relying solely on serum drug levels.

EPIDEMIOLOGY OF ARRHYTHMIAS DURING PREGNANCY

An increased incidence of maternal cardiac arrhythmias is observed during pregnancy. This includes episodes of paroxysmal supraventricular tachycardia (PSVT) in patients with the Wolff-Parkinson-White syndrome (WPW) and new-onset idiopathic ventricular tachycardia (VT) (5–7). The increase in arrhythmias is explained in part by the metabolic, hormonal, and hemodynamic changes of pregnancy. In addition, advances in cardiac surgery have allowed an increased number of women with congenital cardiac malformations to reach reproductive age, and these women are prone to supraventricular and ventricular arrhythmias (8). Arrhythmias may also be the initial presentation of a serious cardiovascular condition that develops or is discovered during pregnancy, such as peripartum cardiomyopathy (9). Fortunately, the most common arrhythmias observed during pregnancy are simply premature ventricular and atrial ectopy, reported in 50–60% of pregnant women and often not correlated with symptoms (6).

SPECIFIC ANTIARRHYTHMIC AGENTS

Experience with antiarrhythmic agents during pregnancy varies among the different classes of drugs (see Tables 1,2). In general, the medications that have been available for longer periods of time have the greatest clinical data regarding safety. Many antiarrhythmic drugs appear to be relatively safe, although there are important exceptions. The majority are United States Food and Drug Administration (USFDA) category C, which means that fetal risk cannot be excluded, either because of animal studies suggesting risk without confirmatory human studies, or the absence of controlled studies in either humans or animals (Table 1).

All antiarrhythmic medications have potential side effects for both the mother and the fetus, so the smallest recommended dose should be used initially, accompanied with regular monitoring of serum drug levels (where appropriate) and clinical response.

Table 1
Definition of FDA Pregnancy Categories
and Antiarrhythmic Agents within Each Category

Pregnancy category	Definition	Antiarrhythmic agents
A	**Controlled studies show no risk.** Adequate, well-controlled studies in pregnant women have failed to demonstrate risk to the fetus in any trimester of pregnancy.	
B	**No evidence of risk in humans.** Adequate, well-controlled studies in pregnant women have not shown increased risk of fetal abnormalities despite adverse findings in animals, or in the absence of adequate human studies, animal studies show no fetal risk. The chance of fetal harm is remote, but remains a possibility.	Lidocaine, sotalol, acebutolol
C	**Risk cannot be ruled out.** Adequate, well-controlled human studies are lacking, and animal studies have shown a risk to the fetus or are lacking as well. There is chance of fetal harm if the drug is administered during pregnancy; but the potential benefits outweigh the risk.	Quinidine, disopyramide, procainamide, mexiletine, flecainide, propafenone, propranolol, metoprolol, bretylium, dofetilide, ibutilide, verapamil, diltiazem, digoxin, adenosine
D	**Positive evidence of risk.** Studies in humans have shown evidence of fetal risk. Nevertheless, the potential benefits from the use of the drug in pregnant women may outweigh the risk.	Phenytoin, amiodarone, atenolol
X	**Contraindicated in pregnancy.** Studies in animals or humans have shown fetal risk, which clearly outweighs any possible benefit to patient.	

(Adapted from: Physicians' Desk Reference. Medical Economics, Inc. Montvale, NJ, 1999.)

The most troubling side effect for the mother is proarrhythmia, which may occur with almost all of the Vaughan Williams class I and III antiarrhythmic agents. These medications should be initiated during inpatient cardiac monitoring. The continued need for the medication should also be reassessed on a regular basis.

Class I (Sodium-Channel-Blocking Agents)

In the Vaughan Williams classification of antiarrhythmic drugs, the sodium-channel-blocking agents are subdivided into class IA (drugs that prolong the action-potential duration), IB (drugs that cause shortening of the action-potential duration), and IC (drugs that cause profound slowing of conduction) *(10)*.

Of the IA agents, quinidine has the longest record of safety during pregnancy, with over 60 years of experience in the management of a variety of maternal and fetal arrhythmias, and in treating maternal malaria *(11–14)*. Although isolated cases of

Table 2
Experience with Antiarrhythmic Drugs During Pregnancy

Drug	Drug class*	FDA class*	Potential adverse effects	Best indication	Use during lactation	Comments
Quinidine	IA	C	Maternal and fetal thrombocytopenia, eighth nerve toxicity, torsades de pointes	Variety of maternal and fetal arrhythmias	Generally compatible, but caution advised	Long record of safety
Procainamide	IA	C	Lupus-like syndrome with long-term use, torsades de pointes	Drug of choice for acute treatment of undiagnosed wide-complex tachycardia	Compatible but long-term therapy should be avoided	Has the advantage of iv dosing, long record of safety
Disopyramide	IA	C	Induction of uterine contractions, torsades de pointes	Limited experience, other alternatives available	Compatible	Limited experience
Lidocaine	IB	B	CNS adverse effects, bradycardia	Maternal VT, arrhythmias caused by digoxin toxicity	Compatible	Long record of safety, avoid if fetal distress occurs
Mexiletine	IB	C	CNS adverse effects, fetal bradycardia, low APGAR	VT	Compatible	Limited experience
Phenytoin	IB	D	Mental and growth retardation, fetal hydantoin syndrome	Arrhythmias caused by digoxin toxicity	Generally compatible, but caution advised	Better alternatives available, avoid if possible
Flecainide	IC	C	Increased mortality in patients with previous myocardial infarction, generally safe in structurally normal hearts	Variety of maternal and fetal VT and SVT	Compatible	First-line option for treating fetal SVT with hydrops
Propafenone	IC	C	Same concerns as flecainide, mild beta-blocker effects	Variety of maternal VT and SVT	Unknown	Limited experience

494

Drug	Class*	Category†	Adverse effects	Indications	Breastfeeding‡	Pregnancy recommendations
Beta-blocking agents	II	B/C/D	Intrauterine growth retardation, fetal bradycardia, hypoglycemia, fetal apnea	Maternal SVT, idiopathic VT, AF rate control	Avoid atenolol. Metoprolol and propranolol are compatible	Generally safe, avoid during first trimester; cardiac selective are preferred
Amiodarone	III	D	Fetal hypothyroidism, prematurity, low birthweight, congenital malformations	Life-threatening ventricular arrhythmias	Avoid, since a large amount of drug is absorbed by the infant	Avoid if possible, especially during first trimester
Sotalol	III	B	Torsades de pointes, beta-blocker effects	Maternal VT and SVT, hypertension in the past	Generally compatible, but caution advised	Limited experience
Dofetilide	III	C	Torsades de pointes	Maternal AF and atrial flutter	Unknown	Avoid because of absence of data
Bretylium	III	C	Maternal hypotension	Maternal VF, VT	Unknown	No experience in pregnancy
Ibutilide	III	C	Torsades de pointes	Acute termination of AF/atrial flutter	Unknown	
Verapamil	IV	C	Maternal hypotension, fetal bradycardia and heart block	Maternal and fetal SVT, idiopathic VT, AF rate control	Compatible	Relatively safe, but safer options are available
Diltiazem	IV	C	Limited experience, same concerns as with verapamil	Maternal SVT, AF rate control	Compatible	Verapamil preferred because of longer record in pregnancy
Adenosine	N/A	C	Dyspnea, bradycardia	Acute termination of maternal SVT	Unknown, but probably safe	First option for acute treatment of SVT
Digoxin	N/A	C	Low birth weight	Fetal and maternal SVT, AF rate contorl	Compatible	Long record of safety

*Vaughan Williams classification of anti-arrhythmic drugs.
† FDA risk category (see Table 1).
‡ Committee on Drugs. Transfer of drugs and other chemicals into human milk. *Pediatrics*. 1994;93:137–150.
N/A = not applicable; SVT = supraventricular tachycardia; VT = ventricular tachycardia; AF = atrial fibrillation.

adverse effects have been reported, such as fetal thrombocytopenia and eighth-nerve toxicity, the drug is considered to be relatively safe when administered in therapeutic doses *(1,15)*. Monitoring of serum levels is mandatory in order to avoid adverse effects. Some authors advise against the use of quinidine by lactating women because of potential accumulation of the drug in the newborn's immature liver *(12)*.

Procainamide has electrophysiologic properties and clinical applications similar to quinidine, but has the advantage of intravenous (iv) dosing. It has proven to be safe and effective in the management of maternal and fetal arrhythmias *(1,16)*, and is an appropriate choice for the acute treatment of undiagnosed wide-complex tachycardia *(17)*. Procainamide is one of the best therapeutic options for arrhythmias that occur in pregnancy. The side-effect profile, when administered over a limited period of time (such as during gestation), has proven to be quite favorable based on general experience. Dose adjustments during different stages of pregnancy may be necessary, and some caution is warranted because of a lupus-like syndrome that occurs with long-term therapy *(15)*.

Disopyramide is also in the IA category, and shares similar antiarrhythmic properties with quinidine and procainamide. However, a lack of experience during pregnancy makes therapy with this agent less attractive than the other class IA drugs.

Care must be taken when administering class IA drugs, because of the risk of potentially fatal ventricular arrhythmias (torsades de pointes) associated with prolongation of the QT interval on electrocardiogram (ECG). All class IA medications must be initiated in the hospital during continuous cardiac monitoring, and serum drug levels should be carefully monitored. Quinidine, procainamide, and disopyramide are considered FDA category C.

The class IB includes lidocaine, mexiletine, tocainide, moricizine, and phenytoin. Lidocaine is used primarily for the acute management of ventricular arrhythmias. It has been widely used during pregnancy, mainly as an anesthetic agent during labor and delivery. Experience with lidocaine as an antiarrhythmic agent during pregnancy is limited, but animal and human registry data suggest that lidocaine is generally safe for both the mother and the fetus *(1,18,19)*. Occasional cases of lidocaine toxicity to the fetus have been reported when large doses are administered for anesthetic purposes *(20)*. The drug is best avoided with prolonged labor or fetal distress; when lidocaine is administered in the presence of fetal acidosis, fetal cardiac and central-nervous-system (CNS) toxicity may occur because of higher free-drug levels *(21)*. Since lidocaine metabolism occurs in the liver, mothers with impaired liver function or heart failure should receive reduced loading and maintenance dosages. Lidocaine is considered FDA category B.

Mexiletine is an oral antiarrhythmic agent similar in structure to lidocaine. Use of mexiletine during pregnancy is much more limited, but it also appears to be safe, even during breastfeeding, since the amount of drug that is excreted in human milk is very small *(21–24)*. Despite reports of safe administration, caution is still advised because of the scarcity of data.

Phenytoin is an anticonvulsant agent that has been used in the past primarily for arrhythmias resulting from digitalis toxicity *(25)*. In recent years it has become of limited value as an antiarrhythmic agent because of the availability of other therapeutic alternatives (including beta-blockers, digoxin-specific antibodies, and lidocaine), and the routine practice of monitoring serum digoxin levels. This drug should be avoided during pregnancy (FDA category D) because of the high risk of congenital malformations and adverse effects to the fetus, including the "fetal hydantoin syndrome," which may occur with drug exposure during the first trimester *(26)*. Nevertheless, phenytoin may be safe when used for short periods of time, especially after the first trimester, and could still be an option for acute management of digitalis-induced arrhythmias that do not respond to other therapies.

Experience with the agents tocainide and moricizine during pregnancy is very limited. Since they offer no unique advantage, it is best to avoid these drugs in favor of agents with better-established utility and safety in pregnancy.

The class IC agents include propafenone and flecainide, two drugs which are useful in the management of VTs and supraventricular tachycardias (SVTs), and appear to be relatively safe during pregnancy. Flecainide is contraindicated in patients with previous myocardial infarctions (MIs) in light of the results of the Cardiac Arrhythmias Suppression Trial (CAST), which showed an increased mortality in post-infarct patients who were treated for suppression of high-grade ventricular ectopy *(27)*. Otherwise, it has proven to be safe and effective in the treatment of diverse maternal arrhythmias, such as atrial tachycardia and VT *(28,29)*. Nevertheless, since the general experience is quite limited, especially during the first trimester, caution is advised.

For the management of fetal arrhythmias, maternally administered flecainide has been shown to be very effective. Allan et al. reported successful termination of supraventricular arrhythmias in 12 of 14 hydropic fetuses within 48 h of therapy initiation, as compared to 2–3 wk with digoxin and verapamil *(30)*. A retrospective analysis showed improved survival when fetuses were treated with flecainide, as compared with digoxin *(31)*. No adverse effects from flecainide were observed in this study. In a different retrospective study involving 127 patients, Simpson et al. confirmed that flecainide worked more rapidly than digoxin and verapamil *(32)*. The drug is excreted in human breast milk, but there is little data regarding pharmacokientics of flecainide in nursing infants. Sporadic cases of adverse effects to the fetus have been reported *(33)*, but generally patients did well when flecainide was administered for fetal arrhythmias. In light of the previously mentioned studies, flecainide should be considered as a first-line alternative in the management of fetal SVT complicated by fetal hydrops.

The use of propafenone is more limited, although no adverse effects to the mother or the fetus have been reported when administered during the third trimester *(34)*. The concerns regarding patients with prior MI may be similar to those with flecainide, because they share similar pharmacologic properties. There are no reports regarding administration of propafenone during the first trimester. Both flecainide and propafenone are considered FDA category C.

Class II (Beta-Adrenergic-Blocking Agents)

The beta-adrenergic blocking agents are useful in the suppression of a variety of maternal and fetal supraventricular and ventricular arrhythmias, and for control of the ventricular response in atrial fibrillation (AF) and atrial flutter. These agents are especially effective in treating pregnant women with idiopathic VT *(7)*. Extensive experience has been accumulated using beta-blockers during pregnancy to treat other conditions, including hypertension, hyperthyroidism, and hypertrophic cardiomyopathy *(1,35)*. The cardiac effects are mediated by $\beta 1$ receptors, and $\beta 2$ receptors act predominantly in bronchi, blood vessels, and uterine relaxation.

Although there have been reports of adverse effects on the fetus such as bradycardia, apnea, hypoglycemia, premature labor, and metabolic abnormalities, the incidence of these complications is low. Prospective randomized trials have failed to show a statistically significant higher incidence of these complications with beta-blockers as compared with placebo (raising the possibility that these reactions occurred as the result of fetal distress in high-risk pregnancies) *(35,36)*.

The main adverse fetal effect associated with beta-blockers—especially propranolol—is intrauterine growth retardation *(37)*, although other studies have failed to confirm this complication. Placebo-controlled studies of atenolol and metoprolol have likewise demonstrated no evidence of growth retardation *(38,39)*. A more recent study reported growth retardation in babies who received atenolol in the first trimester *(40)*. The authors attribute their findings to the dosing of the beta-blocker during the first trimester (and not the second or third trimesters, as was primarily the case in previous studies). Although it is difficult to discern between growth retardation caused by maternal disease vs drug effects, in view of these results, beta-blockers should be avoided during the first trimester if possible. Cardioselective β1 antagonists such as metoprolol are the preferred agents, since they may be less likely to inferfere with β2-mediated peripheral vasodilatation and uterine relaxation *(35)*.

Almost all β antagonists have been shown to be secreted in breast milk, but generally do not cause adverse effects to the nursing infant with normal hepatic and renal function *(41,42)*. However, one case of fetal bradycardia caused by atenolol secretion in breast milk has been reported *(43)*, so caution should be exercised. Propranolol and metoprolol are FDA category C and atenolol is category D.

Class III (Potassium-Channel-Blocking Agents)

The class III agents primarily block potassium channels, causing delay of repolarization and prolonging the QT interval. This class includes amiodarone, bretylium, sotalol, dofetilide, and ibutilide.

Amiodarone is a potent antiarrhythmic agent with properties encompassing class I, II, III and IV agents. It is used for the management of ventricular and, less often, supraventricular arrhythmias. It contains a high concentration of iodine (contributing to some of its side effects), and has a long half-life of 26–107 d.

Multiple adverse effects to the fetus have been reported with amiodarone, including fetal hypothyroidism, low birthweight, prematurity, bradycardia, and QT prolongation *(44–46)*. Concomitant use of amiodarone with beta-blockers should be avoided, in order to prevent excess bradycardia and intrauterine growth retardation *(46)*. Congenital abnormalities have been reported in patients who were exposed to amiodarone during the embryonic period *(46,47)*, so the drug should especially be avoided during the first trimester. Despite the efficacy of amiodarone in treating a number of arrhythmias, the side-effect profile has caused it to be contraindicated during pregnancy (except for life-threatening conditions where other agents have failed and the benefit outweighs the substantial risk). Amiodarone is FDA category D. Relatively high concentrations of amiodarone can be found in breast milk *(48)*, so it is best avoided during lactation.

Sotalol is a class III agent with non-cardiac selective beta-receptor antagonist properties. The most serious side effect is torsades de pointes. Although sotalol has been used successfully during pregnancy, experience is limited, so caution is advised *(28,49)*. Since sotalol crosses the placental barrier freely, concerns have been raised about potential adverse effects to the fetus *(49)*. No adverse events have been reported with nursing, but since a significant amount of the drug is found in human milk, caution is advised during breastfeeding *(1)*. Sotalol is FDA category B.

Dofetilide is a new class III agent indicated for the management of persistent AF and atrial flutter. No data exist regarding dofetilide use during pregnancy, and its use should therefore be avoided. Dofetilide is FDA category C.

Bretylium is an iv class III agent used for refractory VT and ventricular fibrillation (VF). The use of bretylium during pregnancy is rather limited, so it cannot be recommended for routine use except for cases of life-threatening arrhythmias in which other options have failed. It is FDA category C. At present, bretylium is not available in the United States.

Ibutilide is a new class III iv agent that is used for acute termination of AF or atrial flutter. Unlike the other class III agents, ibutilide's mechanism relates in part to an increase in sodium conductance. The main adverse effect of this drug is the occasional (1.7%) induction of sustained torsades de pointes requiring direct current cardioversion *(50)*. There are no case reports of ibutilide use during pregnancy, so although it is labeled as FDA category C, it should be avoided during pregnancy.

Class IV (Calcium-Channel-Blocking Agents)

The calcium-channel-blocking agents with the most important antiarrhythmic action are verapamil and diltiazem. These agents are mainly used in the management of SVTs, for control of the ventricular response in patients with AF or atrial flutter, and in some cases for the treatment of idiopathic VT (IVT) originating from the left ventricle. Favorable results have been reported with verapamil for the acute treatment of SVT in pregnant women, except for the occurrence of maternal hypotension *(51,52)*. Orlandi et al. reported no significant adverse effects when verapamil was used to treat hypertension in 90 patients *(53)*. However, adverse effects to the fetus such as bradycardia, heart block, depression of contractility, hypotension, and death have occurred when verapamil was used in the management of fetal supraventricular arrhythmias *(31,54)*. Overall, the calcium-channel blockers appear to be relatively safe for the treatment of maternal conditions, but because of the reports of adverse effects on the fetus, caution is advised and other alternative therapies should be considered first (such as adenosine and beta-blockers).

The use of diltiazem is more limited than verapamil, so the latter is the calcium antagonist of choice during pregnancy. Both drugs are considered FDA category C, and are compatible with breastfeeding.

ADENOSINE

Adenosine and digoxin do not fit into the Vaughn Williams classification of antiarrhythmic drugs. Adenosine is an endogenous nucleoside with a short half-life (less than 10 s), which has proven to be highly effective in the acute termination of SVT by causing transient conduction block in the atrioventricular (AV) node *(55)*. The drug has been safely used for the termination of SVT in pregnant women, with no significant adverse effects to the mother or fetus *(56)*. The usual dose is a 6-mg rapid iv bolus followed by 12 or even 18 mg if necessary. Safe administration of up to 24 mg has been reported, with no effect on fetal heart rate *(17)*. Minor maternal side effects, such as bradycardia and dyspnea, are usually transient and of no consequence.

The enzyme responsible for adenosine degradation (adenosine deaminase) is reduced in pregnancy by about 25% *(57)*, but the potency of the drug is not usually increased because of expansion in intravascular volume; higher doses than usual may be required *(56)*. Experimental data suggest that significant amounts of adenosine do not cross the placenta *(58)*, probably because of the short half-life. Most of the reports of adenosine administration occurred in the second and third trimester, so caution is advised when administering this drug in the first trimester. Nevertheless, it is the drug of choice for acute termination of SVT during pregnancy *(59)*. Adenosine should not be administered to patients with asthma, since it can induce bronchospasm *(55)*. Adenosine is considered FDA category C.

DIGOXIN

Digoxin is a glycoside that exerts its antiarrhythmic action mainly through vagally mediated AV conduction slowing and block. There is extensive experience with digoxin, and it is probably one of the safest antiarrhythmic drugs for use during pregnancy. Digoxin freely crosses the placenta *(60,61)*, and for many years has been used for the treatment of a variety of maternal and fetal supraventricular arrhythmias *(62,63)*. Direct fetal intramuscular administration of digoxin for the management of fetal SVT has been reported, with good results and no adverse effects *(64)*.

As in nonpregnant patients, the digoxin dose must be adjusted for renal impairment or if there is concomitant administration of drugs that increase the digoxin level *(15)*. Serum drug levels must be monitored, although in the third trimester the serum-concentration measurement may be spuriously high because of a circulating digoxin-like substance that interferes with the radioimmune assay for the drug *(65)*. Despite its safety record, digoxin is considered FDA category C. Digoxin is considered safe for use by lactating mothers *(66)*.

DIAGNOSIS AND MANAGEMENT

Sinus-Node and Atrioventricular Conduction Disturbances

A physiologic increase in heart rate of 10–20 beats per minute (BPM) occurs during pregnancy *(2)*, and sinus-node dysfunction is rare. Rare cases have been attributed to the supine hypotensive syndrome of pregnancy, caused by uterine compression of the inferior vena cava (IVC) blood return with paradoxical sinus slowing *(67)*. In the rare instance when symptomatic bradycardia occurs, this should be treated with a change in position of the mother (usually a left lateral decubitus position). For persistent symptoms, a temporary pacemaker may be necessary. This can be performed safely, especially if the fetus is beyond 8 wk gestation, after which organogenesis is essentially complete and radiation exposure is of minimal risk.

Although the development of high-degree heart block is not associated with pregnancy, congenital complete heart block in the mother is occasionally first recognized during pregnancy. Congenital complete heart block may become manifest during pregnancy, which may be related to the increased level of medical attention in this period or the altered hemodynamic and autonomic state. Any significant symptoms are often related to the severity of the underlying heart disease. Patients with isolated heart block and no other evidence of conduction system or structural heart disease have a favorable outcome, and supportive pacing during pregnancy is usually not necessary. In contrast, during delivery, temporary pacing is recommended for all women with complete heart block because of the high incidence of syncope and bradycardia resulting from Valsalva *(68),* and to allow for adequate heart rate response to increased cardiovascular stress.

For patients with symptoms associated with complete heart block or other bradyarrhythmias during pregnancy, placement of a permanent pacemaker is preferable to prolonged temporary pacing. There are recent reports of permanent pacemaker implantation during pregnancy. Antonelli et al. reported a successful implant of a dual-chamber pacemaker guided by transesophageal echocardiogram *(69).* Other methods employed to minimize radiation exposure include electrocardiographic and transthoracic echocardiogram guidance *(70,71).* The issues regarding radiation exposure are similar to those addressed previously, and radiation risk is low after 8 wk gestation.

Syncope During Pregnancy

In most pregnant patients without structural heart disease, syncope is benign, although occasionally it can be a manifestation of a more serious problem. When syncope occurs late in pregnancy while the patient is supine, it is usually caused by impaired venous return to the heart, the result of IVC compression by the gravid uterus, the "supine hypotensive syndrome" *(72).* Symptoms usually subside when the patient rolls over on her left side, which confirms the diagnosis. Syncope may also occur after standing upright suddenly or after long periods of time, because of a fall in venous return as the result of increased venous pooling associated with pregnancy.

When caval compression or changes in body position cannot explain recurrent syncope, other etiologies must be considered and managed immediately. A complete evaluation of the patient is mandatory, including physical examination, ECG, and laboratory tests. As in nonpregnant patients, multiple potential etiologies must be considered, including tachyarrhythmias, bradyarrhythmias, dehydration, and hypoglycemia, among others. In addition, rare causes reported that are specific to pregnant women include abruptio placenta and bleeding caused by ruptured ectopic pregnancy *(73,74).*

Supraventricular Tachyarrhythmias

Patients with a prior history of SVT should be advised about the possibility of increased symptoms during pregnancy. Sustained SVT should be treated promptly because it can result in impaired fetal blood flow and even fetal demise *(75).* Adenosine is the drug of choice for acute termination of SVT; the initial dose is 6 mg iv, followed by 12 or even 18 mg, as indicated. For patients who require long-term suppressive therapy, β-adrenergic antagonists should be considered because they have the longest record of safety (with the exception of atenolol, which has been reported to cause decreased birthweight when given early during pregnancy) *(40).* Digoxin is safe during pregnancy but is less effective; it is probably most useful in combination with β-adrenergic antagonists, achieving better efficacy while minimizing side effects by allowing lower doses of two drugs. Calcium-channel blockers may also be effective, although the potential for fetal bradyarrhythmias has caused some concern with these agents. Procedures that involve fluoroscopic radiation should be avoided, but can generally be performed at low risk after 8 wk gestation. There is a case report of radiofrequency catheter ablation successfully performed during pregnancy in a patient with the WPW and refractory PSVT, using only 70 s of fluoroscopic time and with no complication or evident adverse effects on the fetus (76).

Anticoagulation for AF During Pregnancy

AF during pregnancy in the absence of structural heart disease is rare. It can be seen occasionally in patients with thyrotoxicosis, pulmonary embolism, congenital heart disease, and cardiomyopathy, but it is most common in the setting of rheumatic heart disease (77). Szekely et al. reported AF to be present in 8% of pregnant women with rheumatic heart disease, and systemic thromboembolism was reported in 27% of them (78). Mendelson et al. reported systemic thromboembolism in 23% of pregnant patients with chronic AF and rheumatic mitral-valve disease (79). Since these are high-risk patients for embolic events, despite the lack of adequate prospective studies targeted to this specific population, we believe that they should be fully anticoagulated throughout pregnancy.

Controversies regarding anticoagulation in pregnant women arise mainly from concerns about safety to the mother vs potential damage to the fetus. Coumarin derivatives cross the placenta and can cause an embryopathy, which consists of nasal hypoplasia and/or stippled epiphyses after exposure during the first trimester, and CNS abnormalities after exposure during any trimester (80). Heparin does not cross the placenta and is safe to the fetus, but prolonged heparin use causes osteoporosis; a reduction in bone density is reported in up to one-third of women who receive heparin (81). Low mol-wt heparins (LMWH) also do not cross the placenta and have benefits over unfractionated heparin, such as longer half-life, more predictable dose-response, and a decreased risk of heparin-induced thrombocytopenia (82,83). A recent study showed LMWH to be safe and effective when used in 61 pregnant women at risk of embolic events, although concerns about bone density were raised in this study (83).

Despite the high risk for thrombotic events in women with mechanical valves, considerable controversy exists on the optimal choice of anticoagulation in this high-risk group (84). The controversy arises from the belief that the superior anticoagulation afforded by warfarin outweighs its risk to the fetus; it should be noted that this apparent superiority can be attributed to prior studies using insufficient heparin dosage in high-risk patients (84). Until more studies are available, we suggest that pregnant women with AF at high risk of embolic events (such as rheumatic heart disease) are treated with full-dose heparin, initiated at doses of 17,000–20,000 subcutaneously every 12 h and adjusted to prolong the activated partial thromboplast in time (APTT) into the therapeutic range (see Table 3). Similar therapy is recommended for patients with mechanical valves (82). Based on limited data, LMWH may be a reasonable alternative (82,83).

Ventricular Tachyarrhythmias and Sudden Cardiac Death

Sustained ventricular tachycardia can also occur during pregnancy. Most commonly described is idiopathic VT originating from the right ventricular outflow tract (RVOT) in women with structurally normal hearts. This group of patients may respond to beta-blockers, such as metoprolol. As recently reported by Rashba et al., an increased incidence of adverse cardiac events is observed during the postpartum period in patients

Table 3
Recommendations for Anticoagulation in Patients with AF During Pregnancy

Subcutaneous (SC) heparin initiated in doses of 17,500–20,000 U q12h and adjusted to
  prolong a 6-h postinjection APTT into the therapeutic range. LMWHs are probably
  reasonable substitutes, but more studies are necessary
  or
Adjusted-dose SC heparin until the 13th wk, warfarin (target INR range 2.5–3.5) until the
  middle of the third trimester, then adjusted-dose SC heparin until delivery

INR = international normalized ratio; APTT = activated partial thromboplastin time; LMWH = low
mol-wt heparin.
(Adapted from: Ginsberg J, Hirsh J. Use of antithrombotic agents during pregnancy. Chest
1998;114: 524S–530S.)

with the long QT syndrome (LQTS) *(85)*. The authors found that therapy with beta-
blockers reduced the incidence of cardiac events, and suggested that patients with
LQTS who become pregnant should be treated continuously with beta-blockers.

When necessary for immediate termination of VT, direct current (DC) cardioversion
has shown to be safe at all stages of pregnancy with no significant ill effects to the
mother or fetus *(86)*. Fetal arrhythmias have been reported, so fetal monitoring is
advised; however, effects on the fetus are rare, perhaps related to the high mammalian
fetal fibrillation threshold, or the fact that the uterus is outside the shocking vector and
receives relatively little electrical current. For acute pharmacologic therapy of VT,
patients with structurally normal hearts may respond to beta-blockers. If a membrane-
stabilizing agent is required, both lidocaine and procainamide have been shown to be
relatively safe. For chronic therapy, a beta-blocker is appropriate for the VTs that occur
in the setting of a structurally normal heart. When class I or III agents are required,
procainamide offers a favorable profile in terms of safety and efficacy.

Therapy with an implantable cardioverter defibrillator (ICD) is a reasonable alternative in patients who have not responded to medical therapy and are at high risk for
sudden cardiac death. A recent series reported the experience of 44 women with ICDs
in place during pregnancy *(87)*. There was no increase in ICD-related complications
or number of ICD discharges during pregnancy, and there were no complications
resulting from ICD shocks. Thus, the ICD should be considered an option for women
with life-threatening arrhythmias who plan to conceive in the future, since exposure
to potentially toxic drugs can be obviated.

The treatment of cardiac arrest during pregnancy (which is fortunately rare, occurring
about once in every 30,000 deliveries) was recently reviewed in a statement from the
International Liaison Committee on resuscitation *(88)*. In addition to the standard causes,
unusual etiologies for arrest should be considered in pregnant women such as amniotic
fluid embolism, pulmonary embolism, bleeding, peripartum cardiomyopathy, and aortic
dissection. If cardiopulmonary resuscitation (CPR) is necessary, it should be performed
as in the nonpregnant state except for modification to avoid compression of the aorta
and inferior vena cava (IVC) by the gravid uterus (*see* Table 4). Thus, it is recommended
that CPR be performed either with the patient in the left lateral decubitus position,
with a wedge placed under the right flank, or with the uterus displaced manually to

Table 4
Management of Cardiac Arrest in Pregnant Women

Key Interventions To Prevent Arrest
  Place the patient in the left lateral position or manually displace uterus
  Give 100% oxygen
  Give fluid bolus
  Evaluate recently administered drugs

Modifications During Cardiac Arrest
  Relieve aortocaval compression by manually displacing gravid uterus, or by using a wedge
    or position the patient's back on the rescuer's thighs
  Consider additional etiologies unique to pregnancy, such as amniotic-fluid embolism or
    pulmonary embolism
  Involve obstetric and neonatal personnel as early as possible
  If all measures are failing and fetal viability exists, consider immediate perimortem
    cesarean section

(Adapted from: Kloeck W, Cummins RO, Chamberlain D, Bossaert L, Callanan V, Carli P, et al. Special resuscitation situations: an advisory statement from the International Liaison Committee on Resuscitation. Circulation 1997;95:2196–2210.)

the left. The patient should be administered 100% oxygen and fluid boluses, and the recent administration of drugs must be evaluated. Cesarean section should be considered and undertaken promptly (ideally within 5 min of the arrest) if the fetus is viable.

CONCLUSION

Most types of ventricular and supraventricular arrhythmias can manifest during pregnancy. For benign arrhythmias, conservative therapies are appropriate. When the arrhythmias jeopardizes the life of the mother or fetus, therapy should be provided without hesitation. Several therapeutic options exist for most arrhythmias, including both pharmacologic therapy and nonpharmacologic procedures. Drug therapy should be avoided during the first trimester of pregnancy, if possible. If necessary, drugs with the longest record of safety should be used as first-line therapy, and should be administered with close and frequent monitoring. Newer agents should also be considered if indicated. The use of an ICD has become a first-line option for women of childbearing potential with life-threatening ventricular arrhythmias. During CPR, compression of the large veins by the gravid uterus should be avoided and prompt cesarean section must be considered.

REFERENCES

1. Cox JL, Gardner MJ. Treatment of cardiac arrhythmias during pregnancy. Prog Cardiovasc Dis 1993;36:137–178.
2. Metcalfe J, Ueland K. Maternal cardiovascular adjustments to pregnancy. Prog Cardiovasc Dis 1974;16:363–374.
3. Dunlop W. Serial changes in renal hemodynamics during normal human pregnancy. Br J Obstet Gynaecol 1981;88:1–9.
4. Mitani R, Steinberg I, Lien E, Harrison E, Elkayam U. The pharmacokinetics of antiarrhythmic agents in pregnancy and lactation. Clin Pharmacokinet 1987;12:253–291.
5. Widerhorn J, Widerhorn AL, Rahimtoola SH, Elkayam U. WPW syndrome during pregnancy: increased incidence of supraventricular arrhythmias. Am Heart J 1992;123:796–798.

6. Shotan A, Ostrzega E, Mehra A, Johnson JV, Elkayam U. Incidence of arrhythmias in normal pregnancy and relation to palpitations, dizziness, and syncope. Am J Cardiol 1997;79:1061–1064.

7. Brodsky M, Doria R, Allen B, Sato D, Thomas G, Sada M. New-onset ventricular tachycardia during pregnancy. Am Heart J 1992;123:933–941.

8. Perloff J. Pregnancy and congenital heart disease. J Am Coll Cardiol 1991;18:340–342.

9. Lee W, Cotton D. Peripartum cardiomyopathy: current concepts and clinical management. Clin Obstet Gynecol 1989;32:54–67.

10. Vaughan Williams EM. A classification of antiarrhythmic actions reassessed after a decade of new drugs. J Clin Pharmacol 1984;24:129–147.

11. Meyer J, Lackner J, Schochet S. Paroxysmal tachycardia in pregnancy. Am Heart J 1931;94:1901–1904.

12. Hill L, Malkasian G. The use of quinidine sulfate throughout pregnancy. Obstet Gynecol 1979;54:366–368.

13. Wladimiroff J, Stewart A. Treatment of fetal cardiac arrhythmias. Br J Hosp Med 1985;34:134–140.

14. Wong R, Murthy A, Mathisen G, Glover N, Thornton P. Treatment of severe falciparum malaria during pregnancy with quinidine and exchange transfusions. Am J Med 1992;92:561–562.

15. Rotmensh H, Elkayam U, Frishman W. Antiarrhythmic drug therapy during pregnancy. Ann Intern Med 1983;98:487–497.

16. Allen NM, Page RL. Procainamide administration during pregnancy. Clin Pharmacol 1993;12:58–60.

17. Page RL. Treatment of arrhythmias during pregnancy. Am Heart J 1995;130:871–876.

18. Schnider S. Choice of anesthesia for labor and delivery. Obstet Gynecol 1981;58:24s–34s.

19. Martin L, Jurand A. The absence of teratogenic effects of some analgesics use in anesthesia: additional evidence from a mouse model. Anaesthesia 1992;47:473–476.

20. Kim W, Pomerance J. Miller A. Lidocaine intoxication in a newborn following local anesthesia for episiotomy. Pediatrics 1979;64:643–645.

21. Brown W, Bell G, Alper M. Acidosis, local anesthesia and the newborn. Obstet Gynecol 1976;48:27–30.

22. Gregg A, Tomich P. Mexiletine use in pregnancy. J Perinatol 1988;8:33–35.

23. Timmis A, Jackson G, Holt D. Mexiletine for control of ventricular dysrrhythmias during pregnancy. Lancet 1980;2:647–648.

24. Lowes H, Ives T. Mexiletine use in pregnancy and lactation. Am J Obstet Gynecol 1987;157:446–447.

25. Atkinson AJ, Davison R. Diphenylhydantoin as an antiarrhythmic drug. Ann Rev Med 1974;25:99–113.

26. Hanson J, Myrianthopoulos N, Sedwick M, Smith D. Risk to the offspring of women treated with hydantoin anticonvulsants, with emphasis on the fetal hydantoin syndrome. J Pediatr 1976;89:662–668.

27. Echt D, Liebson P, Mitchel B, Peters R, Obias-Manno D, Barker A, et al. Mortality and morbidity in patients receiving encainide, flecainide, or placebo. N Engl J Med 1991;324:781–788.

28. Wagner X, Jouglard J, Moulin M, Miller AM, Petitjean J, Pisapia A. Coadministration of flecainide acetate and sotalol during pregnancy: lack of teratogenic effects, passage across the placenta, and excretion in human breast milk. Am Heart J 1990;119:700–702.

29. Ahmed K, Issawi I, Peddireddy R. Use of flecainide for refractory atrial tachycardia of pregnancy. Am J Crit Care 1996;5:306–308.

30. Allan L, Chita S, Sharland G, Maxwell D, Priestley K. Flecainide in the treatment of fetal tachycardias. Br Heart J 1991;65:46–48.

31. Frohn-Mulder IM, Stewart PA, Witsenburg M, Den Hollander NS, Wladimiroff JW, Hess J. The efficacy of flecainide versus digoxin in the management of fetal supraventricular tachycardia. Prenatal Diagn 1995;15:1297–1302.

32. Simpson J, Sharland G. Fetal tachycardias: management and outcome of 127 consecutive cases. Heart 1998;79:576–581.

33. Vanderhal A, Cocjin J, Santulli T, Carlson D, Rosenthal P. Conjugated hyperbilirubinemia in a newborn infant after maternal (transplacental) treatment with flecainide acetate for fetal tachycardia and fetal hydrops. J Pediatr 1995;126:988–990.

34. Capucci A, Boriani G. Propafenone in the treatment of cardiac arrhythmias. A risk-benefit appraisal. Drug Saf 1995;12:55–72.

35. Frishman W, Chesner M. Beta-adrenergic blockers in pregnancy. Am Heart J 1988;115:147–152.

36. Joglar JA, Page RL. Treatment of cardiac arrhythmias during pregnancy: safety considerations. Drug Saf 1999;20:85–94.

37. Pryun S, Phelan J, Buchanan G. Long-term propanolol therapy in pregnancy: maternal and fetal outcome. Am J Obstet Gynecol 1979;135:485–489.

38. Rubin P, Butters L, Clark D. Placebo-controlled trial of atenolol in treatment of pregnancy-associated hypertension. Lancet 1983;2:431–434.

39. Wichman K, Ryulden G, Karberg B. A placebo controlled trial of metoprolol in the treatment of hypertension in pregnancy. Scand J Clin Lab Investig 1984;169:90–94.

40. Lip G, Beevers M, Churchill D, Shaffer L, Beevers D. Effect of atenolol on birth weight. Am J Cardiol 1997;79:1436–1438.

41. Liedholm H, Melander A, Bitzen P-O, Lonnerholm G, Mattiasson I, Nilsson B, et al. Accumulation of atenolol and metoprolol in human breast milk. Eur J Clin Pharmacol 1981;20:229–231.

42. Delvin R, Duchin K, Fleiss P. Nadolol in human serum and breast milk. Br J Clin Pharmacol 1981;12:393–396.

43. Schmimmel M, Eldelman A, Wilschanski M, Shaw D, Oglivie R, Koren G. Toxic effects of atenolol consumed during breast feeding. J Pediatr 1989;114:476–478.

44. Widerhorn J, Bhandari AK, Bughi S, Rahimtoola SH, Elkayam U. Fetal and neonatal adverse effects profile of amiodarone treatment during pregnancy. Am Heart J 1991;122:1162–1166.

45. Wolf DD, Shepper JD, Verhaaren H, Deneyer M, Smitz J, Sacre-Smits L. Congenital hypothyroid goiter and amiodarone. Acta Paediatr Scand 1988;77:616–618.

46. Magee LA, Downar E, Sermer M, Boulton BC, Allen LC, Koren G. Pregnancy outcome after gestational exposure to amiodarone in Canada. Am J Obstet Gynecol 1995;172:1307–1311.

47. Ovadia M, Brito M, Hoyer G, Marcus F. Human experience with amiodarone in the embrionic period. Am J Cardiol 1994;73:316–317.

48. Strunge P, Frandsen J, Andreasen F. Amiodarone during pregnancy. Eur Heart J 1988;9:106–109.

49. O'Hare M, Murnaghan G, Russell C, Leahey W, Varma M. Sotalol as hypotensive agent in pregnancy. Br J Obstet Gynaecol 1980;87:814–820.

50. Kowey P, VanderLugt J, Luderer J. Safety and risk/benefit analysis of ibutilide for acute conversion of atrial fibrillation/flutter. Am J Cardiol 1996;78:46–52.

51. Klein V, Repke J. Supraventricular tachycardia in pregnancy: cardioversion with verapamil. Obstet Gynecol 1984;63:16S–18S.

52. Byerly WG, Hartmann A, Foster DE, Tannenbaum AK. Verapamil in the treatment of maternal paroxysmal supraventricular tachycardia. Ann Emerg Med 1991;20:552–554.

53. Orlandi C, Marlettini M, Cassani A, Trabatti M, Agostini D, Salomone T, et al. Treatment of hypertension during pregnancy with the calcium channel antagonist verapamil. Curr Ther Res 1986;39:884–893.

54. Kleinman C, Copel J, Weinstein E, Santulli T, Hobbins J. Treatment of fetal supraventricular tachyarrhythmias. J Clin Ultrasound 1985;13:265–273.

55. Camm A, Garrat C. Adenosine and supraventricular tachycardia. N Engl J Med 1991;325:1621–1629.

56. Elkayam U, Goodwin TM. Adenosine therapy for supraventricular tachycardia during pregnancy. Am J Cardiol 1995;75:521–523.

57. Jaqueti J, Martinez-Hernandez D, Hernandez-Garcia R, Navarro-Gallar F. Adenosine deaminase in pregnancy serum. Clin Chem 1990;36:2144.

58. Mason B, Ogjunyemi D, Punla O, Koos B. Maternal and fetal cardiorespiratory responses to adenosine in sheep. Am J Obstet Gynecol 1993;168:1558–1561.

59. Page R. Arrhythmias during pregnancy. Cardiac Electrophysiology Review 1997;I278–I282.

60. Chen V, Tse T, Wong V. Transfer of digoxin across the placenta and into breast milk. Br J Obstet Gynaecol 1978;55:605–609.

61. Rogers M, Willerson J, Goldblatt A, Smith T. Serum digoxin concentrations in the human fetus, neonate and infant. N Engl J Med 1972;287:1010–1013.

62. Kerenyi T, Gleicher N, Meller J, Brown E, Stenfeld L, Chitkara U, et al. Transplacental cardioversion of intrauterine supraventricular tachycardia with digitalis. Lancet 1980;2:393–395.

63. King C, Mattioli L, Goertz K, Snodgrass W. Successful treatment of fetal supraventricular tachycardia with maternal digoxin therapy. Chest 1984;85:573–575.

64. Parilla BV, Strasburger JF, Socol ML. Fetal supraventricular tachycardia complicated by hydrops fetalis: a role for direct fetal intramuscular therapy. Am J Perinatol 1996;13:483–486.

65. Gonzalez A, Phelps S, Cochran E, Sibai B. Digitalis-like immunoreactive substance in pregnancy. Am J Obstet Gynecol 1987;157:660–664.

66. Committee on Drugs. Transfer of drugs and other chemicals into human milk. Pediatrics 1994;93:137–150.

67. McAnulty J, Morton M, Ueland K. The heart and pregnancy. Curr Probl Cardiol 1988;13:589–665.

68. Dalvi BV, Chaudhuri A, Kulkarni HL, Kale PA. Therapeutic guidelines for congenital complete heart block presenting in pregnancy. Obstet Gynecol 1992;79:802–804.

69. Antonelli D, Bloch L, Rosenfeld T. Implantation of a permanent dual chamber pacemaker in a pregnant woman by transesophageal echocardiographic guidance. PACE 1999;22:534–535.

70. Guldal M, Kervancioglu C, Oral D, Gurel T, Erol C, Sorrel A. Permanent pacemaker implantation in a pregnant woman with the guidance of ECG and two-dimensional echocardiography. PACE 1987;10:543–545.

71. Jordaens LJ, Vandenbogaerde JF, Van de Bruaene P, Du Buyzere M. Transesophageal echocardiography for insertion of a physiological pacemaker in early pregnancy. PACE 1990;13:955–957.

72. Metcalfe J, McAnulty J, Ueland K. Burwell and Metcalfe's Heart Disease and Pregnancy: Physiology and Management. Little, Brown and Co., Boston, MA, 1986, p. 58.

73. Mechem CC, Knopp RK, Feldman D. Painless abruptio placentae associated with disseminated intravascular coagulation and syncope. Ann Emerg Med 1992;21:883–885.

74. Kniseley RM. Acute internal bleeding as a cause of syncope. American Family Physician 1995;52:1278.

75. Peleg D, Orvieto R, Ferber A, Ben-Rafael Z. Maternal supraventricular tachycardia recorded as apparent fetal heart rate in a case of fetal demise. Acta Obstet Gynecol Scand 1998;77:786–787.

76. Dominguez A, Iturralde P, Hermosillo AG, Colin L, Kershenovich S, Garrido LM. Successful radiofrequency ablation in an accessory pathway during pregnancy. PACE 1999;22:131–134.

77. Ueland K. Rheumatic heart disease and pregnancy. In: Elkayam U, Gleicher N, eds. Cardiac Problems in Pregnancy. Alan R. Liss, New York, NY, 1990, pp. 99–107.

78. Szekely P, Snaith L. Atrial fibrillation and pregnancy. Br Med J 1961;1:1407–1410.

79. Mendelson C. Disorders of the heart beat during pregnancy. Am J Obstet Gynecol 1956;72:1268–1301.

80. Hall J, Paul R, Wilson K. Maternal and fetal sequelae of anticoagulation during pregnancy. Am J Med 1980;68:122–140.

81. Dahlman T, Lindvall N, Hellgren M. Osteopenia in pregnancy during long-term heparin treatment: a radiological study post-partum. Br J Obstet Gynaecol 1990;97:221–228.

82. Ginsberg J, Hirsh J. Use of antithrombotic agents during pregnancy. Chest 1998;114:524s–530s.

83. Nelson-Piercy C, Letsky EA, de Swiet M. Low-molecular-weight heparin for obstetric thromboprophylaxis: experience of sixty-nine pregnancies in sixty-one women at high risk. Am J Obstet Gynecol 1997;176:1062–1068.

84. Dizzon-Townson D, Branch D. Anticoagulation treatment during pregnancy: an update. Semin Thromb Hemost 1998;24:55–63.

85. Rashba EJ, Zareba W, Moss AJ, Hall WJ, Robinson J, Locati EH, et al. Influence of pregnancy on the risk for cardiac events in patients with hereditary long QT syndrome. LQTS Investigators. Circulation 1998;97:451–456.

86. Rosemond R. Cardioversion during pregnancy. JAMA 1993;269:3167.

87. Natale A, Davidson T, Geiger MJ, Newby K. Implantable cardioverter-defibrillators and pregnancy: a safe combination? Circulation 1997;96:2808–2812.

88. Kloeck W, Cummins RO, Chamberlain D, Bossaert L, Callanan V, Carli P, et al. Special resuscitation situations: an advisory statement from the International Liaison Committee on Resuscitation. Circulation 1997;95:2196–2210.

Index